Control of
Communicable
Diseases Manual

David L. Heymann, MD, Editor

Eighteenth Edition   2004

D042414३

An official report of the American Public Health Association

American Public Health Association
800 I Street, NW
Washington, DC 20001-3710

Copyright ©2004 by the
American Public Health Association

All rights reserved. No part of this publication may be reproduced, stored in a retrieval system, or transmitted in any form or by any means, electronic, mechanical, photocopying, recording, scanning, or otherwise, except as permitted under Sections 107 and 108 of the 1976 United States Copyright Act, without either the prior written permission of the Publisher or authorization through payment of the appropriate per-copy fee to the Copyright Clearance Center [222 Rosewood Drive, Danvers, MA 01923 (978) 750-8400, fax (978) 750-4744, www.copyright.com]. Requests to the Publisher for permission should be addressed to the Permissions Department, American Public Health Association, 800 I Street, NW, Washington, DC 20001-3710; fax (202) 777-2531.

American Public Health Association
800 I Street, NW
Washington, DC 20001-3710

Georges C. Benjamin, MD, FACP
Executive Director

Ellen T. Meyer
Director of Publications

Terence Mulligan
Production Manager

Printed and bound in the United States of America

Cover Design: Michele Pryor
Typesetting: Cadmus
Set in: Garamond
Printing and Binding: United Book Press, Inc., Baltimore, Md

Notes on the cover design: The cover illustrates four basic aspects of communicable disease control. Grain—proper nutrition; flask—research; syringe—prevention and treatment; hand and soap—sanitation

ISBN 0-87553-034-6 soft cover
ISBN 0-87553-035-4 hardcover
85M (7/04)
25M (9/05)
20M (3/06)

EDITOR

David L. Heymann, MD
World Health Organization
20 Avenue Appia, 1211 Geneva, SWITZERLAND

ASSOCIATE EDITOR

Michel C. Thuriaux, MD
World Health Organization
20 Avenue Appia, 1211 Geneva, SWITZERLAND

EDITORIAL BOARD

Georges C. Benjamin, MD, FACP
Executive Director
American Public Health Association
800 I Street NW, Washington DC 20001-3710, USA

John Bennett, MD
Head, Clinical Mycology Section
LCI, National Institute for Allergies and Infectious Diseases
National Institutes of Health
Clinical Center Room 11C304
9000 Rockville Pike, Bethesda MD 20892, USA

Johan Giesecke, MD
Professor, Infectious Disease Epidemiology
Karolinska Institute SE-171 77 Stockholm, SWEDEN

Marc Girard, MD
Director General
Fondation Mérieux, 17 rue Bourgelat, 69002 Lyon, FRANCE

Donato Greco, MD
Director, National Epidemiology Centre
Istituto Superiore di Sanità, Viale Regina Elena 299, 00161 Rome, ITALY

Scott B. Halstead, MD
Preventive Medicine and Biostatistics
Uniformed Services University of Health Sciences
5824 Edson Lane N., Bethesda MD 20852, USA

James M. Hughes, MD
Director, National Center for Infectious Diseases
Centers for Disease Control and Prevention
1600 Clifton Road NE, Mailstop C12, Atlanta GA 30333, USA

iii

Jacob John, MD
formerly Professor and Head, Department of Microbiology
Christian Medical College Hospital, Vellore Tamilnadu 632004, INDIA

Omar A. Khan, MD, MMS
Chair, Publications Board
American Public Health Association
800 I Street NW, Washington DC 20001-3710, USA

Ann Marie Kimball, MD, MPH
Professor, Epidemiology and Health Services/Director
Asia Pacific Emerging Infections Network
School of Public Health and Community Medicine
University of Washington
Box 354809, Seattle WA 98195, USA

Mary Ann Lansang, MD, MMSc
Executive Director, The INCLEN Trust
Section E, 5/F Ramon Magsaysay Center
1680 Roxas Boulevard, Malate, Manila 1004, THE PHILIPPINES

Angus Nicoll, MD
Director, PHLS Communicable Disease Surveillance Centre
61 Colindale Avenue, London NW9 5EQ, UNITED KINGDOM

Christophe Paquet, MD, MPH
Département international et tropical
Institut de Veille Sanitaire
12 rue de Val d'Osne, 94415 Saint Maurice, FRANCE

Aileen Plant, MD
Professor of International Health
Centre for International Health, Division of Health Sciences
Curtin University of Technology
GPO U1987, Perth WA, 6845, AUSTRALIA

Stanley A. Plotkin, MD
Emeritus Professor
University of Pennsylvania/Wistar Institute
4650 Wismer Road, Doylestown PA 18901, USA

Guénaël Rodier, MD
Communicable Disease Surveillance & Response
World Health Organization
20 Avenue Appia, 1211 Geneva, SWITZERLAND

Bijan Sadrizadeh, MD
Senior Adviser to the Minister of Health
Ministry of Health and Medical Education
310 Hafez Avenue, Tehran, ISLAMIC REPUBLIC OF IRAN

Robert E. Shope, MD
Professor of Pathology
University of Texas Medical Branch
301 University Blvd., Galveston, TX 77555, USA

Ron St. John, MD
Director General
Centre for Emergency Preparedness & Response
Health Canada, 100 Colonnade, Ottawa ON K1A 0K9, CANADA

Yasuhiro Suzuki, MD, PhD
Secretary of Health
Tochigi Prefecture, 1-1-20 Hanawada Utsunomiya, 320-8501 JAPAN

Pat Troop, MD, CBE, FFPH, FRCP
Chief Executive Officer
Health Protection Agency, 11th Floor, The Adelphi
1-11 John Adam Street, London WC2N 6HT, UNITED KINGDOM

Karl A. Western, MD, DTPH
Assistant Director for International Research
Director, Office of Global Affairs
National Institute for Allergies and Infectious Diseases
Room 2021, 6610 Rockledge Drive, Bethesda, MD 20892-6613, USA

Eng Kiong Yeoh, JP
Secretary for Health Welfare & Food
Health, Welfare, and Food Bureau, Government Secretariat
19/F Murray Building Garden Road Central, Hong Kong, CHINA

COLLABORATORS AND OTHER PRIMARY REVIEWERS

Pierre Busson, PhD
UMR 1598
Centre National de la Recherche Scientifique
Institut Gustave Roussy
rue Camille Desmoulins, 94805 Villejuif CEDEX, FRANCE

Elisabeth Carniel, MD, PhD
WHO CC for Reference and Research on Yersinia
National Laboratory for Plague and other Yersinioses
Institut Pasteru, 28 rue du Dr Roux, 75724 Paris, FRANCE

John Clements, MD
Centre for international Health
Burnet Institute, Melbourne, AUSTRALIA

George Deepe, MD
Director, Infectious Diseases
University of Cincinnati
MSB 7163 POB 670560, Cincinatti, OH 45277-0560, USA

David W. Denning, MBBS
School of Medicine, University of Manchester and Wythenshawe
Hospital
Southmoor Road, Manchester M23NPL, UNITED KINGDOM

Don C. Dragon, PhD
Chemical and Biological Defence Station
Defence Research and Development Canada
Suffield, POB 4000 Station Main, Medicine Hat AB, T1A8K6, CANADA

Ramon Diaz Garcia, MD
Director, Department of Microbiology
Professor of Medical Microbiology.School of Medicine
University of Navarra, Pamplona, SPAIN

J. Stephen Dumler, MD
Director, Medical Microbiology, Dept of Pathology
The Johns Hopkins Medical Institutions
600 N. Wolfe Street, Baltimore, MD 21287, USA

Roderick Hay, MD
Professor (Medicine and Health Sciences)
Room G28A, Queen's University Belfast, Whitla Medical Building
University Road Belfast BT71NN
Northern Ireland, UNITED KINGDOM

Dagmar Hulínská, PhD
Head, National Reference for Borreliosis
Department of Electron Microscopy, Epidemiology and Microbiology
National Institute of Public Health
Šrobarova 48, Prague 10042, CZECH REPUBLIC

Jon Iredell, MD, PhD
Centre for Infectious Diseases and Microbiology
University of Sydney, Westmead Hospital, Sydney 2145, AUSTRALIA

Edward L. Kaplan
Professor, Department of Pediatrics
MMC 296, University of Minnesota Medical School
Room #820-2 Mayo Bldg.,
420 Delaware St SE, Minneapolis MN 55455 USA

Frans van Knapen
Chairman, Department of Public Health and Food Safety
Veterinary Medicine, Urecht University, THE NETHERLANDS

John Mackenzie, MD
Department of Microbiology and Parasitology
School of Molecular and Microbial Sciences
The University of Queensland, Brisbane 4072, AUSTRALIA

Paul Martin, MD
Laboratoire des Listeria
Institut Pasteur, 28 rue du Dr Roux, 75724 Paris, FRANCE

Didier Raoult, MD
Directeur, Laboratoire des Bartonelloses
Université de la Méditerranée
58 Boulevard Charles Livon, 12384 Marseille, FRANCE

Eduardo Salazar-Lindo, MD,
Professor, Department of Pediatrics
Cayetano Heredia University, Lima, PERU

Roberto Salvatella Agrelo, MD
National Adviser/Regional Chagas Disease Focal Point
PAHO/WHO Offices, Av Brasil 2697, CP 11300
Montevideo, URUGUAY

Luiz Carlos Severo, MD, PhD
Associate Professor of Internal Medicine/
Head, Laboratory of Mycology, School of Medicine
Federal University, Rio Grande do Sul, BRAZIL

Anders Sjöstedt, MD
Professor, Department of Clinical Bacteriology
Umeå University
SE-901 85, Umeå, SWEDEN

F. Waldvogel, MD
Professor and Physician-in-chief, Medical Services 2
Hôpital cantonal universitaire de Genève, SWITZERLAND

David H. Walker, MD
Professor and Chairman, Department of Pathology
Executive Director, Center for Biodefense and Emerging Infectious
Diseases
University of Texas Medical Branch,
301 University Boulevard, Keiller Bldg, Galveston, TX 77555-0609, USA

Hiroshi Yanagawa, MD, FFPH,
President, Saitama Prefectural University
820 Sannomiya, Koshigaya-shi, Saitama-ken 343 8540, JAPAN

Centers for Disease Control and Prevention
1600 Clifton Road NE, Mailstop C12, Atlanta, GA 30333, USA

Larry Anderson, MD
C. Ben Beard, PhD
Richard Besser, MD
Anna Bowen, MD, MPH
Chris Braden, MD
Inger Damon, MD, MPH
Amy Dechet, MD
Amy Dubois, MD
Mark Eberhard, PhD
Alicia Fry, MD
Kenneth Gage, PhD

Patricia Griffin, MD
Thomas Ksiazek, MD, DVM
James Maguire, MD, MPH
Eric Mintz, MD, MPH
Lyle Petersen, MD, MPH
Pierre Rollin, MD
Nancy Rosenstein, MD
Jeremy Sobel, MD, MPH
Robert Tauxe, MD, MPH
Cynthia Whitney, MD, MPH

International Agency for Research on Cancer (IARC)
150 cours Albert Thomas, 69008 Lyon, FRANCE

Marilys Corbex, MD
Sylvia Francheschi, MD

David M. Parkin, MD
Bakary Sylla, PhD

World Health Organization
Avenue Appia, CH 1221 Geneva 21, SWITZERLAND

Georg M Antal, MD
Kingsley Asiedu, MD, MPH
R. Bruce Aylward, MD
Sarah Ballance, BSc
Markus Behrend, MD
Eric Bertherat, MD, MPH
Gautam Biswas, MD
Ties Boerma, MD, PhD
Peter Braam, DVM
Claire-Lise Chaignat, MD, MPH
Ottorino Cosivi, DVM
Alya Dabbagh, PhD
Denis Daumerie, MD
Renu Dayal-Drager, PhD
Philippe Desjeux, MD
Philippe Duclos, DVM, PhD
Chris Elliott
Dirk Engels, MD, PhD
Pierre Formenty, DVM, MPH
Pierre Guillet, PhD
Bradley Hersh, MD, MPH

Jean Jannin, MD
Marc Karam, MD
Mary Kindhauser, MA
Daniel Lavanchy, MD
Ivan Lejnev, MD
Karin Leitmeyer, MPH, DTM&H
Ornella Lincetto, MD, MPH
Pam Mari
Gillian Mayers, BSc
Jill Meloni
François-Xavier Meslin, DVM
Antonio Montresor, MD
Francis Ndowa, MD
Tony Pappas, BSc
William Perea, MD, MPH
Poul Erik Petersen, DDS,
    DrOndontSc
Liliana Pievaroli, BSc
Mario Raviglione, MD
Elil Renganathan, MD, PhD
Serge Resnikoff, MD

Susan E. Robertson, MD, MPH

Cathy Roth, PhD

Lorenzo Savioli, MD, MSc

Allan Schapira, MD, DSc

Jorgen Schlundt, DVM, PhD

Nahoko Shindo, MD, PhD

Klaus Stöhr, DVM, PhD

Hajime Toyofuku, DVM, VPH

Julie Symons

Jos Vandelaer, MD, MPH

TABLE OF CONTENTS

FOREWORD

The world of communicable diseases continues to present a challenge to the professionals who track and contain them. These diseases are a leading cause of morbidity and mortality around the world and remain an enigma to many. The new threat of bioterrorism has become a significant security concern of all nations. Emerging and reemerging infectious diseases are also a growing threat. New diseases such as Hantavirus, HIV/AIDS, Ebola, *E. coli* O157:H7 and SARS are but a few of the new threats over the last 30 years. No doubt more are to come. This new version of *Control of Communicable Diseases Manual* (CCDM), the 18th revision of this 87-year-old favorite of the health community, is available to address these important concerns.

The text was initially written in the early 20th century, as a pamphlet for New England health officials, by Dr. Francis Curtis, then the health officer of Newton, Massachusetts. Later, Dr. Robert Hoyt, a health officer from Manchester, New Hampshire, recognized its importance and convinced the American Public Health Association (APHA) at its annual convention in Cincinnati to review, edit, and adopt the text as its own. In 1917, it was published in *Public Health Reports* (32:41:1706–1733), by the United States Public Health Service. Its 30 pages contained disease control measures for the 38 communicable diseases that were then reportable in the United States. It was available from the Government Printing Office for a modest five cents. This manual is now the classic by which all other infectious disease manuals are measured.

CCDM has undergone several rewrites over the years. Even the last word in the title was changed from "Man" to "Manual" to remove the perception of gender bias. There has been a CD-ROM version and this new 18th edition will for the first time be available online. Translations into several languages—currently Bahasa Indonesia, Italian, Korean, Portuguese, Serbian, and Spanish—have made this text a global treasure. It covers over 140 diseases and groups of diseases of importance to communicable disease hunters and researchers.

In its history only five people have served as editors for the CCDM:

Haven Emerson: 1st–7th editions
John Gordon: 8th–10th editions
Abram S. Benenson: 11th–16th editions
James Chin: 17th edition
David L. Heymann: 18th edition

Dr. Heymann and his team at the World Health Organization have assembled an impressive group of experts from around the world to serve as reviewers, authors, and editors. They have completed the transformation of this text into a resource responsive to the needs of the global health

community. I thank them for their work. I also want to thank the many men and women who work silently behind the scenes and on occasion have given their lives to contain the threat of infectious disease.

Finally, I would be remiss in not acknowledging the death during work on this edition of long-time CCDM editor, Dr. Abram S. Benenson, who died December 15, 2003, at his home in Lenox MA. A renowned scientist, research doctor, and professor, Dr. Benenson was editor of CCDM for 28 years, for the 11th–16th editions. Dr. Benenson set a high standard of excellence for CCDM and APHA will always be grateful for his outstanding contributions to the health of the nation and the world, and to the scientific knowledge base of the profession.

Georges C. Benjamin, MD, FACP
Executive Director
American Public Health Association

FOREWORD

The *Control of Communicable Diseases Manual* has long been respected as a major tool in the quest for the control of communicable diseases. It is with great pleasure that WHO has shared in the preparation of this 18th edition with the American Public Health Association, and helped broaden its scope to accommodate the needs of developing countries.

CCDM18, like previous editions, remains compact and easy to use. Our commitment to translate the manual into other languages will make it useful to many countries, and during the coming years we shall work with the WHO Regional Offices and the American Public Health Association to translate it into all official WHO languages.

By making guidance on prevention and control measures available to countries in easy to access format, and by highlighting where drugs and vaccines may be obtained for many of the diseases in this manual, CCDM18 is a public good that will help countries move closer to universal access to and equity in public health.

LEE Jong-wook
Director-General
World Health Organization

PREFACE TO THE EIGHTEENTH EDITION

Communicable diseases kill, maim and surprise. Far from having been conquered, they have resurged dramatically in recent years. The microbial agents that cause them are dynamic, resilient, and well adapted to exploit opportunities for change and spread. Their public health significance in terms of human suffering, deaths, and disability is compounded by the considerable toll they take on economic growth and development. For many important diseases, control is problematic either because of the lack of effective vaccines and therapeutic drugs, or because existing drugs are being rendered ineffective as antimicrobial resistance spreads.

Communicable diseases kill more than 14 million people each year, mainly in the developing world. In these countries, approximately 46% of all deaths are due to communicable diseases, and 90% of these deaths are attributed to acute diarrhoeal and respiratory infections of children, AIDS, tuberculosis, malaria, and measles.

Other diseases, that rarely kill, maim millions. Large populations living in remote areas of the developing world are at risk of disabling diseases, such as poliomyelitis, leprosy, lymphatic filariasis, and onchocerciasis. For these diseases, the toll of suffering and permanent disability is compounded by a double economic burden. The huge number of permanently disabled persons reduces the work force and further undermines the financial security of already impoverished families and communities, who already take on the onus of care and economic support.

Communicable diseases also deliver surprises, whether in the form of new diseases or well-known diseases behaving in new ways. As the emergence of severe acute respiratory syndrome (SARS) so clearly demonstrated, every country is vulnerable, and the economic consequences, exaggerated by public fear of the unknown, can be felt around the world. When severe and poorly understood diseases such as SARS and Ebola emerge, they often take their heaviest toll on health care workers and can jeopardize the capacity of health systems to cope. This situation is likely to be repeated when the next new disease emerges, when the next inevitable influenza pandemic occurs, or following the deliberate release of a pathogen with deliberate intent to harm.

For all these reasons, concern about the impact of communicable diseases has increased, with some encouraging results. Lack of access to effective vaccines and drugs has been a long-standing problem in the developing world. Major new initiatives, including the Global Fund to Fight AIDS, Tuberculosis and Malaria, the Global Alliance for Vaccines and Immunization, and the Roll Back Malaria and Stop TB partnerships, have formed to attack the main communicable diseases that kill and are delivering badly needed drugs and vaccines. The concern of international community is also evident in time-limited drives to eradicate or eliminate polio, leprosy, lymphatic filariasis, onchocerciasis and other diseases that maim. While microbial agents will always deliver surprises, the shock of SARS has encouraged a number of countries to give infrastructures for protecting public health much higher priority. All health care will benefit.

This 18th edition of the *Control of Communicable Diseases Manual* (CCDM18) provides guidance to countries as they give higher priority to the communicable disease threat, and is yet another tool in our collective efforts to protect world populations from communicable diseases— whether rare and exotic or all too common. It has been a privilege to work with the world's experts in communicable disease control as CCDM18 has been updated, and to broaden this edition by adding considerations for developing countries. It was with great sadness, in mid-January of this year, just as the editorial review was completed, that we learned of the death of one of our long time colleagues and fellow editorial board member, Dr Robert E. Shope. Bob Shope was certainly the world's authority on arboviruses, and shared his knowledge with all who asked, including CCDM18 where his final touches to the chapter on arboviruses are yet another memorial to his life and friendship.

David L. Heymann, M.D.

USER'S GUIDE TO CCDM18

Each disease section in CCDM18 is presented in a standardized format that includes the following information:

Disease name: Each disease is identified by the numeric code assigned by the WHO *International Classification of Diseases*, 9th Revision, Clinical Modification (ICD-9 CM) and 10th Revision, ICD-10.

Disease names recommended by the Council for International Organizations of Medical Sciences (CIOMS) and WHO in the *International Nomenclature of Diseases*, Volume II (Part 2, Mycoses, 1st edition, 1982, and Part 3, Viral Diseases, 1st edition, 1983) have been used unless the recommended name has become significantly different from that in current use. In that case, the recommended name is shown as first synonym.

1. **Identification** presents the main clinical features of the disease and differentiates it from others that may have a similar clinical picture. Also noted are those laboratory tests most commonly used to identify or confirm the etiological agent.

2. **Infectious agent** identifies the specific agent or agents causing the disease; classifies the agent(s); and may indicate its (or their) important characteristics.

3. **Occurrence** provides information on where the disease is known to occur and in which population groups it is most likely to occur. Information on past and current outbreaks may also be included.

4. **Reservoir** indicates any person, animal, arthropod, plant, substance—or combination of these—in which an infection agent normally lives and multiplies, on which it depends primarily for survival, and where it reproduces itself in such a manner that it can be transmitted to a susceptible host.

5. **Mode of transmission** describes the mechanisms by which the infectious agent is spread to humans.

6. **Incubation period** is the time interval between initial contact with the infectious organism and the first appearance of symptoms associated with the infection.

7. **Period of communicability** is the time during which an infectious agent may be transferred directly or indirectly from an infected person to another person; from an infected animal to

humans; or from an infected person to animals, including arthropods.

8. **Susceptibility** (including immunity) provides information on human or animal populations at risk of infection, or that are resistant to either infection or disease. Information on subsequent immunity consecutive to infection is also given.

9. **Methods of control** are described under the following headings:

A. **Preventive measures:** for individuals and groups.

B. **Control of patient, contacts and the immediate environment:** measures designed to prevent further spread of the disease from infected persons, and specific best current treatment to minimize the period of communicability and to reduce morbidity and mortality.

- Recommendations for isolation of patients depend first on "universal precautions" with specific measures cited mainly from CDC and WHO guidelines available on the worldwide web.

- CCDM18 is not intended to be a therapeutic guide. However, current clinical management is presented in section 9B7 of each disease. Specific dosages and clinical management are indicated primarily for those diseases where delay in instituting therapy might jeopardize the patient's life.

- Some of the licensed drugs needed for treatment of rare or exotic diseases are available at no cost from WHO, and those which are not licensed may, at times, be available from CDC as Investigational New Drugs (IND).

- Details, including telephone numbers and e-mail addresses are entered in section 9B7 for those diseases where such drugs or biologics may be available.

C. **Epidemic measures:** describes those procedures of an emergency character designed to limit the spread of a communicable disease that has developed widely in a group or community, or within an area, state or nation.

D. **Disaster implications:** given a disaster, indicates the likelihood that the disease might constitute a major problem if preventive actions are not initiated.

E. **International measures:** outlines those interventions designed to protect populations against the known risk of infection from international sources. The WHO Collaborating Centres, the CDC, and other operational institutions can provide national authorities with the services following: laboratory diagnosis, consultation, analysis of information, production and distribution of standard and reference materials and reagents, training, organization of collaborative research, and provision of further information on specific diseases. WHO can be approached directly for further details about these Centres, listed at www.who.int/WHOCC_Net/ for WHO Collaborating Centres dealing specifically with communicable diseases and http://whocc.who.int/ database for all other WHO Collaborating Centres. Outbreaks can be electronically reported 24 hours a day by e-mail at outbreak@who.int.

F. **Measures in case of deliberate use of biological agents to cause harm (formerly bioterrorism measures):** for selected diseases, this new section provides information and guidelines for public health workers who may be confronted with a threatened or actual act of deliberate use with a specific infectious disease agent.

The relevant telephone numbers are:

- +(0041) 22 791 2111 for WHO
- +(001) 770 488 7100/ 404 639 3311/ 404 639 2888 for CDC.

The relevant websites are:

- http://www.who.int/csr/delibepidemics for WHO
- http://www.cdc.gov/

Outbreaks can be electronically reported 24 hours a day:

- outbreak@who.int
- ehheinq@cdc.gov

To update CCDM17, a literature review was done to identify publications during the preceding five-year period for each disease in that edition. These publications were provided to the primary reviewer for use in updating the chapter for CCDM18 (2004); additional chapters were added on Buruli ulcer and on Severe Acute Respiratory Syndrome (SARS). The name of each primary reviewer is provided in square brackets at the end of each disease entry. Some diseases did not undergo major updating for the 18th edition and show no primary reviewer.

REPORTING OF COMMUNICABLE DISEASES

Reporting of some communicable diseases is required within countries and in some instances internationally to WHO. Reporting can take the form of either a case report or an outbreak report.

1. **Case reports:** Case reporting provides diagnosis, age, sex and date of onset for each person with the disease. Sometimes it includes identifying information such as the name and address of the person with the disease. Additional information such as treatment provided and its duration are required for certain case reports.

National guidelines and legislation indicate which diseases must be reported, who is responsible for reporting, the format for reporting, and how case reports are to be entered into and forwarded within the national system. If there is a requirement for international case reporting, national governments report to WHO.

2. **Outbreak reports:** Outbreak reporting provides information about an increase above the expected number of persons with a communicable disease that may be of public concern. The specific disease may not be included in the list of diseases officially reportable, or it may be of unknown etiology if it is newly recognized or emerging.

National guidelines and legislation indicate which type of oubtreak must be reported, who is responsible for reporting, the format for reporting, and how case reports are to be entered into and forwarded within the national system. In general, outbreak reporting is required by the most rapid means of communication available. If there is a requirement for outbreak reporting international, national governments report to WHO.

The diseases listed in CCDM18 are distributed among 5 classes of reporting, referred to by class number throughout the text under section 9B1 of each disease.

Class 1: Case report required internationally to WHO by the *International Health Regulations* or as a disease under surveillance by WHO.

Diseases subject to the *International Health Regulations* (1969):
The *International Health Regulations* (IHR) are the only legally binding instrument requiring international reporting of communicable diseases (currently limited to cholera, plague and yellow fever). WHO is updating and revising the *International Health Regulations* to address the threat of other new and re-emerging infections, and to accommodate

new sources for reporting information on infectious diseases. WHO will formally consult its Member States and constituents on the proposed revisions during 2004 with a target for adoption of the Revised Regulations in 2005. The key proposals in the revision are to:

- Require the establishment of defined core capacities in surveillance and response to public health emergencies.

- Require the international reporting of public health emergencies of international concern as defined by decision-tree analysis under the Regulations.

- Link reporting to specific response actions recommended by WHO and tailored to the epidemiology of the reported event.

- Enhance communication and collaboration during such emergencies through a network of national focal points for the *International Health Regulations*.

Diseases under surveillance by WHO:
Diseases under surveillance by WHO include louse-borne typhus fever, relapsing fever, meningococcal meningitis, paralytic poliomyelitis, malaria, tuberculosis, HIV/AIDS, influenza and SARS.

For both subcategories, case report is required to the WHO through the national health authority. Collective outbreak reports including the number of cases and deaths may be requested on a daily or weekly basis for diseases with outbreak potential such as influenza.

Class 2: Case report regularly required wherever the disease occurs

Diseases of relative urgency require reporting either because identification of contacts is required or because the source of infection must be known in order to begin control measures.

National health authorities generally require reporting of the first recognized case in an area or the first case outside the limits of a known affected local area by the most rapid means available, followed by weekly case reports—examples include diseases under surveillance by WHO (above), typhoid fever and diphtheria. National health authorities may also require reports of infectious diseases caused by agents that may be used deliberately.

Class 3: Selectively reportable in recognized endemic areas

Many national health authorities do not require case reporting of diseases of this class. Reporting may however be required by reason of undue frequency or severity, in order to stimulate control measures or acquire essential epidemiological data. Examples of diseases in this class are scrub typhus, schistosomiasis and fasciolopsiasis.

Class 4: Obligatory report of outbreaks only—no case report required

Many countries require reporting of outbreaks to health authorities by the most rapid means. Information required includes number of cases, date of onset, population at risk and apparent mode of spread. Examples are staphylococcal foodborne intoxication and outbreaks of an unidentified etiology.

Class 5: Official report not ordinarily justifiable

Diseases in this class occur sporadically or are uncommon, often not directly transmissible from person to person (chromoblastomycosis), or of an epidemiological nature that offers no practical measures for control (common cold).

RESPONSE TO AN OUTBREAK REPORT

The response to an outbreak report must be management of those infected, and containment of the outbreak by interrupting transmission of the infectious agent. Steps in an outbreak response are systematic and based on epidemiological evidence despite the fact that public and political reaction, urgency and the local situation may make this difficult. The following steps provide minimal guidance for responding to outbreaks and are sometimes done concurrently:

- Verify the diagnosis

- Confirm the existence of an outbreak

- Identify affected persons and their characteristics
    - Record case histories
    - Identify additional cases

- Define and investigate population at risk

- Formulate a hypothesis as to source and spread of the outbreak

- Contain the outbreak
    - Manage cases
    - Implement control measures to prevent spread
    - Conduct ongoing disease surveillance
    - Prepare a report.

Verify the diagnosis

Initial notification of an outbreak is often made by a health worker who must collect as detailed a history as possible from the initial cases. A tentative differential diagnosis may be made, for example food poisoning or cholera, that enables the investigator to anticipate the diagnostic specimens required and the kind of equipment to be used during the investigation. The laboratory that will analyse the specimens should be alerted at this stage. If initial cases have died, the extent and need for autopsies should be considered. For surveillance and control purposes, investigators must agree on a common *surveillance case definition* (this may not always correspond to the clinical case definition).

Confirm the existence of an outbreak

Some diseases, although long endemic in an area, remain unrecognized; new cases may come to light, for instance, when new treatments attract patients who previously relied on traditional medicines. Such "false outbreaks" must be excluded through attempts at determining the previous incidence or prevalence of the disease.

An outbreak can be demonstrated on a graph of incidence over time and by a map of geographical extension. For endemic diseases, an outbreak is said to have begun when incidence rises above the normally expected level. For diseases showing a cyclical or seasonal variation, the average incidence rates over particular weeks or months of previous years, or average high or low levels over a period of years, may be used as baselines.

Identify affected persons and their characteristics

Record case histories

Information about each confirmed or suspected case must be recorded to obtain a complete understanding of the outbreak. Usually this information includes name, age, sex, occupation, place of residence, recent movements, details of symptoms (including dates and time of onset) and dates of previous immunization against childhood or other diseases. Other details will vary with the differential diagnosis. If the incubation period is known, information on possible source contacts may be sought. This information is best recorded on specially prepared record forms called line lists. The logistics of form duplication, data entry and verification must be worked out in relation to reporting (See Reporting).

Identify additional cases

Initial notification of an outbreak may come from a clinic or hospital; enquiries in health centres, dispensaries and villages in the area may reveal other cases, sometimes with a range of additional symptoms.

Define and investigate population at risk

The population at risk of infection must be identified; this provides the denominator required and ensures that remaining cases can be identified. Overall or specific attack rates (age-specific village-specific) can then be calculated. These calculations may lead to new hypotheses requiring further investigation and development of study designs. In addition the population at risk may require laboratory investigation (e.g. rate of nasal meningococcal carriage in the population). Microbiological typing and susceptibility to antibiotics can then be used to develop appropriate control measures.

Formulate a hypothesis as to source and spread of the outbreak

Determine why the outbreak occurred when it did and what set the stage for its occurrence. Whenever possible the relevant conditions before the outbreak should be determined. For foodborne outbreaks it is necessary to determine source, vehicle, predisposing circumstances and portal of entry. If transmission is widespread this may prove difficult. All links in the process must be considered: i) disease-causing agent in the population and its characteristics; ii) existence of a reservoir; iii) mode of exit from this reservoir or source; iv) mode of transmission to the next host; v) mode of entry; vi) susceptibility of the host.

Contain the outbreak

The key to effective containment of an outbreak is a coordinated investigation and response involving health workers including clinicians, epidemiologists, microbiologists, health educators and the public health authority. The best way to ensure coordination may be to establish an outbreak containment committee early in the outbreak.

Manage cases

Health workers, including clinicians, must assume responsibility for treatment of diagnosed cases. In outbreaks of meningitis, plague or cholera, emergency accommodation may have to be found and additional staff may require rapid essential training. Outbreaks of diseases such as sleeping sickness and cholera may require special treatment and recourse to drugs not normally available. The investigative team must estimate requirements and obtain supplies urgently. Outbreaks such as poliomyelitis may leave in their wake patients with an immediate need for physiotherapy and rehabilitation; timely organization of these services will lessen the impact of the outbreak.

Implement control measures to prevent spread

After the epidemiological characteristics of the outbreak have been better understood, it is possible to implement control measures to prevent further spread of the infectious agent. However, from the very beginning of the investigation the investigative team must attempt to limit the spread and the occurrence of new cases.

Many communicable diseases can be prevented by chemoprophylaxis or vaccination. Immediate isolation of affected persons can prevent spread, and measures to prevent movement in or out of the affected area may be considered. Universal precautions in patient care are essential. Whatever the urgency of the control measures they must also be explained to the community at risk. Population willingness to report new cases, attend vaccination campaigns, improve standards of hygiene or other such activities is critical for successful containment.

If supplies of vaccine or drugs are limited, it may be necessary to identify the groups at highest risk initial for control measures. Once these urgent measures have been put in place, it is necessary to initiate more permanent ones such as health education, improved water supply, vector control or improved food hygiene. It may be necessary to develop and implement long-term plans for continued vaccination after an initial campaign.

Conduct ongoing disease surveillance

During the acute phase of an outbreak it may be necessary to keep persons at risk (e.g. contacts) under surveillance for disease onset. After the outbreak has initially been controlled, continued community surveillance may be needed in order to identify additional cases and to complete containment. Sources of information for surveillance include: i) notifications of illness by health workers, community chiefs, employers, school teachers, heads of families; ii) certification of deaths by medical authorities; iii) data from other sources such as public health laboratories, entomological and veterinary services. It may be necessary to maintain estimates of the immune status of the population when immunization is part of control activities, by relating the amount of vaccine used to the estimated number of persons at risk, including newborns.

Prepare a report

A report should be prepared at intervals during containment if possible, and after the outbreak has been fully contained. Reports may be: i) a popular account for the general public so that they understand the nature of the outbreak and what is required of them to prevent spread or recurrence; ii) an account for planners in the Ministry of Health/local authority so as to ensure that the necessary administrative steps are taken to prevent recurrence: iii) a scientific report for publication in a medical journal or epidemiological bulletin (reports of recent outbreaks are valuable aids when teaching staff about outbreak control).

Undertake experimental verification of agent and mode of transmission

The verification of hypotheses about an outbreak may at times require experimental evidence of biological feasibility. For example, it may be necessary to show that sliced foodstuffs can be contaminated by an infected slicing machine if this has not been proven during the outbreak investigation. Such verification requires more laboratory facilities than are available in the field, and is often not completed until long after the outbreak has been contained.

DELIBERATE USE OF BIOLOGICAL AGENTS TO CAUSE HARM
(BIOTERRORISM, BIOLOGICAL WARFARE)

The deliberate use of biological agents to harm human populations is a public health problem of varying dimensions depending on the size of the target population and the ease with which the agent can infect that population. The response will of necessity involve the intelligence community and law enforcement agencies as well as public health services, and possibly the Defence Ministry as well, especially if the event is considered of non-domestic origin. Difficulties in communication and approaches may arise, since these disciplines do not usually work together.

The risk of deliberate use cannot be quantified or predicted, but the importance of the public health response has been shown in October 2001 in the USA when anthrax spores were deliberately distributed through the postal system, causing 22 infections and five deaths. The public health response included identifying all those at risk of infection through the postal system, and prescribing antibiotics to over 32 000 persons identified as potentially in contact with envelopes contaminated with anthrax spores. The response also involved emergency and law enforcement services in the USA and around the world where numerous false alarms occurred simultaneously. The event and associated hoaxes caused unprecedented demands on public health laboratory services, and several nations had to recruit private laboratories to deal with the overflow.

If the agent is widely dispersed and/or easily transmissible, a surge capacity may be required to accommodate large numbers of patients, and systems must be available for the rapid mobilization and distribution of medicines or vaccines according to the agent released. In the event that the agent is transmissible, additional capacity will be required for contact tracing and active surveillance. Some of the infectious agents of concern include bacteria and rickettsia (anthrax, brucellosis, melioidosis, plague, Q fever, tularemia, and typhus), fungi (coccidioidomycosis) and viruses (arboviruses, filoviruses and variola virus). International threat analysis considers that deliberate use of biological agents to cause harm is a real threat and that it can occur at any time; however, such risk analysis is not generally considered a public health function.

According to national intelligence and defence services, there is evidence that national and international networks have engineered biological agents for use as weapons, in some instances with suggestions of attempts to increase pathogenicity and to develop delivery mechanisms for their deliberate use. Infection of humans may be a one-time occurrence, or may be repeated over a period of time after the initial occurrence. The agent used will determine whether there is a risk of person-to-person transmission after the initial and subsequent attacks; information on this risk is covered in more detail under specific disease agents. Incubation period, period of communicability and susceptibility are agent-specific.

Prevention of the deliberate use of biological agents presupposes accurate and up-to-date intelligence about terrorists and their activities. The agents may be manufactured using equipment necessary for the routine manufacture of drugs and vaccines, and the possibility of dual use of these facilities adds to the complexity of prevention. This has led some analysts to regard a strong public health infrastructure, with rapid and effective detection and response mechanisms for naturally occurring infectious diseases of outbreak potential, as the only reasonable means of responding to the threat of deliberately caused outbreaks of infectious disease.

PREPAREDNESS FOR DELIBERATELY CAUSED OUTBREAKS OF INFECTIOUS DISEASE

Routine national and global surveillance systems for naturally occurring outbreak-prone and emerging infectious diseases enhance the capacity to detect, and respond to, deliberately caused infectious diseases because the public health detection and response mechanisms are the same. Adequate background information on the natural behaviour of infectious diseases will facilitate recognition of an unusual event and help determine whether suspicions of a deliberate use should be investigated.

Preparedness for deliberate use also requires mechanisms that can be immediately called into action to enhance communication and collaboration among the public health authorities, the intelligence community, law enforcement agencies and national defence systems as need may arise. Preparedness should draw on existing plans for responding to large-scale natural disasters, such as earthquakes or industrial or transportation accidents, in which health care facilities are required to deal with a surge of casualties and emergency admissions.

Most health workers will have little or no experience in managing illness arising from several of the potential infectious agents; training in clinical recognition and initial management may therefore be needed for first responders. This training should include methods for infection control, safe handling of diagnostic specimens and body fluids, and decontamination procedures. One of the most difficult issues for the public health system is to decide whether preparedness should include stockpiling of drugs, vaccines and equipment.

CONTROL

One of the routine criteria to be considered for outbreak assessment under the revised *International Health Regulations* is "suspected accidental or deliberate release". The global outbreak alert and response network (GOARN), facilitated by WHO, supports operational implementation of the *International Health Regulations* and will be called into action immediately in case of deliberate use, in order to contribute to a coordinated international response. Outbreaks of international importance, whether naturally occurring or thought to have been deliberately caused, should be reported electronically by national governments to outbreak@who.int

Further information at WHO:

- +004122792531
- http://www.who.int/csr/delibepidemics

ACQUIRED IMMUNODEFICIENCY
SYNDROME   ICD-9 042-044, 279.5; ICD-10 B20-B24
(HIV infection, AIDS)

1. Identification—Acquired Immunodeficiency syndrome (AIDS) is a term first used by epidemiologists concerned about the emergence in 1981 of a cluster of diseases associated with loss of cellular immunity in adults who had no obvious reason for presenting such immune deficiencies. AIDS was subsequently shown to be the late clinical stage of infection with the human immunodeficiency virus (HIV). Within several weeks to several months after infection with HIV, many persons develop an acute self-limited mononucleosis-like illness lasting for a week or two. They may then be free of clinical signs or symptoms for months or years before other clinical manifestations develop. The severity of subsequent HIV-related opportunistic infections or cancers is, in general, directly correlated with the degree of immune system dysfunction.

More than a dozen opportunistic infections and several cancers were considered to be sufficiently specific indicators of the underlying immunodeficiency for inclusion in the initial (1982) case definition of AIDS. If diagnosed by standard histological and/or culture techniques, these diseases were accepted as meeting the surveillance definition of AIDS cases, provided other known causes of immunodeficiency were ruled out.

This definition was broadened in 1987 to include additional indicator diseases and to accept some of the indicator diseases as a presumptive diagnosis if laboratory tests showed evidence of HIV infection. In 1993, a revised surveillance definition of AIDS included additional indicator diseases. In addition, all HIV-infected persons with a CD4+ cell count of under 200/mm^3 or a CD4+ T-lymphocyte percentage of total lymphocytes under 14%, regardless of clinical status, are regarded as AIDS cases. The 1993 definition continues to be generally accepted for clinical use in most industrialized countries; but it is often not used by developing countries, which lack adequate laboratory facilities for CD4+ cell counts or for the histological or culture diagnosis of the surrogate indicator diseases.

The history of WHO AIDS surveillance started with a provisional clinical case definition without serological confirmation and progressed to a revised definition formulated in Bangui, Central African Republic in 1994. Many countries now report new HIV infections rather than new AIDS cases. The revised African AIDS case definition incorporates HIV serological testing, if available, and includes a few indicator diseases (tuberculosis, pneumococcal disease and non-typhoid salmonellosis, which are not diseases of high virulence) as diagnostic in seropositive individuals.

Bacterial pneumonia is one of the commonest presentations. The clinical manifestations of HIV infection in infants and young children overlap with failure to thrive, inherited immunodeficiencies and other childhood health problems. WHO and CDC have published paediatric AIDS case definitions.

The proportion of HIV-infected persons who, in the absence of anti-HIV treatment, will ultimately develop AIDS has been estimated at over 90%. In the absence of effective anti-HIV treatment, the AIDS case-fatality rate is high: survival time in many developing country studies is often under 1 year; in industrialized countries 80%–90% of untreated patients used to die within 3–5 years after diagnosis. Routine use of prophylactic drugs to prevent *Pneumocystis carinii* pneumonia and other opportunistic infections in most industrialized countries significantly postponed the development of AIDS and death seen before effective anti-HIV treatment had become routinely available.

Serological tests for antibodies to HIV have been available commercially since 1985. The most commonly used screening test (EIA or ELISA) is highly sensitive and specific. The testing strategy depends on the purpose of testing. For surveillance purposes different strategies are recommended according to the expected level of HIV prevalence in the population tested. A single test is recommended in populations with a prevalence rate above 10%; lower prevalence levels require a minimum of 2 different tests for reliability. For diagnostic purposes a 3-test strategy for asymptomatic persons is recommended in populations with an HIV prevalence rate under 10% and a 2-test strategy in populations with higher rates. Selection of tests depends on factors such as accuracy and local operational characteristics. Different combinations of testing formats, EIA and rapid tests can be used. Confirmatory testing may include the Western blot or indirect fluorescent antibody (IFA) test. A nonreactive supplemental test negates an initial reactive EIA test; a positive reaction supports it; an indeterminate result in the Western blot test calls for further evaluation. Rapid testing techniques on blood or oral mucosal transudate facilitate delivery of testing and counselling services.

Most persons infected with HIV develop detectable antibodies within 1–3 months after infection. Other tests to detect HIV infection during the period after infection but prior to seroconversion are available; they include tests for circulating HIV antigen (p24) and PCR tests to detect viral nucleic acid sequences. The window period between the earliest possible detection of virus and seroconversion is short (less than 2 weeks). Antibody tests are thus rarely useful in diagnosing early HIV infection. Even for infants born of HIV-infected women these tests are of limited diagnostic value—passively transferred maternal anti-HIV antibodies often cause falsely positive anti-HIV EIA tests in these children even up to the age of 15 months.

The absolute T-helper cell (CD4+) count or percentage is used most often to evaluate the severity of HIV infection and to help clinicians make decisions about treatment. Viral load tests are now available and serve as an additional marker of disease progression and response to treatment. The differential sensitivity of EIA and tests such as p24 antigenaemia has served to identify recent infections. A person reacting positively on the sensitive test and negatively on the less sensitive is likely to have been infected recently.

2. Infectious agent—Human immunodeficiency virus (HIV), a retrovirus. Two serologically and geographically distinct types with similar epidemiological characteristics, HIV-1 and HIV-2, have been identified. The pathogenicity of HIV-2 may be lower than that of HIV-1: they also have genotypic and phenotypic differences, with slower disease progression and lower rates of mother-to-child transmission for HIV-2.

3. Occurrence—AIDS was first recognized as a distinct clinical entity in 1981; in retrospect, however, isolated cases appear to have occurred during the 1970s and even earlier in several areas (Africa, Europe, Haiti, USA). Of the estimated 40 million persons (34–46 million) living with HIV infection or AIDS (HIV/AIDS) worldwide in 2003, the largest elements were estimated at 25–28.2 million in sub-Saharan Africa, 4.6–8.2 million in south and southeastern Asia, 13–1.9 million in Latin America and 800 000–1 million in North America. Globally, AIDS caused an estimated 3.1 million deaths in 2003 (2.5–3.5 million); the epidemic has continued growing, with estimates of 5 million new infections (4.2–5.8 million) and 2.5 million children (2.1–2.9 million) living with HIV/AIDS. HIV-1 is the most prevalent HIV type throughout the world; HIV-2 has been found primarily in western Africa, with cases also in countries linked epidemiologically to western Africa.

In many developing countries numbers of AIDS cases are much higher, but reporting is poor and monitoring efforts have focused on HIV infections rather than AIDS cases. In several industrialized countries, the distribution of AIDS cases by risk behaviours or factors has shifted over the past decade. For example, although the AIDS epidemic in the USA continues to affect primarily men who have sex with men, intravenous drug use (IDU) is the main source of infection in other countries such as the former Soviet Union.

In the USA and other industrialized countries, annual HIV incidence decreased shortly before the mid-1980s and has remained relatively low since then in most groups. However, in the most severely affected countries in sub-Saharan Africa, annual HIV incidence has continued almost unabated at high levels. Outside sub-Saharan Africa, high HIV prevalence rates (more than 1%) in the 15–49 year old population have been noted in the Caribbean and in south and southeastern Asia. China and India, more recently infected, remain of major concern epidemiologically.

4. Reservoir—Humans. HIV is thought to have recently evolved from chimpanzee viruses.

5. Mode of transmission—Person to person transmission through unprotected (heterosexual or homosexual) intercourse; contact of abraded skin or mucosa with body secretions such as blood, CSF or semen; the use of HIV-contaminated needles and syringes, including sharing by intravenous drug users; transfusion of infected blood or its components;

and the transplantation of HIV-infected tissues or organs. The risk of HIV transmission through sexual intercourse is lower than for most other sexually transmitted agents. However, the presence of a concurrent sexually transmitted disease, especially an ulcerative one, can facilitate HIV transmission. The primary determinants of sexual transmission of HIV are patterns and prevalence of sexual risk behaviours such as unprotected intercourse (no condom—a.k.a. unprotected sex) with many concurrent or overlapping sexual partners.

HIV can also be transmitted from mother to child (MTCT or vertical transmission). From 15% to 35% of infants born to HIV-positive mothers are infected through placental processes at birth. HIV-infected women can transmit infection to their infants through breastfeeding and this can account for up to half of mother-to-child HIV transmission. Giving pregnant women antiretrovirals such as zidovudine results in a marked reduction of MTCT.

Up to mid-1999, the only drug shown to reduce the risk of perinatal HIV transmission was azidothymidine (AZT) when administered orally after the 14th week of pregnancy and continued up to delivery; administered intravenously during the intrapartum period; and administered orally to the newborn for the first 6 weeks of life. This chemoprophylactic regimen was shown to reduce the risk of perinatal transmission by 66%. A shorter course of AZT treatment has been shown to reduce the risk of perinatal transmission by about 40%.

After direct exposure of health care workers to HIV-infected blood through injury with needles and other sharp objects, the rate of seroconversion is less than 0.5%, much lower than the risk of hepatitis B virus infection after similar exposures (about 25%). Unsafe injections may account for up to 5% of transmission.

It cannot be sufficiently stressed that carriers are usually asymptomatic; they—and their potential partners—are therefore unaware of their potential infection status.

While the virus has occasionally been found in saliva, tears, urine and bronchial secretions, transmission after contact with these secretions has not been reported. The risk of transmission from oral sex is not easily quantifiable, but is presumed to be low. No laboratory or epidemiological evidence suggests that biting insects have transmitted HIV infection.

6. Incubation period—Variable. Although the time from infection to the development of detectable antibodies is generally 1–3 months, the time from HIV infection to diagnosis of AIDS has an observed range of less than 1 year to 15 years or longer. The median incubation period in infected infants is shorter than in adults. The increasing availability of effective anti-HIV treatment since the mid-1990s has reduced the development of clinical AIDS in most industrialized countries.

There is some evidence that disease progression from HIV infection to AIDS is more rapid in developing countries than in other populations. The only factor that has been consistently shown to affect progression from

HIV infection to the development of AIDS is age at initial infection: adolescent and adults (males and females) who acquire HIV infection at an early age progress to AIDS more slowly than those infected at an older age. Disease progression may also vary somewhat by viral subtype.

7. Period of communicability—Not known precisely; begins early after onset of HIV infection and presumably extends throughout life. Infectivity during the first months is considered to be high; it increases with viral load, with worsening clinical status and with the presence of other STIs. Free or cell-associated virus occurs in secretions and hence ulcerative or inflammatory STIs are a risk factor.

8. Susceptibility—Unknown, but presumed to be general: race, gender and pregnancy status do not appear to affect susceptibility to HIV infection or AIDS. There is increasing evidence of host factors such as chemokine-receptor polymorphisms that may reduce susceptibility. The presence of other STIs, especially if ulcerative, increases susceptibility, as may the fact of not being circumcised as males, a factor possibly related to the general level of penile hygiene. Interactions between HIV and other infectious disease agents have caused great medical and public health concern. The major interaction identified so far is with *Mycobacterium tuberculosis* infection. Persons with latent tuberculous infection who are also infected with HIV develop clinical tuberculosis at an increased rate, with a lifetime risk of developing tuberculosis that is multiplied by a factor of 6–8. This interaction has resulted in a parallel pandemic of tuberculosis: in some urban sub-Saharan African populations where 10%–15% of the adult population have dual infections (*Mycobacterium tuberculosis* and HIV), annual incidence rates for tuberculosis increased 5- to 10-fold during the latter half of the 1990s. No conclusive data indicate that any infection, including *M. tuberculosis* infection, accelerates progression to AIDS in HIV-infected persons. Other adverse interactions with HIV infection include pneumococcal infection, non-Typhi salmonellosis, falciparum malaria and visceral leishmaniasis.

9. Methods of control—

    A. Preventive measures: HIV/AIDS prevention programs can be effective only with full community and political commitment to change and/or reduce high HIV-risk behaviours.

        1) Public and school health education must stress that having multiple and especially concurrent and/or overlapping sexual partners or sharing drug paraphernalia both increase the risk of HIV infection. The specific needs of minorities, persons with different primary languages and those with visual, hearing or other impairments must also be addressed. Students must be taught the skills needed to avoid or reduce risky behaviours. Programs for school-age youth

should address the needs and developmental levels of both students and those who do not attend school.

2) The only absolutely sure way to avoid infection through sex is to abstain from sexual intercourse or to engage in mutually monogamous sexual intercourse only with someone known (preferably through serology) to be uninfected. In other situations, latex condoms must be used correctly every time a person has vaginal, anal or oral sex. Both male and female latex condoms with water-based lubricants have been shown to reduce the risk of sexual transmission.

3) Expansion of facilities for treating drug users reduces HIV transmission. Programs that instruct needle users in decontamination methods and needle exchange have been shown to be effective.

4) HIV testing and counselling is an important intervention for raising awareness of HIV status, promoting behavioural change and diagnosing HIV infection. HIV testing and counselling can be undertaken for:

a) persons who are ill or involved in high-risk behaviours, who may have a test for diagnostic purposes;

b) attenders at antenatal clinics, to diagnose maternal infection and prevent vertical transmission;

c) couple counselling (marital or premarital);

d) anonymous and/or confidential HIV counselling and testing for the "worried well".

5) All pregnant women must be counselled about HIV early in pregnancy and, where culturally and socially appropriate, encouraged to undertake an HIV test as a routine part of standard antenatal care. Those found to be HIV-positive may wish to take a course of ARV treatment, where this is on offer, to reduce the risk of their infant being infected. There is some evidence that *exclusive* breastfeeding is associated with lower transmission rates than partial breastfeeding.

6) All donated units of blood must be tested for HIV antibody; only donations testing negative can be used. People who have engaged in behaviours that place them at increased risk of HIV infection should not donate plasma, blood, organs for transplantation, tissue or cells (including semen for artificial insemination). Organizations that collect plasma, blood or other body fluids or organs should inform potential donors of this recommendation and test all donors. When possible, donations of sperm, milk or bone should be frozen and stored for 3–6 months before use. Donors who test negative after that interval can be considered not to have been infected at the time of donation.

7) Physicians should adhere strictly to medical indications for transfusions. The use of autologous transfusions should be encouraged.

8) Only clotting factor products that have been screened and treated to inactivate HIV must be used.

9) Care must be taken in handling, using and disposing of needles or other sharp instruments. Health care workers should wear latex gloves, eye protection and other personal protective equipment in order to avoid contact with blood or with fluids. Blood should be washed off with soap and water without delay. These precautions must be taken in the care of all patients and in all laboratory procedures

10) WHO recommends immunization of asymptomatic HIV-infected children with the EPI vaccines; those who are symptomatic should not receive BCG vaccine. Live Measles-Mumps-Rubella and polio vaccines are recommended for all HIV-infected children.

B. Control of patient, contacts and the immediate environment:

1) Report to local health authority: Official reporting of AIDS cases is obligatory in most countries. Official reporting of HIV infections is required in some areas, Class 2 (see Reporting). Where nominal reporting is not the rule, care must be taken to protect patient confidentiality.

2) Isolation: Isolation of the HIV-positive person is unnecessary, ineffective and unjustified. Universal precautions apply to all hospitalized patients. Observe additional precautions appropriate for specific infections that occur in AIDS patients.

3) Concurrent disinfection: Of equipment contaminated with blood or body fluids and with excretions and secretions visibly contaminated with blood and body fluids by using bleach solution or germicides effective against *M. tuberculosis*.

4) Quarantine: Not applicable. Patients and their sexual partners should not donate blood, plasma, organs for transplantation, tissues, cells, semen for artificial insemination or breastmilk for human milk banks.

5) Immunization of contacts: Not applicable.

6) Notification of contacts and source of infection: The infected patient should ensure notification of sexual and needle-sharing partners whenever possible. Notification by the health care provider is justified only when the patient, after due counselling, still refuses to notify his/her partner(s), and when health care providers are sure that notification will not entail harm to the index case. Care must be taken to protect patient confidentiality.

7) Specific treatment: Early diagnosis of infection and referral for medical evaluation are indicated. Consult current sources of information for appropriate drugs, schedules and doses, including the WHO and UNAIDS websites.

a) Prior to the development of relatively effective antiretroviral treatment, which, in the industrialized countries, has become routinely available since the mid-1990s, treatment was available only for the opportunistic diseases that complicated HIV infection. Prophylactic use of oral trimethoprim-sufamethoxazole, with aerosolized pentamidine as a less effective backup, is recommended to prevent *P. carinii* pneumonia. All HIV infected persons should receive tuberculin skin tests and be evaluated for active TB. If this is found, patients should be placed on antituberculosis treatment. If no active TB is found, patients who are tuberculin-positive or are anergic but were recently exposed should be offered preventive treatment with isoniazid for 12 months (recommended duration varies).

b) AIDS must be managed as a chronic disease; antiretroviral treatment is complex, involving a combination of drugs: resistance will rapidly appear if a single drug is used. The drugs are toxic and treatment must be lifelong. Adherence is critical for the success of the treatment. A successful treatment is not a cure, although it results in suppression of viral replication. Decisions to initiate or change antiretroviral treatment must be guided by the laboratory parameters of both plasma HIV RNA (viral load) and CD4+ T cell count, and by assessing the clinical condition of the patient. Laboratory results provide important information about the virological and immunological status of the patient and the risk of progression to AIDS. Once the decision to initiate antiretroviral treatment has been made, treatment should be aggressive with the goal of maximal viral suppression. In general, a protease inhibitor and two non-nucleoside reverse transcriptase inhibitors should be used initially. Other regimens may be used but are considered less than optimal. Special considerations apply to adolescents and pregnant women, with specific treatment regimens for these patients.

c) Precautions to minimize the risk of HIV transmission in health care settings must be implemented worldwide. Management of persons, especially health care workers, exposed to blood and other body fluids suspected of containing HIV is complex. The factors to consider before recommending postexposure prophylaxis (PEP) includes the nature of the exposure, whether the exposed worker might be pregnant, and the local occurrence of drug-resistant HIV strains. As of late 1999, recommendations for PEP include a basic 4-week regimen of two drugs (zidovudine and lamivudine) for most HIV exposures, as well as an expanded regimen that includes the addition of a protease inhibitor (indinavir or nelfinavir) for HIV exposures that pose an increased risk of transmission or where resistance to one or more of the antiretroviral agents recommended for PEP is known or suspected. Health care organizations should have protocols that promote and facilitate prompt access to postexposure care and reporting of exposures.

C. *Epidemic measures:* HIV is currently pandemic, with large numbers of infections reported in the Africa, the Americas, southeastern Asia, and Europe. See 9A (Preventive measures) for recommendations.

D. *Disaster implications:* Emergency personnel should follow the same universal precautions as health workers. If latex gloves are not available and skin surfaces comes into contact with blood, this should be washed off as soon as possible. Masks, visors and protective clothing are indicated when performing procedures that may involve spurting or splashing of blood or bloody fluids. Emergency transfusion services should use blood donations screened for HIV antibody; when it is not possible to test donated blood, donations should be accepted only from donors who have engaged in no HIV-risk behaviours and preferably from donors who have previously tested negative for HIV.

E. *International measures:* The United Nations Joint Programme on HIV/AIDS (UNAIDS), which coordinates UN activities, and WHO do not endorse measures such as requirements for AIDS or HIV examinations for foreign travellers prior to entry.

[T. Boerma]

ACTINOMYCOSIS   ICD-9 039; ICD-10 A42

1. **Identification**—A chronic bacterial disease, most frequently localized in the jaw, thorax or abdomen. The lesions, firmly indurated areas of purulence and fibrosis, spread slowly to contiguous tissues; eventually, draining sinuses may appear and penetrate to the surface. In infected tissue, the organism grows in clusters, called "sulfur granules."

Diagnosis is made by demonstrating slim, non-spore-forming, Gram-positive bacilli, with or without branching, or "sulfur granules" in tissue or pus, and by isolating microorganisms from samples of appropriate clinical materials not contaminated with normal flora during collection. Clinical findings and culture allow distinction between actinomycosis and actinomycetoma, which are very different diseases. (See Mycetoma.)

2. Infectious agents—*Actinomyces israelii* is the usual human pathogen; *A. naeslundii*, *A. meyeri*, *A. odontolyticus* and *Propionibacterium propionicus* (*Arachnia propionica* or *Actinomyces propionicus*) are reported to cause human actinomycosis. Rarely, *A. viscosus* has been reported but it is more reliably established as contributing to the etiology of periodontal disease. All species are Gram-positive, non acid-fast, anaerobic to microaerophilic higher bacteria that may be part of normal oral flora.

3. Occurrence—An infrequent human disease, occurring sporadically worldwide. Men and women of all races and age groups may be affected; frequency is maximal between 15 and 35 years; the M:F ratio is approximately 2:1. Cases in cattle, horses and other animals are caused by other *Actinomyces* species.

4. Reservoir—Humans are the natural reservoir of *A. israelii* and other agents. In the normal oral cavity, the organisms grow as saprophytes in dental plaque and in tonsillar crypts, without apparent penetration or cellular response in adjacent tissues. Sample surveys in Sweden, the USA and other countries have demonstrated *A. israelii* microscopically in granules from crypts of 40% of extirpated tonsils, and by anaerobic culture in up to 48% of specimens of saliva or material from carious teeth. *A. israelii* has been found in vaginal secretions of approximately 10% of women using intrauterine devices. No external environmental reservoir such as straw or soil has been demonstrated.

5. Mode of transmission—Presumably the agent passes by contact from person to person as part of the normal oral flora. From the oral cavity, the organism may be aspirated into the lung or introduced into jaw tissues through injury, extraction of teeth or mucosal abrasion. Abdominal disease most commonly originates in the appendix. The source of clinical disease is endogenous.

6. Incubation period—Irregular; probably many years after colonization in the oral tissues, and days or months after precipitating trauma and actual penetration of tissues.

7. Period of communicability—How and when *Actinomyces* and *Arachnia* species become part of normal oral flora is unknown; except for rare instances of human bite, infection is unrelated to specific exposure to an infected person.

8. Susceptibility—Natural susceptibility is low. Immunity following infection has not been demonstrated.

9. Methods of control—

A. *Preventive measures:* Maintenance of oral hygiene, particularly removal of accumulating dental plaque, will reduce risk of oral infection.

B. *Control of patient, contacts and the immediate environment:*

1) Report to local health authority: Official report not ordinarily justifiable, Class 5 (see Reporting).
2) Isolation: Not applicable.
3) Concurrent disinfection: Not applicable.
4) Quarantine: Not applicable.
5) Immmunization of contacts: Not applicable.
6) Investigation of contacts and source of infection: Not beneficial.
7) Specific treatment: No spontaneous recovery. Prolonged administration of penicillin in high doses is usually effective; tetracycline, erythromycin, clindamycin and cephalosporins are alternatives. Surgical drainage of abscesses is often necessary.

C. *Epidemic measures:* Not applicable, a sporadic disease.

D. *Disaster implications:* None.

E. *International measures:* None.

AMOEBIASIS
(Amebiasis)

ICD-9 006; ICD-10 A06

1. Identification—A protozoan parasite infection that exists in 2 forms: the hardy infective cyst and the more fragile potentially pathogenic trophozoite. The parasite may act as a commensal or invade the tissues and give rise to intestinal or extraintestinal disease. Most infections are asymptomatic but may become clinically important under certain circumstances. Intestinal disease varies from acute or fulminating dysentery with fever, chills and bloody or mucoid diarrhea (amoebic dysentery), to mild abdominal discomfort with diarrhea containing blood or mucus, alternating with periods of constipation or remission. Amoebic granulomata (amoeboma), sometimes mistaken for carcinoma, may occur in the wall of the large intestine in patients with intermittent dysentery or colitis of long duration. Ulceration of the skin, usually in the perianal region, occurs rarely by direct extension from intestinal lesions or amoebic liver abscesses; penile lesions may occur in active homosexuals. Dissemination via the bloodstream may occur and produce abscesses of the liver, less commonly of the lung or brain.

Amoebic colitis is often confused with forms of inflammatory bowel disease such as ulcerative colitis; care should be taken to distinguish the two since corticosteroids may exacerbate amoebic colitis. Amoebiasis can also mimic numerous noninfectious and infectious diseases. Conversely, the presence of amoebae may be misinterpreted as the cause of diarrhea in a person whose primary enteric illness is the result of another condition.

Diagnosis is by microscopic demonstration of trophozoites or cysts in fresh or suitably preserved fecal specimens, smears of aspirates or scrapings obtained by proctoscopy or aspirates of abscesses or sections of tissue. The presence of trophozoites containing RBCs is indicative of invasive amoebiasis. Examination should be done on fresh specimens by a trained microscopist since the organism must be differentiated from nonpathogenic amoebae and macrophages. Examination of at least 3 specimens will increase the yield of organisms from 50% in a single specimen to 85%–90%. Stool antigen detection tests have recently become available, but do not distinguish pathogenic from nonpathogenic organisms; assays specific for *Entamoeba histolytica* are also available. Reference laboratory services may be required. Many serological tests are available as adjuncts in diagnosing extraintestinal amoebiasis, such as liver abscess, where stool examination is often negative. Serological tests, particularly immunodiffusion and ELISA, are very useful in the diagnosis of invasive disease. Scintillography, ultrasonography and CAT scanning are helpful in revealing the presence and location of an amoebic liver abscess, and can be considered diagnostic when associated with a specific antibody response to *E. histolytica*.

2. **Infectious agent**—*Entamoeba histolytica*, a parasitic organism not to be confused with *E. hartmanni*, *E. coli or* other intestinal protozoa. In isolates, 9 potentially pathogenic and 13 nonpathogenic zymodemes (classified as *E. dispar*) have been identified. Most asymptomatic cyst passers carry strains of *E. dispar*. Immunological differences and isoenzyme patterns permit differentiation of pathogenic *E. histolytica* from the morphologically identical nonpathogenic *E. dispar*.

3. **Occurrence**—Amoebiasis is ubiquitous. Invasive amoebiasis is mostly a disease of young adults; liver abscesses occur predominantly in males. Amoebiasis is rare below age 5 and especially below age 2, when dysentery is due typically to shigellae. The proportion of cyst passers who have clinical disease is usually low. Published prevalence rates of cyst passage, usually based on cyst morphology, vary from place to place, with rates generally higher in areas with poor sanitation, in mental institutions and among sexually promiscuous male homosexuals (probably *E. dispar*).

In areas with good sanitation, amoebic infections tend to cluster in households and institutions.

4. Reservoir—Humans, usually a chronically ill or asymptomatic cyst passer.

5. Mode of transmission—Mainly through ingestion of fecally contaminated food or water containing amoebic cysts, which are relatively chlorine resistant. Transmission may occur sexually by oral-anal contact. Patients with acute amoebic dysentery probably pose only limited danger to others because of the absence of cysts in dysenteric stools and the fragility of trophozoites.

6. Incubation period—From a few days to several months or years; commonly 2–4 weeks.

7. Period of communicability—During the period *E. histolytica* cysts are passed, which may continue for years.

8. Susceptibility—Susceptibility to infection is general; those harbouring *E. dispar* do not develop disease. Susceptibility to reinfection has been demonstrated but is apparently rare.

9. Methods of control—

   A. Preventive measures:

   1) Educate the general public in personal hygiene, particularly in sanitary disposal of feces and in handwashing after defecation and before preparing or eating food. Disseminate information regarding the risks involved in eating uncleaned or uncooked fruits and vegetables and in drinking water of questionable purity.
   2) Dispose of human feces in a sanitary manner.
   3) Protect public water supplies from fecal contamination. Sand filtration of water removes nearly all cysts and diatomaceous earth filters remove them completely. Water of undetermined quality can be made safe by boiling for 1 minute (at least 10 minutes at high altitudes). Chlorination of water as generally practised in municipal water treatment does not always kill cysts; small quantities of water are best treated with prescribed concentrations of iodine, either liquid (8 drops of 2% tincture of iodine or 12.5 ml of a saturated aqueous solution of iodine crystals per liter or quart of water), or as water purification tablets (1 tablet of tetraglycine hydroperiodide per liter or quart of water). Allow for a contact period of at least 10 minutes (30 minutes if cold) before drinking the water. Portable filters with less than 1.0 micrometer pore sizes are effective.

4) Treat known carriers; stress the need for thorough hand-washing after defecation to avoid reinfection from an infected domestic resident.

5) Educate high-risk groups to avoid sexual practices that may permit fecal-oral transmission.

6) Health agencies should supervise the sanitary practices of people who prepare and serve food in public eating places and the general cleanliness of the premises involved. Routine examination of food handlers as a control measure is impractical.

7) Disinfectant dips for fruits and vegetables are of unproven value in preventing transmission of *E. histolytica*. Thorough washing with potable water and keeping fruits and vegetables dry may help; cysts are killed by desiccation, by temperatures above 50°C (122°F) and by irradiation.

8) Use of chemoprophylactic agents is not advised.

B. Control of patient, contacts and the immediate environment:

1) Report to local health authority: In selected endemic areas; in many countries not reportable, Class 3 (see Reporting).

2) Isolation: For hospitalized patients, enteric precautions in the handling of feces, contaminated clothing and bed linen. Exclusion of individuals infected with *E. histolytica* from food handling and from direct care of hospitalized and institutionalized patients. Release to return to work in a sensitive occupation when chemotherapy is completed.

3) Concurrent disinfection: Sanitary disposal of feces.

4) Quarantine: Not applicable.

5) Immunization of contacts: Not applicable.

6) Investigation of contacts and source of infection: Household members and other suspected contacts should have adequate microscopic examination of feces.

7) Specific treatment: Acute amoebic dysentery should be treated with metronidazole. In cases of extraintestinal amoebiasis or refractory intestinal amoebiasis, metronidazole should be followed by iodoquinol, paromomycin or diloxanide furoate. Dehydroemetine, followed by iodoquinol, paromomycin or diloxanide furoate, is a suitable alternative for severe or refractory intestinal disease. There are concerns with the toxicity of dehydroemetine and the risk of optic neuritis with iodoquinol. Tinidazole and ornidazole are also useful single-dose treatments against luminal and tissue disease (not available in some countries, including the USA).

If a patient with a liver abscess continues to be febrile after 72 hours of metronidazole treatment, nonsurgical aspiration may be indicated. Chloroquine is sometimes added to metronidazole or dehydroemetine for treating a refractory liver abscess. Abscesses may require surgical aspiration if there is a risk of rupture or if the abscess continues to enlarge despite treatment. Asymptomatic carriers may be treated with iodoquinol, paromomycin or diloxanide furoate.

Metronidazole is not recommended for use during the first trimester of pregnancy; however, there has been no proof of teratogenicity in humans. Dehydroemetine is contraindicated during pregnancy.

C. *Epidemic measures:* Any group of possible cases requires prompt laboratory confirmation to exclude false-positive identification of *E. histolytica* or other causal agents and epidemiological investigation to determine source of infection and mode of transmission. If a common vehicle is indicated, such as water or food, appropriate measures should be taken to correct the situation.

D. *Disaster implications:* Disruption of normal sanitary facilities and food management will favor an outbreak of amoebiasis, especially in populations that include large numbers of cyst passers.

E. *International measures:* None.

[L. Savioli]

ANGIOSTRONGYLIASIS   ICD-9 128.8; ICD-10 B83.2
(Eosinophilic meningoencephalitis, Eosinophilic meningitis)

1. Identification—A nematode disease of the CNS with predominantly meningeal involvement. Invasion may be asymptomatic or mildly symptomatic; it is commonly characterized by severe headache, neck and back stiffness and various paresthaesias. Temporary facial paralysis occurs in 5% of patients. Low grade fever may be present. The worm has been found in the CSF and in the eye. CSF usually exhibits pleocytosis with over 20% eosinophils; blood eosinophilia is not always present but has reached 82%. Illness may last a few days to several months. Deaths have rarely been reported.

Differential diagnosis includes cerebral cysticercosis, paragonimiasis, echinococcosis, gnathostomiasis, tuberculous, coccidioidal or aseptic meningitis and neurosyphilis.

The presence of eosinophils in the CSF and a history of eating raw molluscs suggest the diagnosis, especially in endemic areas. Immunodiagnostic tests are presumptive; demonstration of worms in CSF or at autopsy is confirmatory.

2. Infectious agent—*Parastrongylus* (*Angiostrongylus*) *cantonensis*, a nematode (lungworm of rats). The third-stage larvae in the intermediate host (terrestrial or marine molluscs) are infective for humans.

3. Occurrence—The nematode is found as far north as Japan, as far south as Brisbane, Australia, and in Africa as far West as Côte d'Ivoire and also in Egypt, Madagascar, the USA and Puerto Rico. The disease is endemic in China (including Taiwan), Cuba, Indonesia, Malaysia, the Philippines, Thailand, Viet Nam, and Pacific islands including Hawaii and Tahiti.

4. Reservoir—The rat (*Rattus* and *Bandicota* spp.).

5. Mode of transmission—Ingestion of raw or insufficiently cooked snails, slugs or land planarians, which are intermediate or transport hosts harbouring infective larvae. Prawns, fish and land crabs that have ingested snails or slugs may also transport infective larvae. Lettuce and other leafy vegetables contaminated by small molluscs may serve as a source of infection. The molluscs are infected by first-stage larvae excreted by an infected rodent; when third-stage larvae have developed in the molluscs, rodents (and people) ingesting the molluscs are infected. In the rat, larvae migrate to the brain and mature to the adult stage; young adults migrate to the surface of the brain and through the venous system to reach their final site in the pulmonary arteries.

After mating, the female worm deposits eggs that hatch in terminal branches of the pulmonary arteries; first-stage larvae enter the bronchial system, pass up the trachea, are swallowed and passed in the feces.

6. Incubation period—Usually 1-3 weeks; may be longer or shorter.

7. Period of communicability—Not transmitted from person to person.

8. Susceptibility—Susceptibility to infection is general. Malnutrition and debilitating diseases may contribute to an increase in severity, even (rarely) to a fatal outcome.

9. Methods of control—

  A. Preventive measures:

  1) Educate the general public in preparation of raw foods and both aquatic and terrestrial snails.
  2) Control rats.
  3) Boil snails, prawns, fish and crabs for 3-5 minutes, or freeze at −15°C (5°F) for 24 hours; this effectively kills the larvae.
  4) Avoid eating raw foods that may be contaminated by snails or slugs; thorough cleaning of lettuce and other greens to eliminate molluscs and their products does not always elim-

inate infective larvae. Radiation pasteurization would be effective.

B. Control of patient, contacts and the immediate environment:

1) Report to local health authority: Official report not ordinarily justifiable, Class 5 (see Reporting).
2) Isolation: Not applicable.
3) Concurrent disinfection: Not necessary.
4) Quarantine: Not applicable.
5) Immunization of contacts: Not applicable.
6) Investigation of contacts and source of infection: Investigate source of food involved and its preparation.
7) Specific treatment: Mebendazole and albendazole appear effective in treating children.

C. Epidemic measures: Any grouping of cases in a particular geographic area or institution warrants prompt epidemiological investigation and appropriate control measures.

D. Disaster implications: None.

E. International measures: None.

ABDOMINAL ANGIOSTRONGYLIASIS   ICD-9 128.8
INTESTINAL ANGIOSTRONGYLIASIS   ICD-10 B81.3

Since 1967, a syndrome similar to appendicitis has been recognized in Costa Rica, predominantly among children under 13, with abdominal pain and tenderness in the right iliac fossa and flank, fever, anorexia, vomiting, abdominal rigidity, a tumour-like mass in the right lower quadrant and pain on rectal examination. Leukocytosis is generally between 20 000 and 30 000/mm^3 (SI units: 20–30 × 10^9/L), with eosinophils ranging from 11% to 61%. On surgery, yellow granulations are found in the subserosa of the intestinal wall, and eggs and larvae of *Parastrongylus* (*Angiostrongylus*) in lymph nodes, intestinal wall and omentum; adult worms are found in the small arteries, generally in the ileocaecal area. Human infections are also known from Central and South America and the USA.

The reservoir of this parasite is a rodent (the cotton rat, *Sigmodon hispidus*); slugs are the usual intermediate hosts. In the rodent host, adults live in the mesenteric arteries of the ileocoecal area, and eggs are carried into the intestinal wall. On embryonation, first-stage larvae migrate to the lumen, are excreted in the feces and ingested by a slug, where they develop to third stage, which is infective for rats and people. Infective larvae are found in slug slime (mucus) left on soil or other surfaces. When tiny slugs (or perhaps the slime) are ingested by people, infective larvae penetrate the gut wall, maturing in the lymphatic nodes and vessels. Adult worms migrate to the mesenteric arterioles of the ileocoecal region where oviposition occurs. In people, most of the eggs and larvae degenerate and cause a granulomatous reaction. There is no specific treatment; surgical intervention is sometimes necessary.

[L. Savioli]

ANISAKIASIS   ICD-9 127.1; ICD-10 B81.0

1. Identification—A parasitic disease of the human GI tract usually manifested by cramping abdominal pain and vomiting, acquired through ingestion of uncooked or undertreated marine fish containing larval ascaridoid nematodes. The motile larvae burrow into the stomach wall producing acute ulceration with nausea, vomiting and epigastric pain, sometimes with hematemesis. They may migrate upwards and attach in the oropharynx, causing cough. In the small intestine, they cause eosinophilic abscesses, and the symptoms may mimic appendicitis or regional enteritis. At times they perforate into the peritoneal cavity; rarely they involve the large bowel.

Diagnosis is made by recognition of the 2-cm-long larvae invading the oropharynx or by visualizing the larvae through gastroscopic examination or in surgically removed tissue. Serological tests are under development.

2. Infectious agents—Larval nematodes of the subfamily Anisakinae, genera *Anisakis* and *Pseudoterranova*.

3. Occurrence—The disease occurs in individuals who eat uncooked and inadequately treated (frozen, salted, marinated, smoked) saltwater fish, squid or octopus. This is common in Japan, where over 12 000 cases have been described (sushi and sashimi), Scandinavia (gravlax), on the Pacific coast of Latin America (ceviche) and less commonly in the Netherlands (herring). With growing consumption of raw fish, cases are seen with increasing frequency throughout western Europe and the USA.

4. Reservoir—Anisakinae are widely distributed in nature, but only some of those parasitic in sea mammals constitute a major threat to humans. The natural life cycle involves transmission of larvae through predation from small crustaceans to squid, octopus or fish, then to sea mammals, with humans as incidental hosts.

5. Mode of transmission—The infective larvae live in the abdominal mesenteries of fish; after death of the fish host they often invade body muscles. When ingested by humans and liberated through digestion in the stomach, they may penetrate the gastric or intestinal mucosa.

6. Incubation period—Gastric symptoms may develop within a few hours of ingestion. Symptoms referable to the small and large bowel occur within a few days or weeks, depending on the size and location of the larvae.

7. Period of communicability—Direct transmission from person to person does not occur.

8. Susceptibility—Apparently universal susceptibility.

9. Methods of control—

   A. Preventive measures:

   1) Avoid ingestion of inadequately cooked marine fish. Heating to 60°C (140°F) for 10 minutes, blast-freezing to −35°C (−31°F) or below for 15 hours or freezing by regular means at −23°C (−9.4°F) for at least 7 days kills the larvae. The latter control method is used with success in the Netherlands. Irradiation effectively kills the parasite.
   2) Cleaning (evisceration) of fish as soon as possible after they are caught reduces the number of larvae penetrating into the muscles from the mesenteries.
   3) Candling (exposure to a light source) for fishery products where parasites can be visualized.

   B. Control of patient, contacts and the immediate environment:

   1) Report to local health authority: Not ordinarily justifiable, Class 5 (see Reporting). A case or cases recognized in an area not previously known to be involved or where control measures are in effect must be reported.
   2) Isolation: Not applicable.
   3) Concurrent disinfection: Not applicable.
   4) Quarantine: Not applicable.
   5) Immmunization of contacts: Not applicable.
   6) Investigation of contacts and source of infection: Examination of others possibly exposed at the same time may be productive.
   7) Specific treatment: Gastroscopic removal of larval abscesses; excision of lesions.

   C. Epidemic measures: None.

   D. Disaster implications: None.

   E. International measures: None.

[D. Engels]

ANTHRAX   ICD-9 022; ICD-10 A22
(Malignant pustule, Malignant oedema, Woolsorter disease, Ragpicker disease)

1. Identification—An acute bacterial disease that usually affects the skin, but may rarely involve the oropharynx, mediastinum or intestinal tract. In cutaneous anthrax, itching of exposed skin surface occurs first, followed by a lesion that becomes papular, then vesicular and in 2–6 days develops into a depressed black eschar. Moderate to severe and very extensive oedema usually surrounds the eschar, sometimes with small secondary vesicles. Pain is unusual and, if present, is due to oedema or secondary infection. The head, forearms and hands are common sites of infection. The lesion has been confused with human Orf (see Orf virus disease). Obstructive airway disease due to associated oedema may complicate cutaneous anthrax of the face or neck. Untreated infections may spread to regional lymph nodes and the bloodstream with overwhelming septicaemia. The meninges can become involved. Untreated cutaneous anthrax has a case-fatality rate between 5% and 20%; with effective treatment, few deaths occur. The lesion evolves through typical local changes even after the initiation of antibiotherapy.

Initial symptoms of inhalation anthrax are mild and nonspecific and may include fever, malaise and mild cough or chest pain; acute symptoms of respiratory distress, X-ray evidence of mediastinal widening, fever and shock follow in 3–5 days, with death shortly thereafter. Intestinal anthrax is rare and more difficult to recognize; it tends to occur in explosive food poisoning outbreaks where abdominal distress is followed by fever, signs of septicaemia and death in typical cases. An oropharyngeal form of primary disease has been described.

Laboratory confirmation is through demonstration of the causative organism in blood, lesions or discharges by direct polychrome methylene blue (M'Fadyean)-stained smears or by culture, rarely by inoculation of mice, guinea pigs or rabbits. Rapid identification of the organism through immunodiagnostic testing, ELISA and PCR may be available in certain reference laboratories.

2. Causative agent—*Bacillus anthracis*, a Gram-positive, encapsulated, spore forming, nonmotile rod (specifically the anthrax spores of *B. anthracis* are the infectious agent; vegetative *B. anthracis* rarely establish disease.)

3. Occurrence—Primarily a disease of herbivores; humans and carnivores are incidental hosts. In most industrialized countries, anthrax is an infrequent and sporadic human infection; it is an occupational hazard primarily of workers who process hides, hair (especially from goats), bone and bone products and wool; and of veterinarians and agriculture and wildlife workers who handle infected animals. Human anthrax is endemic in the agricultural regions of the world where anthrax in animals is common, such as Africa and Asia, south and central America, southern and eastern Europe. New areas of infection in livestock may develop through introduction of animal feed containing contaminated bone meal. Environmental events such as floods may provoke epizootics. Anthrax has been deliberately used to cause harm; as such, it could present in epidemiologically unusual circumstances.

4. Reservoir—Animals (normally herbivores, both livestock and wildlife) shed the bacilli in terminal hemorrhages or blood at death. On exposure to the air, vegetative cells sporulate and the *B. anthracis* spores, which resist adverse environmental conditions and disinfection, may remain viable in contaminated soil for years. Dormant anthrax spores may be passively redistributed in the soil and adjacent vegetation through the action of water, wind and other environmental forces. Scavengers feeding on infected carcases may also disperse anthrax spores beyond the site of death, either through blood and viscera adhering to their fur or feathers or through excretion of viable anthrax spores in fecal matter. Dried or otherwise processed skins and hides of infected animals may harbour spores for years and are the fomites by which the disease is spread worldwide.

5. Mode of transmission—Contact with tissues of animals (cattle, sheep, goats, horses, pigs and others) dying of the disease; possibly also through biting flies that have partially fed on such animals; contact with contaminated hair, wool, hides or products made from them (e.g. drums, brushes, rugs); or contact with soil associated with infected animals or with contaminated bone meal used in gardening. Inhalation anthrax results from inhalation of spores in risky industrial processes—such as tanning hides and processing wool or bone—with aerosols of *B. anthracis* spores in an enclosed, poorly-ventilated area. Intestinal and oropharyngeal anthrax may arise from ingestion of contaminated undercooked meat; there is no evidence that milk from infected animals transmits anthrax. The disease spreads among grazing animals through contaminated soil and feed; and among omnivorous and carnivorous animals through contaminated meat, bone meal or other feeds derived from infected carcases. Accidental infections may occur among laboratory workers.

In 1979, 66 persons were documented to have died of anthrax and 11 infected persons were known to have survived in an outbreak of largely inhalation anthrax in Yekaterinburg (Sverdlovsk), the Russian Federation; numerous other cases are presumed to have occurred. Investigations disclosed that the cases occurred as the result of a plume emanating from a biological research institute and led to the conclusion that the outbreak had resulted from an accidental aerosol related to biological warfare studies.

6. Incubation period—From 1 to 7 days, although incubation periods up to 60 days are possible. In the Sverdlovsk outbreak, incubation periods extended up to 43 days.

7. Period of communicability—Person-to-person transmission is rare. Articles and soil contaminated with spores may remain infective for several years.

8. Susceptibility—There is some evidence of inapparent infection among people in frequent contact with the infectious agent; second attacks can occur, but reports are rare.

9. Methods of control—

   A. Preventive measures:

   1) Immunize high-risk persons with a cell-free vaccine prepared from a culture filtrate containing the protective antigen (in the USA: Bioport Corporation, 3500 N. Martin Luther King Jr Boulevard, Lansing MI 48909). This vaccine is effective in preventing cutaneous and inhalational anthrax: it is recommended for laboratory workers who routinely work with *B. anthracis* and workers who handle potentially contaminated industrial raw materials. It may also be used to protect military personnel against potential exposure to anthrax used as a biological warfare agent. Annual booster injections are recommended if the risk of exposure continues.
   2) Educate employees who handle potentially contaminated articles about modes of anthrax transmission, care of skin abrasions and personal cleanliness.
   3) Control dust and properly ventilate work areas in hazardous industries, especially those handling raw animal materials. Maintain continuing medical supervision of employees and provide prompt medical care of all suspicious skin lesions. Workers must wear protective clothing; adequate facilities for washing and changing clothes after work must be provided. Locate eating facilities away from places of work. Vaporized formaldehyde has been used for disinfection of workplaces contaminated with *B. anthracis*.
   4) Thoroughly wash, disinfect or sterilize hair, wool and bone meal or other feed of animal origin prior to processing.
   5) Do not sell the hides of animals exposed to anthrax or use their carcasses as food or feed supplements (bone or blood meal).
   6) If anthrax is suspected, do not necropsy the animal but aseptically collect a blood sample for culture. Avoid contamination of the area. If a necropsy is inadvertently performed,

autoclave, incinerate or chemically disinfect/fumigate all instruments or materials used.

Because anthrax spores may survive for years if the carcases are buried, the preferred disposal technique is incineration at the site of death or removal to a rendering plant, ensuring that no contamination occurs en route to the plant. Should these methods prove impossible, bury carcases at the site of death as deeply as possible without digging below the local water table level. Laboratory studies of close relatives of *B. anthracis* in the Bacillus genus have shown that exposure to elevated levels of calcium cations can extend the viable lifespan of spores. The same phenomenon could occur with *B. anthracis* spores and the addition of lye or quicklime to a carcase (originally applied in the—not always confirmed—hope of speeding up putrefaction and discourage scavengers) could actually assist in the survival of anthrax spores.

7) Control effluents and wastes from rendering plants that handle potentially infected animals and from factories that manufacture products from hair, wool, bones or hides likely to be contaminated.

8) Promptly immunize and annually reimmunize all domestic animals at risk. Treat symptomatic animals with penicillin or tetracyclines; immunize them after cessation of treatment. These animals should not be used for food until a few months have passed. Treatment in lieu of immunization may be used for animals exposed to a discrete source of infection, such as contaminated commercial feed.

B. *Control of patient, contacts and the immediate environment:*

1) Report to local health authority: Case report obligatory in many countries, Class 2 (see Reporting). Also report to the appropriate livestock or agriculture authority. Even a single case of human anthrax, especially of the inhalation variety, is so unusual in industrialized countries and large urban centers that it warrants immediate reporting to public health and law enforcement authorities for consideration of deliberate use.

2) Isolation: Standard precautions for the duration of illness for cutaneous and inhalation anthrax. Antibiotherapy sterilizes a skin lesion within 24 hours, but the lesion progresses through its typical cycle of ulceration, sloughing and resolution.

3) Concurrent disinfection: Of discharges from lesions and articles soiled therewith. Hypochlorite is sporicidal and good when organic matter is not overwhelming and the item is not corrodable; hydrogen peroxide, peracetic acid or glutaraldehyde may be alternatives; formaldehyde, ethylene oxide and cobalt irradiation have been used. Spores require steam

sterilization, autoclaving or burning to ensure complete destruction. Fumigation and chemical disinfection may be used for valuable equipment.

4) Quarantine: Not applicable.

5) Immmunization of contacts: Not applicable.

6) Investigation of contacts and source of infection: Search for history of exposure to infected animals or animal products and trace to place of origin. In a manufacturing plant, inspect for adequacy of preventive measures as outlined in 9A. As mentioned in 9B1, it may be necessary to rule out a case of deliberate use for all human cases of anthrax, especially for those with no obvious occupational source of infection.

7) Specific treatment: Penicillin is the drug of choice for cutaneous anthrax and is given for 5–7 days. Tetracyclines, erythromycin and chloramphenicol are also effective. The U.S. military recommends parenteral ciprofloxacin or doxycycline for inhalation anthrax though the duration of treatment is not well defined.

C. *Epidemic measures:* Outbreaks may be an occupational hazard of animal husbandry. Occasional epidemics in the USA and other industrialized countries are local industrial outbreaks among employees who work with animal products, especially goat hair. Outbreaks related to handling and consuming meat from infected cattle have occurred in Africa, Asia, and the former Soviet Union.

D. *Disaster implications:* None, except in case of floods in previously infected areas.

E. *International measures:* Sterilize imported bone meal before use as animal feed. Disinfect wool, hair and other products when indicated and feasible.

F. *Measures in case of deliberate use:* A recent incident of deliberate anthrax use has occurred in the USA in 2001. The general procedures for dealing with such civilian occurrences include the following:

1) Anyone who receives a threat about dissemination of anthrax organisms should notify the relevant local criminal investigative authority immediately. In the USA, the Federal Bureau of Investigation (FBI) has primary responsibility for the investigation of such biological threats.

2) Other agencies must cooperate and provide assistance as requested.

3) Where appropriate, local and state health departments should also be notified and be ready to provide public health management and follow-up as needed.

4) Persons who may have been exposed to anthrax are not contagious, and quarantine is not appropriate.

5) If the threat of exposure to aerosolized anthrax is credible or confirmed, persons at risk should begin postexposure prophylaxis with both an appropriate antibiotic (fluoroquinolones are the drugs of choice; doxycycline is an alternative) and if available an inactivated cell-free vaccine may be considered because of uncertainty as to when or if inhaled spores may germinate or be cleared by the alveolar immune system. Postexposure immunization consists of 3 injections, starting as soon as possible after exposure and at 2 and 4 weeks after exposure. The vaccine has not been evaluated for safety and efficacy in children under 18 or in adults 60 or older.

6) All first responders should follow local protocols for incidents involving biological hazards.

7) Responders can be protected from anthrax spores by donning splash protection, gloves and a full face respirator with high-efficiency particle air (HEPA) filters (Level C) or self-contained breathing apparatus (SCBA) (Level B).

8) Persons who may have been exposed and may be contaminated should be decontaminated with soap and copious amounts of water in a shower. Bleach solutions are usually not required; a 1:10 dilution of household bleach (final hypochlorite concentration 0.5%) should be used only if there is gross contamination with the agent and it is impossible to remove the materials through soap and water decontamination. The bleach solution, to be used only after soap and water decontamination, must be rinsed off after 10 to 15 minutes.

9) All persons who are to be decontaminated should remove clothing and personal effects and place all items in plastic bags, which should be labelled clearly with owner's name, contact telephone number and inventory of contents. Personal items may be kept as evidence in a criminal trial or returned to the owner if the threat is unsubstantiated.

10) If the suspect item associated with an anthrax threat remains sealed (unopened), first responders should not take any action other than notifying the relevant authority and packaging the evidence. Quarantine, evacuation, decontamination and chemoprophylaxis efforts are *not* indicated if the envelope or package remains sealed. For incidents involving possibly contaminated letters, the environment in direct contact with the letter or its contents should be decontaminated with a 0.5% hypochlorite solution following a crime scene investigation. Personal effects may be similarly decontaminated.

[R. Diaz]

ARENAVIRAL HEMORRHAGIC FEVERS IN THE WESTERN HEMISPHERE

ICD-9 078.7;
ICD-10 A96

JUNÍN (ARGENTINIAN) HEMORRHAGIC FEVER	ICD-10 A96.0
MACHUPO (BOLIVIAN) HEMORRHAGIC FEVER	ICD-10 A96.1
GUANARITO (VENEZUELAN) HEMORRHAGIC FEVER	ICD-10 A96.8
SABIÁ (BRAZILIAN) HEMORRHAGIC FEVER	ICD-10 A96.8

1. **Identification**—Acute febrile viral illnesses; duration is 7–15 days. Onset is gradual with malaise, headache, retroorbital pain, conjunctival injection, sustained fever and sweats, followed by prostration. There may be petechiae and ecchymoses, accompanied by erythema of the face, neck and upper thorax. An enanthem with petechiae on the soft palate is frequent. Severe infections result in epistaxis, hematemesis, melaena, hematuria and gingival hemorrhage. Encephalopathies, intention tremors and depressed deep tendon reflexes are frequent. Bradycardia and hypotension with clinical shock are common findings, and leukopenia and thrombocytopenia are characteristic. Moderate albuminuria is present, with cellular and granular casts and vacuolated epithelial cells in the urine. Case-fatality rates range from 15% to 30% in untreated individuals.

Diagnosis is made through virus isolation or antigen detection in blood or organs; by PCR, or serologically by IgM capture ELISA; or through the detection of neutralizing antibody or rises in the titre thereof by ELISA or IFA. Laboratory studies for virus isolation and neutralizing antibody tests require BSL-4.

2. **Infectious agents**—Among the 18 known New World arenaviruses belonging to the Tacaribe complex, 4 have been associated with hemorrhagic fever in humans: Junín for the Argentine disease; the closely related Machupo virus for the Bolivian; Guanarito virus for the Venezuelan; and the Sabiá virus for the Brazilian. These viruses are related to the Old World arenaviruses that include the agents of Lassa fever and lymphocytic choriomeningitis. A further virus, Whitewater Arroyo Virus, has been found in rodents in North America.

3. Occurrence—Argentine hemorrhagic fever was first described among corn harvesters in Argentina in 1955. Since then, the number of cases reported from the endemic areas of the Argentine pampa has ranged from 100 to 4000 per year, with an estimated cumulative total of 30 000 symptomatic cases. The region at risk has been expanding northwards and now potentially affects a population of 5 million. Disease occurs seasonally from late February to October, predominantly in males, 63% in the age group 20–49.

A similar disease, Bolivian hemorrhagic fever, caused by the related virus, occurs sporadically or in epidemics in small villages of rural northeastern Bolivia. In July–September 1994, there were 9 cases with 7 deaths.

In 1989, an outbreak of severe hemorrhagic illness occurred in the municipality of Guanarito, Venezuela; 104 cases with 26 deaths occurred between May 1990 and March 1991 among rural residents in Guanarito and neighboring areas. To date, about 200 confirmed cases have been reported. Although the virus continued circulating in the rodent population, there was an unexplained drop in human cases between 1992 and 2002 (one outbreak with 18 cases).

Sabiá virus caused a fatal illness with hemorrhage and jaundice in Brazil in 1990, a laboratory infection in Brazil in 1992 and a laboratory infection treated with ribavirin in the USA in 1994.

4. Reservoir—In Argentina, wild rodents of the pampas (*Calomys musculinus* and *Calomys laucha*) are the hosts for Junín virus. In Bolivia, *Calomys callosus* is the reservoir animal. Cane rats (*Zygodontomys brevicauda*) were shown to be the main reservoir of Guanarito virus. The reservoir of Sabiá virus is not known, although a rodent host is presumed.

5. Mode of transmission—Transmission to humans occurs primarily by inhalation of small particle aerosols from rodent excreta containing virus, from saliva or from rodents disrupted by mechanical harvesters. Viruses deposited in the environment may also be infective when secondary aerosols are generated by farming and grain processing, when ingested, or by contact with cuts or abrasions. While uncommon, person-to-person transmission of Machupo virus has been documented in health care and family settings. Fatal scalpel accidents during necropsy as well as laboratory infections without further person-to-person transmission have been described.

6. Incubation period—Usually 7–14 days (in extreme cases 5–21 days).

7. Period of communicability—Rarely transmitted directly from person to person, although this has occurred in both Argentine and Bolivian diseases.

8. Susceptibility—All ages appear to be susceptible, but protective immunity of unknown duration follows infection. Subclinical infections occur.

9. Methods of control—

A. *Preventive measures:* Specific rodent control in houses has been successful in Bolivia. In Argentina, human contact most commonly occurs in the fields, and rodent dispersion makes control more difficult. An effective live attenuated Junín vaccine has been administered to more than 150 000 persons in Argentina. In experimental animals, this vaccine is effective against Machupo but not Guanarito virus; it is still not known whether it provides effective cross-protection in humans.

B. *Control of patient, contacts and the immediate environment:*

1) Report to local health authority: In selected endemic areas; in most countries not a reportable disease, Class 3 (see Reporting); category A pathogen list as defined by the CDC.
2) Isolation: Strict isolation during the acute febrile period. Respiratory protection may be desirable along with other barrier methods.
3) Concurrent disinfection: Of sputum and respiratory secretions, and blood-contaminated materials.
4) Quarantine: Not applicable
5) Immunization of contacts: Not applicable.
6) Investigation of contacts and source of infection: Monitoring and, where feasible, control of rodents.
7) Specific treatment: Convalescent serum given within 8 days of onset reduced the case fatality rate in Argentine disease to less than 1%. Ribavirin is likely to be useful in all 4 diseases. Other compounds (inosine-5'monophosphate dehydrogenate inhibitors, phenothiazines and myristic acid analogs) were recently shown to inhibit arenavirus replication in cell culture and animals.

C. *Epidemic measures:* Rodent control; consider immunization.

D. *Disaster implications:* None.

E. *International measures:* None.

[K. Leitmeyer]

ARTHROPOD-BORNE VIRAL
   DISEASES
(Arboviral Diseases)

Introduction

Many arboviruses produce clinical and subclinical infection in humans. There are 4 main clinical syndromes:

1. Acute CNS illness ranging in severity from mild aseptic meningitis to encephalitis, with coma, paralysis and death.

2. Acute benign fevers of short duration, with or without exanthem; some may give rise to more serious illness with CNS involvement or hemorrhages.

3. Hemorrhagic fevers, including acute febrile diseases with extensive hemorrhagic involvement, frequently serious, associated with capillary leakage, shock and high case-fatality rates (all may cause liver damage, most severe in yellow fever and accompanied by frank jaundice).

4. Polyarthritis and rash, with or without fever and of variable duration, benign or with arthralgic sequelae lasting several weeks to months.

Most of these viruses are maintained in zoonotic cycles. Humans are usually an unimportant host in maintaining the cycle; infections in humans are incidental and are usually acquired during blood feeding by an infected arthropod vector. In rare cases such as dengue and yellow fever, humans can serve as the principal source of virus amplification and vector infection. Most viruses are transmitted by mosquitoes, the rest by ticks, sandflies or biting midges. Laboratory infections may occur, including aerosol infections.

Agents differ, but in their transmission cycles these diseases share common epidemiological features (related primarily to their vectors) that are important in control. The diseases selected under each clinical syndrome are arranged in 4 groups: mosquito- and midge-borne; tick-borne; sandfly-borne; unknown. Diseases of major importance are described individually or in groups with similar clinical and epidemiological features.

The main viruses thought to be associated with human disease are listed in the accompanying table with type of vector, predominant character of recognized disease and geographical distribution. In some instances, observed cases of disease due to particular viruses are too few to be certain of the usual clinical course. Some viruses capable of causing disease have only been recognized through laboratory exposure. Viruses in which evidence of human infection is based solely on serological surveys are not included. Those that cause diseases covered in subsequent chapters are marked on the table by an asterisk; some of the less important or less well studied are not discussed or mentioned.

Over 100 viruses currently classified as arboviruses produce disease in humans. Most of these are further classified by antigenic relationships, morphology and replicative mechanisms into families and genera, of which Togaviridae (*Alphavirus*), Flaviviridae (*Flavivirus*) and Bunyaviridae (*Bunyavirus*, *Phlebovirus*, *Nairovirus*) are the best known. These genera contain some agents that predominantly cause encephalitis; others predominantly cause febrile illnesses. Alphaviruses and bunyaviruses are usually mosquito-borne; flaviviruses are either mosquito- or tick-borne, some flaviviruses having no recognized vectors; phleboviruses are generally transmitted by sandflies, apart from Rift Valley fever, transmitted by mosquitoes. Other viruses of the family Bunyaviridae and of several other groups mainly produce febrile diseases or hemorrhagic fevers and may be transmitted by mosquitoes, ticks, sandflies or midges.

DISEASES IN HUMANS CAUSED BY ARTHROPOD-BORNE VIRUSES

Virus family, genus, group	Name of virus	Vector	Disease in humans	Where found
TOGAVIRIDAE *Alphavirus*	*Barmah Forest	Mosquito	Fever, arthralgia, rash	Australia
	*Chikungunya	Mosquito	Fever, arthralgia, rash (hemorrhage rare)	Africa, SE Asia, Philippines
	*Eastern equine encephalomyelitis	Mosquito	Encephalitis	Americas
	*Mayaro (Uruma)	Mosquito	Fever, arthralgia, rash	S America
	*O'nyong-nyong	Mosquito	Fever, arthralgia, rash	Africa
	*Ross River	Mosquito	Fever, arthralgia, rash	Australia, S Pacific
	Semliki Forest	Mosquito	Encephalitis	Africa
	*Sindbis (Ockelbo, Babanki)	Mosquito	Fever, arthralgia, rash	Africa, India, SE Asia, Europe, Philippines, Australia, Russian Federation
	*Venezuelan equine encephalomyelitis	Mosquito	Fever, encephalitis	Americas
	*Western equine encephalomyelitis	Mosquito	Fever, encephalitis	Americas
FLAVIRIDAE *Flavivirus*	*Banzi	Mosquito	Fever	Africa
	Bussuquara	Mosquito	Fever, arthralgia	S America
	*Dengue 1, 2, 3 and 4	Mosquito	Fever, hemorrhage, rash	Throughout tropics
	Edge Hill	Mosquito	Fever, arthralgia	Australia
	Ilhéus	Mosquito	Fever, encephalitis	Central & S America
	*Japanese encephalitis	Mosquito	Encephalitis, fever	Asia, Pacific islands, northern Australia
	Kokobera	Mosquito	Fever, arthralgia	Australia
	Koutango	Fever, rash		Africa
	*Kunjin	Mosquito	Fever, encephalitis	Australia, Sarawak
	*Kyasanur Forest disease	Tick	Hemorrhage, fever, meningoencephalitis	India

* Asterisked groups and viruses are discussed in the text. See index for page numbers.

DISEASES IN HUMANS CAUSED BY ARTHROPOD-BORNE VIRUSES

Virus family, genus, group	Name of virus	Vector	Disease in humans	Where found
FLAVIVIRIDAE *Flavivirus (cont).*	*Louping ill	Tick	Encephalitis	United Kingdom, western Europe
	*Murray Valley encephalitis	Mosquito	Encephalitis	Australia, N. Guinea
	Negishi	Unknown	Encephalitis	Japan
	*Omsk hemorrhagic fever	Tick	Hemorrhage, fever	Russian Federation
	*Powassan	Tick	Encephalitis	Canada, Russian Federation, USA
	Rocio	Mosquito	Encephalitis	Brazil
	Sepik	Mosquito	Fever	Papua New Guinea
	*Spondweni	Mosquito	Fever	Africa
	*St. Louis encephalitis	Mosquito	Encephalitis, hepatitis	Americas
	*Tick-borne encephalitis	Tick	Encephalitis, paralysis	Europe
	*European subtype	Tick	Encephalitis, paralysis	Europe
	*Far Eastern subtype	Tick	Encephalitis	Europe, Asia
	Usutu	Mosquito	Fever, rash	Africa, Europe
	Wesselsbron	Mosquito	Fever	Africa, SE Asia
	*West Nile	Mosquito	Fever, encephalitis, rash	Africa, North America, Indian subcontinent, Middle East, former Soviet Union, Europe
	*Yellow fever	Mosquito	Hemorrhagic fever	Africa, S & Central America
	*Zika	Mosquito	Fever	Africa, SE Asia
BUNYAVIRIDAE *Bunyavirus* *Group C				
	Apeu	Mosquito	Fever	S America
	Caraparu	Mosquito	Fever	S and Central America

*Asterisked groups and viruses are discussed in the text. See index for page numbers.

BUNYAVIRIDAE
Bunyavirus (cont.)

Group	Virus	Vector	Disease	Region
	Itaqui	Mosquito	Fever	S America
	Madrid	Mosquito	Fever	Panama
	Marituba	Mosquito	Fever	S America
	Murutucu	Mosquito	Fever	S America
	Nepuyo	Mosquito	Fever	S and Central America
	Oriboca	Mosquito	Fever	S America
	Ossa	Mosquito	Fever	Panama
	Restan	Mosquito	Fever	Trinidad, Suriname
Bunyamwera group	*Bunyamwera	Mosquito	Fever, rash	Africa
	Germiston	Mosquito	Fever, rash	Africa
	Ilesha	Mosquito	Fever, rash, hemorrhage	Africa
	Tensaw	Unknown	Encephalitis	N America
Bwamba group	*Bwamba	Mosquito	Fever, rash	Africa
California group	*California encephalitis	Mosquito	Encephalitis	USA
	Guaroa	Mosquito	Fever	S America, Panama
	*Jamestown Canyon	Mosquito	Encephalitis	USA, Canada
	*LaCrosse	Mosquito	Encephalitis	USA
	*Snowshoe hare	Mosquito	Encephalitis	Canada, China, Russian Federation, USA
	Tahyna (Lumbo)	Mosquito	Fever	Africa, Asia, Europe
	Trivittatus	Mosquito	Fever	N America
Guama group	Catu	Mosquito	Fever	S America
	Guama	Mosquito	Fever	S America
Simbu group	*Oropouche	Midges (*Culicoides*)	Fever, meningitis	S America, Panama
Phlebovirus (*Sandfly fever group)	Candiru	Unknown	Fever	S. America
	Chagres	Phlebotomine	Fever	Central America
	Sandfly Naples type	Phlebotomine	Fever	Africa, Asia, Europe
	Punta Toro	Phlebotomine	Fever	Panama

*Asterisked groups and viruses are discussed in the text. See index for page numbers.

DISEASES IN HUMANS CAUSED BY ARTHROPOD-BORNE VIRUSES

Virus family, genus, group	Name of virus	Vector	Disease in humans	Where found
BUNYAVIRIDAE				
Nairovirus	Rift Valley fever	Mosquito	Fever, hemorrhage, encephalitis, retinitis	Africa, Arabia
	Sandfly Sicilian type	Phlebotomine	Fever	Africa, Asia, Europe
	Toscana	Phlebotomine	Aseptic meningitis	Italy, Portugal
	*Nairobi sheep disease	Tick	Fever	Africa, India
	*Dughe	Tick	Fever	Africa
	*Crimean-Congo hemorrhagic fever	Tick	Hemorrhagic fever	Africa, central Asia, Europe, Middle East
Unclassified	*Bhanja	Tick	Fever	Africa, Asia, Europe
	Tataguine	Mosquito	Fever, rash	Africa
REOVIRIDAE				
Orbivirus				
*Changuinola group	Changuinola	Phlebotomine	Fever	Central America
*Kemerovo group	Kemerovo	Tick	Fever	Russian Federation
*Colorado tick fever	Colorado tick fever	Tick	Fever	Canada, USA
RHABDOVIRIDAE				
Ungrouped	Orungo	Mosquito	Fever	Africa
Vesicular stomatitis group	*Vesicular stomatitis, Indiana & New Jersey	Phlebotomine	Fever, encephalitis	Americas
	Vesicular stomatitis, Alagoas	Phlebotomine	Fever	S America
	*Chandipura	Mosquito	Fever	Africa, India
ORTHOMYXOVIRIDAE	*Thogoto	Tick	Meningitis	Africa, Europe
NOT CLASSIFIED	*Quaranfil	Tick	Fever	Africa, Arabia

*Asterisked groups and viruses are discussed in the text. See index for page numbers.

[R. Shope, J. Mackenzie]

ARTHROPOD-BORNE VIRAL
ARTHRITIS AND RASH   ICD-9 066.3; ICD-10 B33.1
(Polyarthritis and rash, Ross River fever, Epidemic polyarthritis)

CHIKUNGUNYA VIRUS DISEASE   ICD-10 A92.0
MAYARO VIRUS DISEASE   ICD-10 A92.8
(Mayaro fever, Uruma fever)
O'NYONG-NYONG FEVER   ICD-10 A92.1
SINDBIS (OCKELBO) VIRUS
DISEASE AND OTHERS   ICD-10 A92.8
(Pogosta disease, Karelian fever)

1. Identification—A self-limiting febrile viral disease characterized by arthralgia or arthritis, primarily in the wrist, knee, ankle and small joints of the extremities, lasting days to months. In many patients, onset of arthritis is followed after 1–10 days by a maculopapular rash, usually nonpruritic, affecting mainly the trunk and limbs. Buccal and palatal enanthema may occur. The rash resolves within 7–10 days, and is followed by a fine desquamation. Fever may be absent. Cervical lymphadenopathy is common. Paraesthesias and tenderness of palms and soles occur in a small percentage of cases.

Rash is also common in infections by Mayaro, Sindbis, chikungunya and o'nyong-nyong viruses. Polyarthritis is a characteristic feature of infections with chikungunya, Sindbis and Mayaro viruses.

Minor hemorrhages have been attributed to chikungunya virus disease in southeastern Asia and India (see Dengue hemorrhagic fever). In chikungunya virus disease, leukopenia is common; convalescence is often prolonged.

Serological tests show a rise in titres to alphaviruses; virus may be isolated in newborn mice, mosquitoes or cell culture from the blood of acutely ill patients. Diagnosis may be made by RT-PCR.

2. Infectious agents—Ross River and Barmah Forest viruses; Sindbis, Mayaro, chikungunya and o'nyong-nyong viruses cause similar illnesses.

3. Occurrence—Major outbreaks of Ross River virus disease (epidemic polyarthritis) have occurred in Australia, chiefly from January to May. Sporadic cases occur in other coastal regions of Australia and Papua New Guinea. In 1979, an outbreak in Fiji spread to other Pacific islands, including American Samoa, the Cook Islands, and Tonga. Barmah Forest virus infection has been reported from Queensland, the Northern Territory and western Australia. Chikungunya virus occurs in Africa, southeastern Asia, India, and the Philippines; Sindbis virus throughout the eastern hemisphere. O'nyong-nyong virus is known only from Africa; epidemics in 1959–1963 and 1996–1997 involved millions of cases throughout eastern Africa. Mayaro occurs in northern South America and Trinidad.

4. Reservoir—Unknown for most viruses. Transovarian transmission of Ross River virus has been demonstrated in *Aedes vigilax*, making an insect reservoir a possibility. Similar transmission cycles may occur with other viruses of the group. Birds are a source of mosquito infection for Sindbis virus.

5. Mode of transmission—Ross River virus is transmitted by *Culex annulirostris*, *Ae. vigilax*, *Ae. polynesiensis* and other *Aedes* spp.; chikungunya virus by *Ae. aegypti* and possibly others; o'nyong-nyong virus by *Anopheles* spp.; Sindbis virus by various *Culex* spp., especially *C. univittatus* and *C. morsitans* and *Ae. communis*; Mayaro virus by *Mansonia* and *Haemagogus* spp.

6. Incubation period—From 3 to 11 days.

7. Period of communicability—No evidence of direct person-to-person transmission.

8. Susceptibility—Recovery is universal and followed by lasting homologous immunity; second attacks are unknown. Inapparent infections are common, especially in children, among whom the overt disease is rare. In epidemic polyarthritis, arthritis occurs most frequently among adult females and in people with HLA DR7 Gm $a^+x^+b^+$ phenotypes.

9. Methods of control—

  A. *Preventive measures:* General measures applicable to mosquito-borne viral encephalitides (see Arthropod-borne viral encephalitides, I9A, 1–5 and 8).

  B. *Control of patient, contacts and the immediate environment:*

   1) Report to local health authority: In selected endemic areas; in many countries, not a reportable disease, Class 3 (see Reporting).
   2) Isolation: To avoid further transmission, protect patients from mosquitoes.
   3) Concurrent disinfection: Not applicable.
   4) Quarantine: Not applicable.
   5) Immmunization of contacts: Not applicable.
   6) Investigation of contacts and source of infection: Search for unreported or undiagnosed cases where the patient lived during the 2 weeks prior to onset; check all family members serologically.
   7) Specific treatment: None.

C. *Epidemic measures:* Same as for arthropod-borne viral fevers (see Dengue fever, 9C).

D. *Disaster implications:* None.

E. *International measures:* WHO Collaborating Centres.

[R. Shope, J. Mackenzie]

ARTHROPOD-BORNE VIRAL ENCEPHALITIDES

I. MOSQUITO-BORNE VIRAL ENCEPHALITIDES	ICD-9 062
JAPANESE ENCEPHALITIS	ICD-10 A83.0
WESTERN EQUINE ENCEPHALITIS	ICD-10 A83.1
EASTERN EQUINE ENCEPHALITIS	ICD-10 A83.2
ST. LOUIS ENCEPHALITIS	ICD-10 A83.3
MURRAY VALLEY ENCEPHALITIS (AUSTRALIAN ENCEPHALITIS)	ICD-10 A83.4
LACROSSE ENCEPHALITIS	ICD-10 A83.5
CALIFORNIA ENCEPHALITIS	ICD-10 A83.5
ROCIO ENCEPHALITIS	ICD-10 A83.6
JAMESTOWN CANYON ENCEPHALITIS	ICD-10 A83.8

1. Identification—A group of acute inflammatory viral diseases of short duration involving parts of the brain, spinal cord and meninges. Signs and symptoms of these diseases are similar but vary in severity and rate of progress. Most infections are asymptomatic; mild cases often occur as febrile headache or aseptic meningitis. Severe infections are usually marked by acute onset, headache, high fever, meningeal signs, stupor, disorientation, coma, tremors, occasional convulsions (especially in infants) and spastic (rarely flaccid) paralysis. Case-fatality rates range from 0.3% to 60%, rates for Japanese encephalitis (JE), Murray Valley (MV) and eastern equine encephalomyelitis (EEE) are among the highest. Neurological sequelae occur with variable frequency depending on age and infecting agent; they tend to be most severe in infants infected with JE, western equine encephalomyelitis (WEE) and EEE viruses. Mild leukocytosis is usual; leukocytes in the CSF, predominantly lymphocytes, range from 50 to 500/mm^3 (SI units: 50 to 500 x 106/L) and may be 1000/mm^3 or greater (SI units: 1000 x 106/L or greater) in infants infected with EEE virus. The elderly are at greatest risk of encephalitis with St. Louis encephalitis (SLE) or EEE virus infection, while children under 15 are at greatest risk from LaCrosse virus infection and may develop seizures.

These diseases require differentiation from tick-borne encephalitides (see below); encephalitic and nonparalytic poliomyelitis; rabies; mumps meningoencephalitis; lymphocytic choriomeningitis; aseptic meningitis due to enteroviruses; herpes encephalitis; postvaccinal or postinfection encephalitides; and bacterial, mycoplasmal, protozoal, leptospiral and mycotic meningitides or encephalitides. Venezuelan equine encephalomyelitis, Rift Valley fever and West Nile viruses primarily produce fever (see Arthropod-borne viral fevers), but may sometimes cause encephalitis. This is especially true of West Nile virus infection, which has become the most common cause of arboviral encephalitis since 1999 in the U.S.A.

Identification is made by demonstrating specific IgM, specific nucleic acid by RT-PCR in acute-phase serum or CSF, or rises in antibody titres between early and late serum specimens by neutralization, CF, HI, FA, ELISA or other serological tests. Cross-reactions may occur within a virus group. Virus may occasionally be isolated from the brain tissue of fatal cases, rarely from blood or CSF by inoculation of suckling mice or cell culture after symptoms have appeared; histopathological changes are not specific for individual viruses.

2. Infectious agents—Each disease is caused by a specific virus in one of 3 genera: EEE and WEE for the alphaviruses (Togaviridae, *Alphavirus*); JE, Kunjin, MV encephalitis, SLE and Rocio encephalitis in the flaviviruses (Flaviviridae, *Flavivirus*); and LaCrosse, California encephalitis, Jamestown Canyon and snowshoe hare viruses in the California group of bunyaviruses (Bunyaviridae, *Bunyavirus*).

3. Occurrence—EEE occurs in eastern, Gulf, and north central USA and adjacent Canada, in scattered areas of central and South America and in the Caribbean islands; WEE in western and central USA, Canada and parts of South America; JE in western Pacific islands from the Republic of Korea to the Philippines and to Pakistan through southern and southeastern Asia, extending to North Queensland. Kunjin and MV encephalitis occur in parts of Australia and Papua New Guinea; SLE in most of the USA, in Canada and in central America and Brazil; Rocio encephalitis in Brazil; LaCrosse encephalitis in the USA from Minnesota and Texas to New York and Georgia; snowshoe hare encephalitis in Canada, China and the Russian Federation. Cases due to these viruses occur in temperate latitudes in summer and early fall and are commonly limited to areas and years of high temperature and many mosquitoes.

4. Reservoir—California group viruses overwinter in *Aedes* eggs; the true reservoir or means of winter carryover for other viruses is unknown, possibly birds, rodents, bats, reptiles, amphibians or survival in mosquito eggs or adults; the mechanisms probably differ for each virus.

5. Mode of transmission—Bite of infective mosquitoes. Most important vectors:

- EEE in the USA and Canada: probably *Culiseta melanura* from bird to bird, and one or more *Aedes* or *Coquillettidia* spp. from birds or other animals to humans
- WEE in western USA and Canada: *Culex tarsalis*
- JE: *C. tritaeniorhynchus*, *C. vishnui* complex and in the tropics, *C. gelidus*;
- MV: probably *C. annulirostris*
- SLE in the USA, *C. tarsalis*, the *C. pipiens-quinquefasciatus* complex and *C. nigripalpus*
- LaCrosse: *Ae. triseriatus.*

Mosquitoes, if not transovarially infected, acquire virus from wild birds or small mammals; pigs, as well as birds, are important for JE. LaCrosse virus is transovarially and venereally transmitted in *Ae. triseriatus* mosquitoes.

6. Incubation period—Usually 5–15 days.

7. Period of communicability—No direct person-to-person transmission. Virus not usually demonstrable in human blood after onset of disease. Mosquitoes remain infective for life. Viraemia in birds usually lasts 2–5 days, but may be prolonged in bats, reptiles and amphibia, particularly if interrupted by hibernation. Horses develop active disease with the two equine viruses and with JE, but viraemia is rarely present in high titre or for long periods; therefore, humans and horses are uncommon sources of mosquito infection.

8. Susceptibility—Susceptibility to clinical disease is usually highest in infancy and old age; inapparent or undiagnosed infection is more common at other ages. Susceptibility varies with virus, e.g. LaCrosse encephalitis is usually a disease of children, while severity of SLE increases with age. Infection results in homologous immunity. In highly endemic areas, adults are largely immune to local strains by reason of mild and inapparent infection; susceptibles are mainly children.

9. Methods of control—

    A. Preventive measures:

        1) Educate the public as to the modes of spread and control.
        2) Destroy larvae and eliminate breeding places of known and suspected vector mosquitoes.
        3) Kill mosquitoes through space and residual spraying of human habitations (see Malaria, 9A1-5).
        4) Screen sleeping and living quarters; use bednets, preferably impregnated.
        5) Avoid exposure to mosquitoes during hours of biting, or use repellents (see Malaria, 9A2-4).

6) In endemic areas, immunize domestic animals or house them away from living quarters, e.g. pigs in JE endemic areas.

7) Mouse-brain inactivated vaccine against JE encephalitis is used for children in India, Japan, the Republic of Korea, Taiwan (China), and Thailand: it is commercially available and is recommended for those travelling to endemic areas for extended visits to rural areas. Live attenuated and formalin-inactivated primary hamster kidney cell vaccines are licensed and widely used in China.

For those under continued intensive exposure in laboratory situations, EEE and WEE vaccines (inactivated, dried) may be available by special arrangement from U.S. Army Medical Research and Material Command, Fort Detrick, Frederick, MD 21702-5009 (301-619-2051).

8) Protect accidentally exposed laboratory workers passively with human or animal immune serum.

B. Control of patient, contacts and the immediate environment:

1) Report to local health authority: Case report obligatory in several countries, Class 2 (see Reporting). Report under appropriate disease; or as "encephalitis, other forms"; or "aseptic meningitis," specify cause or clinical type when known.

2) Isolation: Not applicable; virus not usually found in blood, secretions or discharges during clinical disease. Enteric precautions appropriate until enterovirus meningoencephalitis (see Viral meningitis) is ruled out.

3) Concurrent disinfection: Not applicable.

4) Quarantine: Not applicable.

5) Immmunization of contacts: Not applicable.

6) Investigation of contacts and source of infection: Search for missed cases and the presence of vector mosquitoes; test for viraemia in both febrile and asymptomatic family members. Primarily a community vector control problem (see 9C).

7) Specific treatment: None.

C. Epidemic measures:

1) Identification of infection among horses or birds and recognition of human cases in the community have epidemiological value by indicating frequency of infection and areas involved. Immunization of horses probably does not limit spread of the virus in the community; immunization of pigs against JE should have a significant effect.

2) Fogging or spraying from aircraft with suitable insecticides has shown promise for aborting urban epidemics of SLE.

D. *Disaster implications:* None.

E. *International measures:* Spray with insecticide those air-planes arriving from recognized areas of prevalence. WHO Collaborating Centres.

II. TICK-BORNE VIRAL ENCEPHALITIDES — ICD-9 063; ICD-10 A84

FAR EASTERN TICK-BORNE ENCEPHALITIS — ICD-10 A84.0
(Russian spring-summer encephalitis)

CENTRAL EUROPEAN TICK-BORNE ENCEPHALITIS — ICD-10 A84.1

LOUPING ILL — ICD-10 A84.8

POWASSAN VIRUS ENCEPHALITIS — ICD-10 A84.8

1. **Identification**—A group of viral diseases clinically resembling the mosquito-borne encephalitides except that the Far Eastern tick-borne subtype (FE) is often associated with focal epilepsy, flaccid paralysis (particularly of the shoulder girdle) and other residua. Central European tick-borne encephalitis (CEE), also called diphasic milk fever or diphasic meningoencephalitis, produces a milder disease but has a longer course averaging 3 weeks. The initial febrile stage of CEE is not associated with symptoms referable to the CNS; the second phase of fever and meningo-encephalitis follows 4–10 days after apparent recovery; death and severe residua are less frequent than for the FE tick-borne disease. Powassan encephalitis (PE) has a similar clinical course with a 10% case-fatality rate and neurological sequelae among 50% of survivors. Louping ill in humans also has a diphasic pattern and is relatively mild.

Specific identification is made through demonstration of specific IgM or nucleic acid in acute phase serum or CSF, serological tests of paired sera, or virus isolation from blood during acute illness or from brain postmortem (inoculation of suckling mice or cell culture). Common serological tests distinguish the group from most other similar diseases but differentiating within this group requires DNA analysis.

2. **Infectious agents**—A complex within the flaviviruses; minor antigenic differences exist, more with Powassan than others, but viruses causing these diseases are closely related.

3. **Occurrence**—Disease of the CNS caused by this complex is distributed spottily over much of the former Soviet Union, other parts of eastern and central Europe, Scandinavia and the United Kingdom. FE subtype found predominantly in the extreme eastern regions of the former Soviet Union, CEE predominating in Europe, louping ill chiefly in the

United Kingdom and Ireland, but recently recognized in western Europe. Powassan virus present in Canada, the Russian Federation, and the USA. Seasonal incidence depends on density of the tick vectors. *Ixodes persulcatus* in eastern Asia is usually active in spring and early summer; *I. ricinus* bites occur in Europe in both early summer and early autumn; in Canada and the USA, human bites by *I. cookei* peak from June to September.

Areas of highest incidence are those where humans have intimate association with large numbers of infected ticks, generally rural or forested areas, but also urban populations. Local epidemics of CEE have occurred among people consuming unpasteurized milk and dairy products from goats and sheep, hence the name "diphasic milk fever". The age pattern varies in different regions and is influenced by opportunity for exposure to ticks, consumption of milk from infected animals or previously acquired immunity. Laboratory infections are common, some with serious sequelae, including death.

4. Reservoir—The tick or ticks and mammals in combination appear to be the true reservoir; transovarian tick passage of some tick-borne encephalitis viruses has been demonstrated. Sheep and deer are the primary vertebrate hosts for louping ill, while rodents and other small mammals and birds serve as sources of tick infections with FE, CEE and PE viruses.

5. Mode of transmission—Bites of infective ticks or consumption of milk from certain infected animals. *Ixodes persulcatus* is the main vector in the eastern areas of the Russian Federation, *I. ricinus* in the western areas thereof and in other parts of Europe (it is also the vector of louping ill of sheep in Scotland). *I. cookei* is the main vector in eastern Canada and USA. Larval ticks ingest virus by feeding on infected vertebrates, including rodents, other mammals or birds. CEE may be acquired through consumption of infected raw milk.

6. Incubation period—Usually 7–14 days.

7. Period of communicability—No direct person-to-person transmission. A tick infected at any stage remains infective for life. Viraemia may last for days in vertebrates; in humans, up to 7–10 days.

8. Susceptibility—Men and women of all ages are susceptible. Infection, whether inapparent or overt, leads to immunity.

9. Methods of control—

    A. Preventive measures:

        1) See Lyme Disease, 9A, for measures against ticks.
        2) Inactivated virus vaccines have been used extensively in Europe and the former Soviet Union with reported safety and effectiveness.

3) Boil or pasteurize milk of susceptible animals in areas where diphasic meningoencephalitis (CEE) occurs.

B. Control of patient, contacts and the immediate environment:

1) Report to local health authority: In selected endemic areas; in most countries not a reportable disease, Class 3 (see Reporting).
2) Isolation: None, after tick removal.
3) Concurrent disinfection: Not applicable.
4) Quarantine: Not applicable.
5) Immmunization of contacts: Not applicable.
6) Investigation of contacts and source of infection: Search for missed cases, presence of tick vectors and animals excreting virus in milk.
7) Specific treatment: None.

C. Epidemic measures: See Lyme disease, 9C.

D. Disaster implications: None.

E. International measures: WHO Collaborating Centres.

[R. Shope, J. Mackenzie]

ARTHROPOD-BORNE VIRAL FEVERS

I. MOSQUITO-BORNE AND CULICOIDES-BORNE VIRAL FEVERS:

(Yellow fever and dengue are presented separately.)

I.A. VENEZUELAN EQUINE ENCEPHALOMYELITIS VIRUS DISEASE   ICD-9 066.2; ICD-10 A92.2

(Venezuelan equine encephalitis, Venezuelan equine fever)

1. Identification—Clinical manifestations of this viral infection are influenza-like, with abrupt onset of severe headache, chills, fever, myalgia, retroorbital pain, nausea and vomiting. Conjunctival and pharyngeal congestion are the only physical signs. Most infections are relatively mild, with symptoms lasting 3–5 days. Some cases may have a diphasic fever course; after a few days of fever, particularly in children, CNS involvement may range from somnolence to frank encephalitis with disorientation, convulsions, paralysis, coma and death.

Presumptive diagnosis is based on clinical and epidemiological grounds (exposure in an area where an equine epizootic is in progress) and confirmed by virus isolation, rise in antibody titres, detection of specific IgM or DNA. Virus can be isolated in cell culture or in newborn mice from blood and nasopharyngeal washings during the first 72 hours of symptoms; acute and convalescent sera drawn 10 days apart can show rising antibody titres. Laboratory infections may occur in the absence of proper containment facilities.

2. Infectious agent—Venezuelan equine encephalomyelitis (VEE) virus, an alphavirus (Togaviridae, *Alphavirus*), with enzootic subtypes and epizootic varieties of subtype 1.

3. Occurrence—Endemic in northern South America, Trinidad and central America. The disease appears as epizootics, mainly in northern and western South America; and in 1971 spread temporarily into the southern part of the USA.

4. Reservoir—Enzootic subtypes of VEE are maintained in a rodent-mosquito cycle. Epizootic varieties of subtype 1 are believed to arise periodically from enzootic VEE 1D viruses in northern South America. During outbreaks, epizootic VEE virus is transmitted in a cycle involving horses, which serve as the major source of virus, to mosquitoes, which in turn infect humans. Humans also develop sufficient viraemia to serve as hosts in a human-mosquito-human transmission cycle.

5. Mode of transmission—Bite of an infected mosquito. VEE viruses have been isolated from *Culex* (*Melanoconion*), *Aedes*, *Mansonia*, *Psorophora*, *Haemagogus*, *Sabethes*, *Deinocerites* and *Anopheles* mosquitoes, *Simulium* and possibly ceratopogonid gnats. Infection by aerosol transmission is common; primarily in laboratories; there is no evidence of horses-to-humans transmission.

6. Incubation period—Usually 2-6 days; can be as short as 1 day.

7. Period of communicability—Infected humans and horses are infectious for mosquitoes for up to 72 hours; infected mosquitoes probably transmit virus throughout life.

8. Susceptibility—General. Mild infections and subsequent immunity occur frequently in endemic areas. Children are at greatest risk for developing CNS infection.

9. Methods of control —

   A. Preventive measures:

   1) Use general mosquito control procedures.
   2) Avoid forested endemic areas, especially at night.
   3) Live attenuated virus (TC-83) and inactivated vaccines for VEE have been used to protect laboratory workers and other adults at high risk (U.S. Army Medical Research and Material

Command, Fort Detrick, Frederick, MD 21702-5009; 301-619-2051). Vaccine for use in horses is commercially available.

B. Control of patient, contacts and the immediate environment:

1) Report to local health authority: In selected endemic areas; in most countries, not a reportable disease, Class 3 (see Reporting).
2) Isolation: Blood and body fluid precautions. Patients should be treated in a screened room or in quarters treated with a residual insecticide for at least 5 days after onset, or until afebrile.
3) Concurrent disinfection: Not applicable.
4) Quarantine: Not applicable.
5) Immmunization of contacts: Not applicable.
6) Investigation of contacts and source of infection: Search for unreported or undiagnosed cases.
7) Specific treatment: None.

C. Epidemic measures:

1) Determine extent of the infected areas; immunize horses and/or restrict their movement from the affected area.
2) Use approved mosquito repellents for those exposed.
3) Conduct a community survey to determine density of vector mosquitoes, their breeding places and effective control measures.
4) Identify infected horses, prevent mosquitoes from feeding on them and intensify mosquito control efforts in the affected area.

D. Disaster implications: None.

E. International measures: Immunize animals and restrict their movement from epizootic areas to areas free of the disease.

I.B. OTHER MOSQUITO-BORNE AND CULICOIDES-BORNE FEVERS

	ICD-9 066.3
BUNYAMWERA VIRAL FEVER	ICD-10 A92.8
BWAMBA VIRUS DISEASE	ICD-10 A92.8
RIFT VALLEY FEVER	ICD-10 A92.4
WEST NILE FEVER	ICD-10 A92.3
GROUP C VIRUS DISEASE	ICD-10 A92.8
OROPOUCHE VIRUS DISEASE	ICD-10 A93.0

1. Identification—A group of viruses that cause febrile illnesses usually lasting a week or less, many of which are dengue-like. Initial symptoms include fever, headache, malaise, arthralgia or myalgia, and occasionally nausea and vomiting; generally, there is some conjunctivitis and photophobia. Fever may or may not be diphasic. Rash is common in infections with West Nile virus.

Meningoencephalitis is an occasional complication of West Nile and Oropouche virus infections. It has been recognized since 1999 in the USA and later in Canada as a prominent complication of West Nile virus infection, especially among the elderly. Persons with Rift Valley fever (RVF) may develop retinitis, encephalitis or hepatitis associated with hemorrhages that may be fatal. Several group C viruses are reported to produce weakness in the lower limbs; they are not fatal. Epidemics of RVF and Oropouche fever may involve thousands of patients.

Serological tests differentiate other fevers of viral or unknown origin, and the diagnosis may be facilitated by DNA analysis. Virus isolation by inoculation into suckling mice or cell culture of blood drawn during the febrile period may be possible. Laboratory infections may occur with many of these viruses.

2. Infectious agents—Each disease is caused by a distinct virus with the same name as the disease. West Nile, Banzi, Kunjin, Spondweni and Zika viruses are flaviviruses; the group C bunyaviruses are Apeu, Caraparu, Itaqui, Madrid, Marituba, Murutucu, Nepuyo, Oriboca, Ossa and Restan. Oropouche is a bunyavirus of the Simbu group. RVF is a phlebovirus.

3. Occurrence—West Nile virus is widespread in Africa, North America, Europe, the Middle East and India; it has caused outbreaks in Canada, the Czech Republic, Egypt, France, India, Israel, Romania and the USA. Bwamba and Bunyamwera fevers have been identified only in Africa. West Nile virus also causes equine encephalitis and a fatal encephalitis in some birds, especially the American crow. The first epidemic of Rift Valley fever outside Africa occurred in 2000 in the Arabian peninsula (probable vector *Ae. vexans arabiensis*). Group C virus fevers occur in tropical South America, Panama and Trinidad; Oropouche fever in Brazil, Panama, Peru and Trinidad; Kunjin virus in Australia. Seasonal incidence depends on vector density. Occurrence is primarily rural, although occasionally Oropouche, RVF, and West Nile have been involved in explosive urban and suburban outbreaks.

4. Reservoir—Unknown for many of these viruses; some may be maintained in a continuous vertebrate-mosquito cycle in tropical environments. Oropouche virus may be transmitted by *Culicoides*. Birds are a source of mosquito infection for West Nile virus; rodents serve as reservoirs for group C viruses.

5. Mode of transmission—In most instances, bite of an infective mosquito:

- West Nile: *Culex univittatus* in southern Africa, *C. modestus* in France, *C. pipiens molestus* in Israel; *C. pipiens*, *C. quinquefasciatus*, *C. tarsalis* and *Ae. albopictus* in North America; virus also isolated from *Aedes* and *Mansonia*, and from ticks.

- Bunyamwera: *Aedes* spp.;
- Group C viruses: *Aedes* and *Culex* (*Melanoconion*);
- Rift Valley (in sheep and other animals): potential vectors include *Aedes* mosquitoes; *Ae. mcintoshi* may be infected transovarially and account for maintenance of RVF virus in enzootic foci. *C. pipiens* was implicated in a 1977 epidemic of RVF in Egypt with at least 600 deaths. Mechanical transmission by hematophagous flies and transmission by aerosols or contact with highly infective blood may contribute to RVF outbreaks. Many human infections of RVF are associated with the handling of animal tissues during necropsy or butchering. Other arthropods may be vectors, such as *Culicoides paraensis* for the Oropouche virus.

6. Incubation period—Usually 3–12 days.

7. Period of communicability—No direct person-to-person transmission. Infected mosquitoes probably transmit virus throughout life. Viraemia, essential for vector infection, often occurs during early clinical illness in humans.

8. Susceptibility—Susceptibility appears to be general in both sexes at all ages. Inapparent infections and mild disease are common. Since infection leads to immunity, susceptibles in endemic areas are mainly young children.

9. Methods of control—

A. Preventive measures:

1) Follow measures applicable to mosquito-borne viral encephalitides (see 9A1–6 and 9A8). For RVF, precautions in care and handling of infected animals and their products, as well as human acute phase blood, are important.
2) An inactivated cell culture RVF vaccine is available for humans as an investigational new drug; live and inactivated vaccines are available for sheep, goats and cattle.

B. Control of patient, contacts and the immediate environment:

1) Report to local health authority: In selected endemic areas; in most countries, not a reportable disease, Class 3 (see Reporting). For RVF, notify WHO, FAO and the International Office of Epizootics in Paris.
2) Isolation: Blood and body fluid precautions. Keep patient in screened room or in quarters treated with an insecticide for at least 5 days after onset or until afebrile. Blood of RVF patients may be infectious. Screen blood for West Nile nucleic acid in North America during summer and fall, before transfusion.
3) Concurrent disinfection: Not applicable.

    4) Quarantine: Not applicable.

    5) Immmunization of contacts: Not applicable.

    6) Investigation of contacts and source of infection: Determine patient's place of residence during fortnight before onset. Search for unreported or undiagnosed cases.

    7) Specific treatment: None.

C. *Epidemic measures:*

    1) Use approved mosquito repellents for people exposed to bites of vectors.

    2) Do not slaughter sick or dying domestic animals suspected of being infected with RVF.

    3) Determine density of vector mosquitoes; identify and destroy their breeding places.

    4) Immunize sheep, goats and cattle against RVF.

    5) Identification of infected sheep and other animals (Rift Valley) and serological surveys of birds (West Nile) or rodents (group C viruses) provide information on prevalence of infection and areas involved.

D. *Disaster implications:* None.

E. *International measures:* For RVF, immunize animals and restrict their movement from enzootic areas to clean areas; do not butcher sick animals; for others, none except enforcement of international agreements designed to prevent transfer of mosquitoes by ships, airplanes and land transport. WHO Collaborating Centres.

II. TICK-BORNE VIRAL FEVERS   ICD-9 066.1
COLORADO TICK FEVER AND   ICD-10 A93.2
OTHER TICK-BORNE FEVERS   ICD-10 A93.8

    1. Identification—Colorado tick fever (CTF) is an acute febrile (often diphasic) viral disease with infrequent rash. After initial onset, a brief remission is usual, followed by a second bout of fever lasting 2–3 days; neutropenia and thrombocytopenia almost always occur on the 4th to 5th day of fever. Characteristically, CTF is a moderately severe disease, with occasional encephalitis, myocarditis or tendency to bleed. Deaths are rare. Bhanja virus can cause severe neurological disease and death; CNS infections also occur with Kemerovo and Thogoto viruses (the latter may cause hepatitis).

    Laboratory confirmation of CTF is made by isolation of virus from blood inoculated into suckling mice or cell cultures or by demonstration of antigen in erythrocytes by IF (CTF virus may persist in erythrocytes for up to 120 days). IFA detects serum antibodies as early as 10 days after onset of illness. Diagnostic methods for confirming other tick-borne viral fevers vary only slightly, except that serum is used for virus isolation instead of erythrocytes.

2. Infectious agents—Colorado tick fever, Nairobi sheep disease (Ganjam), Kemerovo, Lipovnik, Quaranfil, Bhanja, Thogoto and Dugbe viruses.

3. Occurrence—Colorado tick fever is endemic in the mountainous regions above 1500 meters (5000 feet) in Canada and the western USA. Virus has been isolated from *Dermacentor andersoni* ticks in Alberta and British Columbia (Canada). It occurs most frequently in those with recreational or occupational exposure (hiking, fishing) in enzootic loci; seasonal incidence parallels the period of greatest tick activity (April-June in the Rocky Mountains of the USA). Geographic distribution of other viruses is shown in the introductory table.

4. Reservoir—Reservoirs for CTF include small mammals such as ground squirrels, porcupines, chipmunks and *Peromyscus* spp.; also ticks, principally *D. andersoni*.

5. Mode of transmission—By bite of an infective tick. Immature ticks (*D. andersoni*) acquire CTF virus by feeding on viraemic animals; they pass the virus transstadially and transmit virus to humans when feeding as adult ticks.

6. Incubation period—Usually 4–5 days.

7. Period of communicability—Not directly transmitted from person to person except by transfusion. The wildlife cycle is maintained by ticks, which remain infective throughout life. Virus is present in blood during the febrile stage and in CTF, in erythrocytes from 2 to 16 weeks or more after onset.

8. Susceptibility—Susceptibility apparently universal. Second attacks are rare.

9. Methods of control—

    A. Preventive measures: Personal protective measures to avoid tick bites; control of ticks and rodent hosts (see Lyme disease, 9A).

    B. Control of patient, contacts and the immediate environment:

        1) Report to local health authority: In endemic areas (USA); in most states and countries, not a reportable disease, Class 3 (see Reporting).
        2) Isolation: Blood and body fluid precautions. No blood donations for 4 months.
        3) Concurrent disinfection. Remove ticks from patients.

4) Quarantine: Not applicable.
5) Immmunization of contacts: Not applicable.
6) Investigation of contacts and source of infection: Identification of tick-infested areas.
7) Specific treatment: None.

C. Epidemic measures: Not applicable.

D. Disaster implications: None.

E. International measures: WHO Collaborating Centres.

III. PHLEBOTOMINE-BORNE VIRAL FEVERS

SANDFLY FEVER   ICD-9 066.0; ICD-10 A93.1
(Phlebotomus fever, Papatasi fever)

CHANGUINOLA VIRUS
   DISEASE   ICD-9 066.0; ICD-10 A93.8
(Changuinola fever)

VESICULAR STOMATITIS VIRUS
   DISEASE   ICD-9 066.8; ICD-10 A93.8
(Vesicular stomatitis fever)

1. Identification—A group of arboviral diseases with headache; fever of 38.3°C–39.5°C (101°F–103°F), sometimes higher; retrobulbar pain on motion of the eyes; injected sclerae; malaise; nausea and pain in the limbs and back. Pharyngitis, oral mucosal vesicular lesions and cervical adenopathy are characteristic of vesicular stomatitis virus (VSV) infections. Leukopenia is usual on the 4th to 5th day after onset of fever. Symptoms may be alarming, but death is very rare. Complete recovery may be preceded by prolonged mental depression. Encephalitis may occur following Toscana and Chandipura virus infections.

A presumptive diagnosis is based on the clinical picture and the occurrence of multiple similar cases. Diagnoses may be confirmed serologically by detection of specific IgM antibodies or by antibody titre rise, or isolation of virus from blood inoculated into newborn mice or cell culture; for VSV infections, from throat swabs and vesicular fluid.

2. Infectious agents—The sandfly fever group of viruses (Bunyaviridae, *Phlebovirus*); several related immunological types have been isolated from humans and differentiated. In addition, Changuinola virus (an orbivirus) and VSV of the Indiana type (a rhabdovirus), both of which produce febrile disease in humans, have been isolated from *Lutzomyia* spp. sandflies. Chandipura virus is a rhabdovirus.

3. Occurrence—A disease of subtropical and tropical areas with long periods of hot, dry weather in Europe, Asia and Africa, and rainforests in

Western Hemisphere tropics, distributed in a belt extending around the Mediterranean and eastward into China and Myanmar. The disease is seasonal in temperate zones north of the equator, occurring between April and October, and is prone to affect military personnel and travellers from nonendemic areas.

4. Reservoir—The main reservoir is the sandfly, in which the virus is maintained transovarially. Arboreal rodents and nonhuman primates may harbour VSV. Rodents (gerbils) have been implicated as a reservoir for Eastern Hemisphere sandfly viruses.

5. Mode of transmission—Bite of an infective sandfly. The vector of the classic virus is a small, hairy, blood-sucking midge (*Phlebotomus papatasi*, the common sandfly), which bites at night and has a limited flight range. Sandflies of the genus *Sergentomyia* have also been found to be infected and may be vectors. Members of the genus *Lutzomyia* are involved in central and South America.

6. Incubation period—Up to 6 days, usually 3–4 days, rarely less.

7. Period of communicability—Virus is present in the blood of an infected person at least 24 hours before and 24 hours after onset of fever. Phlebotomines become infective about 7 days after biting an infected person and remain so for their normal life span of about 1 month.

8. Susceptibility—Susceptibility is universal; homologous acquired immunity is probably lasting. Relative resistance of native populations in sandfly areas is probably attributable to infection early in life.

9. Methods of control—

 A. ***Preventive measures:*** Personal protective measures to prevent sandfly feeding; control of sandflies is the principal objective (see Leishmaniasis, cutaneous and mucosal, 9A2).

 B. ***Control of patient, contacts and the immediate environment:***

   1) Report to local health authority: In selected endemic areas; in most countries, not a reportable disease, Class 3 (see Reporting).
   2) Isolation: None; consider preventing access of sandflies to infected individuals for the first few days of illness by very fine screening or mosquito bednets (10–12 mesh/cm or 25–30 mesh/inch, aperture size not more than 0.085 cm or 0.035 inch) and by spraying quarters with insecticide.
   3) Concurrent disinfection: Destroy sandflies in residences.
   4) Quarantine: Not applicable.
   5) Immunization of contacts: Not currently available.
   6) Investigation of contacts and source of infection: In the eastern Hemisphere, search for breeding areas of sandflies

around dwellings, especially in rubble heaps, in masonry cracks and under stones.

7) Specific treatment: None.

C. Epidemic measures:

1) Educate the public about conditions leading to infection and the importance of preventing sandfly bites by use of repellents, particularly after sundown.

2) Use insecticides to control sandflies in and about human habitations, community wide.

D. Disaster implications: None.

E. International measures: WHO Collaborating Centres.

[R. Shope, J. Mackenzie]

ARTHROPOD-BORNE VIRAL HEMORRHAGIC FEVERS

I. MOSQUITO-BORNE DISEASES
(Dengue hemorrhagic fever and yellow fever are presented separately.)
II. TICK-BORNE DISEASES
II.A. CRIMEAN-CONGO HEMORRHAGIC FEVER   ICD-9 065.0; ICD-10 A98.0
(Central Asian hemorrhagic fever)

1. Identification—A viral disease with sudden onset of fever, malaise, weakness, irritability, headache, severe pain in limbs and loins and marked anorexia. Vomiting, abdominal pain and diarrhea occur occasionally. Flush on face and chest and conjunctival injection develop early. hemorrhagic enanthem of soft palate, uvula and pharynx, and a fine petechial rash spreading from the chest and abdomen to the rest of the body are generally associated with the disease, sometimes with large purpuric areas.

There may be bleeding from gums, nose, lungs, uterus and intestine, but only in serious or fatal cases does this occur in large amounts, often associated with severe liver damage. Hematuria and albuminuria are common but usually not massive. Fever is constantly elevated for 5–12 days or may be biphasic; it falls rapidly by lysis. Convalescence is prolonged. Other findings are leukopenia, with lymphopenia more marked than neutropenia. Thrombocytopenia is common. The reported case-fatality rate ranges from 2% to 50%. In the Russian Federation, an estimated 5 infections occur for each hemorrhagic case.

Diagnosis is through isolation of virus from blood (inoculation of cell cultures or suckling mice) or PCR. Serological diagnosis is by ELISA, reverse passive HI, IFA, CF, immunodiffusion or plaque-reduction neutralization test. Specific IgM may be present during the acute phase; convalescent sera often have low neutralization antibody titres.

2. **Infectious agent**—The Crimean-Congo hemorrhagic fever virus (Bunyaviridae, *Nairovirus*).

3. **Occurrence**—Observed in the steppes of western Crimea and in the Rostov and Astrakhan regions of the Russian Federation, as well as in Afghanistan, Albania, Bosnia and Herzegovina, Bulgaria, western China, the Islamic Republic of Iran, Iraq, Kazakhstan, Pakistan, South Africa, Turkey, Uzbekistan, the Arabian Peninsula and sub-Saharan Africa. Most patients are animal husbandry workers or medical personnel. Seasonal occurrence in the Russian Federation is from June to September, the period of vector activity.

4. **Reservoir**—In nature, believed to be hares, birds and *Hyalomma* spp. of ticks in Eurasia and South Africa; reservoir hosts remain undefined in tropical Africa, but *Hyalomma* and *Boophilus* ticks, insectivores and rodents may be involved. Domestic animals (sheep, goats and cattle) may act as amplifying hosts.

5. **Mode of transmission**—Bite of infective adult *Hyalomma marginatum* or *H. anatolicum*, or by crushing those ticks. Immature ticks are believed to acquire infection from the animal hosts and by transovarian transmission. Nosocomial infection of medical workers, occurring after exposure to blood and secretions from patients, has been important in recent outbreaks; tertiary cases have occurred in family members of medical workers. Infection is also associated with butchering infected animals.

6. **Incubation period**—Usually 1 to 3 days, with a range of 1–12 days.

7. **Period of communicability**—Highly infectious in the hospital setting. Nosocomial infections are common after exposure to blood and secretions.

8. **Susceptibility**—Immunity after infection probably lifelong.

9. **Methods of control**—

    A. *Preventive measures:* See Lyme disease, 9A, for preventive measures against ticks. An inactivated mouse brain vaccine has been used in eastern Europe and the former Soviet Union (not available in the USA).

B. Control of patient, contacts and the immediate environment:

1) Report to local health authority: In selected epidemic areas; in most countries, not a reportable disease, Class 3 (see Reporting).
2) Isolation: Blood and body fluid precautions.
3) Concurrent disinfection: Bloody discharges are infective; decontaminate by heat or chlorine disinfectants.
4) Quarantine: Not applicable.
5) Immunization: Not applicable, except in eastern Europe.
6) Investigation of contacts and source of infection: Search for missed cases and the presence of infective animals and possible vectors.
7) Specific treatment: Intravenous ribavirin and convalescent plasma with a high neutralizing antibody titre are regarded as useful.

C. Epidemic measures: See Lyme disease, 9C.

D. Disaster implications: None.

E. International measures: WHO Collaborating Centres.

ARTHROPOD-BORNE VIRAL HEMORRHAGIC FEVERS
II.B. OMSK HEMORRHAGIC FEVER ICD-9 065.1; ICD-10 A98.1
KYASANUR FOREST DISEASE ICD-9 065.2; ICD-10 A98.2

1. Identification—These two viral diseases have marked similarities: Onset is sudden with chills, headache, fever, pain in lower back and limbs and severe prostration, often associated with conjunctivitis, diarrhea and vomiting by the 3rd or 4th day. A papulovesicular eruption on the soft palate, cervical lymphadenopathy and conjunctival suffusion are usually present. Confusion and encephalopathic symptoms may occur in patients with Kyasanur Forest disease (KFD); often there is a biphasic course of illness and fever, and the CNS abnormalities develop after an afebrile period of 1–2 weeks.

Severe cases are associated with hemorrhages but with no cutaneous rash. Bleeding occurs from gums, nose, GI tract, uterus and lungs (rarely from the kidneys), sometimes for many days and, when severe, results in shock and death; shock may also occur without manifest hemorrhage. The febrile period ranges from 5 days to 2 weeks, at times with a secondary rise in the third week. Estimated case-fatality rate is from 1% to 10%. Leukopenia and thrombocytopenia are marked. Convalescence tends to be slow and prolonged.

Diagnosis is made through isolation of virus from blood in suckling mice or cell cultures (virus may be present up to 10 days following onset) or through serological tests.

2. Infectious agents—The Omsk hemorrhagic fever (OHF) and KFD viruses are closely related; they belong to the tick-borne encephalitis-louping ill complex of flaviviruses and are similar antigenically to the other viruses in the complex.

3. Occurrence—In the Kyasanur Forest of the Shimoga and Kanara districts of Karnataka, India, principally in young adult males exposed in the forest during the dry season, from November to June. In 1983, there were 1155 cases with 150 deaths, the largest epidemic of KFD ever reported. OHF occurs in the forest steppe regions of western Siberia, within the Omsk, Novosibirsk, Kurgan and Tjumen regions. The Novosibirsk district reported 2 to 41 cases per year between 1989 and 1998, mostly in muskrat trappers. Seasonal occurrence in each area coincides with vector activity. Laboratory infections are common with both viruses.

4. Reservoir—In KFD, probably rodents, shrews, and monkeys in combination with ticks; in OHF, rodents, muskrats and ticks.

5. Mode of transmission—Bite of infective (especially nymphal) ticks, probably *Haemaphysalis spinigera* in KFD. In OHF, infective ticks possibly are *Dermacentor reticulatus (pictus)* and *D. marginatus*; direct transmission from muskrat to human occurs, with disease in the families of muskrat trappers.

6. Incubation period—Usually 3–8 days.

7. Period of communicability—Not directly transmitted from person to person. Infected ticks remain so for life.

8. Susceptibility and resistance—Men and women of all ages are probably susceptible; previous infection leads to immunity.

9. Methods of control—See Tick-borne viral encephalitides and Lyme disease, 9. A formalinized mouse-brain virus vaccine has been reported for OHF; tick-borne encephalitis vaccine also has been used to protect against OHF without proof of efficacy. An experimental vaccine has been used to prevent KFD in endemic areas of India.

[R. Shope, P. Formenty, J. Mackenzie]

ASCARIASIS   ICD-9 127.0; ICD-10 B77
(Roundworm infection, Ascaridiasis)

1. Identification—A helminthic infection of the small intestine generally associated with few or no overt clinical symptoms. Live worms, passed in stools or occasionally from the mouth, anus, or nose, are often the first recognized sign of infection. Some patients have pulmonary manifestations (pneumonitis, Löffler syndrome) caused by larval migration (mainly during reinfections) and characterized by wheezing, cough, fever, eosinophilia and pulmonary infiltration. Heavy parasite burdens may aggravate nutritional deficiency and, if chronic, may affect work and school performance. Serious complications, sometimes fatal, include bowel obstruction by a bolus of worms, particularly in children; or obstruction of bile duct, pancreatic duct or appendix by one or more adult worms. Reports of ascaris pancreatitis are increasing.

Diagnosis is made by identifying eggs in feces, or adult worms passed from the anus, mouth or nose. Intestinal worms may be visualized by radiological and sonographic techniques; pulmonary involvement may be confirmed by identifying ascarid larvae in sputum or gastric washings.

2. Infectious agent—*Ascaris lumbricoides*, the large intestinal roundworm of humans. *A. suum*, a similar parasite of pigs, rarely, if ever, develops to maturity in humans, although it may cause larva migrans.

3. Occurrence—Common and worldwide, with greatest frequency in moist tropical countries where prevalence often exceeds 50%. Prevalence and intensity of infection are usually highest in children between 3 and 8 years.

4. Reservoir—Humans; ascarid eggs in soil.

5. Mode of transmission—Ingestion of infective eggs from soil contaminated with human feces or from uncooked produce contaminated with soil containing infective eggs, but not directly from person to person or from fresh feces. Transmission occurs mainly in the vicinity of the home, where children, in the absence of sanitary facilities, fecally pollute the area; heavy infections in children are frequently the result of ingesting soil (pica). Contaminated soil may be carried long distances on feet or footwear into houses and conveyances; transmission of infection by dust is also possible.

Eggs reach the soil in the feces, then undergo development (embryonation); at summer temperatures they become infective after 2–3 weeks and may remain infective for several months or years in favorable soil. Ingested embryonated eggs hatch in the intestinal lumen; the larvae penetrate the gut wall and reach the lungs via the circulatory system. Larvae grow and develop in the lungs, pass into the alveoli 9–10 days after infection, ascend the trachea and are swallowed to reach the small intestine 14-20 days after infection, where they grow to maturity, mate and begin laying eggs 45-60 days after initial ingestion of the embryonated eggs. Eggs passed by gravid females are discharged in feces.

6. **Incubation period**—The life cycle requires 4-8 weeks to be completed.

7. **Period of communicability**—As long as mature fertilized female worms live in the intestine. Usual life span of adult worms is 12 months; maximum may reach 24 months. The female worm can produce more than 200 000 eggs a day. Under favorable conditions, embryonated eggs can remain viable in soil for years.

8. **Susceptibility**—Susceptibility is general.

9. **Methods of control**—

   A. *Preventive measures:*

   1) Educate the public in the use of toilet facilities.
   2) Provide adequate facilities for proper disposal of feces and prevent soil contamination in areas immediately adjacent to houses, particularly in children's play areas.
   3) In rural areas, construct latrines that prevent dissemination of ascarid eggs through overflow, drainage or otherwise. Treating human feces by composting for later use as fertilizer may not kill all eggs.
   4) Encourage satisfactory hygienic habits on the part of children; in particular, train them to wash hands before eating and handling food.
   5) In endemic areas, protect food from dirt. Food that has been dropped on the floor should not be eaten unless washed or reheated.
   6) WHO recommends a strategy focused on high-risk groups for the control of morbidity due to soil-transmitted helminths, including community treatment (also against *Trichuris trichiura* and hookworm), differentiated according to prevalence and severity of infections: i) universal medication of women (once a year, including pregnant women) and preschool children over 1 (twice or thrice a year) if schoolchildren show 10% or more of heavy infections (50 000+ *Ascaris* eggs per gram of feces) whatever the prevalence; ii) yearly community medication targeted to risk groups (including pregnant women) if prevalence >50% and schoolchildren show <10% of heavy infections; iii) individual case management if prevalence <50% and schoolchildren show <10% of heavy infections. Extensive monitoring has shown no significant ill effects of administration to pregnant women under these circumstances.

B. Control of patient, contacts and the immediate environment:

1) Report to local health authority: Official report not ordinarily justifiable, Class 5 (see Reporting).
2) Isolation: Not applicable.
3) Concurrent disinfection: Sanitary disposal of feces.
4) Quarantine: Not applicable.
5) Immmunization of contacts: Not applicable.
6) Investigation of contacts and source of infection: Determine others who should be treated. Environmental sources of infection should be sought, particularly on premises of affected families.
7) Specific treatment: Single-dose oral mebendazole (500 mg), albendazole (400 mg, half dose for children 12–24 months); on theoretical grounds, both are contraindicated during the first trimester of pregnancy unless there are specific medical or public health indications. Erratic migration of ascarid worms has been reported following mebendazole therapy; this may also occur with other medications, or spontaneously in heavy infections. Single-dose pyrantel pamoate (10 mg/kg) or levamisole (2.5 mg/kg) also effective (also against hookworm, but not against *T. trichiura*).

C. Epidemic measures: Survey for prevalence in highly endemic areas, educate the community in environmental sanitation and in personal hygiene and provide treatment facilities. Community treatment for high-risk groups, especially children or for the whole population.

D. Disaster implications: None.

E. International measures: None.

[L. Savioli]

ASPERGILLOSIS   ICD-9 117.3; ICD-10 B44

1. Identification—A fungal disease that may present with a variety of clinical syndromes produced by several of the *Aspergillus* species. Allergic bronchopulmonary aspergillosis, with symptoms similar to those of asthma, is an allergy to the spores of *Aspergillus* moulds. Up to 5% of adult asthmatics may develop it at some time during their lives; it is also common in cystic fibrosis patients reaching adolescence and adulthood. Some patients have central bronchiectasis. In the long term, allergic bronchopulmonary aspergillosis can lead to permanent lung damage (fibrosis) if untreated. Increasing evidence suggests that fungal allergy is associated with increasing severity of asthma. The diagnosis can be made by X-ray or by sputum, positive *Aspergillus* skin-prick testing, the detection of elevated IgE (>1000 IU/ml) or positive *Aspergillus* precipitins.

Aspergilloma (and chronic cavitary pulmonary aspergillosis) is a different disease also caused by *A. fumigatus* and *A. niger*. The fungus grows within a previously damaged cavity of the lung (e.g. during tuberculosis or sarcoidosis) or other cavity-causing lung disease. The spores penetrate the cavity and germinate therein, forming a fungal ball. Cavities may sometimes be formed by *Aspergillus* and no fungal ball is present (chronic cavitary pulmonary aspergillosis). Symptoms may initially be absent. Weight loss, chronic cough, feeling rundown and tired are common symptoms later, and almost universal in chronic cavitary disease. Hemoptysis can occur in up to 80% of affected people. The diagnosis is made by X-rays, lung scans and *Aspergillus* precipitins testing.

Acute *Aspergillus* sinusitis (a form of invasive aspergillosis) may occur in cases of neutropenia or following a bone marrow/stem cell transplant. Symptoms include fever, facial pain, nasal discharge and headaches. Diagnosis is made by finding the fungus in sinus fluid or tissue and with scans.

Invasive aspergillosis is usually clinically diagnosed in immunosuppressed persons (bone marrow/stem cell transplant, neutropenia, HIV infection, solid organ transplantation or major burns). A rare inherited condition (chronic granulomatous disease) puts affected people at moderate risk. Symptoms usually include fever, cough, chest pain or discomfort or breathlessness that do not respond to standard antibiotics. X-rays and CT scans are abnormal. Bronchoscopy may confirm the diagnosis, together with microscopy and culture. Sputum cultures have low sensitivity and specificity. Antigen tests on blood, CSF and respiratory fluids may help confirm the diagnosis.

In up to 40% of infected people with poor immune systems, hematogenous dissemination to the brain or to other organs, including the eye, the heart, the kidneys and the skin occurs, with worsening of the prognosis. In some cases however, skin infection allows an earlier diagnosis and treatment. *Aspergillus* spp. may cause keratitis after minor injury to the cornea, often leading to unilateral blindness. The organisms may infect the implantation site of a cardiac prosthetic valve or other surgical sites.

2. Infectious agents—Of the 180-odd species of *Aspergillus*, about 40 cause disease, only 5 commonly causing invasive infection: *A. flavus*, *A. fumigatus*, *A. nidulaus*, *A. niger*, and *A. terreus*. Common allergenic species include *A. fumigatus*, *A. clavatus* and *A. versicolor*. *A. fumigatus* causes most cases of fungus ball; *A. niger* is the commonest fungal cause of external otitis.

3. Occurrence—Worldwide; uncommon and sporadic; no distinctive differences in incidence by race or gender. Infections are more common during the colder months of the year. On certain foods, many isolates of *A. flavus* and *A. parasiticus* (occasionally other species) will produce aflatoxins or other mycotoxins that cause disease in animals and fish and are highly carcinogenic for experimental animals. An association between high aflatoxin levels in foods and hepatocellular cancer has been noted in Africa and southeastern Asia. Outbreaks of acute aflatoxicosis (liver necrosis with ascites) have been described in humans in India and Kenya, and in animals.

4. Reservoir—*Aspergillus* species are ubiquitous in nature, particularly in decaying vegetation, such as in piles of leaves or compost piles. Conidia are commonly present in the air both outdoors and indoors and in all seasons of the year. Hospital water may be infected, as may foods such as pepper.

5. Mode of transmission—Inhalation of airborne conidia.

6. Incubation period—Probably between 2 days and 3 months.

7. Period of communicability—No person-to-person transmission.

8. Susceptibility—The ubiquity of *Aspergillus* species and the usual occurrence of the disease as a secondary infection suggest that most people are naturally immune and do not develop disease caused by *Aspergillus*. Immunosuppressive or cytotoxic therapy increase susceptibility, and invasive disease is seen primarily in those with prolonged neutropenia or corticosteroid treatment. Patients with HIV infection or chronic granulomatous disease of childhood are also susceptible.

9. Methods of control—

    A. Preventive measures: High efficiency particulate air (HEPA) filtered room air can decrease the incidence of invasive aspergillosis in hospitalized patients with profound and prolonged neutropenia.

    B. Control of patient, contacts and the immediate environment:

       1) Report to local health authority: Official report not ordinarily justifiable, Class 5 (see Reporting).
       2) Isolation: Not applicable.
       3) Concurrent disinfection: Ordinary cleanliness. Terminal cleaning.
       4) Quarantine: Not applicable.
       5) Immmunization of contacts: Not applicable.
       6) Investigation of contacts: Not ordinarily indicated.
       7) Specific treatment: Allergic bronchopulmonary aspergillosis is treated with steroids by aerosol or by mouth, especially during attacks, and treatment is usually prolonged. Itraconazole is useful in reducing the amount of steroids needed.

         Surgical resection, if possible, is the treatment of choice for patients with aspergilloma who cough blood, but it is best reserved for single cavities. Asymptomatic patients may require no treatment; oral itraconazole (400 mg/day) or the newer voriconazole may help symptoms but do not kill the fungi. Voriconazole (IV or orally) is useful in tissue-invasive forms. Alternatives are itraconazole or amphotericin B IV. Caspofungin (IV only) is used as a rescue treatment. Immunosuppressive therapy should be discontinued or reduced as much as possible. Endobronchial colonization should be treated by measures to improve bronchopulmonary drainage. In sinusitis, surgery may help in eradicating the fungus. Treatment with amphotericin B, caspofungin, voriconazole or itraconazole is usually effective, although relapse is common.

C. Epidemic measures: Not generally applicable; a sporadic disease.

D. Disaster implications: None. Aflatoxin is one possible substance that could be used deliberately and added to water and/or food.

E. International measures: None.

[D. Denning]

BABESIOSIS   ICD-9 088.8; ICD-10 B60.0

1. Identification—A potentially severe and sometimes fatal disease caused by infection with a protozoan parasite of red blood cells. Clinical syndrome may include fever, chills, myalgia, fatigue and jaundice secondary to a hemolytic anaemia that may last from several days to a few months. Seroprevalence studies indicate that most infections are asymptomatic. In some cases, symptomless parasitaemia may last months or even years. Dual infection with *Borrelia burgdorferi*, causal agent of Lyme disease, may increase the severity of both diseases.

Diagnosis is through identification of the parasite within red blood cells on a thick or thin blood film. Demonstration of specific antibodies by serological analysis (IFA babesial DNA [PCR]) or isolation in appropriate laboratory animals provides supportive evidence for the diagnosis. Differentiation from *Plasmodium falciparum* may be difficult in patients who have been in malarious areas or who may have acquired infection by blood transfusion; if diagnosis is uncertain, manage as if it were a case of malaria and send thick and thin blood films to an appropriate reference laboratory.

2. Infectious agents—Several species are known to cause disease in humans. *Babesia microti* is the most common in the eastern and midwestern USA, while Babesia isolate type WA1 parasites are most common on the western coast. *B. divergens* is the most common species in Europe.

3. **Occurrence**—Worldwide, scattered. In the USA, the geographic distribution of *B. microti* infection has increased with the range of the tick vector, *Ixodes scapularis* (formerly *I. dammini*). Babesiosis is endemic on several eastern coastal islands and in southern Connecticut. Infection has also been reported from Wisconsin and Minnesota. Babesia isolate type WA1 and other species have caused human cases reported in California, Washington and Missouri states in the USA, and in Mexico. In Europe, human infections caused by *B. divergens* have been reported from France, Germany, Ireland, the Russian Federation, Serbia and Montenegro (formerly the Federal Republic of Yugoslavia), Spain, Sweden and the United Kingdom (Scotland). Human infections with less well-characterized species have been reported from China (including Taiwan), Egypt, Japan, Spain (Canary Islands), and South Africa.

4. **Reservoir**—Rodents for *B. microti* and cattle for *B. divergens*. Reservoirs for Babesia isolate type WA1 and MO1 (Missouri) are unknown.

5. **Mode of transmission**—*B. microti* is transmitted primarily during summer through the bite of nymphal Ixodes ticks (*I. scapularis*) that have fed on infected deer mice (*Peromyscus leucopus*) and other small mammals (e.g. voles, *Microtus pennsylvanicus*). The adult tick is normally found on deer (which are not infected by the parasite) but may also feed on other mammalian and avian hosts. The vector of *B. divergens* in Europe appears to be *I. ricinus*. Blood transfusion from asymptomatic parasitaemic donors has occasionally induced cases of babesiosis. Patients usually do not recall a tick bite. Two cases of mother-to-infant transmission have been reported.

6. **Incubation period**—Variable; 1 week to 8 weeks has been reported after discrete exposures. Recrudescence of symptoms after prolonged asymptomatic parasitaemia may occur months to more than a year after initial exposure.

7. **Period of communicability**—No person-to-person transmission except through blood transfusion. Asymptomatic blood donors may be infectious for as long as 12 months after initial infection.

8. **Susceptibility**—Susceptibility to *B. microti* is assumed to be universal; immunocompromised, asplenic and elderly persons are at particular risk of symptomatic infection.

9. **Methods of control**—

    A. ***Preventive measures:*** Educate the public about the mode of transmission and means for personal protection. Control rodents around human habitation and use tick repellents.

B. Control of patient, contacts and the immediate environment:

1) Report to local health authority: Reporting of newly suspected cases in some countries, particularly in areas not previously known to be endemic, Class 3 (see Reporting).
2) Isolation: Blood and body fluid precautions.
3) Concurrent disinfection: Not applicable.
4) Quarantine: Not applicable.
5) Protection of contacts: Household members possibly exposed at the same time as the patient should be evaluated for infection and observed for fever.
6) Investigation of contacts and source of infection: Cases occurring in a new area deserve careful study. Blood donors in transfusion-related cases must be investigated promptly and refrain from future donations.
7) Specific treatment: The combination of clindamycin and quinine has been effective in experimental animal studies and in most patients with *B. microti* infections. Infection does not respond to chloroquine. Azithromycin, alone or in combination with quinine or with clindamycin and doxycycline, has been effective in some cases, and azithromycin in combination with atovaquone can be used for non life-threatening babesiosis in immunocompetent patients or in those who cannot tolerate clindamycin or quinine. Pentamidine in combination with trimethoprim-sufamethoxazole was effective in one reported case of *B. divergens*. Exchange transfusion may be envisaged in patients with a high proportion of parasitized red blood cells. Dialysis may be necessary for patients with renal failure.

C. Epidemic measures: None.

D. Disaster implications: None.

E. International measures: None.

[F. Meslin, K. Western]

BALANTIDIASIS   ICD-9 007.0; ICD-10 A07.0
(Balantidiosis, Balantidial dysentery)

1. Identification—A protozoan infection of the colon characteristically producing diarrhea or dysentery, accompanied by abdominal colic, tenesmus, nausea and vomiting. Occasionally the dysentery resembles that due to amoebiasis, with stools containing much blood and mucus but relatively little pus. Peritoneal or urogenital invasion is rare.

Diagnosis is made by identifying the trophozoites or cysts of *Balantidium coli* in fresh feces, or trophozoites in material obtained by sigmoidoscopy.

2. Infectious agent—*Balantidium coli*, a large ciliated protozoan.

3. Occurrence—Worldwide; the incidence of human disease is low. Waterborne epidemics occasionally occur in areas of poor environmental sanitation. Environmental contamination with swine feces may result in a higher incidence. Laboratory pigs may carry this parasite. A large epidemic occurred in frontier areas of Ecuador in 1978.

4. Reservoir—Swine and possibly other animals, such as rats and nonhuman primates.

5. Mode of transmission—Ingestion of cysts from feces of infected hosts; in epidemics, mainly through fecally contaminated water. Sporadic transmission is by transfer of feces to mouth by hands or contaminated water or food.

6. Incubation period—Unknown; may be only a few days.

7. Period of communicability—As long as the infection persists.

8. Susceptibility—People appear to have a high natural resistance. In individuals debilitated from other diseases the infection may be serious and even fatal.

9. Methods of control—

   A. Preventive measures:

   1) Educate the general public in personal hygiene.
   2) Educate and supervise food handlers through health agencies.
   3) Dispose of feces in a sanitary manner.
   4) Minimize contact with swine feces.
   5) Protect public water supplies against contamination with swine feces. Diatomaceous earth and sand filters remove all cysts, but ordinary water chlorination does not destroy cysts. Small quantities of water are best treated by boiling.

   B. Control of patient, contacts and the immediate environment:

   1) Report to local health authority: Official report not ordinarily justifiable, Class 5 (see Reporting).
   2) Isolation: Not applicable.
   3) Concurrent disinfection: Sanitary disposal of feces.
   4) Quarantine: Not applicable.

5) Immunization of contacts: Not applicable.
6) Investigation of contacts and source of infection: Microscopic examination of feces of household members and suspected contacts. Also investigate contact with swine; consider treating infected pigs with tetracycline.
7) Specific treatment: Tetracyclines eliminate infection; metronidazole may also be effective.

C. Epidemic measures: Any grouping of several cases in an area or institution requires prompt epidemiological investigation, especially of environmental sanitation.

D. Disaster implications: None.

E. International measures: None.

[L. Savioli]

BARTONELLOSIS   ICD-9 088.0; ICD-10 A44
(Oroya fever, Verruga peruana, Carrión disease)

1. Identification—A bacterial infection with two clinical forms: a febrile anaemia (Oroya fever, ICD-10 A44.0) and a benign dermal eruption (Verruga peruana, ICD-10 A44.1). Asymptomatic infection and a carrier state may both occur. Oroya fever is characterized by irregular fever, headache, myalgia, arthralgia, pallor, severe hemolytic anaemia (macro- or normocytic, usually hypochromic) and generalized nontender lymphadenopathy. Verruga peruana has a pre-eruptive stage characterized by shifting pains in muscles, bones and joints; the pain, often severe, lasts minutes to several days at any one site. The dermal eruption may be miliary with widely disseminated small hemangioma-like nodules, or nodular with fewer but larger deep-seated lesions, most prominent on the extensor surfaces of the limbs. Individual nodules, particularly near joints, may develop into tumour-like masses with an ulcerated surface.

Verruga peruana may be preceded by Oroya fever or by an asymptomatic infection, with an interval of weeks to months between the stages. The case-fatality rate of untreated Oroya fever ranges from 10% to 90%; death is often associated with protozoal and bacterial superinfections, including salmonella septicaemia. Verruga peruana has a prolonged course but seldom results in death.

Diagnosis is through demonstration by Giemsa staining of the infectious agent adherent to or within RBCs during the acute stage, in sections of skin lesions during the eruptive stage or again through blood culture on special media during either stage. PCR and a number of serological techniques have been used to establish the diagnosis.

2. Infectious agent—*Bartonella bacilliformis.*

3. Occurrence—Limited to mountain valleys of southwestern Colombia, of Ecuador and of Peru, at altitudes between 600 and 2800 meters (2000 to 9200 ft), where the sandfly vector is present; no special predilection for age, race or gender.

4. Reservoir—Humans with the agent present in the blood. In endemic areas, the asymptomatic carrier rate may reach 5%. There is no known animal reservoir.

5. Mode of transmission—Through the bite of sandflies of the genus *Lutzomyia*. Species are not identified for all areas; *Lutzomyia verrucarum* is important in Peru. These insects feed only from dusk to dawn. Blood transfusion, particularly during the Oroya fever stage, may transmit infection.

6. Incubation period—Usually 16–22 days, occasionally 3–4 months.

7. Period of communicability—No direct person-to-person transmission other than by transfused blood. Humans are infectious for the sandfly for a long period; the agent may be present in blood weeks before and up to several years after clinical illness. Duration of infectivity of the sandfly is unknown.

8. Susceptibility—Susceptibility is general, the disease is milder in children than in adults. Inapparent infections and carriers are known. Recovery from untreated Oroya fever almost invariably gives permanent immunity to this form; the Verruga stage may recur.

9. Methods of control—

    A. Preventive measures:

        1) Control sandflies (see Leishmaniasis, cutaneous, 9A).
        2) Avoid known endemic areas after sundown; otherwise apply insect repellent to exposed parts of the body and use fine-mesh bednets, preferably insecticide-treated.
        3) Blood from residents of endemic areas should not be used for transfusions until it has tested negative.

    B. Control of patient, contacts and the immediate environment:

        1) Report to local health authority: In selected endemic areas; in most countries not a reportable disease, Class 3 (see Reporting).
        2) Isolation: Blood and body fluid precautions. The infected individual should be protected from sandfly bites (see 9A).
        3) Concurrent disinfection: Not applicable.
        4) Quarantine: Not applicable.

5) Immmunization of contacts: Not applicable.
6) Investigation of contacts and source of infection: Identification of sandflies, particularly in localities where the infected person was exposed after sundown during the preceding 3–8 weeks.
7) Specific treatment: Penicillin, streptomycin, chloramphenicol and tetracyclines are all effective in reducing fever and bacteraemia in the acute stages. Ampicillin and chloramphenicol are also effective against the frequent secondary complication, salmonellosis. They do not prevent evolution to Verruga peruana. The latter must be treated by streptomycin or rifampicin.

C. Epidemic measures: Intensify case-finding and systematically spray houses with a residual insecticide.

D. Disaster implications: Only if refugee centers are established in an endemic locus.

E. International measures: None.

[D. Raoult]

BLASTOMYCOSIS   ICD-9 116.0; ICD-10 B40
(North American blastomycosis, Gilchrist disease)

1. Identification—A granulomatous mycosis, primarily of the lungs, skin, bone and/or genitourinary tract with hematogenous dissemination. Pulmonary blastomycosis may be acute or chronic. Acute infection is rarely recognized but presents with the sudden onset of fever, cough and a pulmonary infiltrate on chest X-ray. The acute disease resolves spontaneously after 1–3 weeks of illness. During or after the resolution of pneumonia, some patients exhibit extrapulmonary infection. More commonly, there is an indolent onset that evolves into chronic disease.

Cough and chest ache may be mild or absent so that patients may present with infection already spread to other sites, particularly the skin, less often to bone, prostate or epididymis. Cutaneous lesions begin as erythematous papules that become verrucous, crusted or ulcerated and spread slowly. Most commonly, cutaneous lesions are located on the face and distal extremities. Weight loss, weakness and low-grade fever are often present; pulmonary lesions may cavitate. Untreated disseminated or chronic pulmonary blastomycosis eventually progresses to death.

Direct microscopic examination of unstained smears of sputum and lesional material shows characteristic "broad-based" budding forms of the fungus, often dumbbell-shaped, which can be isolated through culture.

Serological tests are not useful. There is no commercially available skin test.

2. Infectious agent—*Blastomyces dermatitidis* (teleomorph, *Ajellomyces dermatitidis*), a dimorphic fungus that grows as a yeast in tissue and in enriched culture media at 37°C (98.6°F), and as a mould at room temperature (25°C/77°F).

3. Occurrence—Uncommon. Occurs sporadically in Africa (Democratic republic of the Congo, South Africa, the United Republic of Tanzania), Canada, India, Israel, Saudi Arabia, central and southeastern USA. Rare in children; more frequent in males than females. Disease in dogs is frequent; it has also been reported in cats, a horse, a captive African lion and a sea lion.

4. Reservoir—Moist soil, particularly wooded areas along waterways and undisturbed places, e.g. under porches or sheds.

5. Mode of transmission—Conidia, typical of the mould or saprophytic growth form, inhaled in spore-laden dust.

6. Incubation period—Indefinite; probably weeks to months. For symptomatic infections, median is 45 days.

7. Period of communicability—No direct person-to-person or animal-to-person transmission.

8. Susceptibility—Unknown. Inapparent pulmonary infections are probable but of unknown frequency. Cell-mediated immunity plays a role in controlling lung infection. The rarity of the natural disease and of laboratory-acquired infections suggests humans are relatively resistant.

9. Methods of control—

   A. Preventive measures: Unknown.

   B. Control of patient, contacts and the immediate environment:

   1) Report to local health authority: Official report not ordinarily justifiable, Class 5 (see Reporting).
   2) Isolation: Not applicable.
   3) Concurrent disinfection: Sputum, discharges and all contaminated articles. Terminal cleaning.
   4) Quarantine: Not applicable.
   5) Immmunization of contacts: Not applicable.
   6) Investigation of contacts and source of infection: Not beneficial unless clusters of disease occur.
   7) Specific treatment: Itraconazole is the drug of choice; amphotericin B is indicated in patients severely ill or with brain lesions.

C. Epidemic measures: Not applicable, a sporadic disease.

D. Disaster implications: None.

E. International measures: None.

[L. Severo]

BOTULISM

INTESTINAL BOTULISM
FORMERLY INFANT
BOTULISM   ICD-9 005.1; ICD-10 A05.1

1. Identification—Human botulism is a serious but relatively rare intoxication caused by potent preformed toxins produced by *Clostridium botulinum*. Of the 7 recognized types of *Clostridium botulinum*, types A, B, E, rarely F and possibly G cause human botulism.

There are 3 forms of botulism: foodborne (the classic form), wound, and intestinal (infant and adult) botulism. The site of toxin production differs for each form but all share the flaccid paralysis that results from botulinum neurotoxin. The name "intestinal botulism" is now used instead of infant botulism.

Foodborne botulism is a severe intoxication resulting from ingestion of preformed toxin present in contaminated food. The characteristic early symptoms and signs are marked fatigue, weakness and vertigo, usually followed by blurred vision, dry mouth, and difficulty in swallowing and speaking. Vomiting, diarrhea, constipation and abdominal swelling may occur. Neurological symptoms always descend through the body: shoulders are first affected, then upper arms, lower arms, thighs, calves, etc. Paralysis of breathing muscles can cause loss of breathing and death unless assistance with breathing (mechanical ventilation) is provided. There is no fever and no loss of consciousness. Similar symptoms usually appear in individuals who shared the same food. Most cases recover, if diagnosed and treated promptly, including early administration of antitoxin and intensive respiratory care. The case-fatality rate in the USA is 5%–10%. Recovery may take months.

Intestinal (infant) botulism is rare; it affects children below 1 and (rarely) adults with altered GI anatomy and microflora. Ingested spores germinate and produce bacteria that reproduce in the gut and release toxin. In most adults and children over 6 months, germination would not happen because natural defences prevent germination and growth of *Clostridium botulinum*. Clinical symptoms in infants include constipation, loss of appetite, weakness, an altered cry, and a striking loss of head control. Infant botulism has in some cases been associated with ingestion of honey contaminated with botulism spores, and mothers are warned not to feed raw honey to their infants.

Infant botulism ranges from mild illness with gradual onset to sudden infant death; some studies suggest that it may cause an estimated 5% of cases of sudden infant death syndrome (SIDS). The case fatality rate of hospitalized cases is less than 1%; it is much higher without access to hospitals with paediatric intensive care units.

Wound botulism, a rare disease, occurs when spores get into an open wound and reproduce in an anaerobic environment. Symptoms are similar to the foodborne form, but may take up to 2 weeks to appear.

Diagnosis of foodborne botulism is made by demonstration of botulinum toxin in serum, stool, gastric aspirate or incriminated food; or through culture of *C. botulinum* from gastric aspirate or stool in a clinical case. Identification of organisms in suspected food is helpful but not diagnostic because botulinum spores are ubiquitous; the presence of toxin in suspect food source is more significant. The diagnosis may be accepted in a person with the clinical syndrome who had consumed a food item incriminated in a laboratory-confirmed case. Toxin in serum or positive wound culture confirms the diagnosis of wound botulism. Electromyography with rapid repetitive stimulation can corroborate the clinical diagnosis for all forms of botulism.

Identification of *C. botulinum* and/or toxin in patient's feces or in autopsy specimens helps establish the diagnosis of intestinal botulism. Toxin is rarely detected in the sera of patients.

2. Infectious agent—Foodborne botulism is caused by toxins produced by *Clostridium botulinum*, a spore-forming obligate anaerobic bacillus. A few nanograms of the toxin can cause illness. Most human outbreaks are due to types A, B, E and rarely F; type G has been isolated from soil and autopsy specimens but a causal role in botulism is not established. Type E outbreaks are usually related to *Clostridium botulinum* fish, seafood and meat from marine mammals. Proteolytic (A, some B and F) and nonproteolytic (E, some B and F) groups differ in water activity, temperature, pH and salt requirements for growth.

Toxin is produced in improperly processed, canned, low acid or alkaline foods, and in pasteurized and lightly cured foods held without refrigeration, especially in airtight packaging. Toxin is destroyed by boiling (e.g. 80°C/176°F for 10 minutes or longer); inactivation of spores requires much higher temperatures. Type E toxin can be produced slowly at temperatures as low as 3°C (37.4°F), lower than that of ordinary refrigeration.

Most cases of infant botulism are caused by type A or B. A few cases (E and F) have been reported from neurotoxigenic clostridia *C. butyricum* and *C. baratii*, respectively.

3. Occurrence—Worldwide; sporadic cases, family and general outbreaks occur where food is prepared or preserved by methods that do not destroy spores and permit toxin formation. Cases rarely result from commercially processed products; outbreaks have occurred from contamination through cans damaged after processing. Cases of intestinal botulism have been reported from the Americas, Asia, Australia and Europe. Actual incidence and distribution of intestinal botulism are unknown because physician awareness and diagnostic testing remain limited. The vast majority of global cases were reported by the USA, with close to half of those reported by California. Internationally, about 150 cases have been detected in Argentina; less than 20 each in Australia and Japan; less than 15 in Canada; and about 30 from Europe (mostly Italy and the United Kingdom), with scattered reports from Chile, China, Egypt, the Islamic Republic of Iran, Israel, and Yemen.

4. Reservoir—Spores, ubiquitous in soil worldwide, are frequently recovered from agricultural products, including honey, and also found in marine sediments and in the intestinal tract of animals, including fish.

5. Mode of transmission—Foodborne botulism occurs when *C. botulinum* is allowed to grow and produce toxin in food which is then eaten without sufficient heating or post-production cooking to inactivate the toxin. Growth of this anaerobic bacteria and formation of toxin tend to occur in products with low oxygen content and the right combination of storage temperature and preservative parameters, as is most often the case in lightly preserved foods such as fermented, salted or smoked fish and meat products and in inadequately processed home-canned or home-bottled low acid foods such as vegetables. The food implicated reflects local eating habits and food-preservation procedures. Occasionally, commercially prepared foods are involved.

Poisonings are often due to home-canned vegetables and fruits; meat is an infrequent vehicle. Several outbreaks have occurred following consumption of uneviscerated fish, baked potatoes, improperly handled commercial potpies, sautéed onions, minced garlic in oil. Some of these recent outbreaks originated in restaurants. Garden foods such as tomatoes, formerly considered too acidic to support growth of *C. botulinum*, may no longer be considered low-hazard foods for home-canning.

In Canada and Alaska, outbreaks have been associated with seal meat, smoked salmon and fermented salmon eggs. In Europe, most cases are due to sausages and smoked or preserved meats; in Japan, to seafood. These differences have been attributed in part to the greater use of sodium nitrite for preserving meats in the USA.

Inhalation botulism, following inhalation of the toxin (aerosol), has occurred in laboratory workers. In these cases, neurological symptoms may be the same as in foodborne botulism, but the incubation period may be longer.

Waterborne botulism could theoretically also result from the ingestion of the preformed toxin. Since water treatment processes inactivate the toxin, the risk is considered low.

Wound botulism often results from contamination of wounds by ground-in soil or gravel or from improperly treated open fractures. It has been reported among chronic drug abusers (primarily in dermal abscesses from subcutaneous injection of heroin and also from sinusitis in cocaine "sniffers").

Intestinal botulism arises from ingestion of spores that germinate in the colon, rather than through ingestion of preformed toxin. Possible sources of spores for infants include foods and dust. Honey, fed on occasion to infants, can contain *C. botulinum* spores.

6. **Incubation period**—Neurological symptoms of foodborne botulism usually appear within 12–36 hours, sometimes several days after eating contaminated food. The shorter the incubation period, the more severe the disease and the higher the case-fatality rate. The incubation period of intestinal botulism in infants is unknown, since the precise time of ingestion often cannot be determined.

7. **Period of communicability**—Despite excretion of *C. botulinum* toxin and organisms at high levels (about 10^6 organisms/gram) in the feces of intestinal botulism patients weeks to months after onset of illness, no instance of secondary person-to-person transmission has been documented. Foodborne botulism patients typically excrete the toxin for shorter periods.

8. **Susceptibility**—Susceptibility is general. Almost all patients hospitalized with intestinal botulism are between 2 weeks and 1 year old; 94% are less than 6 months; the median age at onset was 13 weeks. Adults with special bowel problems leading to unusual GI flora (or with a flora unintentionally altered by antibiotic treatment for other purposes) may be susceptible to intestinal botulism.

9. **Methods of control**—

    A. Preventive measures: Good practices in food preparation (particularly preservation) and hygiene; inactivation of bacterial spores in heat-sterilized, canned products or inhibition of growth in all other products. Commercial heat pasteurization (vacuum-packed pasteurized products, hot smoked products) may not suffice to kill all spores and the safety of these products must be based on preventing growth and toxin production. Refrigeration combined with control of salt content and/or acidity will prevent the growth or formation of toxin. If exposure to the toxin via an aerosol is suspected, the patient's clothing must be removed and stored in plastic bags until it can be washed with soap and water. The patient must shower thoroughly.

Food and water samples associated with suspect cases must be obtained immediately, stored in sealed containers and sent to reference laboratories.

B. *Control of patient, contacts and the immediate environment:*

1) Report to local health authority: Case report of suspected and confirmed cases obligatory in most countries, Class 2 (see Reporting); immediate telephone report indicated.

2) Isolation: Not required; handwashing indicated after handling soiled material including diapers.

3) Concurrent disinfection: Detoxify implicated food(s) by boiling before discarding, or break the containers and bury them deeply in soil to prevent ingestion by animals. Sterilize contaminated utensils by boiling or by chlorine disinfection to inactivate any remaining toxin. Usual sanitary disposal of feces from infant cases. Terminal cleaning.

4) Quarantine: Not applicable.

5) Management of contacts: None for simple direct contacts. Those known to have eaten the incriminated food should be purged with cathartics, given gastric lavage and high enemas and kept under close medical observation. The decision to provide presumptive treatment with polyvalent (equine type AB or ABE) antitoxin to asymptomatic exposed individuals should be weighed carefully: balance potential protection of antitoxin administered early (within 1–2 days after ingestion) against the risk of adverse reactions and sensitization to horse serum.

6) Investigation of contacts and source of toxin: Study recent food history of those ill, and recover all suspected foods for appropriate testing and disposal. Search for other cases of botulism to rule out foodborne botulism.

7) Specific treatment: Intravenous administration of 1 vial of polyvalent (AB or ABE) botulinum antitoxin as soon as possible, obtained from national or international sources (in USA, CDC, 404-639-2206 or 770-488-7100) is part of routine treatment. Serum should be collected to identify the specific toxin before antitoxin is administered, but antitoxin should not be withheld pending test results. Immediate access to an intensive care unit is essential so that respiratory failure, the usual cause of death, can be anticipated and managed promptly. For wound botulism, in addition to antitoxin, the wound should be debrided and/or drainage established, with appropriate antibiotics (e.g. penicillin).

In intestinal botulism, meticulous supportive care is essential. Equine botulinum antitoxin is not used because of the hazard of sensitization and anaphylaxis. In the USA, an investigational human derived botulinal immune globulin (BIG) is available for the treatment of infant botulism patients under an FDA approved open-label from the California Department of Health Services (510-540-2646). Antibiotics do not improve the course of the disease, and aminoglycoside antibiotics in particular may worsen it by causing a synergistic neuromuscular blockade. They should be used only to treat secondary infections. Assisted respiration may be required.

There is a vaccine against botulism, but its effectiveness and side-effects have not been fully evaluated.

C. **Epidemic measures:** Suspicion of a single case of botulism should immediately raise the question of a group outbreak involving a family or others who have shared a common food. Home-preserved foods are the prime suspect until ruled out, although restaurant foods or widely distributed commercially preserved foods are occasionally identified as the source of intoxication and pose a greater public health threat.

Recent outbreaks have implicated unusual food items, and even unlikely foods should be considered. Any food implicated by epidemiological or laboratory findings requires immediate recall, as is immediate search for people sharing the suspect food and for any remaining food from the same source. Any remaining food may be similarly contaminated; if found, it should be submitted for laboratory examination. Sera, gastric aspirates and stool from patients and (when indicated) from others exposed but not ill should be collected and forwarded immediately to a reference laboratory before administration of antitoxin.

D. **Disaster implications:** None with exception of large-scale deliberate use (see F).

E. **International measures:** Commercial products may have been distributed widely; international efforts may be required to recover and test implicated foods. International common source outbreaks have occurred.

F. **Measures in case of deliberate use:** There have been attempts to use botulinum toxin as a bioweapon. Although the greatest threat may be aerosol use, the more common threat may be through use in food and drink. The occurrence of even a single case of botulism, especially if there is no obvious source of improperly preserved food, raises the possibility of deliberate use of botulinum toxin. All such cases must be reported immediately so that appropriate investigations can be initiated without delay.

Sensible precautions, coupled with strong surveillance and response capacity, constitute the most efficient and effective way of countering all such potential assaults, including food terrorism. The WHO document entitled *Terrorist threats to food: guidance for establishing and strengthening prevention and response systems* http://whqlibdoc.who.int/publications/2002/9241545844.pdf provides guidance on integrating consideration of deliberate food sabotage into existing programs for controlling the production of safe food. It also provides guidance on strengthening communicable disease control systems to ensure that surveillance, preparedness and response systems are sufficiently sensitive. Such systems and programs will increase the capacity to reduce the burden of foodborne illness and to address the threat of food terrorism.

[H. Toyofuku]

BRUCELLOSIS   ICD-9 023; ICD-10 A23
(Undulant fever, Malta fever, Mediterranean fever)

1. Identification—A systemic bacterial disease of acute or insidious onset, with continued, intermittent or irregular fever of variable duration; headache; weakness; profuse sweating; chills; arthralgia; depression; weight loss and generalized aching. Localized suppurative infections of organs, including liver and spleen, as well as chronic localized infections may occur; subclinical disease has been reported. The disease may last days, months or occasionally a year or more if not adequately treated.

Osteoarticular complications occur in 20%–60% of cases; sacroiliitis is the most frequent joint manifestation. Genitourinary involvement is seen in 2%–20% of cases, with orchitis and epididymitis as common manifestations. Recovery is usual but disability is often pronounced. The case-fatality rate of untreated brucellosis is 2% or less and usually results from endocarditis caused by *Brucella melitensis* infections. Part or all of the original syndrome may reappear as relapses. A neurotic symptom complex is sometimes misdiagnosed as chronic brucellosis.

Laboratory diagnosis is through appropriate isolation of the infectious agent from blood, bone marrow or other tissues, or from discharges. Current serological tests allow a precise diagnosis in over 95% of cases, but it is necessary to combine a test (Rose Bengal and seroaglutination) detecting agglutinating antibodies (IgM, IgG and IgA) with others detecting non-agglutinating antibodies (Coombs–IgG or ELISA-IgG) developing in later stages. These methods do not apply for *B. canis*, where diagnosis requires tests detecting antibodies to rough-lipopolysaccharide antigens.

2. Infectious agents—*Brucella abortus*, biovars 1–6 and 9; *B. melitensis*, biovars 1–3; *B. suis*, biovars 1–5; *B. canis*.

3. Occurrence—Worldwide, especially in Mediterranean countries (Europe and Africa), Middle East, Africa, central Asia, central and South America, India, Mexico. Sources of infection and responsible organism vary according to geographic area. Brucellosis is predominantly an occupational disease of those working with infected animals or their tissues, especially farm workers, veterinarians and abattoir workers; hence it is more frequent among males. Sporadic cases and outbreaks occur among consumers of raw milk and milk products (especially unpasteurized soft cheese) from cows, sheep and goats. Isolated cases of infection with *B. canis* occur in animal handlers from contact with dogs. The disease is often unrecognized and unreported.

4. Reservoir—Cattle, swine, goats and sheep. Infection may occur in bison, elk, caribou and some species of deer. *B. canis* is an occasional problem in laboratory dog colonies and kennels; a small percentage of pet dogs and a higher proportion of stray dogs have positive *B. canis* antibody titres. Coyotes have been found to be infected.

5. Mode of transmission—Contact through breaks in the skin with animal tissues, blood, urine, vaginal discharges, aborted fetuses and especially placentas; ingestion of raw milk and dairy products (unpasteurized cheese) from infected animals. Airborne infection occurs in pens and stables for animals, and for humans in laboratories and abattoirs. A small number of cases have resulted from accidental self-inoculation of strain 19 Brucella vaccine; the same risk is present when Rev-1 vaccine is handled.

6. Incubation period—Variable and difficult to ascertain; usually 5–60 days; 1–2 months commonplace; occasionally several months.

7. Period of communicability—No evidence of person-to-person communicability.

8. Susceptibility—Severity and duration of clinical illness vary. Duration of acquired immunity uncertain.

9. Methods of control—The control of human brucellosis rests on the elimination of the disease among domestic animals.

　　A. Preventive measures:

　　　　1) Educate the public (especially tourists) regarding the risks associated with drinking untreated milk or eating products made from unpasteurized or otherwise untreated milk.

　　　　2) Educate farmers and workers in slaughterhouses, meat processing plants and butcher shops as to the nature of the disease and the risk in handling carcases and products from potentially infected animals, together with proper operation

of abattoirs to reduce exposure (especially appropriate ventilation).

3) Educate hunters to use protective outfits (gloves, clothing) in handling feral swine and to bury the remains.

4) Search for infection among livestock by serological testing and by ELISA or testing of cows' milk ("ring test"); eliminate infected animals (segregation and/or slaughtering). Infection among swine usually requires slaughter of the herd. In high-prevalence areas, immunize young goats and sheep with live attenuated Rev-1 strain of *B. melitensis*, and calves and sometimes adult animals with strain 19, *B. abortus*. Since 1996, strain RB51 of *B. abortus* has largely replaced strain 19 for immunization of cattle against *B. abortus*, although the usefulness of this vaccine is increasingly questioned. RB51 vaccine appears to be less virulent for humans than strain 19 when accidentally injected.

5) Rev 1 is resistant to streptomycin, and RB51 to rifampicin. This must be taken into account when treating human cases of animal vaccine infections, which are otherwise to be treated like other human cases of brucellosis.

6) Pasteurize milk and dairy products from cows, sheep and goats. Boiling milk is effective when pasteurization is impossible.

7) Exercise care in handling and disposal of placenta, discharges and fetuses. Disinfect contaminated areas.

B. Control of patient, contacts and the immediate environment:

1) Report to local health authority: Case report obligatory in most countries, Class 2 (see Reporting).

2) Isolation: Draining and secretion precautions if there are draining lesions; otherwise none.

3) Concurrent disinfection: Of purulent discharges.

4) Quarantine: Not applicable.

5) Immmunization of contacts: Not applicable.

6) Investigation of contacts and source of infection: Trace infection to the common or individual source, usually infected domestic goats, swine or cattle, or raw milk or dairy products from cows and goats. Test suspected animals and remove reactors.

7) Specific treatment: A combination of rifampicin (600–900 mg daily) or streptomycin (1 gram daily), and doxycycline (200 mg daily) for at least 6 weeks is the treatment of choice. In severely ill toxic patients, corticosteroids may be helpful. Tetracycline should preferably be avoided in children under 7 to avoid tooth staining. Trimethoprim-sufamethoxazole is effective, but relapses are common (30%). Relapses occur in

about 5% of patients treated with doxycycline and rifampicin and are due to sequestered rather than resistant organisms; patients should be treated again with the original regimen. Arthritis may occur in recurrent cases.

C. *Epidemic measures:* Search for common vehicle of infection, usually raw milk or milk products, especially cheese, from an infected herd. Recall incriminated products; stop production and distribution unless pasteurization is instituted.

D. *Disaster implications:* None.

E. *International measures:* Control of domestic animals and animal products in international trade and transport. WHO Collaborating Centres.

F. *Measures in the case of deliberate use:* Their potential to infect humans and animals through aerosol exposition is such that Brucella species may be used as potent biological weapons.

[D. Dragon]

BURULI ULCER   ICD-9 031.1; ICD-10 A31.1

1. Identification—Classically, Buruli ulcer presents as a chronic essentially painless skin ulcer with undermined edges and a necrotic whitish or yellowish base ("cotton wool" appearance). Most lesions are located on the extremities and occur among children living near wetlands in rural tropical environments. Buruli ulcer often starts as a painless nodule or a papule, which eventually ulcerates; other presentations, such as plaques and indurated oedematous lesions, represent a rapidly disseminated form that does not pass through a nodular stage. Bones and joints may be affected by direct spread from an overlying cutaneous lesion of Buruli ulcer or through the blood stream; osteomyelitis due to *Mycobacterium ulcerans* is being reported with increasing frequency. Long-neglected or poorly managed patients usually present with scars—sometimes hypertrophic or keloid, with partially healed areas or disabling contractures, especially for lesions that cross joints. Marjolin ulcers (squamous cell carcinoma) may develop in unstable or chronic non-pigmented scars.

In experienced hands and in endemic areas, diagnosis can usually be made on clinical grounds. Smears and biopsy specimens can be sent to the laboratory for confirmation by the Ziehl-Neelsen stain for acid-fast bacilli, culture, PCR and histopathology. Histopathological features of active disease include the contiguous coagulation necrosis of subcutaneous fat and demonstration of acid-fast bacilli. The differential diagnosis of *M. ulcerans* disease includes the following: minor infections: insect bites and a variety of dermatological conditions; nodules: cysts, lipomas, boils, onchocercomas, lymphadenitis and mycoses; plaques: leprosy, cellulitis, mycoses and psoriasis; oedematous forms: cellulitis, elephantiasis, actinomycosis; ulcers: tropical phagedenic ulcer, leishmaniasis, neurogenic ulcer, yaws, squamous cell carcinoma, pyoderma gangrenosum, noma.

2. **Infectious agent**—The infectious agent, *M. ulcerans* is an acid-fast bacillus, a slow-growing environmental mycobacterium. It can be identified through culture (in 6 weeks), and genetic sequence analysis using PCR. *M. ulcerans* secretes a polyketide macrolide toxin, mycolactone, an apparent virulence factor that destroys tissues and has local immunosuppressive activity. Molecular analysis defines 4 strains of *M. ulcerans*: African, American, Asian, and Australian. Mycolactone production varies with the different groups and is maximal in the African strain.

3. **Occurrence**—*M. ulcerans* infection is an emerging disease, and has been reported in over 30 countries worldwide, mostly tropical. The global burden of the disease is yet to be determined. Africa is the continent most affected. Numbers of reported cases have been increasing over the last 25 years, most strikingly in western Africa, where M. *ulcerans* disease is second only to tuberculosis in terms of mycobacterial disease prevalence (in some endemic districts and communities, it is the most prevalent mycobacterial disease).

4. **Reservoir**—Some evidence points to the environment of the fauna and flora and other ecological factors in the wetlands. Water-dwelling insects, snails and fish are naturally infected and may serve as natural hosts for *M. ulcerans*. In Australia, it has been described not only in humans but also in native animals including the koala (*Phascolarctos cinereus*), the brushtail and ringtail possum (family Phalangeridae) and the long-footed potoroo (*Potorous longipes*). There has been a case reported in a domesticated alpaca (*Lama pacos*); all of these except for those in the potoroo occurred in the focal areas where human cases occurred.

5. **Mode of transmission**—In most studies a significant number of patients had antecedent trauma at the site of the lesion. Circumstances suggest that trauma introduces the causal agent into the skin. Recent evidence suggests that aquatic insects (Naucoridae) may be natural reservoirs and their bite may transmit the disease to humans. Snails belonging to the families of *Ampullariidae* and *Planorbidae* could be contaminated after feeding on aquatic plants covered by a biofilm of *M. ulcerans*. Aerosols arising from stagnant waters may disseminate *M. ulcerans*.

Environmental changes that promote flooding, such as deforestation, dam construction and irrigation systems, are often associated with outbreaks of Buruli ulcer. Population increases in rural wetlands place increasing populations at risk during manual farming activities. Lack of protected water supplies contributes to dependence on pond water for domestic use.

6. Incubation period—Incubation period is about 2−3 months; anecdotal observations suggest that *M. ulcerans* infections may have long periods of latency. As for tuberculosis, it is believed that only a small proportion of infected people develop the disease.

7. Period of communicability—Interhuman transmission of Buruli ulcer in the field is exceptional; rare cases have developed in caretakers of Buruli ulcer patients.

8. Susceptibility—In all probability all persons can be infected. Most, however, are believed to abort the disease in a preclinical stage and others show only small lesions that are rapidly self-healing. Residence or travel to the permanent wetlands of endemic areas, regular contact with the contaminated aquatic environment, and local trauma to the skin are known risk factors. Factors that probably determine the type of disease are dose of agent, depth of inoculation of the agent, host immunological response. BCG neonatal vaccination, for example, appears to protect against *M. ulcerans* osteomyelitis in patients with skin lesions. HIV infection is not a risk factor but may exacerbate the clinical course of the disease.

9. Methods of control—

   A. Preventive measures:

   1) Wear clothing that covers the extremities.
   2) Provide a protected water supply.
   3) Provide health education on the disease for populations at risk.
   4) BCG neonatal vaccination provides short-term prophylaxis.
   5) Early detection and early treatment of suspicious skin lesion helps avoid complications and deformities.

   B. Control of patients, contacts and immediate environment:

   1) Report to local health authority: Although neither a notifiable nor a contagious disease, it is recommended that cases be reported to local health authorities because of its emerging nature.
   2) Isolation: Not applicable.
   3) Concurrent disinfection: Not applicable.
   4) Quarantine: Not applicable.
   5) Immunization of contacts: Not applicable.
   6) Investigation of contacts and source of infection: Investigation of possible places where the patient has been over the last 3 months or longer.
   7) Specific treatment: Surgical excision and primary suturing, or skin graft depending on the severity of the disease. Specific antibiotics—rifampicin and an aminoglycoside

(streptomycin or amikacin)— given for at least 4 weeks and not more than 12 weeks. Antibiotics should be started 1 or 2 days before the initial surgery to minimize *M. ulcerans* bacteraemia. Clinical improvements will dictate continuation of antibiotherapy or further surgical intervention.

C. *Epidemic measures.* Epidemics are very uncommon and call for education, cleanliness, early reporting, and the provision of wound care materials.

D. *Disaster implications:* During wars and other conflicts, diagnosis and treatment of patients is neglected because the health care infrastructure needed to treat patients is disrupted or destroyed. This may lead to severe superinfection of lesions.

E. *International measures:* Endemic countries should coordinate efforts across borders. Health workers in non-endemic areas must be aware of the disease and its management because of international travel. Further information on http://www.who.int/gtb-buruli; WHO Collaborating Centres.

[K. Asiedu]

CAMPYLOBACTER ENTERITIS
(Vibrionic enteritis)

ICD-9 008.4; ICD-10 A04.5

1. Identification—An acute zoonotic bacterial enteric disease of variable severity characterized by diarrhea (frequently with bloody stools), abdominal pain, malaise, fever, nausea and/or vomiting. Symptoms usually occur 2–5 days after exposure and may persist for a week. Prolonged illness and/or relapses may occur in adults. Gross or occult blood with mucus and WBCs is often present in liquid stools. Less common forms include a typhoid-like syndrome, febrile convulsions, meningeal syndrome; rarely, post-infectious complications include reactive arthritis, febrile convulsions or Guillain-Barré syndrome. Cases may mimic acute appendicitis or inflammatory bowel disease. Many infections are asymptomatic and occasionally self-limited.

Diagnosis is based on isolation of the organisms from stools using selective media, reduced oxygen tension and incubation at 43°C (109.4°F). Visualization of motile and curved, spiral or S-shaped rods similar to those of *Vibrio cholerae* by stool phase contrast or darkfield microscopy can provide rapid presumptive evidence for *Campylobacter* enteritis.

2. **Infectious agents**—*Campylobacter jejuni* and, less commonly, *C. coli* are the usual causes of *Campylobacter* diarrhea in humans. At least 20 biotypes and serotypes occur; their identification may be helpful for epidemiological purposes. Other *Campylobacter* organisms, including *C. larii* and *C. fetus* subsp. *fetus*, have been associated with diarrhea in normal hosts; standard culture methods may not detect *C. fetus*.

3. **Occurrence**—These organisms are an important cause of diarrheal illness in all age groups, causing 5%–14% of diarrhea worldwide. They are an important cause of travellers' diarrhea. In industrialized countries; children under 5 and young adults have the highest incidence of illness. Persons who are immunocompromised show an increased risk for infection and recurrences, more severe symptoms and a greater likelihood of being chronic carriers. In developing countries, illness is confined largely to children under 2, especially infants. Common-source outbreaks have occurred, most often associated with foods, especially undercooked poultry, unpasteurized milk and nonchlorinated water. The largest numbers of sporadic cases in temperate areas occur in the warmer months.

4. **Reservoir**—Animals, most frequently poultry and cattle. Puppies, kittens, other pets, swine, sheep, rodents and birds may also be sources of human infection. Most raw poultry meat is contaminated with *C. jejuni*.

5. **Mode of transmission**—Ingestion of the organisms in undercooked meat, contaminated food and water, or raw milk; from contact with infected pets (especially puppies and kittens), farm animals or infected infants. Contamination of milk usually occurs from intestinal carrier cattle; people and food can be contaminated from poultry, especially from common cutting boards. The infective dose is often low. Person-to-person transmission with *C. jejuni* appears uncommon.

6. **Incubation period**—Usually 2 to 5 days, with a range of 1–10 days, depending on dose ingested.

7. **Period of communicability**—Throughout the course of infection; usually several days to several weeks. Individuals not treated with antibiotics may excrete organisms for 2–7 weeks. The temporary carrier state is probably of little epidemiological importance, except for infants and others who are incontinent of stool. Chronic infection of poultry and other animals constitutes the primary source of infection.

8. **Susceptibility**—Immune mechanisms are not well understood, but lasting immunity to serologically related strains follows infection. In developing countries, most people develop immunity in the first 2 years of life.

9. **Methods of control—**

A. *Preventive measures:*

1) Control and prevention measures at all stages of the food-chain, from agricultural production on the farm to processing, manufacturing and preparation of foods in both commercial establishments and the domestic environment.

2) Pasteurize all milk and chlorinate or boil water supplies. Use irradiated foods or thoroughly cook all animal foodstuffs, particularly poultry. Avoid common cutting boards and re-contamination from uncooked foods within the kitchen after cooking is completed.

3) Reduce incidence of *Campylobacter* on farms through specific interventions. Comprehensive control programs and hygienic measures (change of boots and clothes; thorough cleaning and disinfection) to prevent spread of organisms in poultry and animal farms. Good slaughtering and handling practices will reduce contamination of carcases and meat products. Further reduction of contamination through freezing poultry.

4) Recognize, prevent and control *Campylobacter* infections among domestic animals and pets. Puppies and kittens with diarrhea are possible sources of infection; erythromycin may be used to treat their infections, reducing risk of transmission to children. Stress handwashing after animal contact.

5) Minimize contact with poultry and their feces; wash hands when this cannot be avoided.

B. *Control of patient, contacts and the immediate environment:*

1) Report to local health authority: Obligatory case report in several countries, Class 2 (see Reporting).

2) Isolation: Enteric precautions for hospitalized patients. Exclude symptomatic individuals from food handling or care of people in hospitals, custodial institutions and day care centres; exclude asymptomatic convalescent stool-positive individuals only for those with questionable handwashing habits. Stress proper handwashing.

3) Concurrent disinfection: Cleaning of areas and articles soiled with stools. In communities with an adequate sewage disposal system, feces can be discharged directly into sewers without preliminary disinfection. Terminal cleaning required.

4) Quarantine: Not applicable.

5) Immunization of contacts: Not applicable.

6) Investigation of contacts and source of infection: Useful only to detect outbreaks; investigate outbreaks to identify impli-

cated food, water or raw milk to which others may have been exposed.

7) Specific treatment: None generally indicated except rehydration and electrolyte replacement (see Cholera, 9B7). *C. jejuni* or *C. coli* organisms are susceptible in vitro to many antimicrobial agents, including erythromycin, tetracyclines and quinolones, but these are of value only early in the illness and when the identity of the infecting organism is known, in invasive cases, or to eliminate the carrier state. In some areas (USA) quinolone resistance of campylobacter is increasing.

C. Epidemic measures: Report groups of cases, e.g. in a classroom, to the local health authority, with search for vehicle and mode of spread.

D. Disaster implications: A risk when mass feeding and poor sanitation coexist.

E. International measures: WHO Collaborating Centres; see also *Joint FAO/WHO Expert Committee on Risk Assessment of (. . .) Campylobacter spp. in broiler chickens,* 2001, http://whglibdoc.who.int/hq/2001/WHO_SDE_PHE_FOS_01.4.pdf.

[H. P. Braam]

CANDIDIASIS   ICD-9 112; ICD-10 B37
(Moniliasis, Thrush, Candidosis)

1. **Identification**—A mycosis usually confined to the superficial layers of skin or mucous membranes, presenting clinically as oral thrush, intertrigo, vulvovaginitis, paronychia or onychomycosis. Ulcers or pseudomembranes may form in the oesophagus, stomach or intestine. Candidemia commonly arises from intravascular catheters and may produce lesions in many organs: oesophagus, CNS, kidneys, vagina, spleen, endocardium, liver, eyes, meninges, respiratory and urinary tracts and native cardiac valves (or around prosthetic cardiac valves).

Diagnosis requires both laboratory and clinical evidence of candidiasis. The single most valuable laboratory test is microscopic demonstration of pseudohyphae and/or yeast cells in infected tissue or body fluids. Culture confirmation is important, but isolation from sputum, bronchial washings, stool, urine, mucosal surfaces, skin or wounds is not proof of a causal relationship to the disease. Severe or recurrent oropharyngeal infection in an adult with no obvious underlying cause should suggest the possibility of HIV infection.

2. Infectious agents—*Candida albicans, C. tropicalis, C. dubliniensis* and occasionally other species of *Candida. Candida (Torulopsis) glabrata* is distinguished from other causes of candidiasis by lack of pseudohyphae formation in tissue.

3. Occurrence—Worldwide. *C. albicans* is often part of the normal human flora.

4. Reservoir—Humans.

5. Mode of transmission—Contact with secretions or excretions of mouth, skin, vagina and feces, from patients or carriers; by passage from mother to neonate during childbirth; and by endogenous spread.

6. Incubation period—Variable, 2-5 days for thrush in infants.

7. Period of communicability—Presumably while lesions are present.

8. Susceptibility—The frequent isolation of *Candida* species from sputum, throat, feces and urine in the absence of clinical evidence of infection suggests a low level of pathogenicity or widespread immunity Oral thrush is a common, usually benign condition during the first few weeks of life. Clinical disease occurs when host defences are low. Local factors contributing to superficial candidiasis include interdigital intertrigo and paronychia on hands with excessive water exposure (e.g. cannery and laundry workers) and intertrigo in moist skinfolds of obese individuals. Repeated clinical skin or mucosal eruptions are common.

Prominent among systemic factors predisposing to superficial candidiasis are diabetes mellitus, HIV infection and treatment with broad-spectrum antibiotics or supraphysiological doses of adrenal corticosteroids. Women in the third trimester of pregnancy are prone to vulvovaginal candidiasis. Factors predisposing to deep candidiasis include immunosuppression (including that due to HIV infection), indwelling intravenous catheters, neutropenia, hematological malignancies, burns, postoperative complications and very low birthweight in neonates. Urinary tract candidiasis usually arises as a complication of prolonged catheterization of the bladder or renal pelvis. Most adults and older children have a delayed dermal hypersensitivity to the fungus and possess humoral antibodies.

9. Methods of control—

  A. *Preventive measures:* Early detection and local treatment of any infection in the mouth, oesophagus or urinary bladder of those with predisposing systemic factors (see Susceptibility) to prevent systemic spread. Fluconazole chemoprophylaxis decreases the incidence of deep candidiasis during the first 2 months following allogenic bone marrow transplantation. Antifungal agents that are absorbed fully (fluconazole, ketoconazole, itraconazole) or partially (miconazole, clotrimazole) from the gastrointestinal tract have been found to be effective in preventing oral candidiasis in cancer patients receiving chemotherapy.

B. *Control of patient, contacts and the immediate environment:*

1) Report to local health authority: Official report not ordinarily justifiable, Class 5 (see Reporting).
2) Isolation: Not applicable.
3) Concurrent disinfection: Of secretions and contaminated articles.
4) Quarantine: Not applicable.
5) Immmunization of contacts: Not applicable.
6) Investigation of contacts and source of infection: Not beneficial in sporadic cases.
7) Specific treatment: Ameliorating the underlying causes of candidiasis, e.g. removal of indwelling central venous catheters, often facilitates cure. Topical nystatin or an azole (miconazole, clotrimazole, ketoconazole, fluconazole) is useful in many forms of superficial candidiasis. Oral clotrimazole troches or nystatin suspension are effective for treatment of oral thrush. Itraconazole suspension or fluconazole is effective in oral and oesophageal candidiasis. Vaginal infection may be treated with oral fluconazole or topical clotrimazole, miconazole, butoconazole, terconazole, tioconazole or nystatin. Amphotericin B IV, with or without 5-fluorocytosine, is the drug of choice for visceral or invasive candidiasis. Lipid formulations of amphotericin B are probably also effective. Fluconazole is an effective alternative to amphotericin B.

C. *Epidemic measures:* Outbreaks are most frequently due to contaminated intravenous solutions and thrush in nurseries for newborns. Concurrent disinfection and terminal cleaning comparable to that used for epidemic diarrhea in hospital nurseries (see Diarrhea, section IV, 9A).

D. *Disaster implications:* None.

E. *International measures:* None.

[F. Ndowa]

CAPILLARIASIS

Three types of nematodes of the superfamily Trichuroidea, genus *Capillaria*, produce disease in humans.

I. CAPILLARIASIS DUE TO *CAPILLARIA PHILIPPINENSIS*   ICD-9 127.5; ICD-10 B81.1
(Intestinal capillariasis)

1. Identification—First described in Luzon, Philippines, in the early 1960s, the disease is clinically an enteropathy with massive protein loss and a malabsorption syndrome leading to progressive weight loss and emaciation. Fatal cases are characterized by the presence of great numbers of parasites in the small intestine together with ascites and pleural transudate. Case-fatality rates of 10% have been reported. Subclinical cases also occur, but usually become symptomatic over time.

Diagnosis is based on clinical findings plus the identification of eggs or larval or adult parasites in the stool. The eggs resemble those of *Trichuris trichiuria*. Jejunal biopsy may show worms in the mucosa.

2. Infectious agent—*Capillaria philippinensis*.

3. Occurrence—Intestinal capillariasis is endemic in the Philippines and in Thailand; cases have been reported from Egypt, Japan, the Republic of Korea and Taiwan (China). Isolated cases have also been reported from Colombia, India, Indonesia, and the Islamic Republic of Iran. In Luzon (Philippines), more than 1800 cases have been seen since 1967. Males between the ages of 20 and 45 appear to be particularly at risk.

4. Reservoir—Unknown; possibly aquatic birds. Fish are considered intermediate hosts.

5. Mode of transmission—A history of ingestion of raw or inadequately cooked small fish eaten whole is usually obtained from patients. Experimentally, infective larvae develop in the intestines of freshwater fish that ingest eggs; monkeys, Mongolian gerbils and some birds fed these fish become infected, the parasite maturing within their intestines.

6. Incubation period—Unknown in humans; in animal studies, about a month or more.

7. Period of communicability—Not transmitted directly from person to person.

8. Susceptibility—Susceptibility appears to be general in those geographic areas in which the parasite is prevalent. Attack rates are often high.

9. Methods of control—

A. *Preventive measures:*

1) Avoid eating uncooked fish or other aquatic animal life in known endemic areas.
2) Provide adequate facilities for the disposal of feces.

B. *Control of patient, contacts and the immediate environment:*

1) Report to local health authority: Case report by most practicable means, Class 3 (see Reporting).
2) Isolation: Not applicable.
3) Concurrent disinfection: Sanitary disposal of feces.
4) Quarantine: Not applicable.
5) Immmunization of contacts: Not applicable.
6) Investigation of contacts and source of infection: Stool examination for all members of family groups and others with common exposure to raw or undercooked fish, with treatment of infected individuals.
7) Specific treatment: Mebendazole or albendazole as drugs of choice.

C. *Epidemic measures:* Prompt investigation of cases and contacts; treatment of cases as indicated. Education on the need to cook all fish prior to eating.

D. *Disaster implications:* None.

E. *International measures:* None.

II. CAPILLARIASIS DUE TO
CAPILLARIA HEPATICA   ICD-9 128.8; ICD-10 B83.8
(Hepatic capillariasis)

1. Identification—An uncommon and occasionally fatal disease in humans due to the presence of adult *Capillaria hepatica* in the liver. The picture is that of an acute or subacute hepatitis with marked eosinophilia resembling that of visceral larva migrans; the organism can disseminate to the lungs and other viscera.

Diagnosis is made by demonstrating eggs or the parasite in a liver biopsy or at necropsy.

2. Infectious agent—*Capillaria hepatica* (*Hepaticola hepatica*).

3. Occurrence—Since identification as a human disease in 1924, about 30 cases have been reported from Africa, North and South America, Asia, Europe and the Pacific area.

4. Reservoir—Primarily rats (as many as 86% infected in some reports) and other rodents, but also a large variety of domestic and wild mammals. The adult worms live and produce eggs in the liver.

5. Mode of transmission—The adult worms produce fertilized eggs that remain in the liver until the death of the host animal. When infected liver is eaten, the eggs are freed by digestion, reach the soil in the feces and develop to the infective stage in 2-4 weeks. When ingested by a suitable host, embryonated eggs hatch in the intestine; larvae migrate through the wall of the gut and are transported via the portal system to the liver, where they mature and produce eggs. Spurious infection in humans may be detected when eggs are found in stools after consumption of infected liver, raw or cooked; since these eggs are not embryonated, infection cannot be established.

6. Incubation period—From 3 to 4 weeks.

7. Period of communicability—Not directly transmitted from person to person.

8. Susceptibility—Susceptibility is universal; malnourished children appear more often infected.

9. Methods of control—

A. Preventive measures:

1) Avoid ingestion of dirt, directly (pica) or in contaminated food or water or on hands.
2) Protect water supplies and food from soil contamination.

B. Control of patient, contacts and the immediate environment:

1) Report to local health authority: Official report not ordinarily justifiable, Class 5 (see Reporting).
2) Isolation: Not applicable.
3) Concurrent disinfection: Not applicable.
4) Quarantine: Not applicable.
5) Immmunization of contacts: Not applicable.
6) Investigation of contacts and source of infection: Not applicable.
7) Specific treatment: Thiabendazole and albendazole effectively kill the worms in the liver.

C. Epidemic measures: Not applicable.

D. Disaster implications: None.

E. International measures: None.

III. PULMONARY
CAPILLARIASIS ICD-9 128.8; ICD-10 B 83.8

A pulmonary disease manifested by fever, cough and asthmatic breathing, caused by *Capillaria aerophila* (*Thominx aerophila*), a nematode parasite of cats, dogs and other carnivorous mammals. Pneumonitis may be severe; heavy infections may be fatal. The worms live in tunnels in the epithelial lining of the trachea, bronchi and bronchioles; fertilized eggs are sloughed into the air passages, coughed up, swallowed and discharged from the body in the feces. In the soil, larvae develop in the eggs and remain infective for a year or longer. Infection is acquired mainly by children, through ingestion of infective eggs in soil or in soil-contaminated food or water. Eggs may appear in the sputum in 4 weeks; symptoms may appear earlier or later. Human cases have been recorded from the Islamic Republic of Iran, Morocco and the former Soviet Union; animal infection has been reported in North and South America, Europe, Asia and Australia.

[D. Engels]

CAT-SCRATCH DISEASE ICD-9 078.3; ICD-10 A28.1
(Cat-scratch fever, Benign lymphoreticulosis)

1. Identification—A subacute, usually self-limited bacterial disease characterized by malaise, granulomatous lymphadenitis and variable patterns of fever. Often preceded by a cat scratch, lick or bite that produces a red papular lesion with involvement of a regional lymph node, usually within 2 weeks; may progress to suppuration. The papule at the inoculation site can be found in 50%–90% of cases. Parinaud oculoglandular syndrome (granulomatous conjunctivitis with pretragal adenopathy) can occur after direct or indirect conjunctival inoculation; neurological complications such as encephalopathy and optic neuritis can also occur. Prolonged high fever may be accompanied by osteolytic lesions and/or hepatic and splenic granulomata. Bacteraemia, hepatic extravasation of blood (peliosis hepatis) and bacillary angiomatosis due to this infection may occur among young children and among immunocompromised persons, particularly those with HIV infection.

Cat-scratch disease can be clinically confused with other diseases that cause regional lymphadenopathies, e.g. tularaemia, brucellosis, tuberculosis, plague, pasteurellosis and lymphoma.

Diagnosis is based on a consistent clinical picture combined with serological evidence of antibody to *Bartonella*. A titre of 1:64 or greater by IFA assay is considered positive.

Histopathological examination of affected lymph nodes may show consistent characteristics but is not diagnostic. Pus obtained from lymph nodes is usually bacteriologically sterile by conventional techniques. Immunodetection and PCR are highly efficient in detecting *Bartonella* in biopsies of lymph nodes. *Bartonella* has been grown from blood and from lymph node aspirates after prolonged incubation on rabbit blood agar in 5% CO2 at 36°C (96.8°F).

2. Infectious agent—*Bartonella* (formerly *Rochalimaea*) *henselae* has been implicated epidemiologically, bacteriologically and serologically as the causal agent of most cat-scratch disease. Related Bartonellae, such as *B. quintana* and *B. clarridgeiae*, may also produce illnesses among immunocompromised hosts, but do not cause cat-scratch disease. *Afipia felis*, a previously described candidate organism, plays a minor role if any.

3. Occurrence—Worldwide, but uncommon; equally affects men and women, cat-scratch disease is more common in children and young adults. Familial clustering rarely occurs. Most cases are seen during in the late summer, autumn and winter months.

4. Reservoir—Domestic cats are the main vectors and reservoirs for *B. henselae*; no evidence of clinical illness in cats even when chronic bacteraemia has been demonstrated. Cat fleas and ticks may be infected.

5. Mode of transmission—Over 90% of patients give a history of scratch, bite, lick or other exposure to a healthy, usually young cat or kitten. Dog scratch or bite, monkey bite or contact with rabbits, chickens or horses has been reported prior to the syndrome, but cat involvement was not excluded in all cases. Cat fleas (*Ctenocephalides felis*) transmit *B. henselae* among cats, but play no clear role in direct transmission to humans.

6. Incubation period—Variable, usually 3−14 days from inoculation to primary lesion and 5–50 days from inoculation to lymphadenopathy.

7. Period of communicability—Not directly transmitted from person to person.

8. Susceptibility—Unknown.

9. Methods of control—

    A. Preventive measures: Thorough cleaning of cat scratches and bites may help. Flea control is very important to prevent infection of cats.

    B. Control of patient, contacts and the immediate environment:

      1) Report to local health authority: Official report not ordinarily justifiable, Class 5 (see Reporting).
      2) Isolation: Not applicable.
      3) Concurrent disinfection: Of discharges from purulent lesions.

    4), 5) and 6) Quarantine, Immunization of contacts and Investigation of contacts and source of infection: Not applicable.

    7) Specific treatment: Treatment of uncomplicated disease in immunocompetent patients is not indicated, but all immunocompromised patients must be treated for 1-3 months. Prolonged administration (at least 1 month) of antibiotics such as erythromycin, rifampicin, ciprofloxacin or gentamicin is effective in the disseminated forms seen in persons with HIV infection. Needle aspiration of suppurative lymphadenitis may be required for relief of pain, but incisional biopsy of lymph nodes should be avoided.

C. Epidemic measures: Not applicable.

D. Disaster implications: None.

E. International measures: None.

[D. Raoult]

CHANCROID   ICD-9 099.0; ICD-10 A57
(Ulcus molle, Soft chancre)

1. Identification—An acute bacterial infection localized in the genital area and characterized clinically by single or multiple painful, necrotizing ulcers at site of infection, frequently accompanied by painful swelling and suppuration of regional lymph nodes. Minimally symptomatic lesions may occur on the vaginal wall or cervix; asymptomatic infections may occur in women. Extragenital lesions have been reported. Chancroid ulcers, like other genital ulcers, are associated with increased risk of HIV infection.

Diagnosis is by isolation of the organism from lesion exudate on a selective medium incorporating vancomycin into chocolate, rabbit or horse blood agar enriched with fetal calf serum. Gram stains of lesion exudates may suggest the diagnosis if numerous Gram-negative coccobacilli are seen "streaming" between leukocytes. PCR and immunofluorescence for direct detection of organisms in ulcers, and serology, are available on a research basis.

2. Infectious agent—*Haemophilus ducreyi*, the Ducrey bacillus.

3. Occurrence—More often diagnosed in men, especially clients of sex workers. Most prevalent in tropical and subtropical regions, where incidence may be higher than that of syphilis and approach that of gonorrhoea in men. With an exclusively human reservoir, chancroid has disappeared from many regions with increased access to condoms and antimicrobial agents and in response to the AIDS threat. The disease is much less common in temperate zones and may occur in small outbreaks. In the USA and other industrialized countries, outbreaks and some endemic transmission have occurred, principally among migrant farm workers and poor inner city residents.

4. Reservoir—Humans.

5. Mode of transmission—Direct sexual contact with discharges from open lesions and pus from buboes. Auto-inoculation to non-genital sites may occur in infected persons. Beyond the neonatal period, sexual abuse must be considered when chancroid is found in children.

6. Incubation period—From 3 to 5 days, up to 14 days.

7. Period of communicability—Until healed and as long as infectious agent persists in the original lesion or discharging regional lymph nodes— up to several weeks or months without antibiotherapy. Antibioherapy eliminates *H. ducreyi* and lesions heal in 1-2 weeks.

8. Susceptibility—Susceptibility is general; the uncircumcised are at higher risk than the circumcised. There is no evidence of natural resistance.

9. Methods of control—

A. Preventive measures:

1) See Syphilis, 9A.
2) Serological follow-up for syphilis and HIV in all patients with nonherpetic genital ulcerations.

B. Control of patient, contacts and the immediate environment:

1) Report to local health authority: Case report obligatory in many countries, Class 2 (see Reporting).
2) Isolation: Avoid sexual contact until all lesions are healed.
3) Concurrent disinfection: Not applicable.
4) Quarantine: Not applicable.
5) Immmunization of contacts: Not applicable.
6) Investigation of contacts and source of infection: Examine and treat all sexual contacts within the 10 days preceding onset of symptoms. Women without visible signs may, rarely, be carriers. Sexual contacts even without signs should receive prophylactic treatment.
7) Specific treatment: Ceftriaxone, erythromycin, azithromycin or, for adults only, ciprofloxacin. Alternatives include amoxicillin with clavulanic acid. Fluctuant inguinal nodes must be aspirated through intact skin to prevent spontaneous rupture.

C. *Epidemic measures:* Persistent occurrence or increased incidence is an indication for stricter application of measures outlined in 9A and 9B above. When compliance with treatment is a problem, consideration should be given to a single dose of ceftriaxone or azithromycin. Empirical therapy to high-risk groups with or without lesions, including sex workers, to clinic patients reporting contact with sex workers, and to clinic patients with genital ulcers and negative darkfields may be required to control an outbreak. Interventions providing periodic presumptive treatment covering sex workers and their clients have an impact on chancroid and provide valuable information for strategies to eliminate the disease in areas of high prevalence.

D. *Disaster implications:* None.

E. *International measures:* See Syphilis, 9E.

[F. Ndowa]

CHICKENPOX/HERPES ZOSTER

(Varicella/Shingles)

ICD-9 052-053;
ICD-10 B01-B02

1. Identification—Chickenpox (varicella) is an acute, generalized viral disease with sudden onset of slight fever, mild constitutional symptoms and a skin eruption that is maculopapular for a few hours, vesicular for 3–4 days and leaves a granular scab. The vesicles are unilocular and collapse on puncture, in contrast to the multilocular, noncollapsing vesicles of smallpox. Lesions commonly occur in successive crops, with several stages of maturity present at the same time; they tend to be more abundant on covered than on exposed parts of the body. Lesions may appear on the scalp, high in the axilla, on mucous membranes of the mouth and upper respiratory tract and on the conjunctivae; they tend to occur in areas of irritation, such as sunburn or diaper rash. They may be so few as to escape observation. Mild, atypical and inapparent infections occur. Occasionally, especially in adults, the fever and constitutional manifestations may be severe. Although varicella is usually a benign childhood disease, and rarely rated as an important public health problem, varicella zoster virus may induce pneumonia or encephalitis, sometimes with persistent sequelae or death. Secondary bacterial infections of the vesicles may leave disfiguring scars or result in necrotizing fasciitis or septicaemia.

The case-fatality rate in the USA is lower for children (1:100 000 infected in the 5–9 age group) than for adults (1:5000). Serious complications include pneumonia (viral and bacterial), secondary bacterial infections, hemorrhagic complications and encephalitis. Children with acute leukae-mia, including those in remission after chemotherapy, are at increased risk of disseminated disease, fatal in 5%–10% of cases. Neonates who develop varicella between ages 5 and 10 days are at increased risk of developing severe generalized chickenpox, as are those whose mothers develop the disease 5 days prior to or within 2 days after delivery; prior to the availability of effective viral drugs, the case-fatality rate in neonates reached 30%, but is likely to be lower now. Infection early in pregnancy may be associated with congenital varicella syndrome in 0.7% of cases, and at 13–20 weeks gestation with a 2% risk. Clinical chickenpox was a frequent antecedent of Reye syndrome before the association of Reye syndrome with aspirin use for viral infections was identified.

Herpes zoster (shingles) is a local manifestation of reactivation of latent varicella infection in the dorsal root ganglia. Vesicles with an erythematous base are restricted to skin areas supplied by sensory nerves of a single or associated group of dorsal root ganglia. Lesions may appear in irregular crops along nerve pathways; they are histologically identical to those of chickenpox but usually unilateral, deeper seated and more closely aggre-gated. Severe pain and paraesthesia are common, and herpes zoster may result in permanent neurological damage such as cranial nerve palsy and contralateral hemiplegia, or visual impairment following zoster ophthal-mia. Nearly 15% of zoster patients have pain or parasthaesias in the affected dermatome for at least several weeks and sometimes permanently (postherpetic neuralgia). The incidence of both zoster and postherpetic neuralgia increase with age; there is some evidence that almost 10% of children being treated for a malignant neoplasm are prone to develop zoster, and persons with HIV infection are also at increased risk for zoster. In the immunosuppressed and those with diagnosed malignancies, but also in otherwise normal individuals with fewer lesions, extensive chick-enpox-like lesions may appear outside the dermatome. Intrauterine infec-tion and varicella before 2 are also associated with zoster at an early age. Occasionally, a varicelliform eruption follows shortly after herpes zoster, and rarely there is a secondary eruption of zoster after chickenpox.

Laboratory tests such as visualization of virus by EM; virus isolation in cell cultures; demonstration of viral antigen in smears using FA, of viral DNA by PCR, or of a rise in serum antibodies are not routinely required but are useful in complicated cases and in epidemiological studies. In the vaccine era, viral strain identification may be needed (e.g. to document whether herpes zoster in a vaccine recipient is due to vaccine or wild virus). Several antibody assays are now commercially available, but they are not sensitive enough to be used for post-immunization testing of immunity. Multinucleated giant cells may be detected in Giemsa-stained scrapings from the base of a lesion; these are not found in vaccinia lesions but do occur in herpes simplex lesions. They are not specific for varicella infections, and the availability of rapid direct fluorescent antibody testing has limited their value for clinical testing.

2. Infectious agent—Human (alpha) herpesvirus 3 (varicella-zoster virus, VZV), a member of the *Herpesvirus* group.

3. Occurrence—Worldwide. Infection with human (alpha) herpesvirus 3 is nearly universal. In temperate climates, at least 90% of the population has had chickenpox by age 15 and at least 95% by young adulthood. In temperate zones, chickenpox occurs most frequently in winter and early spring. The epidemiology of varicella in tropical countries differs from temperate climates, with a higher proportion of cases occurring among adults. Zoster occurs more commonly in older people.

4. Reservoir—Humans.

5. Mode of transmission—Person-to-person by direct contact, droplet or airborne spread of vesicle fluid or secretions of the respiratory tract of cases or of vesicle fluid of patients with herpes zoster; indirectly through articles freshly soiled by discharges from vesicles and mucous membranes of infected people. In contrast to vaccinia and variola, scabs from varicella lesions are not infective. Chickenpox is one of the most readily communicable of diseases, especially in the early stages of the eruption; zoster has a lower rate of transmission (varicella seronegative contacts of herpes zoster patients develop chickenpox). Susceptibles have an 80%–90% risk of infection after household exposure to varicella.

6. Incubation period—2 to 3 weeks; commonly 14–16 days; may be prolonged after passive immunization against varicella (see 9A2) and in the immunodeficient.

7. Period of communicability—As long as 5 but usually 1–2 days before onset of rash, and continuing until all lesions are crusted (usually about 5 days). Contagiousness may be prolonged in patients with altered immunity. The secondary attack rate among susceptible siblings is 70%–90%. Patients with zoster may be infectious for a week after the appearance of vesiculopustular lesions. Susceptible individuals should be considered infectious for 10–21 days following exposure.

8. Susceptibility—Susceptibility to chickenpox is universal among those not previously infected; ordinarily a more severe disease of adults than of children. Infection usually confers long immunity; second attacks are rare in immunocompetent persons but have been documented; subclinical reinfection is common. Viral infection remains latent; disease may recur years later as herpes zoster in about 15% of older adults, and sometimes in children.

Neonates whose mothers are not immune and patients with leukaemia may suffer severe, prolonged or fatal chickenpox. Adults with cancer—especially of lymphoid tissue, with or without steroid therapy—immunodeficient patients and those on immunosuppressive therapy may have an increased frequency of severe zoster, both localized and disseminated.

9. **Methods of control—**

   A. *Preventive measures:*

   1) A live attenuated varicella virus vaccine has been licensed for use in Japan, the Republic of Korea, the United States and several countries in Europe. A single 0.5 ml SC dose is recommended for routine immunization of children aged 12 to 18 months and for children up to 12 years who have not had varicella. This vaccine has a cumulative preventive efficacy estimated at 70%–90% in children followed for up to 6 years. If an immunized person does get "break-through varicella", it is usually a mild case with fewer lesions (up to 50, frequently not vesicular), mild or no fever and shorter duration. The protection against zoster induced by varicella vaccine, administered either in childhood or in adult populations, is not yet sufficiently documented. If administered within 3 days of exposure, varicella vaccine is likely to prevent or at least modify disease in a case contact.

   Varicella vaccine is also recommended for susceptible persons over 13, e.g. those with no history of varicella during childhood (even though serological tests often reveal they have in fact been infected). Vaccination is often offered without confirmation of seronegativity. Priority groups for adult immunization include close contacts of persons at high risk for serious complications, persons who live or work in environments where transmission of varicella is likely (e.g. teachers of young children, day care employees, residents and staff in institutional settings), or where transmission can occur (e.g. college students, inmates and staff members of correctional institutions and military personnel), nonpregnant women of childbearing age, adolescents and adults in households with children and international travellers.

   In immunocompromised persons, including persons with advanced HIV infection, varicella vaccination is currently contraindicated. Other contraindications for varicella vaccination include a history of anaphylactic reactions to any component of the vaccine (including neomycin), pregnancy (theoretical risk to the fetus—pregnancy should be avoided for 4 weeks following vaccination), ongoing severe illness, and advanced immune disorders.

   Except for patients with acute lymphatic leukaemia in stable remission, ongoing treatment with systemic steroids (adults >20mg/day, children >1mg/kg/day) is considered a contraindication for varicella vaccination. A history of congenital immune disorders in close family members is a relative contraindication. Routine childhood immunization against varicella may be considered in countries where the disease is a public health and socioeconomic problem, where immunization is affordable and where sustained high vaccine coverage (85%–90%) can be achieved. Persons over 13 require 2 doses of vaccine 4–8 weeks apart.

A mild varicella-like rash at the site of vaccine injection or at distant sites has been observed in 2%–4% of children and about 5% of adults. Rare occasions of mild zoster following vaccination show that the currently used vaccine strains may induce latency, with the subsequent risk of reactivation, although the rate seems to be lower than after natural disease. Duration of immunity is unknown, but antibodies have persisted for at least 10 years; persistence of antibody has occurred in the presence of circulating wild virus.

2) Protect high-risk individuals who cannot be immunized, e.g. nonimmune neonates and the immunodeficient, from exposure by immunizing household or other close contacts.

3) Varicella-zoster immune globulin (VZIG), prepared from the plasma of normal blood donors with high VZV antibody titre, effectively modifies or prevents disease if given within 96 hours after exposure (see 9B5).

B. Control of patient, contacts and the immediate environment:

1) Report to local health authority: In many countries, not a reportable disease; varicella-related deaths became nationally notifiable in the USA on January 1, 1999; Class 3 (see Reporting).

2) Isolation: Exclude children from school, medical offices, emergency rooms or public places until vesicles become dry, usually after 5 days in unimmunized children and 1–4 days with breakthrough varicella in immunized children; exclude infected adults from workplace and avoid contact with susceptibles. In hospital, strict isolation because of the risk of varicella in susceptible immunocompromised patients.

3) Concurrent disinfection: Articles soiled by discharges from the nose and throat.

4) Quarantine: Usually none. However, in places where susceptible children with known recent exposure must remain for medical reasons, the risk of spread to steroid treated or immunodeficient patients may justify quarantine of known contacts for at least 10–21 days after exposure (up to 28 days if varicella zoster IG was given).

5) Protection of contacts: Varicella vaccine is effective in preventing illness or modifying severity if used within 3 days,

and possibly up to 5 days, of exposure; it is recommended for susceptible persons following exposure to varicella.

Varicella zoster IG within 96 hours of exposure may prevent or modify disease in susceptible close contacts of cases. It is available in several countries for high-risk persons exposed to chickenpox and indicated for newborns of mothers who develop chickenpox within 5 days prior to or within 2 days after delivery. There is no assurance that administering VZIG to a pregnant woman will prevent congenital malformations in the fetus, but it may modify varicella severity in the pregnant woman.

Antiviral drugs such as acyclovir appear useful in preventing or modifying varicella in exposed individuals if given within a week of exposure. A dose of 80 mg/kg/day in 4 divided doses has been used, but no regimen is as yet generally recommended for this purpose.

6) Investigation of contacts and source of infection: The source of infection may be a case of varicella or herpes zoster. All contacts, especially if ineligible for postexposure immunization, should be evaluated promptly for administration of varicella zoster IG. Infectious patients should be isolated until all lesions are crusted; exposed susceptibles eligible for immunization should receive vaccine immediately to control or prevent an outbreak.

7) Specific treatment: While both vidarabine (adenine arabinoside) and acyclovir are moderately effective in treating varicella-zoster infections, acyclovir is considered the agent of choice for treatment of varicella. Oral valacyclovir or famciclovir are effective and well-tolerated for herpes zoster, These drugs help shorten the duration of the infection and possibly that of postherpetic neuralgia; they may shorten the duration of symptoms and pain of zoster in the normal older patient, especially if administered within 24 hours of rash onset.

C. **Epidemic measures:** Outbreaks of varicella are common in schools and other institutional settings; they may be protracted, disruptive and associated with complications. Infectious cases should be isolated and susceptible contacts immunized promptly (or referred to their health care provider for immunization). Persons ineligible for immunization, such as susceptible pregnant females and those at high risk for severe disease (as above), should be evaluated immediately for administration of Varicella zoster IG.

D. **Disaster implications:** Outbreaks of chickenpox may occur among children crowded together in emergency housing situations.

E. **International measures:** See C.

[D. Lavanchy]

CHLAMYDIAL INFECTIONS

As laboratory techniques improve, chlamydial organisms are increasingly implicated as causes of human disease. Chlamydiae are obligate intracellular bacteria that differ from viruses and rickettsiae but, like the latter, are sensitive to broad-spectrum antimicrobials. Those that cause human disease are classified into 3 species:

1) *Chlamydia psittaci*, the etiologic agent of psittacosis (q.v.);

2) *C. trachomatis*, including serotypes that cause trachoma (q.v.), genital infections (see below), chlamydial conjunctivitis (q.v.) and infant pneumonia (q.v.), and other serotypes that cause lymphogranuloma venereum (q.v.); and

3) *C. pneumoniae*, the cause of respiratory disease including pneumonia (q.v.) and implicated in coronary artery disease.

Chlamydiae are increasingly recognized as important pathogens responsible for several sexually transmitted infections, with infant eye and lung infections consequent to maternal genital infection.

GENITAL INFECTIONS,
CHLAMYDIAL   ICD-9 099.8; ICD-10 A56

1. Identification—Sexually transmitted genital infection is manifested in males primarily as a urethritis, and in females as a cervical infection. Clinical manifestations of urethritis are often difficult to distinguish from gonorrhoea and include moderate or scanty mucopurulent discharges, urethral itching, and burning on urination. Asymptomatic infection may be found in 1%–25% of sexually active men. Possible complications or sequelae of male urethral infections include epididymitis, infertility and Reiter syndrome. In homosexual men, receptive anorectal intercourse may result in chlamydial proctitis.

In the female, the clinical manifestations may be similar to those of gonorrhoea and may present as a mucopurulent endocervical discharge, with oedema, erythema and easily induced endocervical bleeding caused by inflammation of the endocervical columnar epithelium. Up to 70% of sexually active women with chlamydial infections are asymptomatic. Complications and sequelae include salpingitis with subsequent risk of infertility, ectopic pregnancy or chronic pelvic pain. Asymptomatic chronic infections of endometrium and fallopian tubes may lead to the same outcome. Less frequent manifestations include Bartholinitis, urethral syndrome with dysuria and pyuria, perihepatitis (Fitz-Hugh-Curtis syndrome) and proctitis. Infection during pregnancy may result in premature rupture of membranes and preterm delivery, and conjunctival and pneumonic infection of the newborn. Endocervical chlamydial infection has been associated with increased risk of acquiring HIV infection.

Chlamydial infections may be acquired concurrently with gonorrhoea and persist after gonorrhoea has been treated successfully. Because gonococcal and chlamydial cervicitis are often difficult to distinguish clinically, treatment for both organisms is recommended when one is suspected.

Diagnosis of nongonococcal urethritis (NGU) or cervicitis is usually based on the failure to demonstrate *Neisseria gonorrhoeae* by smear and culture; chlamydial etiology is confirmed by examination of intraurethral or endocervical swab material by direct IF test with monoclonal antibody, EIA, DNA probe, nucleic acid amplification test (NAAT) or cell culture. NAATs can be used with urine specimens. The intracellular organisms are less readily recoverable from the discharge itself. For other agents, see Urethritis, nongonococcal.

2. Infectious agent—*Chlamydia trachomatis*, immunotypes D through K, has been identified in approximately 35%–50% of cases of nongonococcal urethritis in the USA.

3. Occurrence—Common worldwide; recognition has increased steadily in the last two decades.

4. Reservoir—Humans.

5. Mode of transmission—Sexual intercourse.

6. Incubation period—Poorly defined, probably 7–14 days or longer.

7. Period of communicability—Unknown. Relapses are probably common.

8. Susceptibility—Susceptibility is general. No acquired immunity has been demonstrated; cellular immunity is immunotype-specific.

9. Methods of control—

  A. Preventive measures:

   1) Health and sex education; same as for syphilis (see Syphilis, 9A), with emphasis on use of a condom when engaging in sexual intercourse.
   2) Annual screening of sexually active adolescent girls should be routine. Screening of adult women should also be considered if they are under 25, have multiple or new sex partners, and/or use barrier contraceptives inconsistently. Newer tests for *C. trachomatis* infection that also enable screening of adolescent and young adult males may be used on urine specimens.

  B. Control of patient, contacts and the immediate environment:

   1) Report to local health authority: Case report is required in many industrialized countries, Class 2 (see Reporting).

2) Isolation: Universal precautions, as appropriate for hospitalized patients. Appropriate antibiotherapy renders discharges noninfectious; patients should refrain from sexual intercourse until treatment of index patient and current sexual partners is completed.

3) Concurrent disinfection: Care in disposal of articles contaminated with urethral and vaginal discharges.

4) Quarantine: Not applicable.

5) Immunization of contacts: Not applicable.

6) Investigation of contacts and source of infection: Presumptive treatment of sexual partners is recommended. As a minimum, concurrent treatment of regular sex partners is a practical approach to management. If neonates born to infected mothers have not received systemic treatment, chest X-rays at 3 weeks of age and again after 12–18 weeks may be considered to exclude subclinical chlamydial pneumonia.

7) Specific treatment: Doxycycline (PO), 100 mg twice daily for 7 days or azithromycin (PO), 1 gram in a single dose. Tetracycline (PO), 500 mg 4 times daily for 7 days is an alternative but is cumbersome in terms of frequency and the need to avoid food and milk products before ingestion, thus negatively affecting patient compliance. Erythromycin is an alternative drug of choice for newborn and for women with a known or suspected pregnancy.

C. *Epidemic measures:* None.

D. *Disaster implications:* None.

E. *International measures:* None.

URETHRITIS, NONGONOCOCCAL AND NONSPECIFIC (NGU, NSU)   ICD-9 099.4; ICD-10 N34.1

While chlamydiae are the most frequently isolated causal agents in cases of non-gonococcal urethritis, other agents are involved in a significant number of cases. *Ureaplasma urealyticum* is considered the causal agent in approximately 10%–20% of NGU cases and *Mycoplasma genitalium* has been implicated in some studies. Herpesvirus simplex type 2 is rarely implicated; *Trichomonas vaginalis*, though rarely implicated, has been shown to be a significant cause of urethritis in some high prevalence settings. If laboratory facilities for demonstration of chlamydia are not available, all cases of NGU (together with their sexual partners) are best managed as though their infections were due to chlamydia, especially since many chlamydia-negative cases also respond to antibiotherapy.

[F. Ndowa]

CHOLERA AND OTHER VIBRIOSES
ICD-9 001; ICD-10 A00

I. *VIBRIO CHOLERAE* SEROGROUPS
O1 AND O139

1. Identification—An acute bacterial enteric disease characterized in its severe form by sudden onset, profuse painless watery stools (rice-water stool), nausea and profuse vomiting early in the course of illness. In untreated cases, rapid dehydration, acidosis, circulatory collapse, hypoglycaemia in children, and renal failure can rapidly lead to death. In most cases infection is asymptomatic or causes mild diarrhea, especially with organisms of the El Tor biotype; asymptomatic carriers can transmit the infection. In severe dehydrated cases (cholera gravis), death may occur within a few hours, and the case-fatality rate may exceed 50%. With proper and timely rehydration, this can be less than 1%.

Diagnosis is confirmed by isolating *Vibrio cholerae* of the serogroup O1 or O139 from feces. *V. cholerae* grows well on standard culture media, the most widely used of which is TCBS agar. The strains are further characterized by O1 and O139 specific antisera. Strains that agglutinate in O1 antisera are further characterized for serotype. If laboratory facilities are not nearby or immediately available, Cary Blair transport medium can be used to transport or store a fecal or rectal swab. For clinical purposes, a quick presumptive diagnosis can be made by darkfield or phase microscopic visualization of the vibrios moving like "shooting stars", inhibited by preservative-free, serotype-specific antiserum. For epidemiological purposes, a presumptive diagnosis can be based on the demonstration of a significant rise in titre of antitoxic and vibriocidal antibodies. In nonendemic areas, organisms isolated from initial suspected cases should be confirmed in a reference laboratory through appropriate biochemical and serological reactions and by testing the organisms for cholera toxin production or for the presence of cholera toxin genes. A one-step dipstick test for rapid detection of *V. cholerae* O1 and O139 has been developed and should soon be available on the market to improve application of effective public health interventions. In epidemics, once laboratory confirmation and antibiotic sensitivity have been established, it becomes unnecessary to confirm all subsequent cases. Shift should be made to using primarily the clinical case definition proposed by WHO as follows:

- Disease unknown in area: severe dehydration or death from acute watery diarrhea in a patient aged 5 or more
- Endemic cholera: acute watery diarrhea with or without vomiting in a patient aged 5 or more

- Epidemic cholera: acute watery diarrhea with or without vomiting in any patient.

However, monitoring an epidemic should include laboratory confirmation and antimicrobial sensitivity testing of a small proportion of cases on a regular basis.

2. **Infectious agent**—Only *Vibrio cholerae* serogroups O1 and O139 are associated with the epidemiological characteristics and clinical picture of cholera. Serogroup O1 occurs as two biotypes–classical and El Tor–each of which occurs as 3 serotypes (Inaba, Ogawa and rarely Hikojima). The clinical pictures of illness caused by *V. cholerae* O1 of either biotype and *V. cholerae* O139 are similar because an almost identical enterotoxin is elaborated by these organisms. In any single epidemic, one particular serogroup and biotype tends to be dominant. The current seventh pandemic is characterized by the O1 serogroup El Tor biotype. *V. cholerae* O1 or classical biotype has not been diagnosed over recent years and *V. cholerae* O139 remains confined to South East Asia.

Prior to 1992, non-O1 strains were recognized as causing sporadic cases and rare outbreaks of diarrheal disease, but were not associated with large epidemics. However, in 1992−1993, large-scale epidemics of cholera-like disease were reported in India and Bangladesh, caused by a new organism, *V. cholerae* O139 serogroup. This organism elaborates the same cholera toxin but differs from O1 strains in lipopolysaccharide (LPS) structure and in the production of capsular antigen. The clinical and epidemiological picture of illness caused by this organism is typical of cholera, and cases should be reported as such. The epidemic O139 strain, which possesses the virulence factors of *V. cholerae* O1 El Tor, was apparently derived by a deletion in the genes that encode the O1 lipopolysaccharide antigen of an El Tor strain, followed by the acquisition of a large fragment of new DNA encoding the enzymes that allow synthesis of O139 lipopolysaccharide and capsule.

The reporting as cholera of *V. cholerae* other than O1 is inaccurate and leads to confusion.

3. **Occurrence**—Cholera is one of the oldest and best understood epidemic diseases. Epidemics and pandemics are strongly linked to the consumption of unsafe water, poor hygiene, poor sanitation and crowded living conditions. Conditions leading to epidemics exist in many developing countries where cholera is either endemic or a recurring problem in a large number of areas. Typical settings for cholera are periurban slums where basic urban infrastructure is missing. Outbreaks of cholera can also occur on a seasonal basis in endemic areas of Asia and Africa. For example, KwaZulu-Natal, South Africa, experienced an outbreak in 2000−2001 that resulted in more than 125 000 cases with a low case fatality rate of less than 0.5%—a low rate that had never been observed in an outbreak of that magnitude.

Man-made or natural disasters such as complex emergencies and floods resulting in population movements as well as overcrowded refugee camps are conducive to explosive outbreaks with high case fatality rates. An outbreak of *V. cholerae* El Tor among Rwandan refugees in Goma (Zaire as it was then known, now the Democratic Republic of the Congo) in July 1994 resulted in more than 50 000 cases and 24 000 deaths over the course of little more than one month.

Cholera is one of the 3 diseases requiring notification under the *International Health Regulations*. In 2002, 52 countries officially reported 142 311 cases (of which 36 imported cases) and 4564 deaths—an overall case fatality rate of 3.2%. Low case fatality rate values were observed in several countries including South Africa. Elsewhere, case fatality rates remain high and can reach up to $30-40\%$ among vulnerable populations in high risk areas who are not correctly rehydrated. The actual number of cholera cases, however, is likely to be much higher because of underreporting and poor surveillance systems.

During the 19th century, cholera spread repeatedly through 6 pandemic waves from the Gulf of Bengal to most of the world. During the first half of the 20th century, the disease was confined largely to Asia, except for a severe epidemic in Egypt in 1947. During the latter half of the 20th century, the epidemiology of cholera has been marked by: 1) the relentless global spread of the seventh pandemic of cholera caused by *V. cholerae* O1 El Tor; 2) recognition of environmental reservoirs of cholera such as on the shore of the Gulf of Bengal and along the Gulf of Mexico coast of the USA; 3) the appearance for the first time of large explosive epidemics of cholera caused by *V. cholerae* organisms of a serogroup other than O1 (*V. cholerae* O139)

During the current (seventh) pandemic that started in 1961, *V. cholerae* of the El Tor biotype has spread worldwide from Indonesia to the Asian mainland in $1963-1969$, to western Africa in 1970 and spread rapidly throughout the African continent in large parts of which it became endemic, reaching Madagascar in 1999. Cholera reached Latin America in 1991 after nearly a century of absence; it caused explosive epidemics along the Pacific coast of Peru and hence in neighboring countries—by 1994, approximately one million cholera cases had been recorded in Latin America. Although the clinical disease was as severe as in other regions of the world, the overall case fatality rate in Latin America was kept at a remarkably low 1%, except in highly rural areas in the Andes and Amazon region where patients were often far from medical care.

In late 1992, the new serogroup of *V. cholerae* designated O139 Bengal emerged in Southern India and Bangladesh and spread rapidly throughout the region over the next few months, infecting several hundred thousand. During this epidemic period, *V. cholerae* O139 almost completely replaced *V. cholerae* O1 strains in hospitalized cholera patients and in samples of surface water. The epidemic continued to spread through 1994, with cases of O139 cholera reported from 11 countries in Asia. This new strain was soon introduced into other continents by infected travellers, but secondary spread outside of Asia has not been reported and *V. cholerae* O139 remains confined to the southeastern areas of the Asian continent. No evidence is currently available as to whether this new strain has the potential to generate a new pandemic and therefore requires continued international surveillance.

Cases of cholera are regularly imported into industrialized countries. Several prospective studies using optimized bacteriological methods (TCBS medium) have shown that the incidence of traveller's cholera in USA and Japanese travellers is considerably higher than previously estimated. However, safe water and adequate sanitation limit the potential for outbreaks.

The occurrence of laboratory and sporadic cases in the USA since 1911 over many years in the Gulf coast area, all due to a single indigenous strain, has led to the identification of an environmental reservoir of *V. cholerae* O1 El Tor Inaba in the Gulf of Mexico.

4. Reservoir—The main reservoir is humans. Observations in the Australia, Bangladesh and the USA have shown that environmental reservoirs exist, apparently in association with copepods or other zooplankton in brackish water or estuaries.

5. Mode of transmission—Cholera is acquired through ingestion of an infective dose of contaminated food or water and can be transmitted through many mechanisms. Water usually is contaminated by feces of infected individuals and can itself contaminate, directly or through the contamination of food. Contamination of drinking water occurs usually at source, during transportation or during storage at home. Food may also be contaminated by soiled hands during preparation or while eating. In funeral ceremonies transmission may occur through consumption of food and beverages prepared by family members after they handled the corpse for burial. *V. cholerae* O1 and O139 can persist in water for long periods and multiply in moist leftover food.

When epidemic El Tor cholera appeared in Latin America in 1991, faulty municipal water systems, contaminated surface waters, and unsafe domestic water storage methods resulted in extensive waterborne transmission of cholera. Beverages prepared with contaminated water and sold by street vendors, ice and even commercial bottled water have been incriminated as vehicles in cholera transmission, as have cooked grains with sauces. *V. cholerae* introduced by a food handler into one of these foods and stored unrefrigerated can increase by several logs within 8–12 hours. Vegetables and fruit "freshened" with untreated sewage wastewater have also served as vehicles of transmission. Outbreaks or epidemics as well as sporadic cases are often attributed to raw or undercooked seafood. In other instances, sporadic cases of cholera follow the ingestion of raw or inadequately cooked seafood from nonpolluted waters. Cases have been traced to eating shellfish from coastal and estuarine waters where a natural reservoir of *V. cholerae* O1, serotype Inaba, exists in an estuarine environment not characterized by sewage contamination. Clinical cholera in endemic areas is usually confined to the lowest socioeconomic groups.

6. **Incubation period**—From a few hours to 5 days, usually 2−3 days.

7. **Period of communicability**—As long as stools are positive, usually only a few days after recovery. Occasionally the carrier state may persist for several months. Antibiotics known to be effective against the infecting strains (e.g. tetracycline or doxycycline) shorten the period of communicability but are not recommended for treatment. Rarely, chronic biliary infection lasting for years, associated with intermittent shedding of vibrios in the stool, has been observed in adults.

8. **Susceptibility**—Variable; gastric achlorhydria increases the risk of illness, and breastfed infants are protected. Cholera occurs significantly more often among persons with blood group O. Infection with either *V. cholerae* O1 or O139 results in a rise in agglutinating and antitoxic antibodies, and increased resistance to reinfection. Serum vibriocidal antibodies, which are readily detected following O1 infection (but for which comparably specific, sensitive and reliable assays are not available for O139 infection), are the best immunological correlate of protection against O1 cholera. Field studies show that an initial clinical infection by *V. cholerae* O1 of the classical biotype confers protection against either classical or El Tor biotypes; in contrast an initial clinical infection caused by biotype El Tor results in only a modest level of long-term protection that is limited to El Tor infections. In endemic areas, most people acquire antibodies by early adulthood. However, infection with O1 strains affords no protection against O139 infection and vice-versa. In experimental challenge studies in volunteers, an initial clinical infection due to *V. cholerae* O139 conferred significant protection against diarrhea upon rechallenge with *V. cholerae* O139.

9. **Methods of control**—

   A. *Preventive measures:*

   1) See Typhoid fever, 9A1-10.
   2) Traditional injectable cholera vaccines based on killed whole cell microorganisms provide only partial protection (50% efficacy) of short duration (3−6 months) they do not prevent asymptomatic infection and are associated with adverse effects. Their use has never been recommended by WHO.

      Two oral cholera vaccines (OCV) that are safe and provide significant protection for several months against cholera caused by O1 strains have become available on the international market. These vaccines are mainly used by travellers from industrialized countries. One is a single-dose live vaccine (strain CVD 103-HgR); the other is a killed vaccine consisting of inactivated vibrios plus B-subunit of the cholera toxin, given on a 2-dose regimen. As of 2003, these vaccines were not licensed in the USA. These vaccines are currently under consideration for use as an additional public health tool for cholera control activities, especially in complex emergencies and among refugees. The first large-scale trial is under way in Mozambique (2003−2004).

3) Measures that inhibit or otherwise compromise the movement of people, foods or other goods are not epidemiologically justified and have never proved effective to control cholera.

B. Control of patient, contacts and the immediate environment:

1) Report to local health authority: Case report universally required by *International Health Regulations*; Class 1 (see Reporting).

2) Isolation: Hospitalization with enteric precautions is desirable for severely ill patients; strict isolation is not necessary. Less severe cases can be managed on an outpatient basis with oral rehydration and an appropriate antimicrobial agent to prevent spread. Cholera wards can be operated even when crowded without hazard to staff and visitors, provided standard procedures are observed for hand washing and cleanliness and for the circulation of staff and visitors. Fly control should be practised.

3) Concurrent disinfection: Of feces and vomit and of linens and articles used by patients, using heat, carbolic acid or other disinfectant. In communities with a modern and adequate sewage disposal system, feces can be discharged directly into the sewers without preliminary disinfection. Terminal cleaning.

4) Quarantine: Not applicable.

5) Management of contacts: Surveillance of persons who shared food and drink with a cholera patient for 5 days from last exposure. If there is evidence or high likelihood of secondary transmission within households, household members can be given chemoprophylaxis; in adults, tetracycline (500 mg 4 times daily) for 3 days or doxycycline a single dose of 300 mg, unless local strains are known or believed to be resistant to tetracycline. Children may also be given tetracycline (50 mg/kg/day in 4 divided doses for 3 days or doxycycline as a single dose of 6 mg/kg). There is no risk of staining teeth with such short courses of tetracyclines. Alternative prophylactic agents that may be useful where *V. cholerae* O1 strains are resistant to tetracycline include: furazolidone (100 mg 4 times daily for adults and

1.25 mg/kg 4 times daily for children); and erythromycin (paediatric dosage 40 mg/kg/day in 4 divided doses; adult dosage 250 mg 4 times daily). Mass chemoprophylaxis of whole communities is never indicated, is a waste of resources and can lead to antibiotic resistance.

6) Investigation of contacts and source of infection: Investigate possibilities of infection from polluted drinking water and contaminated food. Meal companions for the 5 days prior to onset should be interviewed. A search by stool culture for unreported cases is recommended only among household members or those exposed to a possible common source in a previously uninfected area.

7) Specific treatment: The cornerstone of cholera treatment is timely and adequate rehydration. Patients presenting mild dehydration can be treated successfully by oral rehydration therapy using ORS. Only severely dehydrated patients need rehydration through intravenous routes to repair fluid and electrolyte loss through diarrhea. As rehydration therapy becomes increasingly effective, patients who survive from hypovolaemic shock and severe dehydration may manifest certain complications, such as hypoglycaemia, that must be recognized and treated promptly.

Most patients with mild or moderate fluid loss can be treated entirely with oral rehydration solutions that contain glucose 75 mmol/L; NaCl 75 mmol/L; KCl 20 mmol/L; and trisodium citrate dihydrate 10 mmol/L. This new formula of ORS was approved by a WHO expert committee in June 2002; it has a total osmolarity of 245 mOsm/L and is particularly efficacious for treatment of children with acute non-cholera diarrhea in both developing and industrialized areas. Mild and moderate volume depletion should be corrected with oral solutions, replacing over 4−6 hours a volume matching the estimated fluid loss (approximately 5% of body weight for mild and 7% for moderate dehydration). Continuing losses are replaced by giving, over 4 hours, a volume of oral solution equal to 1.5 times the stool volume lost in the previous 4 hours.

Severely dehydrated patients or patients in shock should be given rapid IV rehydration with a balanced multielectrolyte solution containing approximately 130 mEq/L of Na+, 25−48 mEq/L of bicarbonate, acetate or lactate ions, and 10−15 mEq/L of K+. Useful solutions include Ringer lactate (4 grams NaCl, 1 gram KCl, 6.5 grams sodium acetate and 8 grams glucose/L), and "Dacca solution" (5 grams NaCl, 4 grams NaHCO3 and 1 gram KCl/L), which can be prepared locally in an emergency.

The initial fluid replacement should be 30 mL/kg in the first hour for infants and in the first 30 minutes for persons over 1 year, after which the patient should be reassessed. After circulatory collapse has been effectively reversed, most patients can continue on oral rehydration to complete the 10% initial fluid deficit replacement and to match continuing fluid loss.

In severe cases, appropriate antimicrobial agents can shorten the duration of diarrhea, reduce the volume of rehydration solutions required, and shorten the duration of vibrio excretion. Adults are given tetracycline 500 mg 4 times a day, and children 12.5 mg/kg 4 times daily, for 3 days. For adults a single dose of 300mg of doxyxycline is a good alternative treatment. Where tetracycline-resistant strains of *V. cholerae* are prevalent, alternative antimicrobial regimens include furazolidone (100 mg 4 times daily for adults and 1.25 mg/kg 4 times daily for children, for 3 days); or erythromycin (250 mg 4 times daily for adults and 30 mg/kg 4 times daily for children, for 3 days). Ciprofloxacin, 250 mg once daily for 3 days, is also a useful regimen for adults. *V. cholerae* O1 and O139 strains are resistant to trimethoprim-cotrimoxazole. Since individual strains of *V. cholerae* O1 or O139 may be resistant to any of these antimicrobials, knowledge of the sensitivity of local strains to these agents, if available, should be used to guide the choice of the antimicrobial therapy.

C. Epidemic measures:

1) Educate the population at risk concerning the need to seek appropriate treatment without delay.
2) Provide effective treatment facilities.
3) Adopt emergency measures to ensure a safe water supply. Chlorinate public water supplies, even if the source water appears to be uncontaminated. Chlorinate or boil water used for drinking, cooking and washing dishes and food containers unless the water supply is adequately chlorinated and subsequently protected from contamination.
4) Ensure careful preparation and supervision of food and drinks. After cooking or boiling, protect against contamination by flies and insanitary handling; leftover foods should be thoroughly reheated (70°C— or 158°F—for at least 15 minutes) before ingestion. Persons with diarrhea should not prepare food or haul water for others. Food served at funerals of cholera victims may be particularly hazardous if the body has been prepared for burial by the participants

without stringent precautions and this practice should be discouraged during epidemics.

5) Initiate a thorough investigation designed to find the vehicle of infection and circumstances (time, place, person) of transmission, and plan control measures accordingly.

6) Provide appropriate safe facilities for sewage disposal.

7) Parenteral whole cell vaccine is not recommended.

8) Use of the currently available oral cholera vaccines is under study in Mozambique as an additional public health tool.

D. Disaster implications: Outbreak risks are high in endemic areas if large groups of people are crowded together without safe water in sufficient quantity, adequate food handling or sanitary facilities.

E. International measures:

1) Governments are required to report cholera cases due to *V. cholerae* O1 and O139 to WHO. In the USA, suspected cases are reported to the State epidemiologist, State health departments then notify the CDC, which confirms the case and notifies WHO.

2) Measures applicable to ships, aircraft and land transport arriving from cholera areas are specified in *International Health Regulations* (1969), Third Annotated Edition 1983, updated and reprinted 1992, WHO, Geneva.

3) International travellers: Immunization with the parenteral whole cell vaccine is not recommended by WHO. No country requires proof of cholera vaccination as a condition of entry and the International Certificate of Vaccination no longer provides a specific space for the recording of cholera vaccination. Immunization with either of the new oral vaccines can be recommended for individuals from industrialized countries travelling to areas of endemic or epidemic cholera. In countries where the new oral vaccines are already licensed, immunization is particularly recommended for travellers with known risk factors such as hypochlorhydria (consequent to partial gastrectomy or medication) or cardiac disease (e.g. arrhythmia), and for the elderly or individuals of blood group O.

4) WHO Collaborating Centres. Further information on http://www.who.int/csr/disease/cholera or http://www.who.int/emc/diseases/cholera.

II. *VIBRIO CHOLERAE*
SEROGROUPS OTHER THAN
O1 AND O139   ICD-9 005.8; ICD-10 A05.8

1. **Identification**—Of the more than 200 *V. cholerae* serogroups that exist, only O1 and O139 are associated with the clinical syndrome of cholera and can cause large epidemics. Organisms of *V. cholerae* serogroups other than O1 and O139 have been associated with sporadic cases of foodborne outbreaks of gastroenteritis, but have not spread in epidemic form. They have been associated with wound infection and also, rarely, isolated from patients (usually immunocompromised hosts) with septicemic disease.

2. **Infectious agent**—*V. cholerae* pathogens of serogroups other than O1 and O139.

Serogroups of *V. cholerae* have been defined on the basis of their surface antigen (lipopolysaccharide O antigen). Vibrios that are biochemically indistinguishable but do not agglutinate in *V. cholerae* serogroup O1 or O139 antisera (non-O1 nonO139 strains, formerly known as nonagglutinable vibrios [NAGs] or noncholera vibrios [NCVs]) are now included in the species *V. cholerae*. Some strains elaborate cholera enterotoxin, but most do not.

As with all *V. cholerae*, growth is enhanced in an environment of 1% NaCl. Rarely do non-O1/non-O139 *V. cholerae* strains elaborate cholera toxin or harbour the colonization factors of O1 and O139 epidemic strains. Some non-O1/non-O139 strains produce a heat-stable enterotoxin (so-called NAG-ST). Epidemiological and volunteer challenge studies have documented the pathogenicity of strains producing NAG-ST. The non-O1/non-O139 strains isolated from blood of septicemic patients have been heavily encapsulated.

The reporting of nontoxinogenic *V. cholerae* O1 or of non-O1/non-O139 *V. cholerae* infections as cholera is inaccurate and leads to confusion.

3. **Occurrence**—Non-O1/non-O139 *V. cholerae* strains are associated with 2%–3% of cases (including travellers) of diarrheal illness in tropical developing countries. Isolation rates are higher in coastal areas. Most non-O1 non-O139 *V. cholerae* are of little public health importance.

4. **Reservoir**—Non-O1/non-O139 *V. cholerae* are found in aquatic environments worldwide, particularly in mildly brackish waters where they constitute indigenous flora. Although halophilic, they can also proliferate in fresh water (e.g. lakes). Vibrio counts vary with season and peak in warm seasons. In brackish waters they are found adherent to chitinous zooplankton and shellfish. Isolates of *V.cholerae* other than O1 and O139 are able to survive and multiply in a variety of foodstuffs.

5. Mode of transmission—Cases of non-O1/non-O139 gastroenteritis are usually linked to consumption of raw or undercooked seafood, particularly shellfish. In tropical endemic areas, some infections may be due to ingestion of surface waters. Wound infections arise from environmental exposure, usually to brackish water or from occupational accidents among fishermen, shellfish harvesters, etc. In high-risk hosts septicemia may result from a wound infection or from ingestion of contaminated seafood.

6. Incubation period—Short, 12–24 hours in outbreaks and an average of 10 hours in experimental challenge of volunteers (range 5.5–96 hours).

7. Period of communicability—It is not known whether in nature these infections can be transmitted from person to person or by humans contaminating food vehicles. If the latter indeed occurs, the period of potential communicability would likely be limited to the period of vibrio excretion, usually several days.

8. Susceptibility—All humans are believed to be susceptible to gastroenteritis if they ingest a sufficient number of non-O1/non-O139 *V. cholerae* in an appropriate food vehicle or to develop a wound infection if the wound is exposed to vibrio-containing water or shellfish. Septicaemia develops only in hosts such as those who are immunocompromised, have chronic liver disease or severe malnutrition.

9. Methods of control—

    A. Preventive measures:

        1) Educate consumers about the risks associated with eating raw seafood unless it has been irradiated or well cooked for 15 minutes at 70°C/158°F

        2) Educate seafood handlers and processors on the following preventive measures:

            a) Ensure that cooked seafood reaches temperatures adequate to kill the organism by heating for 15 minutes at 70°C/158°F (organisms may survive at 60°C/140°F for up to 15 minutes and at 80°C/176°F for several minutes).

            b) Handle cooked seafood in a manner that precludes contamination from raw seafood or contaminated seawater.

            c) Keep all seafood, raw and cooked, adequately refrigerated before eating.

            d) Avoid use of seawater in food handling areas, e.g. on cruise ships.

B., C. and **D. Control of patient, contacts and immediate environment; Epidemic measures** and **Disaster implications:** See Staphylococcal food intoxication (section I, 9B except for B2, 9C and 9D). Isolation: Enteric precautions.

Patients with liver disease or who are immunosuppressed (because of treatment or underlying disease) and alcoholics should be warned not to eat raw seafood. When disease occurs in these individuals, a history of eating seafood and especially the presence of bullous skin lesions justify early institution of antibioherapy, with a combination of oral minocycline (100 mg every 12 h) and intravenous cefotaxime (2 grams every 8 h) as the treatment regimen of choice. Tetracyclines and ciprofloxacin are also effective.

III. *VIBRIO PARAHAEMOLYTICUS* ENTERITIS   ICD-9 005.4; ICD-10 A05.3
(*Vibrio parahaemolyticus* infection)

1. Identification—An intestinal disorder characterized by watery diarrhoea and abdominal cramps in nearly all cases, usually with nausea, vomiting, fever and headache. About one quarter of patients experience a dysentery-like illness with bloody or mucoid stools, high fever and high WBC count. Typically, it is a disease of moderate severity lasting 1–7 days; systemic infection and death rarely occur.

Diagnosis is confirmed by isolating *Vibrio parahaemolyticus* from the patient's stool on appropriate media (typically TCBS media); or identifying 10^5 or more organisms per gram of an epidemiologically incriminated food (usually seafood).

2. Infectious agent—*Vibrio parahaemolyticus*, a halophilic vibrio. Twelve different O antigen groups and approximately 60 different K antigen types have been identified. Pathogenic strains are generally (but not always) capable of producing a characteristic hemolytic reaction (the "Kanagawa phenomenon"). Newer methods use DNA gene probes for a thermostable direct hemolysin (TDH) and thermostable direct related hemolysin (TRH) in order to determine virulence.

3. Occurrence—Sporadic cases and common-source outbreaks have been reported from many parts of the world, particularly Japan, southeastern Asia and the USA. Several large foodborne outbreaks have occurred in the USA in which undercooked seafood was the food vehicle; consumption of raw or undercooked clams or oysters is often implicated in individual cases. Cases occur primarily in warm months.

4. Reservoir—Marine coastal environs are the natural habitat. During the cold season, organisms are found in marine silt; during the warm season, they are found free in coastal waters and in fish and shellfish.

5. Mode of transmission—Ingestion of raw or inadequately cooked seafood, or any food contaminated by handling raw seafood, or by rinsing with contaminated water.

6. Incubation period—Usually between 12 and 24 hours, but can range from 4 to 30 hours.

7. Period of communicability—Not normally communicable from person to person (except fecal-oral transmission).

8. Susceptibility and resistance—Most people are probably susceptible, especially in case of liver disease, decreased gastric acidity, diabetes, peptic ulcer or immunosuppression.

9. Methods of control—

A. *Preventive measures: See non toxigenic* V. *cholerae* infections; monitor shellfish and coastal waters for pathogenic V. *parahaemolyticus*.

B., C. and *D. Control of patient, contacts and immediate environment; Epidemic measures* and *Disaster implications:* See Staphylococcal food intoxication (section I, 9C and 9D). Isolation: Enteric precautions. Reporting of outbreaks mandatory in some areas.

1) Specific treatment: Rehydration as appropriate. If septicemia, effective antimicrobials (aminoglycosides, third-generation cephalosporins, fluoroquinolones, tetracycline).

IV. INFECTION WITH *VIBRIO VULNIFICUS*   ICD-9 005.8; ICD-10 A05.8

1. Identification—Infection with *Vibrio vulnificus* produces septicemia in persons with chronic liver disease, chronic alcoholism or hemochromatosis, or those who are immunosuppressed. The disease appears 12 hours to 3 days after eating raw or undercooked seafood, especially oysters. One-third of patients are in shock when they present for care or develop hypotension within 12 hours after hospital admission. Three-quarters of patients have distinctive bullous skin lesions; thrombocytopenia is common and there is often evidence of disseminated intravascular coagulation. Over 50% of patients with primary septicemia die; the case-fatality rate exceeds 90% among those who become hypotensive. *V. vulnificus* can also infect wounds sustained in coastal or estuarine waters; wounds range from mild, self-limited lesions to rapidly progressive cellulitis and myositis that can mimic clostridial myonecrosis in the rapidity of spread and destructiveness.

2. Infectious agent—A halophilic, usually lactose-positive (85% of isolates) marine Vibrio that is biochemically quite similar to *V. parahae-*

molyticus. Confirmation of species identity sometimes requires use of DNA probes or numerical taxonomy in a reference laboratory. *V. vulnificus* expresses a polysaccharide capsule, of which there are multiple antigenic types on its surface.

3. Occurrence—*V. vulnificus* is the most common agent of serious infections caused by the genus Vibrio in the USA. In coastal areas the annual incidence of *V. vulnificus* disease is about 0.5 cases per 100 000 population; approximately two-thirds of these cases are primary septicemia. *V. vulnificus* infection has been reported from many areas of the world (e.g. Israel, Japan, the Republic of Korea, Spain, Taiwan (China) and Turkey).

4. Reservoir—*V. vulnificus* is a free-living autochthonous element of flora of estuarine environments. It is recovered from estuarine waters and from shellfish, particularly oysters. During warm summer months it can be isolated routinely from most cultured oysters.

5. Mode of transmission—Among persons at high risk, including those who are immunocompromised or have chronic liver disease, infection is acquired through ingestion of raw or undercooked seafood. In immunocompetent normal hosts, infections typically occur after exposure of wounds to estuarine water (e.g. boating accidents) or from occupational wounds (oyster shuckers, fishermen).

6. Incubation period—Usually 12 to 72 hours after eating raw or undercooked seafood.

7. Period of communicability—This is not considered to be an infection that is transmitted from person to person, either directly or via contamination of food except as described in I.5 above.

8. Susceptibility—Persons with cirrhosis, hemochromatosis and other chronic liver disease and immunocompromised hosts (from either underlying disease or medication) are at increased risk for the septicemic form of disease. For the period 1981–1992 the annual incidence of *V. vulnificus* illness among adults with liver disease in Florida (USA) who ate raw oysters was 7.2 per 100 000 versus 0.09 for adults without known liver disease.

9. Methods of control—

   A. *Preventive measures:* The same as those for prevention of non-O1/non-O139 *V. cholerae* infections.

V. INFECTION WITH OTHER VIBRIOS ICD-9 005.8; ICD-10 A05.8

Infection with certain other Vibrio species has been associated with sporadic cases of diarrheal disease and rarely with outbreaks. These include *V. cholerae* of serogroups other than O1 and O139, *V. mimicus* (some strains elaborate an enterotoxin indistinguishable from that produced by *V. cholerae* O1 and O139), *V. fluvialis*, *V. furnissii* and *V. hollisae*. Septicaemic disease in hosts with underlying liver disease, severe malnutrition or immunocompetence has, rarely, been associated with *V. hollisae*. *V. alginolyticus* and *V. damsela* have been associated with wound infections.

Vibrio species other than O1 and O139 have never been associated with large outbreaks. The clinical picture of infections with these strains is different from cholera and does not deserve reporting as such.

[C. Chaignat]

CHROMOMYCOSIS ICD-9 117.2; ICD-10 B43
(Chromoblastomycosis, Dermatitis verrucosa)

1. Identification—A chronic spreading mycosis of the skin and subcutaneous tissues, usually of a lower extremity. Progression to contiguous tissues is slow, over a period of years, with eventual large verrucous or even cauliflower-like masses and lymphatic stasis. Rarely a cause of death.

Microscopic examination of scrapings or biopsies from lesions shows characteristic large, brown, thick-walled rounded cells that divide by fission in two planes. Confirmation of the diagnosis should be made by biopsy and attempted cultures of the fungus.

2. Infectious agents—*Phialophora verrucosa*, *Fonsecaea* (*Phialophora*) *pedrosoi*, *F. compacta*, *Cladosporium carrionii*, *Rhinocladiella aquaspersa*, *Botryomyces caespitatus*, *Exophiala spinifera* and *E. jeanselmei*.

3. Occurrence—Worldwide; sporadic cases in widely scattered areas, but mainly southern USA, central America, Latin America, Caribbean islands, South Pacific islands, Africa (including Madagascar), Australia, Japan. Primarily a disease of rural barefoot agricultural workers in tropical regions, probably because of frequent penetrating wounds of feet and limbs not protected by shoes or clothing. The disease is most common in men aged 30–50 years; women are rarely infected.

4. **Reservoir**—Wood, soil and decaying vegetation.

5. **Mode of transmission**—Minor penetrating trauma, usually a sliver of contaminated wood or other material.

6. **Incubation period**—Unknown; probably months.

7. **Period of communicability**—Not transmitted from person to person.

8. **Susceptibility**—Unknown; rarity of disease and absence of laboratory acquired infections suggest that humans are relatively resistant.

9. **Methods of control**—

  A. *Preventive measures:* Protect against small puncture wounds by wearing shoes or protective clothing.

  B. *Control of patient, contacts and the immediate environment:*

    1) Report to local health authority: Official report not ordinarily justifiable, Class 5 (see Reporting).
    2) Isolation: Not applicable.
    3) Concurrent disinfection: Of discharges from lesions and articles soiled therewith.
    4) Quarantine: Not applicable.
    5) Immunization of contacts: Not applicable.
    6) Investigation of contacts and source of infection: Not indicated.
    7) Specific treatment: Oral 5-fluorocytosine or itraconazole benefit some patients. Large lesions may respond better when 5-fluorocytosine is combined with amphotericin B IV. Small lesions are sometimes cured by excision.

  C. *Epidemic measures:* Not applicable; a sporadic disease.

  D. *Disaster implications:* None.

  E. *International measures:* None.

[L. Savioli]

CLONORCHIASIS　　　　ICD-9 121.1; ICD-10 B66.1
(Chinese or oriental liver fluke disease)

1. **Identification**—A trematode disease of the bile ducts. Clinical complaints may be slight or absent in light infections; symptoms result from local irritation of bile ducts by the flukes. Loss of appetite, diarrhea and a sensation of abdominal pressure are common early symptoms.

Rarely, bile duct obstruction producing jaundice may be followed by cirrhosis, enlargement and tenderness of the liver, with progressive ascites and oedema. It is a chronic disease, sometimes of 30 years duration or longer, but rarely a direct or contributing cause of death and often completely asymptomatic. However, it is a significant risk factor for development of cholangiocarcinoma.

Diagnosis is made by finding the characteristic eggs in feces or duodenal drainage fluid, to be differentiated from those of other flukes. Serological diagnosis by ELISA can be performed, but is not always specific. "Antigenic cocktails" for serodiagnosis are under development.

2. **Infectious agent**—*Clonorchis sinensis*, the Chinese liver fluke.

3. **Occurrence**—Present throughout China (including Taiwan) except in the northwestern areas and highly endemic in southeastern China; occurs in Japan (rarely), the Republic of Korea, Viet Nam and probably in Cambodia and Lao Democratic Republic, principally in the Mekong River delta. In other parts of the world, imported cases may be recognized in immigrants from Asia. In most endemic areas highest prevalence is among adults over the age of 30.

4. **Reservoir**—Humans, cats, dogs, swine, rats and other animals.

5. **Mode of transmission**—People are infected by eating raw or undercooked freshwater fish containing encysted larvae. During digestion, larvae are freed from cysts and migrate via the common bile duct to biliary radicles. Eggs deposited in the bile passages are evacuated in feces. Eggs in feces contain fully developed miracidia; when ingested by a susceptible operculate snail (e.g. *Parafossarulus*), they hatch in its intestine, penetrate the tissues and asexually generate larvae (cercariae) that emerge into the water. On contact with a second intermediate host (about 110 species of freshwater fish belonging mostly to the family Cyprinidae), cercariae penetrate the host fish and encyst, usually in muscle, occasionally on the underside of scales. The complete life cycle, from person to snail to fish to person, requires at least 3 months.

6. **Incubation period**—Unpredictable, as it varies with the number of worms present; flukes reach maturity within 1 month after encysted larvae are ingested.

7. **Period of communicability**—Infected individuals may pass viable eggs for as long as 30 years; infection is not directly transmitted from person to person.

8. **Susceptibility and resistance**—Susceptibility is universal.

9. **Methods of control—**

A. *Preventive measures:*

1) Thoroughly cook or irradiate all freshwater fish. Freezing at -10°C (14°F) for at least 5 days; storage for several weeks in a saturated salt solution has been recommended but remains unproven.
2) In endemic areas, educate the public to the dangers of eating raw or improperly treated fish and the necessity for sanitary disposal of feces to avoid contaminating sources of food fish. Prohibit disposal of night soil and animal waste (excreta) in fishponds.

B. *Control of patient, contacts and the immediate environment:*

1) Report to local health authority: Official report not ordinarily justifiable, Class 5 (see Reporting).
2) Isolation: Not applicable.
3) Concurrent disinfection: Sanitary disposal of feces.
4) Quarantine: Not applicable.
5) Immunization of contacts: Not applicable.
6) Investigation of contacts and source of infection: Of the individual case, not usually indicated. A community problem (see C).
7) Specific treatment: The drug of choice is praziquantel. Albendazole is under investigation.

C. *Epidemic measures:* Locate source of infected fish. Shipments of dried or pickled fish are the likely source in nonendemic areas, as are fresh or chilled freshwater fish brought from endemic areas.

D. *Disaster implications:* None.

E. *International measures:* Control of fish or fish products imported from endemic areas.

OPISTHORCHIASIS ICD-9 121.0; ICD-10 B66.0

Opisthorchiasis is caused by small liver flukes of cats and some other fish eating mammals. *Opisthorchis felineus* occurs in Europe and Asia, and has infected 2 million people in the former Soviet Union; *O. viverrini* is endemic in southeastern Asia, especially Thailand, where approximately 8 million are infected. These worms are the leading cause of cholangiocarcinoma throughout the world; in northern Thailand, rates for the latter are as high as 85/10 000 population. The biology of these flatworms, the characteristics of the disease and methods of control are essentially the same as those for clonorchiasis. Eggs cannot be easily distinguished from those of *Clonorchis*.

[D. Engels]

COCCIDIOIDOMYCOSIS   ICD-9 114; ICD-10 B38
(Valley fever, San Joaquin fever, Desert fever, Desert rheumatism, Coccidioidal granuloma)

1. Identification A deep mycosis that generally begins as a respiratory infection. The primary infection may be entirely asymptomatic or resemble an acute influenzal illness with fever, chills, cough and (rarely) pleuritic pain. About 1 in 5 clinically recognized cases (an estimated 5% of all primary infections) develops erythema nodosum, most common in Caucasian females and rarest in American males of African origin. Primary infection may heal completely without detectable sequelae; may leave fibrosis, a pulmonary nodule that may or may not have calcified areas; may leave a persistent thin-walled cavity; or most rarely, may progress to the disseminated form of the disease.

An estimated 1 out of every 1000 cases of symptomatic coccidioidomycosis becomes disseminated. Disseminated coccidioidomycosis is a progressive, uncommon, frequently fatal granulomatous disease characterized by lung lesions and abscesses throughout the body, especially in subcutaneous tissues, skin, bone and the CNS. Coccidioidal meningitis resembles tuberculous meningitis but runs a more chronic course.

Diagnosis is made through demonstration of fungus on microscopic examination or through culture of sputum, pus, urine, CSF or biopsies of skin lesions or organs. Handling cultures of the mould form is extremely hazardous and must be carried out in a BSL-2 or BSL-3 facility. A positive skin test to spherulin appears from 2–3 days to 3 weeks after onset of symptoms. Precipitin and CF tests are usually positive within the first 3 months of clinical disease. The precipitin test detects IgM antibody, which appears 1–2 weeks after symptoms appear and persists for 3–4 months. Complement fixation tests detect mostly IgG antibody, which appears 1–2 months after clinical symptoms start and persists for 6–8 months. Serial skin and serological tests may be necessary to confirm a recent infection or indicate dissemination; skin tests are often negative in disseminated disease, and serological tests may be negative in the immunocompromised.

2. Infectious agent—*Coccidioides immitis*, a dimorphic fungus. It grows in soil and culture media as a saprophytic mould that reproduces by arthroconidia; in tissues and under special conditions, the parasitic form grows as spherical cells (spherules) that reproduce by endospore formation.

3. Occurrence—Primary infections are common only in arid and semi-arid areas of the Western Hemisphere: the USA from California to southern Texas; northern Argentina, Brazil (Nordeste), Colombia, Mexico, Paraguay, Venezuela and central America. Elsewhere, dusty fomites from endemic areas can transmit infection; disease has occurred in people who have merely travelled through endemic areas. The disease affects all ages and all races. More than half the patients with symptomatic infection are between 15 and 25; men are affected more frequently than women, probably because of occupational exposure. Infection is most frequent in summers following a rainy winter or spring, especially after wind and dust storms. It is an important disease among migrant workers, archaeologists and military personnel from nonendemic areas who move into endemic areas. Since 1991, a marked increase of coccidioidomycosis has been reported in California.

4. Reservoir—Soil; especially in and around Indian middens and rodent burrows, in regions with appropriate temperature, moisture and soil requirements; infects humans, cattle, cats, dogs, horses, burros, sheep, swine, wild desert rodents, coyotes, chinchillas, llamas and other animal species.

5. Mode of transmission—Inhalation of infective arthroconidia from soil and in laboratory accidents from cultures. While the parasitic form is normally not infective, accidental inoculation of infected pus or culture suspension into the skin or bone can result in granuloma formation.

6. Incubation period—In primary infection, 1 to 4 weeks. Dissemination may develop insidiously years after the primary infection, sometimes without recognized symptoms of primary pulmonary infection.

7. Period of communicability—No direct person-to-person or animal-to-human transmission. *C. immitis* on casts and dressings may rarely change from the parasitic to the infective saprophytic form after 7 days.

8. Susceptibility—Frequency of subclinical infection is indicated by the high prevalence of positive coccidioidin or spherulin reactors in endemic areas; recovery is generally followed by solid, lifelong immunity. Reactivation can occur in those who become immunosuppressed therapeutically or through HIV infection. Susceptibility to dissemination is greater in Americans of African origin, Asians, pregnant women and those with AIDS or other types of immunosuppression. Sporadic coccidioidal meningitis cases occur more commonly among Caucasian males.

9. **Methods of control—**

A. *Preventive measures:*

1) In endemic areas: Planting grass, oiling unpaved airfields, and other dust control measures (including facemasks, air-conditioned cabs and wetted soil).
2) Individuals from nonendemic areas should preferably not be recruited to dusty occupations, such as road building. Skin testing could be used to screen out those susceptible.

B. *Control of patient, contacts and the immediate environment:*

1) Report to local health authority: Case report of recognized cases, especially outbreaks, in selected endemic areas; in many countries, not a reportable disease, Class 3 (see Reporting).
2) Isolation: Not applicable.
3) Concurrent disinfection: Discharges and soiled articles must be disinfected. Terminal cleaning.
4) Quarantine: Not applicable.
5) Immunization of contacts: Not applicable.
6) Investigation of contacts and source of infection: Not recommended except in cases appearing in nonendemic areas, where residence, work exposure and travel history should be obtained.
7) Specific treatment: Primary coccidioidomycosis usually resolves spontaneously without therapy. Amphotericin B IV is beneficial in severe infections. Fluconazole is currently the agent of choice for meningeal infection. Ketoconazole and itraconazole have been useful in chronic, nonmeningeal coccidioidomycosis.

C. *Epidemic measures:* Outbreaks occur when groups of susceptibles are infected by airborne conidia. Institute dust control measures where feasible (see 9A1).

D. *Disaster implications:* Possible hazard if large groups of susceptibles are forced to move through or to live under dusty conditions in areas where the fungus is prevalent.

E. *International measures:* None.

F. *Measures in case of deliberate use:* C. immitis arthrospores have potential use as a weapon. See Anthrax, section F, for general measures to be taken when confronted with a threat such as that posed by C. immitis arthrospores.

[L. Severo]

CONJUNCTIVITIS/KERATITIS ICD-9 372.0-372.3, 370; ICD-10 H10, H16

I. ACUTE BACTERIAL
CONJUNCTIVITIS ICD-9 372.0; ICD-10 H10.0-H10.3
(Pinkeye, "Sticky eye", Brazilian purpuric fever [ICD-10 A48.4])

1. Identification—A clinical syndrome beginning with lacrimation, irritation and hyperaemia of the palpebral and bulbar conjunctivae of one or both eyes, followed by oedema of eyelids and mucopurulent discharge. In severe cases, ecchymoses of the bulbar conjunctiva and marginal infiltration of the cornea with mild photophobia may occur. Nonfatal (except as noted below), the disease may last from 2 days to 2–3 weeks; many patients have no more than hyperaemia of the conjunctivae and slight exudate for a few days.

Confirmation of clinical diagnosis through microscopic examination of a stained smear or culture of the discharge is required to differentiate bacterial from viral or allergic conjunctivitis, or adenovirus/enterovirus infection. Inclusion conjunctivitis (see below), trachoma and gonococcal conjunctivitis are described separately.

2. Infectious agents—*Haemophilus influenzae* biogroup *aegyptius* (Koch-Weeks bacillus) and *Streptococcus pneumoniae* appear to be the most important; *H. influenzae* type b, *Moraxella* and *Branhamella* spp., *Neisseria meningitidis* and *Corynebacterium diphtheriae* may also produce the disease. *H. influenzae* biogroup *aegyptius*, gonococci (see Gonoccocal infections), *S. pneumoniae*, *S. viridans*, various Gram-negative enteric bacilli and, rarely, *Pseudomonas aeruginosa* may produce the disease in newborn infants.

3. Occurrence—Widespread and common worldwide, particularly in warmer climates; frequently epidemic. In North America, infection with *H. influenzae* biogroup *aegyptius* is confined largely to southern rural areas from Georgia to California, primarily during summer and early autumn; in North Africa and the Middle East, infections occur as seasonal epidemics. Infection due to other organisms occurs throughout the world, often associated with acute viral respiratory disease during cold seasons. Occasional cases of systemic disease have occurred among children in several communities in Brazil, 1–3 weeks after conjunctivitis due to a unique invasive clone of *Haemophilus influenzae* biogroup *aegyptius*. This severe Brazilian purpuric fever (BPF), had a 70% case-fatality rate among more than 100 cases recognized over a wide area of Brazil including 4 states; it may be clinically indistinguishable from meningococcaemia. The causal agent has been isolated from conjunctival, pharyngeal and blood cultures. The disease has been restricted essentially to Brazil; 2 cases in Australia were similar clinically, but the organism differed from the Brazilian strain.

4. Reservoir—Humans. Carriers of *H. influenzae* biogroup *aegyptius* and *S. pneumoniae* are common in many areas during interepidemic periods.

5. Mode of transmission—Contact with discharges from conjunctivae or upper respiratory tracts of infected people; contaminated fingers, clothing and other articles, including shared eye makeup applicators, multiple dose eye medications and inadequately sterilized instruments such as tonometers. Eye gnats or flies may transmit the organisms mechanically in some areas, but their importance as vectors is undetermined and probably differs from area to area.

6. Incubation period—Usually 24–72 hours.

7. Period of communicability—During the course of active infection.

8. Susceptibility—Children under 5 are most often affected; incidence decreases with age. The very young, the debilitated and the aged are particularly susceptible to staphylococcal infections. Immunity after attack is low grade and varies with the infectious agent.

9. Methods of control—

A. *Preventive measures:* Personal hygiene, hygienic care and treatment of affected eyes.

B. *Control of patient, contacts and the immediate environment:*

1) Report to local health authority: Obligatory report of epidemics; no case report for classic disease, Class 4; for systemic disease, Class 2 (see Reporting).
2) Isolation: Drainage and secretion precautions. Children should not attend school during the acute stage.
3) Concurrent disinfection: Of discharges and soiled articles. Terminal cleaning.
4) Quarantine: Not applicable.
5) Immmunization of contacts: Not applicable.
6) Investigation of contacts and source of infection: Usually not beneficial for conjunctivitis; but must be undertaken for Brazilian purpuric fever.
7) Specific treatment: Local application of an ointment or drops containing a sulfonamide such as sodium sulfacetamide, gentamicin or combination antibiotics such as polymyxin B

with neomycin or trimethoprim is generally effective. For BPF, systemic treatment is required; isolates are sensitive to both ampicillin and chloramphenicol and resistant to tri-methoprim-sufamethoxazole. Oral rifampicin (20 mg/kg/day for 2 days) may be more effective than local chloramphenicol in eradication of the causal clone and may be useful in prevention among children with Brazilian purpuric fever clone conjunctivitis. (See Gonococcal conjunctivitis, 9B7.)

C. Epidemic measures:

1) Prompt and adequate treatment of patients and their close contacts.
2) In areas where insects are suspected of mechanically trans-mitting infection, measures to prevent access of eye gnats or flies to eyes of sick and well people.
3) Insect control, according to the suspected vector.

D. Disaster implications: None.

E. International measures: None.

II. KERATOCONJUNCTIVITIS, ADENOVIRAL ICD-9 077.1; ICD-10 B30.0
(Epidemic keratoconjunctivitis [EKC], Shipyard conjunctivitis, Shipyard eye)

1. **Identification**—An acute viral disease of the eye, with unilateral or bilateral inflammation of conjunctivae and oedema of the lids and perior-bital tissue. Onset is sudden with pain, photophobia, blurred vision and occasionally low-grade fever, headache, malaise and tender preauricular lymphadenopathy. Approximately 7 days after onset in about half the cases, the cornea exhibits several small round subepithelial infiltrates; these may eventually form punctate erosions that stain with fluorescein. Duration of acute conjunctivitis is about 2 weeks; it may continue to evolve, leaving discrete subepithelial opacities that may interfere with vision for a few weeks. In severe cases permanent scarring may result.

Diagnosis is confirmed by recovery of virus from appropriate cell cultures inoculated with eye swabs or conjunctival scrapings; virus may be visualized through FA staining of scrapings or through IEM; viral antigen may be detected by ELISA testing. Serum neutralization or HAI tests may identify type-specific titre rises.

2. **Infectious agents**—Typically, adenovirus types 8, 19 and 37 are responsible, though other adenovirus types have been involved. Most severe disease has been found in infections caused by types 8, 5 and 19.

3. Occurrence—Presumably worldwide. Both sporadic cases and large outbreaks have occurred in Asia, Europe, Hawaii and North America.

4. Reservoir—Humans.

5. Mode of transmission—Direct contact with eye secretions of an infected person and, indirectly, through contaminated surfaces, instruments or solutions. In industrial plants, epidemics are centered in first-aid stations and dispensaries where treatment is frequently administered for minor trauma to the eye; transmission occurs through fingers, instruments and other contaminated items. Similar outbreaks have originated in eye clinics and medical offices. Dispensary and clinic personnel acquiring the disease may act as sources of infection. Family spread is common, with children typically introducing the infection.

6. Incubation period—Between 5 and 12 days, but in many instances this duration is exceeded.

7. Period of communicability—From late in the incubation period to 14 days after onset. Prolonged viral shedding has been reported.

8. Susceptibility—There is usually complete type-specific immunity after adenoviral infections. Trauma, even minor, and eye manipulation increase the risk of infection.

9. Methods of control—

  A. Preventive measures:

  1) Educate patients about personal cleanliness and the risk associated with use of common towels and toilet articles. Educate patients to minimize hand-to-eye contact.
  2) Avoid shared use of eyedroppers, medicines, eye makeup, instruments or towels.
  3) During ophthalmological procedures in dispensaries, clinics and offices, asepsis should include vigorous handwashing before examining each patient and systematic sterilization of instruments after use; high-level disinfection is recommended for instruments that will be in contact with the conjunctivae or eyelids. Gloves should be worn for examining eyes of patients with possible or confirmed epidemic keratoconjunctivitis. Any ophthalmic medicines or droppers that have come in contact with eyelids or conjunctivae must be discarded. Medical personnel with overt conjunctivitis should not have physical contact with patients.
  4) With persistent outbreaks, patients with epidemic keratoconjunctivitis should be seen in physically separate facilities.
  5) Use safety measures such as goggles in industrial plants.

B. *Control of patient, contacts and the immediate environment:*

1) Report to local health authority: Obligatory report of epidemics in some countries; no individual case report, Class 4 (see Reporting).

2) Isolation: Drainage and secretion precautions; patients must use separate towels and linens during the acute stage. Infected medical personnel or patients should not come in contact with uninfected patients.

3) Concurrent disinfection: Of conjunctival and nasal discharges and articles soiled therewith. Terminal cleaning.

4) Quarantine: Not applicable.

5) Immmunization of contacts: Not applicable.

6) Investigation of contacts and source of infection: In outbreaks, the source of infection should be identified and precautions taken to prevent further transmission.

7) Specific treatment: None during the acute phase. If residual opacities interfere with the patient's ability to work, topical corticosteroids may be administered by a qualified ophthalmologist.

C. *Epidemic measures:*

1) Strictly apply recommendations in 9A.

2) Organize convenient facilities for prompt diagnosis, with no or minimal contact between infected and uninfected individuals.

D. *Disaster implications:* None.

E. *International measures:* WHO Collaborating Centres.

III. ADENOVIRAL HEMORRHAGIC
CONJUNCTIVITIS ICD-9 077.2; ICD-10 B30.1
(Pharyngoconjunctival fever)
ENTEROVIRAL HEMORRHAGIC
CONJUNCTIVITIS ICD-9 077.4; ICD-10 B30.3
(Apollo 11 disease, Acute hemorrhagic conjunctivitis)

1. Identification—In adenoviral conjunctivitis, lymphoid follicles usually develop, the conjunctivitis lasts 7–15 days and there are frequently small subconjunctival hemorrhages. In one adenoviral syndrome, pharyngoconjunctival fever, there is upper respiratory disease and fever with minor degrees of corneal epithelial inflammation (epithelial keratitis).

In enteroviral acute hemorrhagic conjunctivitis (AHC), onset is sudden with redness, swelling and pain often in both eyes; the course of the inflammatory disease is 4–6 days, during which subconjunctival hemorrhages appear on the bulbar conjunctiva as petechiae that enlarge to form confluent subconjunctival hemorrhages. Large hemorrhages gradually resolve over 7-12 days. In major outbreaks of enteroviral origin, there has been a low incidence of a polio-like paralysis, including cranial nerve palsies, lumbosacral radiculomyelitis and lower motor neuron paralysis. Neurological complications start a few days to a month after conjunctivitis and often leave residual weakness.

Laboratory confirmation of adenovirus infections is through isolation of the virus from conjunctival swabs in cell culture, rising antibody titres, detection of viral antigens through IF or identification of viral nucleic acid with a DNA probe. Enterovirus infection is diagnosed by isolation of the agent, immunofluorescence, demonstration of a rising antibody titre or PCR

2. Infectious agents—Adenoviruses and picornaviruses. Most adeno-viruses can cause PCF, but types 3, 4 and 7 are the most common causes.

The most prevalent picornavirus type has been designated as enterovi-rus 70; this and a variant of coxsackievirus A24 have caused large outbreaks of AHC.

3. Occurrence—PCF occurs during outbreaks of adenovirus associ-ated respiratory disease or as summer epidemics associated with swim-ming pools. Adenoviral hemorrhagic conjuctivitis was first recognized in Ghana in 1969 and Indonesia in 1970; numerous epidemics have occurred since then in tropical areas of Asia, Africa, Central and South America, the Caribbean, the Pacific islands and parts of Florida and Mexico. An outbreak in American Samoa in 1986 due to coxsackievirus A24 variant affected an estimated 48% of the population. Smaller outbreaks have occurred in Europe, usually associated with eye clinics. Cases have also occurred among southeastern Asian refugees in the USA and travellers returning to the USA from affected areas.

4. Reservoir—Humans.

5. Mode of transmission—Direct or indirect contact with discharge from infected eyes. Person-to-person transmission is most noticeable in families, where high attack rates often occur. Adenovirus can be transmit-ted in poorly chlorinated swimming pools and has been reported as "swimming pool conjunctivitis"; it is also transmitted through respiratory droplets. Large AHC epidemics are often associated with overcrowding and low hygienic standards. Schoolchildren have been implicated in the rapid dissemination of AHC throughout a community.

6. Incubation period—For adenovirus infection, 4-12 days with an average of 8 days. For picornavirus infection, 12 hours to 3 days.

7. Period of communicability—Adenovirus infections may be com-municable up to 14 days after onset, picornavirus at least 4 days after onset.

8. Susceptibility—Infection can occur at all ages. Reinfections and/or relapses have been reported. The role and duration of the immune response are not yet clear.

9. Methods of control—

A. *Preventive measures:* No effective treatment; prevention is critical. Personal hygiene should be emphasized, including use of non-shared towels and avoidance of overcrowding. Maintain strict asepsis in eye clinics; wash hands before examining each patient. Eye clinics must ensure high level disinfection of potentially contaminated equipment. Adequate chlorination of swimming pools. Closing schools may be necessary.

B. *Control of patient, contacts and the immediate environment:*

1) Report to local health authority: Obligatory report of epidemics; no case report, Class 4 (see Reporting).
2) Isolation: Drainage and secretion precautions; restrict contact with cases while disease is active; e.g. children should not attend school.
3) Concurrent disinfection: Of conjunctival discharges and articles and equipment soiled therewith. Terminal cleaning.
4) Quarantine: Not applicable.
5) Immmunization of contacts: Not applicable.
6) Investigation of contacts and source of infection: Locate other cases to determine whether a common source of infection is involved.
7) Specific treatment: None.

C. *Epidemic measures:*

1) Organize adequate facilities for the diagnosis and symptomatic treatment of cases.
2) Improve standards of hygiene and limit overcrowding wherever possible.

D. *Disaster implications:* None.

E. *International measures:* WHO Collaborating Centres.

IV. CHLAMYDIAL CONJUNCTIVITIS   ICD-9 077.0; ICD-10 A74.0
(Inclusion conjunctivitis, Paratrachoma, Neonatal inclusion blennorrhoea, "Sticky eye")
(See separate chapter for Trachoma.)

1. Identification—In the newborn, an acute conjunctivitis with purulent discharge, usually recognized within 5–12 days after birth. The acute stage usually subsides spontaneously in a few weeks; inflammation of the eye may persist for more than a year if untreated, with mild scarring of the conjunctivae and infiltration of the cornea (micropannus). Chlamydial pneumonia (see Pneumonia, chlamydial) occurs in some infants with concurrent nasopharyngeal infection. Gonococcal infection must be ruled out.

In children and adults, an acute follicular conjunctivitis is seen typically with preauricular lymphadenopathy on the involved side, hyperaemia, infiltration and a slight mucopurulent discharge, often with superficial corneal involvement. In adults, there may be a chronic phase with scant discharge and symptoms that sometimes persist for more than a year if untreated. The agent may cause symptomatic infection of the urethral epithelium in men and women and the cervix in women, with or without associated conjunctivitis.

Laboratory methods to assist diagnosis include isolation in cell culture, antigen detection using IF staining of direct smears, EIA methods, DNA probe.

2. **Infectious agents**—*Chlamydia trachomatis* of serovars D through K. Feline strains of *C. psittaci* have caused acute follicular keratoconjunctivitis in humans.

3. **Occurrence**—Sporadic cases of conjunctivitis are reported worldwide among sexually active adults. Neonatal conjunctivitis due to *C. trachomatis* is common and occurs in 15%–35% of newborns exposed to maternal infection. Among adults with genital chlamydial infection, 1 in 300 develops chlamydial eye disease.

4. **Reservoir**—Humans for *C. trachomatis*, cats for *C. psittaci*.

5. **Mode of transmission**—Generally transmitted during sexual intercourse; the genital discharges of infected people are infectious. In the newborn, conjunctivitis is usually acquired by direct contact with infectious secretions during transit through the birth canal. In utero infection may also occur. The eyes of adults become infected by the transmission of genital secretions to the eye, usually by the fingers. Older children may acquire conjunctivitis from infected newborns or other household members; they should be assessed for sexual abuse as appropriate. Outbreaks reported among swimmers in nonchlorinated pools have not been confirmed by culture and may be due to adenoviruses or other known causes of "swimming pool conjunctivitis."

6. **Incubation period**—In newborns, 5–12 days, ranging from 3 days to 6 weeks; adults 6–19 days.

7. **Period of communicability**—While genital or ocular infection persists; carriage on mucous membranes has been observed as long as 2 years after birth.

8. **Susceptibility**—There is no evidence of resistance to reinfection, although the severity of the disease may be decreased.

9. **Methods of control—**

   A. *Preventive measures:*

   1) Correct and consistent use of condoms to prevent sexual transmission; prompt treatment of persons with chlamydial urethritis and cervicitis.
   2) General preventive measures as for other STIs (see Syphilis, 9A).
   3) Identification of infection in high-risk pregnant women, by culture or antigen detection. Treatment of cervical infection in pregnant women will prevent subsequent transmission to the infant. Erythromycin base, 500 mg 4 times daily for 7 days, is usually effective, but frequent GI side-effects interfere with compliance. Evaluation and treatment of sexual partners should also be undertaken.
   4) Routine prophylaxis for gonococcal ophthalmia neonatorum is effective against chlamydial infection and should be practised. The method of choice is either a single application into the eyes of the newborn of povidone-iodine (2.5% solution), tetracycline 1% eye ointment, erythromycin 0.5% eye ointment or silver nitrate eye drops (1%) within 1 hour after delivery. All methods give comparable results in preventing gonococcal conjunctivitis; in field studies povidone-iodine was significantly more effective in preventing neonatal eye infections. Ocular prophylaxis does not prevent nasopharyngeal colonization and risk of subsequent chlamydial pneumonia. Penicillin is ineffective against chlamydiae.

   B. *Control of patient, contacts and the immediate environment:*

   1) Report to local health authority: Case report of neonatal cases obligatory in many countries, Class 2 (see Reporting).
   2) Isolation: Drainage and secretion precautions for the first 96 hours after starting treatment.
   3) Concurrent disinfection: Aseptic techniques and handwashing by personnel appear to be adequate to prevent nursery transmission.
   4) Quarantine: Not applicable.
   5) Immunization of contacts: Not applicable.
   6) Investigation of contacts and source of infection: All sexual contacts of adult cases, and mothers and fathers of neonatally infected infants should be examined and treated. Infected adults should be investigated for evidence of ongoing infection with gonorrhoea or syphilis.
   7) Specific treatment: For ocular and genital infections of adults, a tetracycline, erythromycin or ofloxacin is effective when

given by mouth for 2 weeks. Azithromycin is an effective single dose therapy.

Oral treatment of neonatal ocular infections with erythromycin for 2 weeks is recommended to eliminate the risk of chlamydial pneumonia as well; the dose is 10 mg/kg, given every 12 hours during the first week of life and every 8 hours thereafter.

C. Epidemic measures: Sanitary control of swimming pools; ordinary chlorination suffices.

D. Disaster implications: None.

E. International measures: WHO Collaborating Centres.

[S. Resnikoff]

COXSACKIEVIRUS DISEASES ICD-9 074; ICD-10 B34.1

The coxsackieviruses, members of the enterovirus group of the family Picornaviridae, are the causal agents of a group of diseases discussed here, as well as epidemic myalgia, enteroviral hemorrhagic conjunctivitis and meningitis (see under individual disease listings) and coxsackievirus carditis (see below). They cause disseminated disease in newborns; there is evidence suggesting their involvement in the etiology of juvenile onset insulin-dependent diabetes.

I.A. ENTEROVIRAL VESICULAR PHARYNGITIS ICD-9 074.0; ICD-10 B08.5
(Herpangina, Aphthous pharyngitis)

I.B. ENTEROVIRAL VESICULAR STOMATITIS WITH EXANTHEM ICD-9 074.3; ICD-10 B08.4
(Hand, foot and mouth disease)

I.C. ENTEROVIRAL LYMPHONODULAR PHARYNGITIS ICD-9 074.8; ICD-10 B08.8
(Acute lymphonodular pharyngitis, Vesicular pharyngitis)

1. Identification—Vesicular pharyngitis (herpangina) is an acute, self-limited, viral disease characterized by sudden onset, fever, sore throat and small (1-2 mm), discrete, greyish papulovesicular pharyngeal lesions on an erythematous base, gradually progressing to slightly larger ulcers. These lesions usually occur on the anterior pillars of the tonsillar fauces, soft palate, uvula and tonsils, and may persist 4-6 days after the onset of illness. No fatalities have been reported. In one series, febrile convulsions occurred in 5% of cases.

Vesicular stomatitis with exanthem (hand, foot and mouth disease) differs from vesicular pharyngitis in that oral lesions are more diffuse and may occur on the buccal surfaces of the cheeks and gums and on the sides of the tongue. Papulovesicular lesions, which may persist from 7 to 10 days, also occur commonly as an exanthem, especially on the palms, fingers and soles; maculopapular lesions occasionally appear on the buttocks. Although the disease is usually self-limited, rare cases have been fatal in infants.

Acute lymphonodular pharyngitis also differs from vesicular pharyngitis in that the lesions are firm, raised, discrete, whitish to yellowish nodules, surrounded by a 3-6 mm zone of erythema. They occur predominantly on the uvula, anterior tonsillar pillars and posterior pharynx, with no exanthem.

Stomatitis due to herpes simplex virus requires differentiation; it has larger, deeper, more painful ulcerative lesions, commonly located in the front part of the mouth. These diseases are not to be confused with vesicular stomatitis caused by the vesicular stomatitis virus, normally of cattle and horses, which in humans usually occurs among dairy workers, animal husbandrymen and veterinarians. Foot-and-mouth disease of cattle, sheep and swine rarely affects laboratory workers handling the virus; however, humans can be a mechanical carrier of the virus and the source of animal outbreaks. A virus not serologically differentiable from coxsackievirus B-5 causes vesicular disease in swine, which may be transmitted to humans.

Differentiation of the related but distinct coxsackievirus syndromes is facilitated during epidemics. Virus may be isolated from lesions and nasopharyngeal and stool specimens through cell cultures and/or inoculation to suckling mice. Since many serotypes may produce the same syndrome and common antigens are lacking, serological diagnostic procedures are not routinely available unless the virus is isolated for use in the serological tests.

2. Infectious agents—For vesicular pharyngitis, coxsackievirus, group A, types 1-10, 16 and 22. For vesicular stomatitis with or without exanthem (hand, foot and mouth disease), coxsackievirus, group A, type A16 predominantly and types 4, 5, 9 and 10; group B, types 2 and 5; and (less often) enterovirus 71. For acute lymphonodular pharyngitis, coxsackievirus, group A, type 10. Other enteroviruses have occasionally been associated with these diseases.

3. Occurrence—Probably worldwide for vesicular pharyngitis and vesicular stomatitis, both sporadically and in epidemics; maximal incidence in summer and early autumn; mainly in children under 10, but adult cases (especially young adults) are not unusual. Isolated outbreaks of acute lymphonodular pharyngitis, predominantly in children, may occur in summer and early autumn. These diseases frequently occur in outbreaks among groups of children (e.g. in nursery schools, childcare centers).

4. Reservoir—Humans.

5. Mode of transmission—Direct contact with nose and throat discharges and feces of infected people (who may be asymptomatic) and by aerosol droplet spread; no reliable evidence of spread by insects, water, food or sewage.

6. Incubation period—Usually 3–5 days for vesicular pharyngitis and vesicular stomatitis; 5 days for acute lymphonodular pharyngitis.

7. Period of communicability—During the acute stage of illness and perhaps longer, since viruses persist in stool for several weeks.

8. Susceptibility—Susceptibility to infection is universal. Immunity to the specific virus is probably acquired through clinical or inapparent infection; duration unknown. Second attacks may occur with group A coxsackievirus of a different serological type.

9. Methods of control—

　　A. Preventive measures: Limit person-to-person contact, where practicable, by measures such as crowd reduction and ventilation. Promote handwashing and other hygienic measures in the home.

　　B. Control of patient, contacts and the immediate environment:

　　　　1) Report to local health authority: Obligatory report of epidemics in some countries; no case report, Class 4 (see Reporting).
　　　　2) Isolation: Enteric precautions.
　　　　3) Concurrent disinfection: Of nose and throat discharges. Wash or discard articles soiled therewith. Give careful attention to prompt handwashing when handling discharges, feces and articles soiled therewith.
　　　　4) Quarantine: Not applicable.
　　　　5) Immmunization of contacts: Not applicable.
　　　　6) Investigation of contacts and source of infection: Of no practical value except to detect other cases in groups of preschool children.
　　　　7) Specific treatment: None.

　　C. Epidemic measures: Give general notice to physicians of increased incidence of the disease, together with a description of onset and clinical characteristics. Isolate diagnosed cases and all children with fever, pending diagnosis, with special attention to respiratory secretions and feces.

D. Disaster implications: none.

E. International measures: WHO Collaborating Centres.

[D. Lavanchy]

II. COXSACKIEVIRUS
   CARDITIS   ICD-9 074.2; ICD-10 B33.2
(Viral carditis, Enteroviral carditis)

1. Identification—An acute or subacute viral myocarditis or pericarditis occurring (occasionally with other manifestations) as a manifestation of infection with enteroviruses, especially group B coxsackievirus.

The myocardium is affected, particularly in neonates, in whom fever and lethargy may be followed rapidly by heart failure with pallor, cyanosis, dyspnoea, tachycardia and enlargement of heart and liver. Heart failure may be progressive and fatal, or recovery may take place over a few weeks; some cases run a relapsing course over months and may show residual heart damage. In young adults, pericarditis is the more common manifestation, with acute chest pain, disturbance of heart rate, and often dyspnoea. It may mimic myocardial infarction but is frequently associated with pulmonary or pleural manifestations (pleurodynia). The disease may be associated with aseptic meningitis, hepatitis, orchitis, pancreatitis, pneumonia, hand, foot and mouth disease, rash or epidemic myalgia (see Myalgia, epidemic).

Serological studies or virus isolation from feces usually help diagnosis, but such results are inconclusive; a significant rise in specific antibody titres is diagnostic. Virus is rarely isolated from pericardial fluid, myocardial biopsy or postmortem heart tissue; such an isolation provides a definitive diagnosis.

2. Infectious agents—Group B coxsackievirus (types 1-5); occasionally group A coxsackievirus (types 1, 4, 9, 16, 23) and other enteroviruses.

3. Occurrence—An uncommon disease, mainly sporadic, but increased during epidemics of group B coxsackievirus infection. Institutional outbreaks, with high case-fatality rates in newborns, have been described in maternity units.

4., 5., 6., 7., 8. and **9. Reservoir—Mode of transmission, Incubation period, Period of communicability, Susceptibility** and **Methods of control**—See Epidemic myalgia.

[D. Lavanchy]

CRYPTOCOCCOSIS   ICD-9 117.5; ICD-10 B45
(Torula)

1. Identification—Infection with *Cryptococcus* starts through inhalation into the lungs, but tends to hematogenic spread to the brain, usually presenting as a subacute or chronic meningitis; infection of lungs, kidneys, prostate and bone may occur. The skin may show acneiform lesions, ulcers or subcutaneous tumour-like masses. Occasionally, the causal agent *Cryptococcus neoformans* may act as an endobronchial saprophyte in patients with other lung diseases. Untreated meningitis terminates fatally within weeks to months.

Diagnosis of cryptococcal meningitis is aided by the evidence of encapsulated budding forms on microscopic examination of CSF mixed with India ink; urine or pus may also contain these forms. Tests for antigen in serum and CSF are often helpful. Diagnosis is confirmed through histopathology or culture (media containing cycloheximide inhibit the agent and should not be used) Mayer mucicarmine stains most cryptococci in tissue deep red, aiding histopathological diagnosis.

2. Infectious agents—*Cryptococcus neoformans* var. *neoformans* and var. *grubii* and *C. bacillusporus* (= *C. neoformans* var. *gattii*) the latter more frequent in tropical or subtropical climates. The perfect (sexual) states of these fungi are called *Filobasidiella neoformans* and *F. bacillispora*; Fontana-Masson stain for melanin is useful to identify capsule-deficient *Cryptococci*.

3. Occurrence—Sporadic cases occur worldwide. Mainly adults are infected, males more frequently than females. Patients with advanced HIV infection have increased susceptibility to cryptococcosis, almost always *C. neoformans*. Infection also occurs in cats, dogs, horses, cows, monkeys and other animals.

4. Reservoir—Saprophytic growth in the external environment. *C. neoformans* can be isolated consistently from old pigeon nests and pigeon droppings and from soil in many parts of the world. Foilage and bark of certain species of eucalyptus have yielded *C. bacillusporus*.

5. Mode of transmission—Presumably by inhalation.

6. Incubation period—Unknown. Pulmonary disease may precede brain infection by months or years.

7. Period of communicability—No person-to-person or animal-to-person transmission.

8. Susceptibility—All races are susceptible; the frequency of

C. neoformans in the external environment and the rarity of infection suggest that humans have appreciable resistance. Susceptibility is increased during corticosteroid therapy, immune deficiency disorders (especially HIV infection) and disorders of the reticuloendothelial system, particularly Hodgkin disease and sarcoidosis.

9. **Methods of control—**

   A. *Preventive measures:* While there have been no case clusters traced to exposure to pigeon droppings, the ubiquity of *C. neoformans* in weathered droppings suggests that removal of large accumulations be preceded by chemical decontamination, such as by an iodophor, or thorough wetting to prevent aerosolization of the agent.

   B. *Control of patient, contacts and the immediate environment:*

   1) Report to local health authority: Official report required in some jurisdictions as a possible manifestation of AIDS, Class 2 (see Reporting).
   2) Isolation: Not applicable.
   3) Concurrent disinfection: Of discharges and contaminated dressings. Terminal cleaning.
   4) Quarantine: Not applicable.
   5) Immmunization of contacts: Not applicable.
   6) Investigation of contacts and source of infection: None.
   7) Specific treatment: Amphotericin B IV is effective in many cases; 5-fluorocytosine is useful in combination with amphotericin B. The combination is often the therapy of choice but has substantial toxicity. In AIDS patients cryptococcosis is difficult to cure; fluconazole, continued indefinitely, is useful after an initial course of amphotericin B.

   C. *Epidemic measures:* None.

   D. *Disaster implications:* None.

   E. *International measures:* None.

[L: Severo]

CRYPTOSPORIDIOSIS   ICD-9 136.8; ICD-10 A07.2

1. **Identification**—A parasitic infection of medical and veterinary importance affecting epithelial cells of the human GI, biliary and respiratory tracts, as well as over 45 different vertebrate species including poultry and other birds, fish, reptiles, small mammals (rodents, cats, dogs) and large mammals (particularly cattle and sheep). Asymptomatic infections

are common and constitute a source of infection for others. The major symptom in human patients is diarrhea, which may be profuse and watery, preceded by anorexia and vomiting in children. The diarrhea is associated with cramping abdominal pain. General malaise, fever, anorexia, nausea and vomiting occur less often. Symptoms often wax and wane but remit in less than 30 days in most immunologically healthy people. In immunodeficient persons, especially those infected with HIV, who may be unable to clear the parasite, the disease has a prolonged and fulminant clinical course contributing to death. Symptoms of cholecystitis may occur in biliary tract infections; the relationship between respiratory tract infections and clinical symptoms is unclear.

Diagnosis is generally through identification of oocysts in fecal smears or of life cycle stages of the parasites in intestinal biopsy sections. Oocysts are small (4–6 micrometers) and may be confused with yeast unless appropriately stained. Most commonly used stains include auramine-rhodamine, a modified acid-fast stain, and safranin-methylene blue. More sensitive immunobased ELISA assays have recently become available. A fluorescein-tagged monoclonal antibody is useful for detecting oocysts in stool and in environmental samples. Infection with this organism is not easily detected unless looked for specifically. Serological assays may help in epidemiological studies, but it is not known when the antibody appears and how long it lasts after infection.

2. Infectious agent—*Cryptosporidium parvum*, a coccidian protozoon, is the species associated with human infection.

3. Occurrence—Worldwide. *Cryptosporidium* oocysts have been identified in human fecal specimens from more than 50 countries. In industrialized countries, prevalence of infection is less than 1% to 4.5% of individuals surveyed by stool examination. In developing regions, prevalence ranges from 3% to 20%. Children under 2, animal handlers, travellers, men who have sex with men and close personal contacts of infected individuals (families, health care and day care workers) are particularly prone to infection. Outbreaks have been reported in day care centers around the world, and have also been associated with: drinking water (at least 3 major outbreaks involved public water supplies); recreational use of water including waterslides, swimming pools and lakes; and consumption of contaminated beverages.

4. Reservoir—Humans, cattle and other domesticated animals.

5. Mode of transmission—Fecal-oral, which includes person-to-person, animal-to-person, waterborne and foodborne transmission. The parasite infects intestinal epithelial cells and multiplies initially by schizogony, followed by a sexual cycle resulting in fecal oocysts that can survive under adverse environmental conditions for long periods of time. Oocysts are highly resistant to chemical disinfectants used to purify drinking water. One or more autoinfectious cycles may occur in humans.

6. **Incubation period**—Not known precisely; 1–12 days is the likely range, with an average of about 7 days.

7. **Period of communicability**—Oocysts, the infectious stage, appear in the stool at the onset of symptoms and are infectious immediately upon excretion. Excretion continues in stools for several weeks after symptoms resolve; outside the body, oocysts may remain infective for 2–6 months in a moist environment.

8. **Susceptibility**—Immunocompetent people may have asymptomatic or self-limited symptomatic infections; it is not clear whether reinfection and latent infection with reactivation can occur. Immunodeficient individuals generally clear their infections when factors of immunosuppression (including malnutrition or intercurrent viral infections such as measles) are removed. In those with HIV infection, the clinical course may vary and asymptomatic periods may occur, but the infection usually persists throughout the illness; approximately 2% of AIDS patients reported to CDC were infected with cryptosporidiosis when AIDS was diagnosed; hospital experience indicates that 10%–20% of AIDS patients develop infection at some time during their illness.

9. **Methods of control—**

   A. *Preventive measures:*

   1) Educate the public in personal hygiene.
   2) Dispose of feces in a sanitary manner; use care in handling animal or human excreta.
   3) Have those in contact with calves and other animals with diarrhea (scours) wash their hands carefully.
   4) Boil drinking water supplies for 1 minute; chemical disinfectants are not effective against oocysts in drinking water. Only filters capable of removing particles 0.1–1.0 micrometers in diameter should be considered.
   5) Remove infected persons from jobs that require handling food that will not be subsequently cooked.
   6) Exclude infected children from day care facilities until diarrhea stops.

   B. *Control of patient, contacts and the immediate environment:*

   1) Report to local health authority: Case report in some countries by most practicable means, Class 3 (see Reporting).
   2) Isolation: For hospitalized patients, enteric precautions in the handling of feces, vomitus and contaminated clothing and bed linen; exclusion of symptomatic individuals from food handling and from direct care of hospitalized and institutionalized patients; release to return to work in sensitive occupations when asymptomatic. Stress proper handwashing.

3) Concurrent disinfection: Of feces and articles soiled there-with. In communities with modern and adequate sewage disposal systems, feces can be discharged directly into sewers without preliminary disinfection. Terminal cleaning. Heating to 45°C (113°F) for 5–20 minutes, 60°C (140°F) for 2 minutes, or chemical disinfection with 10% formalin or 5% ammonia solution is effective.

4) Quarantine: Not applicable.

5) Immmunization of contacts: Not applicable.

6) Investigation of contacts and source of infection: Micro-scopic examination of feces in household members and other suspected contacts, especially if symptomatic. Con-tact with cattle or domestic animals warrants investigation. If waterborne transmission is suspected, large volume water sampling filters can be used to look for oocysts in the water.

7) Specific treatment: No treatment other than rehydration, when indicated, has been proven effective; administration of passive antibodies and antibiotics is under study. If the individual is taking immunosuppressive drugs, these should be stopped or reduced wherever possible.

C. *Epidemic measures:* Epidemiological investigation of clus-tered cases in an area or institution to determine source of infection and mode of transmission; search for common vehicle, such as recreational water, drinking water, raw milk or other potentially contaminated food or drink; institute applicable prevention or control measures. Control of person-to-person or animal-to-person transmission requires emphasis on personal cleanliness and safe disposal of feces.

D. *Disaster implications:* None.

E. *International measures:* None.

DIARRHEA CAUSED BY
CYCLOSPORA   ICD-10 A07.8

This diarrheal disease is caused by *Cyclospora cayetanensis*, a sporu-lating coccidian protozoon infecting the upper small bowel. The clinical syndrome consists of watery diarrhea, nausea, anorexia, abdominal cramps, fatigue and weight loss; fever is rare. The median incubation period is about 1 week. Diarrhea in the immunocompetent can be prolonged but is self-limited; mean duration of organism shedding was 23 days in Peruvian children. In the immunocompromised, diarrhea lasted for months in some patients. It has also been associated with diarrhea in travellers to Asia, the Caribbean, Mexico and Peru.

Diagnosis is made by identification in the stools of the 8–10 micrometer size oocysts, about twice the size of *Cryptosporidium parvum* in wet mount under phase contrast microscopy. A modified acid-fast stain or modified safranin technique can be used. Organisms autofluoresce under ultraviolet illumination.

Cyclospora is endemic in many developing countries. Transmission can be food- or waterborne and occurs either through drinking—or swimming in—contaminated water or through consumption of contaminated fresh fruits and vegetables. *Cyclospora* oocysts in freshly excreted stool are not infectious. They require days to weeks outside the host to sporulate and become infectious. *C. cayetanensis* was responsible for multiple foodborne outbreaks in North America linked to various types of fresh produce imported from developing countries. Raspberries, basil and lettuce are among the incriminated vehicles.

Produce should be washed thoroughly before it is eaten, although this practice does not eliminate the risk of cyclosporiasis. *Cyclospora* is resistant to chlorination.

Cyclosporiasis can be treated with a 7-day course of oral trimethoprim-sulfamethoxazole (for adults, 160 mg trimethoprim plus 800 mg sulfamethoxazole twice daily; for children, 5 mg/kg trimethoprim plus 25 mg/kg sulfamethoxazole twice daily). In patients who are not treated, illness can be protracted, with remitting and relapsing symptoms. Treatment regimens for patients who cannot tolerate sulfa drugs have not been identified.

Health care providers should consider the diagnosis of *Cyclospora* infection in persons with prolonged diarrheal illness and request stool specimens so that specific tests for this parasite can be made. In jurisdictions where formal reporting mechanisms are not yet established, clinicians and laboratory workers who identify cases of cyclosporiasis are encouraged to inform the appropriate health departments.

[L. Savioli]

CYTOMEGALOVIRUS INFECTIONS
CYTOMEGALOVIRUS DISEASE   ICD-9 078.5; ICD-10 B25
CONGENITAL CYTOMEGALOVIRUS INFECTION   ICD-9 771.1; ICD-10 P35.1

1. Identification—While infection with cytomegalovirus (CMV) is common, it often passes undiagnosed as a febrile illness without specific characteristics. Serious manifestations of infection vary depending on the age and immunocompetence of the individual at the time of infection.

The most severe form of the disease develops in 5%–10% of infants infected in utero. These show signs and symptoms of severe generalized infection, especially involving the CNS and liver. Lethargy, convulsions, jaundice, petechiae, purpura, hepatosplenomegaly, chorioretinitis, intracerebral calcifications and pulmonary infiltrates may occur. Survivors show mental retardation, microcephaly, motor disabilities, hearing loss and evidence of chronic liver disease. Death may occur in utero; the neonatal case-fatality rate is high for severely affected infants. Neonatal CMV infection occurs in 0.3%–1% of births, making it one of the most common congenital infections; 90%–95% of these intrauterine infections are inapparent but 15%–25% of these infants eventually manifest some degree of neurosensory disability. Fetal infection may occur during either primary or reactivated maternal infections; primary infections carry a much higher risk for symptomatic disease and sequelae. Seronegative newborns who receive blood transfusions from seropositive donors may also develop severe disease.

Infection acquired later in life is generally inapparent but may cause a syndrome clinically and hematologically similar to Epstein-Barr virus mononucleosis, distinguishable by virological or serological tests and the absence of heterophile antibodies. CMV causes up to 10% of all cases of mononucleosis seen among university students and hospitalized adults aged 25–34. It is the most common cause of mononucleosis following transfusion to nonimmune individuals; many posttransfusion infections are clinically inapparent. Disseminated infection, with pneumonitis, retinitis, GI tract disorders (gastritis, enteritis, colitis) and hepatitis, occurs in immunodeficient and immunosuppressed patients—this is a serious manifestation of AIDS.

CMV is also the most common cause of posttransplant infection, both for solid organ and bone marrow transplants; in the former, this is particularly so with a seronegative recipient and a seropositive (carrier) donor, whereas reactivation is a common cause of disease after bone marrow transplant. In both cases, serious disease occurs in about 1 of 4 cases.

Optimal diagnosis in the newborn is through virus isolation or PCR, usually from urine. Positive tests for IgM antibodies to CMV are also helpful. Diagnosis of CMV disease in the adult is made difficult by the high frequency of asymptomatic and relapsing infections. Multiple diagnostic modalities should be used if possible. Virus isolation, CMV antigen detection (which can be done within 24 hours) and CMV DNA detection by PCR or in situ hybridization can be used to demonstrate virus in organs, blood, respiratory secretions or urine. Serological studies should be done to demonstrate the presence of CMV specific IgM antibody or a 4-fold rise in antibody titre. Interpretation of the results requires knowledge of the patient's clinical and epidemiological background.

2. Infectious agent—Human (beta) herpesvirus 5 (human CMV), a member of the subfamily Betaherpesvirus of the family Herpesviridae;

includes 4 major genotypes and many strains, although there often is cross-antigenicity among genotypes and strains.

3. Occurrence—Worldwide. In the USA, intrauterine infection occurs in 0.5%–1% of pregnancies, usually as the result of a primary infection. In Europe, intrauterine infection is slightly less common. The situation in developing countries is not well described, but infection generally occurs early in life and most intrauterine infections are due to reactivation or reinfection of maternal infection. Serum antibody prevalence in young adults varies from 40% in highly industrialized countries to almost 100% in some developing countries; it is higher in women than in men and is inversely related to socioeconomic status within the USA; in the United Kingdom, antibody prevalence is related to race rather than social class. In various population groups, 8%–60% of infants begin shedding virus in the urine during their first year of life as a result of infection acquired from the mother's cervix or breastmilk.

4. Reservoir—Humans are the only known reservoir of human CMV; strains found in many animal species are not infectious for humans.

5. Mode of transmission—Intimate exposure through mucosal contact with infectious tissues, secretions and excretions. CMV is excreted in urine, saliva, breastmilk, cervical secretions and semen during primary and reactivated infections. Persistent excretion may occur in infected newborns and immunosuppressed individuals. The fetus may be infected in utero from either a primary or reactivated maternal infection; serious fetal infection with manifest disease at birth occurs most commonly during a mother's primary infection, but infection (usually without disease) may develop even when maternal antibodies existed prior to conception. Postnatal infection occurs more commonly in infants born to mothers shedding CMV in cervical secretions at delivery; thus, transmission of the virus from the infected cervix at delivery is a common means of neonatal infection. Virus can be transmitted to infants through infected breastmilk, an important source of infection but not of disease, except when milk from a surrogate mother is given to seronegative infants. Viraemia may be present in asymptomatic people, so the virus may be transmitted by blood transfusion, probably associated with leukocytes. Many children in day care centers excrete CMV; this may represent a community reservoir. Transmission through sexual intercourse is common and is reflected by the almost universal infection of men who have many male sexual partners.

6. Incubation period—Illness following a transplant or transfusion with infected blood begins within 3–8 weeks. Infection acquired during birth is first demonstrable 3–12 weeks after delivery.

7. Period of communicability—Virus is excreted in urine and saliva for many months and may persist or be episodic for several years following primary infection. After neonatal infection, virus may be excreted for 5–6 years. Adults appear to excrete virus for shorter periods, but the virus persists as a latent infection. Fewer than 3% of healthy adults are pharyngeal excreters. Excretion recurs with immunodeficiency and immunosuppression.

8. Susceptibility—Infection is ubiquitous. Fetuses, patients with debilitating diseases, those on immunosuppressive drugs and especially organ allograft recipients (kidney, heart, bone marrow) and patients with AIDS are more susceptible to overt and severe disease.

9. Methods of control—

A. Preventive measures:

1) Take care in handling diapers; wash hands after diaper changes and toilet care of newborns and infants.
2) Women of childbearing age who work in hospitals (especially delivery and pediatric wards) should use "universal precautions". Workers in day care centers and preschools (especially those dealing with mentally retarded populations) should observe strict standards of hygiene, including handwashing.
3) Avoid transfusing neonates of seronegative mothers with blood from CMV-seropositive donors.
4) Avoid transplanting organs from CMV-seropositive donors to seronegative recipients. If unavoidable, hyperimmune IG or prophylactic administration of antivirals may be helpful. Antivirals are also helpful in seropositive bone-marrow transplant recipients, who carry latent CMV.

B. Control of patient, contacts and the immediate environment:

1) Report to local health authority: Official report not ordinarily justifiable, Class 5 (see Reporting).
2) Isolation: Secretion precautions may be applied while in hospital for patients known to excrete virus.
3) Concurrent disinfection: Discharges from hospitalized patients and articles soiled therewith.
4) Quarantine: Not applicable.
5) Immmunization of contacts: Not applicable.
6) Investigation of contacts and source of infection: None, because of the high prevalence of asymptomatic shedders in the population.
7) Specific treatment: Ganciclovir, IV and orally, cidofovir IV (together with probenecid) and foscarnet IV have been approved for the treatment of CMV retinitis in immunocompromised persons. They may also be helpful, especially when combined with anti-CMV immune globulin, for pneu-

monitis and possibly GI disease in immunocompromised persons. These drugs and valaciclovir are licensed for use in CMV infections occurring after organ transplantation.

C. Epidemic measures: None.

D. Disaster implications: None.

E. International measures: None.

[D. Lavanchy]

DENGUE FEVER ICD-9 061; ICD-10 A90
(Breakbone fever)

1. Identification—An acute febrile viral disease characterized by sudden onset, fever for 2–7 days (sometimes biphasic), intense headache, myalgia, arthralgia, retro-orbital pain, anorexia, nausea, vomiting and rash. Early generalized erythema occurs in some cases. A generalized maculo-papular rash may appear about the time of defervescence. Rash is frequently not visible in dark-skinned patients. Minor bleeding phenomena, such as petechiae, epistaxis or gum bleeding may occur at any time during the febrile phase. With underlying conditions, adults may have major bleeding phenomena, such as GI hemorrhage in peptic ulcer cases or menorrhagia. These should be differentiated from dengue infections and DHF with increased vascular permeability, bleeding manifestations and involvement of specific organs. Recovery may be associated with prolonged fatigue and depression. Lymphadenopathy and leukopenia with relative lymphocytosis are usual; mild thrombocytopenia (less than 100×10^3 cells per mm^3; or 100 SI units $\times 10^9$ per L) and elevated transaminases occur less frequently. Epidemics are explosive, but fatalities are rare.

Differential diagnosis includes chikungunya and other epidemiologically relevant diseases listed under arthropod-borne viral fevers, influenza, measles, rubella, malaria, leptospirosis, typhoid, scrub typhus and other systemic febrile illnesses, especially those accompanied by rash.

Laboratory confirmation of dengue infection is through detection of virus either in acute phase blood/serum within 5 days of onset or of specific antibodies in convalescent phase serum obtained 6 days or more after onset of illness. Virus is isolated from blood by inoculation to mosquitoes, or by culture in mosquito cell lines, then identified through immunofluorescence with serotype-specific monoclonal antibodies. These procedures provide a definitive diagnosis, but practical considerations limit their use in endemic countries. The IgM capture ELISA is the most commonly used serological procedure for diagnosis and is particularly suitable for high-volume testing. IgM antibody, indicating current or recent infection, is usually detectable by day 6-7 after onset of illness. A positive test result in a single serum indicates presumptive recent infection; a definitive diagnosis requires increased antibody levels in paired sera. Reverse transcriptase PCR amplification protocols using dengue oligonucleotide primers can detect dengue virus RNA in patient serum and tissue from fatal cases. PCR with specific primers can distinguish among the dengue virus serotypes; PCR with nucleotide sequencing and restriction enzyme analysis can characterize dengue strains and genotypes. Since these assays are costly, demand meticulous technique, and are highly prone to false-positives through contamination, they are not yet applicable for wide use in all settings.

2. **Infectious agent**—The viruses of dengue fever are flaviviruses and include serotypes 1, 2, 3 and 4 (dengue-1, -2, -3, -4). The same viruses are responsible for dengue hemorrhagic fever (see below).

3. **Occurrence**—Dengue viruses of multiple types are endemic in most countries in the tropics. In Asia, 2-5 year dengue/DHF epidemic cycles are established in southern Cambodia, China, Indonesia, Lao Democratic Republic, Malaysia, Myanmar, the Philippines, Thailand and Viet Nam, with increasing epidemic activity and geographic spread in Bangladesh, India, Maldives, Pakistan, and Sri Lanka, and lower endemicity in New Guinea, Singapore and Taiwan (China). Dengue viruses of several types have regularly been reintroduced into the Pacific and into northern Queensland, Australia, since 1981.

Dengue-1, -2, -3 and -4 are endemic in Africa. In large areas of western Africa, dengue viruses are probably transmitted epizootically in monkeys; urban dengue involving humans is also common in this area. In recent years, outbreaks of dengue fever have occurred on the eastern coast of Africa from Ethiopia to Mozambique and on offshore islands such as the Comoros and the Seychelles, with a small number of dengue and DHF-like cases reported from the Arabian peninsula.

Successive introduction and circulation of all 4 serotypes in tropical and subtropical areas of the Americas has occurred since 1977; dengue entered Texas in 1980, 1986, 1995 and 1997. As of the late 1990s, two or more dengue viruses are endemic or periodically epidemic in virtually all of the Caribbean and Latin America including Brazil, Bolivia, Colombia, Ecuador, the Guyanas, Mexico, Paraguay, Peru, Suriname, Venezuela, and central America. Dengue was introduced into Easter Island, Chile in 2002 and reintroduced into Argentina at the northern border with Brazil. Epidemics may occur wherever vectors are present and virus is introduced, whether in urban or rural areas.

4. **Reservoir**—The viruses are maintained in a human/*Aedes aegypti* mosquito cycle in tropical urban centers; a monkey/mosquito cycle may serve as a reservoir in the forests of southeastern Asia and western Africa.

5. **Mode of transmission**—Bite of infective mosquitoes, principally

Ae. aegypti. This is a day biting species, with increased biting activity for 2 hours after sunrise and several hours before sunset. Dengue outbreaks have been attributed to *Ae. albopictus*, an urban species abundant in Asia, that has now spread to Latin America and the USA, Caribbean and the Pacific, parts of southern Europe and Africa. *Ae. albopictus* is less anthropophilic than *Ae. aegypti* and hence is a less efficient epidemic vector. In Polynesia, one of the *Ae. scutellaris* spp. complex serves as the vector. In Malaysia, *Ae. nivaeus* complex and in western Africa *Ae. furcifer-taylori* complex mosquitoes are involved in enzootic monkey/mosquito transmission.

6. **Incubation period**—From 3 to 14 days, commonly 4–7 days.

7. **Period of communicability**—No direct person-to-person transmission. Patients are infective for mosquitoes from shortly before the febrile period to the end thereof, usually 3–5 days. The mosquito becomes infective 8–12 days after the viraemic blood-meal and remains so for life.

8. **Susceptibility**—Susceptibility in humans is universal, but children usually have a milder disease than adults. Recovery from infection with one serotype provides lifelong homologous immunity but only short-term protection against other serotypes and may exacerbate disease upon subsequent infections (see Dengue hemorrhagic fever).

9. **Methods of control**—

   A. *Preventive measures:*

   1) Educate the public and promote behaviours to remove, destroy or manage mosquito vector larval habitats, which for *Ae. aegypti* are usually artificial water-holding containers close to or inside human habitations e.g. old tires, flowerpots, discarded containers for food or water storage.
   2) Survey the community to determine the abundance of vector mosquitoes, identify the most productive larval habitats, promote and implement plans for their elimination, management or treatment with appropriate larvicides.
   3) Personal protection against day biting mosquitoes through repellents, screening and protective clothing (see Malaria, 9A3 and 9A4).

   B. *Control of patient, contacts and the immediate environment:*

   1) Report to local health authority: Obligatory report of epidemics; case reports, Class 4 (see Reporting).
   2) Isolation: Blood precautions. Until the fever subsides, prevent access of day biting mosquitoes to patients by screening the sickroom or using a mosquito bednet, preferably insecticide-impregnated, for febrile patients, or by spraying quarters with a knockdown adulticide or residual insecticide.

3) Concurrent disinfection: Not applicable.
4) Quarantine: Not applicable.
5) Immmunization of contacts: Not applicable. If dengue occurs near possible jungle foci of yellow fever, immunize the population against yellow fever because the urban vector for the two diseases is the same.
6) Investigation of contacts and source of infection: Determine patient's place of residence during the 2 weeks before onset of illness and search for unreported or undiagnosed cases.
7) Specific treatment: Supportive, including oral rehydration. Acetylsalicylic acid (aspirin) is contraindicated because of its hemorrhagic potential.

C. Epidemic measures:

1) Search for and destroy *Aedes* mosquitoes in sites of human habitation, and eliminate or apply larvicide to all potential *Ae. aegypti* larval habitats.
2) Use mosquito repellents for people exposed to vector mosquitoes.

D. Disaster implications: Epidemics can be extensive and affect a high percentage of the population.

E. International measures: Enforce international agreements designed to prevent the spread of *Ae. aegypti* via ships, airplanes and land transport. Improve international surveillance and exchange of data between countries. WHO Collaborating Centres.

Further information on http://www.who.int/denguenet and http://www.who.int/health_topics/dengue/en

DENGUE HEMORRHAGIC FEVER/ DENGUE SHOCK SYNDROME
(DHF/DSS)   ICD-9 065.4; ICD-10 A91

1. Identification—A severe mosquito-transmitted viral illness endemic in much of southern and southeastern Asia, the Pacific and Latin America, characterized by increased vascular permeability, hypovolaemia and abnormal blood clotting mechanisms. It is recognized principally in children but occurs also in adults. The WHO proposed case definition for DHF is: (1) fever or history of recent fever lasting 2–7 days; (2) thrombocytopenia; $100 \times 10^3/mm^3$ or less (SI units $100 \times 10^9/L$ or less); (3) at least 1 of the following hemorrhagic manifestations: positive tourniquet test, petechiae/ ecchymoses/purpura/hematemesis/melaena, other overt bleeding; (4) evidence of plasma leakage by at least 1 of the following: (>20% rise in hematocrit or >20% drop in hematocrit following volume replacement, pleural effusion, ascites, hypoproteinaemia). Dengue shock syndrome (DSS) includes all above criteria plus signs of shock: (1) rapid, weak pulse; (2) narrow pulse pressure (less than 20 mm Hg); (3) hypotension for age; (4) cold, clammy skin and restlessness. Prompt oral or intravenous fluid therapy may reduce hematocrit rise and require alternate observations to document increased plasma leakage.

Illness begins abruptly with fever and, in children, mild upper respiratory complaints, often anorexia, facial flush and mild GI disturbances. Coincident with defervescence and decreasing platelet count, the patient's condition suddenly worsens in severe cases, with marked weakness, restlessness, facial pallor and often diaphoresis, severe abdominal pain and circumoral cyanosis. The liver may be enlarged, with occasional tenderness just before shock. Warning signs include intense continuous abdominal pain with persistent vomiting.

Hemorrhagic phenomena occur frequently (see earlier). GI hemorrhage is an ominous sign that usually follows a prolonged period of shock. In severe cases, findings include accumulation of fluids in serosal cavities, low serum albumin, elevated transaminases, a prolonged prothrombin time and low levels of C3 complement protein. DHF cases with severe liver damage (with or without encephalopathy) have been observed during large epidemics of dengue-3 in Indonesia and Thailand. Case-fatality rates in mistreated shock have been as high as 40%–50%; with good physiological fluid replacement therapy, rates should be 1%–2%.

Serological tests show a rise in antibody titre against dengue viruses. IgM antibody, indicating a current or recent flavivirus infection, is usually detectable by day 6–7 after onset of illness. Viruses can be isolated from blood during the acute febrile stage of illness by inoculation to mosquitoes or cell cultures. Inoculation to mosquitoes improves the chances of isolating viruses from organs at autopsy; PCR may detect virus-specific nucleic acid sequences.

Infection with dengue viruses with or without hemorrhagic manifestations is covered above. The related yellow fever and other hemorrhagic fevers are presented separately.

2. Infectious agent—See Dengue fever. All 4 dengue serotypes (in descending order of frequency: types 2, 3, 4 and 1) can cause DHF/DSS.

3. Occurrence—Recent epidemics of DHF have occurred in Asia (Cambodia, China, India, Indonesia, Lao People's Democratic Republic, Malaysia, Maldives, Myanmar, New Caledonia, Pakistan, Philippines, Singapore, Sri Lanka, Tahiti, Thailand and Viet Nam) and in the Americas (Brazil, Colombia, Cuba, Ecuador, El Salvador, French Guiana, Guatemala, Honduras, Nicaragua, Puerto Rico, Suriname and Venezuela). In an unprecedented pandemic in 1998, 56 countries reported 1.2 million cases of dengue and DHF. In tropical Asia, DHF/DSS is observed primarily among children of the local population under 15. In outbreaks in the Americas, the disease is observed in all age groups although two-thirds of fatalities occur among children. Malaysia, the Philippines, and Thailand report an increase in the number of DHF adult cases. Occurrence is greatest during the rainy season and in areas of high *Ae. aegypti* prevalence.

4., 5., 6. and **7. Reservoir, Mode of transmission, Incubation period** and **Period of communicability**—See Dengue fever.

8. Susceptibility—The best-described risk factor is the circulation of heterologous dengue antibody, acquired passively in infants or actively from an earlier infection. Such antibodies may enhance infection of mononuclear phagocytes through the formation of infectious immune complexes. Geographic origin of dengue strain, age, gender and human genetic susceptibility are also important risk factors.

In the 1981 Cuban outbreak caused by a southeastern Asian dengue-2 virus, DHF/DSS was observed 5 times more often in white than in black patients. In Myanmar, Burmese and Indians were equally susceptible to DHF.

9. Methods of control—

    A. *Preventive measures:* See Dengue fever.

    B. *Control of patient, contacts and immediate environment:*

        1), 2), 3), 4), 5) and 6) Report to local health authority, Isolation, Concurrent disinfection, Quarantine, Immunization of contacts and Investigation of contacts and source of infection: See Dengue fever.

        7) Specific treatment: Hypovolaemic shock resulting from plasma leakage often responds to oxygen therapy and rapid replacement with fluid and electrolyte solution (lactated Ringer solution or physiological saline at 10–20 ml/kg/hour). In more severe cases of shock, plasma and/or plasma expanders should be used. The rate of fluid administration must be judged by estimates of loss, usually through serial microhematocrit urine output and clinical monitoring. A continued rise in hematocrit value in the presence of vigorous IV fluid administration indicates a need for plasma or other colloid. Care must be taken to watch for and avoid overhydration. Blood transfusions are indicated for massive bleeding or in cases with unstable signs or a true fall in hematocrit. The use of heparin to manage clinically significant hemorrhage occurring in the presence of well-documented disseminated intravascular coagulation is high-risk and of no proven benefit. Fresh plasma, fibrinogen and

platelet concentrate may be used to treat severe hemorrhage. Aspirin is contraindicated because of its hemorrhagic
potential.

C., D. and **E. Epidemic measures, Disaster implications** and
International measures: See Dengue fever.

[R. Dayal-Drager]

DERMATOPHYTOSIS ICD-9 110; ICD-10 B35
(Tinea, Ringworm, Dermatomycosis, Epidermophytosis,
Trichophytosis, Microsporosis)

Dermatophytosis and tinea are general terms, essentially synonymous,
applied to fungal infection of keratinized areas of the body (hair, skin and
nails). Various genera and species of fungi known collectively as the
dermatophytes are causative agents. The dermatophytoses are subdivided
according to the site of infection.

I. TINEA BARBAE AND TINEA
 CAPITIS ICD-9 110.0; ICD-10 B35.0
(Ringworm of the beard and scalp, Kerion, Favus)

1. Identification—A fungal disease that begins as a small area of
erythema and/or scaling and spreads peripherally, leaving scaly patches of
temporary baldness. Infected hairs become brittle and break off easily.
Occasionally, boggy, raised suppurative lesions develop, called kerions.

Favus of the scalp (ICD-9 110.0; ICD-10 B35.0) is a variety of tinea capitis
caused by *Trichophyton schoenleinii*. It is characterized by a mousy smell
and by the formation of small, yellowish, cuplike crusts (scutulae) that
amalgamate to form a pale or yellow visible mat on the scalp surface.
Affected hairs do not break off but become grey and lustreless, eventually
falling out and leaving baldness that may be permanent.

Tinea capitis is easily distinguished from black piedra, a fungus infection
of the hair occurring in tropical areas of South America, southeastern Asia
and Africa. This is characterized by black, hard "gritty" nodules on hair
shafts, caused by *Piedraia hortai*. There is a white form in which
Trichosporon beigelii, now called *T. ovoides* or *T. inkin*, produces white,
soft pasty nodules.

Examination of the scalp under UV light (Wood lamp) for yellow-green
fluorescence is helpful in diagnosing tinea capitis caused by *Microsporum*
species such as *M. canis* and *M. audouinii*; *Trichophyton* species do not
fluoresce. In infections caused by *Microsporum* spp., microscopic examination of scales and hair in 10% potassium hydroxide or under UV
microscopy of a calcofluor white preparation reveals characteristic non-

pigmented ectothrix (outside the hair) arthrospores; many *Trichophyton* spp. present an endothrix (inside the hair) pattern of invasion; *T. verrucosum*, the cause of cattle ringworm, produces large ectothrix spores. Confirmation of the diagnosis requires culture of the fungus. Genetic identification methods are still largely experimental.

2. Infectious agents—Various species of *Microsporum* and *Trichophyton*. Species and genus identification is important for epidemiological, prognostic and therapeutic reasons.

3. Occurrence—Tinea capitis caused by *Trichophyton tonsurans* can be epidemic in urban areas in Australia, Mexico, the United Kingdom, eastern USA and Puerto Rico as well as in many developing countries. *M. canis* infections occur in rural and urban areas wherever infected cats and dogs are present. *M. audouinii* is endemic in western Africa and was formerly widespread in Europe and the USA, particularly in urban areas; *T. verrucosum* and *T. mentagrophytes* var. *mentagrophytes* infections occur primarily in rural areas where the disease exists in cattle, horses, rodents and wild animals.

4. Reservoir—Humans for *T. tonsurans*, *T. schoenleinii* and *M. audouinii*; animals, especially dogs, cats and cattle, harbour the other organisms noted above.

5. Mode of transmission—Direct skin-to-skin or indirect contact, especially from the backs of seats, barber clippers, toilet articles (combs, hairbrushes), clothing and hats that are contaminated with hair from infected people or animals. Infected humans can generate considerable aerosols of infective arthrospores

6. Incubation period—Usually 10 to 14 days.

7. Period of communicability—Viable fungus and infective arthrospores may persist on contaminated materials for long periods.

8. Susceptibility—Children below the age of puberty are highly susceptible to *M. canis*; all ages are subject to *Trichophyton* infections. Reinfections mainly occur for infections spread amongst humans.

9. Methods of control—

    A. Preventive measures:

        1) Educate the public, especially parents, to the danger of acquiring infection from infected individuals as well as from dogs, cats and other animals.

        2) In the presence of epidemics or in hyperendemic areas where non-*Trichophyton* species are prevalent, survey heads of young children by UV light (Wood lamp) before school entry.

B. Control of patient, contacts and the immediate environment:

1) Report to local health authority: Obligatory report of epidemics in some countries; no individual case report, Class 4 (see Reporting). Outbreaks in schools must be reported to school authorities.

2) Isolation: Not applicable.

3) Concurrent disinfection: In mild cases, daily washing of scalp removes loose hair. Selenium sulfide or ketoconazole shampoos help remove scale. In severe cases, wash scalp daily and cover hair with a cap, which should be boiled after use.

4) Quarantine: Not practical.

5) Immmunization of contacts: Not applicable.

6) Investigation of contacts and source of infection: Study household contacts, pets and farm animals for evidence of infection; treat if infected. Some animals, especially cats, may be inapparent carriers. With some agent (e.g. *T. tonsurans*) children may have mild infections accompanied by hair invasion; careful clinical examination of contacts is required.

7) Specific treatment: Topical agents are ineffective in true infections. Oral griseofulvin for at least 4 weeks is effective. Terbinafine and itraconazole are also effective. Terbinafine is more active than griseofulvin against agents such as *T. tonsurans* but higher doses of this drug should be used in *Microsporum* infections. Systemic antibacterial agents are useful if lesions become secondarily infected by bacteria; in the case of kerions, also use an antiseptic cream and remove scaly crusts from the scalp by gentle soaking. Examine regularly and take cultures; when cultures become negative, complete recovery may be assumed.

C. Epidemic measures: In school or other institutional epidemics, educate children and parents as to mode of spread, prevention and personal hygiene. If more than 2 infected children are present in a class, examine the others. Enlist services of physicians and nurses for diagnosis; carry out follow-up surveys.

D. Disaster implications: None.

E. International measures: None.

II. TINEA CRURIS   ICD-9 110.3; ICD-10 B35.6
(Ringworm of groin and perianal region)
TINEA CORPORIS   ICD-9 110.5; ICD-10 B35.4
(Ringworm of the body)

1. Identification—A fungal disease of the skin other than of the scalp, bearded areas and feet, characteristically appearing as flat, spreading, ring-shaped or circular lesion with a characteristic raised edge around all or part of the lesion. This periphery is usually reddish, vesicular or pustular and may be dry and scaly or moist and crusted. As the lesion progresses peripherally, the central area often clears, leaving apparently normal skin. Differentiation from inguinal candidiasis, often distinguished by the presence of "satellite" pustules outside the lesion margins, is necessary because treatment differs.

Presumptive diagnosis is made by taking scrapings from the advancing lesion margins, clearing in 10% potassium hydroxide and examining microscopically or under UV microscopy of calcofluor white preparations for segmented, branched non-pigmented fungal filaments. Final identification is through culture.

2. Infectious agents—Most species of *Microsporum* and *Trichophyton*; also *Epidermophyton floccosum*.

3. Occurrence—Worldwide and relatively frequent. Males are infected more often than females.

4. Reservoir—Humans, animals and soil.

5. Mode of transmission—Direct or indirect contact with skin and scalp lesions of infected people, lesions of animals; contaminated floors, shower stalls, benches and similar articles.

6. Incubation period—Usually 4 to 10 days.

7. Period of communicability—As long as lesions are present and viable fungus persists on contaminated materials.

8. Susceptibility—Susceptibility is widespread, aggravated by friction and excessive perspiration in axillary and inguinal regions, and when environmental temperatures and humidity are high. All ages are susceptible.

9. Methods of control—

A. *Preventive measures:* Launder towels and clothing with hot water and/or fungicidal agent; general cleanliness in public showers and dressing rooms (repeated washing of benches; frequent hosing and rapid draining of shower rooms). A fungicidal agent such as cresol should be used to disinfect benches and floors.

B. *Control of patient, contacts and the immediate environment:*

1) Report to local health authority: Obligatory report of epidemics in some countries; no individual case report, Class 4 (see Reporting). Report infections of schoolchildren to school authorities.

2) Isolation: While under treatment, infected persons should be excluded from swimming pools and activities likely to lead to exposure of others.
3) Concurrent disinfection: Effective and frequent laundering of clothing.
4) Quarantine: Not applicable.
5) Immmunization of contacts: Not applicable.
6) Investigation of contacts and source of infection: Examine school and household contacts, household pets and farm animals; treat infections as indicated.
7) Specific treatment: Thorough bathing with soap and water, removal of scabs and crusts and application of an effective topical fungicide (miconazole, ketoconazole, clotrimazole, econazole, naftifine, terbinafine, tolnaftate or ciclopirox) may suffice. Oral griseofulvin is effective; as are oral itraconazole and oral terbinafine.

C. *Epidemic measures:* Educate children and parents about the infection, its mode of spread and the need to maintain good personal hygiene. Outbreaks are common amongst military personnel.

D. *Disaster implications:* None.

E. *International measures:* None.

III. TINEA PEDIS   ICD-9 110.4; ICD-10 B35.3
(Ringworm of the foot, Athlete foot)

1. Identification—This fungal disease presents with characteristic scaling or cracking of the skin, especially between the toes (interdigital), diffuse scaling over the sole of the foot (dry type) or blisters containing a thin watery fluid; commonly called athlete foot. In severe cases, vesicular lesions appear on various parts of the body, especially the hands; these dermatophytids do not contain the fungus but are an allergic reaction to fungus products.

Presumptive diagnosis is verified by microscopic examination of potassium hydroxide-or calcofluor white-treated scrapings from lesions that reveal septate branching filaments. Clinical appearance is not diagnostic; final identification is through culture. Note that bacteria, including Gram-negative organisms and coryneforms, as well as *Candida* and *Scytalidium* species, may produce similar lesions. Itching is often a clue that dermatophyte fungi are present. *Scytalidium* can also cause similar dry lesions on the sole.

2. Infectious agents—*Trichophyton rubrum*, *T. mentagrophytes var. interdigitale* and *Epidermophyton floccosum*.

3. Occurrence—Common worldwide. Adults are more often affected than children, males more than females. Infections are more frequent and more severe in hot weather. They are also common in industrial workers, schoolchildren, athletes and military personnel who share shower or bathing facilities.

4. Reservoir—Humans.

5. Mode of transmission—Direct or indirect contact with skin lesions of infected people or with contaminated floors, shower stalls and other articles used by infected people.

6. Incubation period—Unknown.

7. Period of communicability—As long as lesions are present and viable spores persist on contaminated materials.

8. Susceptibility—Susceptibility is variable and infection may be inapparent. Repeated attacks and chronic infections are frequent.

9. Methods of control—

A. *Preventive measures:* See *Tinea corporis.* Educate the public to maintain strict personal hygiene; take special care in drying between toes after bathing; regularly use a dusting powder or cream containing an effective antifungal on the feet and particularly between the toes. Occlusive shoes may predispose to infection and disease.

B. *Control of patient, contacts and the immediate environment:*

   1) Report to local health authority: Obligatory report of epidemics in some countries; no individual case report, Class 4 (see Reporting). Report high incidence in schools to school authorities.
   2) Isolation: Not applicable.
   3) Concurrent disinfection: Launder socks of heavily infected individuals to prevent reinfection.
   4) Quarantine: Not applicable.
   5) Immmunization of contacts: Not applicable.
   6) Investigation of contacts and source of infection: Not applicable.
   7) Specific treatment: Topical antifungals (miconazole, clotrimazole, ketoconazole, terbinafine, ciclopirox or tolnaftate). Expose feet to air by wearing sandals; use dusting powders. Oral terbinafine, or itraconazole may be indicated in severe, extensive or protracted disease; griseofulvin, although less active, is an alternative.

C. *Epidemic measures:* Thoroughly clean and wash floors of showers and similar sources of infection; disinfect with a fungicidal agent such as cresol. Educate the public about the mode of spread.

D. Disaster implications: None.

E. International measures: None.

IV. ONYCHOMYCOSIS DUE TO DERMATOPHYTES   ICD-9 110.1; ICD-10 B35.1
(Tinea unguium Ringworm of the nails, Onychomycosis)

1. Identification—A chronic fungal disease involving one or more nails of the hands or feet. The nail gradually becomes detached from the nail bed, thickens, and becomes discolored and brittle, an accumulation of soft keratinous material forms beneath the nail or the nail becomes chalky and disintegrates.

Diagnosis is made by microscopic examination of potassium hydroxide preparations of the nail and of detritus beneath the nail for hyaline fungal elements. Etiology should be confirmed by culture.

2. Infectious agents—Various species of *Trichophyton*. Rarely other dermatophytes. *Scytalidium hyalinum* and *S. dimidiatum* cause an almost identical disease (not strictly speaking a tinea infection), differentiated through culture on cycloheximide-free media.

3. Occurrence—Common.

4. Reservoir—Humans; rarely animals or soil.

5. Mode of transmission—Presumably through extension from skin infections acquired by direct contact with skin or nail lesions of infected people, or from indirect contact (contaminated floors and shower stalls) with a low rate of transmission, even to close family associates.

6. Incubation period—Unknown.

7. Period of communicability—As long as an infected lesion is present.

8. Susceptibility—Susceptibility variable. Reinfection is frequent.

9. Methods of control—

   A. Preventive measures: Cleanliness and use of a fungicidal agent such as cresol for disinfecting floors in common use; frequent hosing and rapid draining of shower rooms.

   B. Control of patient, contacts and the immediate environment:

   1) Report to local health authority: Official report not ordinarily justifiable, Class 5 (see Reporting).

2), 3), 4), 5) and 6) Isolation, Concurrent disinfection, Quarantine, Immunization of contacts and Investigation of contacts and source of infection: Not practical.

7) Specific treatment: Oral itraconazole and terbinafine are the drugs of choice. Oral griseofulvin is less effective. Treatment to be given until nails grow out (about 3−6 months for fingernails, 12−18 months for toenails). At present there is no effective treatment for *Scytalidium* infections.

C., D. and **E. Epidemic measures, Disaster implications** and **International measures:** Not applicable.

[R. Hay]

DIARRHEA, ACUTE   ICD-9 001-009; ICD-10 A09

Diarrhea is often accompanied by other clinical signs and symptoms including vomiting, fever, dehydration and electrolyte disturbances. It is a symptom of infection by many different bacterial, viral and parasitic enteric agents. The specific diarrheal diseases—cholera, shigellosis, salmonellosis, *Escherichia coli* infections, yersiniosis, giardiasis, Campylobacter enteritis, cryptosporidiosis and viral gastroenteropathy—are each described in detail under individual listings elsewhere in this book. Diarrhea can also occur in association with other infectious diseases such as malaria and measles, as well as chemical agents. Change in the enteric flora induced by antibiotics may produce acute diarrhea by overgrowth and toxin production by *Clostridium difficile*.

Approximately 70%–80% of the vast number of sporadic diarrheal episodes in people visiting treatment facilities in less industrialized countries could be diagnosed etiologically if the complete battery of newer laboratory tests were available and utilized. In the USA, where 5 million cases per year are estimated to occur and approximately 4 million are seen by a health care provider, the comparable figure is about 45% of cases. From a practical clinical standpoint, diarrheal illnesses can be divided into 3 clinical presentations:

1) Acute watery diarrhea (including cholera), lasting several hours or days; the main danger is dehydration; weight loss occurs if feeding is not continued. For severe dehydration (one or more of the following: child lethargic or unconscious, drinking poorly or not at all, eyes very sunken and dry, mouth very dry, very slow skin pinch—corresponding to a fluid deficit >10% of body weight), the preferred treatment is rapid intravenous therapy followed by oral rehydration; in other cases (no or some dehydration) give oral rehydration solution (ORS) by mouth;

2) Acute bloody diarrhea (dysentery), caused by organisms such as *Shigella*, *E. coli* O157:H7 and other organisms; the main dangers are intestinal damage, sepsis and malnutrition; other complications including dehydration may occur.

3) Persistent diarrhea, lasting 14 days or longer; the main danger is malnutrition and serious extraintestinal infection; dehydration may also occur.

The details pertaining to the individual diseases are presented in separate chapters.

[O. Fontaine]

DIARRHEA CAUSED BY
ESCHERICHIA COLI
ICD-9 008.0;
ICD-10 A04.0-A04.4

Six major categories of *Escherichia coli* strains cause diarrhea: 1) enterohemorrhagic; 2) enterotoxigenic; 3) enteroinvasive; 4) enteropathogenic; 5) enteroaggregative; and 6) diffuse-adherent. Each has a different pathogenesis, possesses distinct virulence properties, and comprises a separate set of O:H serotypes. Different clinical syndromes and epidemiological patterns may also be seen. Transmission is usually through contaminated food, water or hands; an outbreak in 2003 in Ohio was attributed to respiratory transmission via contaminated sawdust.

I. DIARRHEA CAUSED BY
ENTEROHEMORRHAGIC
STRAINS
ICD-9 008.0; ICD-10 A04.3
(EHEC, Shiga toxin producing *E. coli* [STEC], *E. coli* O157:H7, Verotoxin producing *E. coli*) [VTEC]

1. Identification—This category of diarrhea-causing *E. coli* was recognized in 1982 when an outbreak of hemorrhagic colitis occurred in the USA and was shown to be due to an unusual serotype, *E. coli* O157:H7, not previously incriminated as an enteric pathogen. The diarrhea may range from mild and nonbloody to stools that are virtually all blood. Lack of fever in most patients can help to differentiate this infection from that due to other enteric pathogens. The most severe clinical manifestation of EHEC infection is the hemolytic uraemic syndrome (HUS) (sometimes diagnosed as thrombotic thrombocytopenic purpura (TTP) in adults). About 8% of persons with *E. coli* O157:H7 diarrhea progress to this syndrome. Rates are likely to vary for other serotypes. EHEC elaborate potent cytotoxins called Shiga toxins 1 and 2 (also called verocytotoxins and previously called Shiga-like toxins). Shiga toxin 1 is identical to the toxin elaborated by *Shigella dysenteriae* 1; HUS is also a complication of *S. dysenteriae* 1 infection. The structural genes for the toxins are found on chromosomally-encoded phages. Most EHEC strains have a chromosomal pathogenicity island containing multiple virulence genes, including those encoding proteins that cause attaching and effacing lesions.

In North America most strains of the most common EHEC serotype, O157:H7, can be identified in stool cultures on sorbitol-MacConkey media by their inability to ferment sorbitol. Because most other EHEC strains ferment sorbitol, other techniques must be used, among which are demonstrating the ability to elaborate Shiga toxins (a commercial assay is available), or the use of DNA probes that identify the toxin genes. All EHEC strains should sent to the state health department laboratory for serotyping to monitor the frequency of various serotypes and to help detect outbreaks. In addition, *E. coli* O157:H7 strains are subtyped by pulsed-field gel electrophoresis to help detect outbreaks.

2. Infectious agent—The main EHEC serotype in North America is *E. coli* O157:H7; this serotype is thought to cause over 90% of cases of diarrhea-associated HUS. The other most common serogroups in the United States are O26, O111, O103, O45, and O121.

3. Occurrence—These infections are an important problem in North America, Europe, Japan, the southern cone of South America and southern Africa. Their importance in the rest of the world is less well established.

4. Reservoir—Cattle are the most important reservoir of EHEC; humans may also serve as a reservoir for person-to-person transmission. Other animals, including deer, may also carry EHEC.

5. Mode of transmission—Mainly through ingestion of food contaminated with ruminant feces. Serious outbreaks, including cases of hemorrhagic colitis, HUS, and some deaths have occurred in the USA from beef (usually as inadequately cooked hamburgers), produce (including melons, lettuce, coleslaw, apple cider, and alfalfa sprouts), and unpasteurized dairy milk. Direct person-to-person transmission occurs in families, child care centers and custodial institutions. Waterborne transmission occurs both from contaminated drinking water and from recreational waters.

6. Incubation period—Relatively long, 2–10 days, with a median of 3–4 days.

7. Period of communicability—The duration of excretion of the pathogen is typically 1 week or less in adults but 3 weeks in one-third of children. Prolonged carriage is uncommon.

8. Susceptibility—The infectious dose is very low. Little is known about differences in susceptibility and immunity, but infections occur in persons of all ages. Children under 5 years old are most frequently diagnosed with infection and are at greatest risk of developing HUS. The elderly also appear to be at increased risk of complications.

9. **Methods of control—**

   A. *Preventive measures:* The potential severity of this disease and the importance of infection in vulnerable groups such as children and the elderly calls for early involvement of local health authorities to identify the source and apply appropriate preventive measures. As soon as the diagnosis is suspected, it is of paramount importance to block person-to-person transmission by instructing family members about the need for frequent (especially postdefecatory) handwashing with soap and water, disposal of soiled diapers and human waste, and prevention of food and beverage contamination. Measures likely to reduce the incidence of illness include the following:

   1) Manage slaughterhouse operations to minimize contamination of meat by animal intestinal contents.
   2) Pasteurize milk and dairy products. Irradiate beef, especially ground beef.
   3) Decrease the carriage and excretion of *E. coli* O157:H7 in cattle on farms, and especially in the days just before slaughter. Decrease the contamination with animal feces of foods consumed with no or minimal cooking
   4) Wash fruits and vegetables carefully, particularly if eaten raw. They should preferably be peeled.
   5) Wash hands thoroughly and frequently using soap, in particular after contact with farm animals or the farm environment.
   6) Heat beef adequately during cooking, especially ground beef, preferably to an internal temperature of 68°C (155°F) for at least 15–16 seconds. Reliance on cooking until all pink color is gone is not as reliable as using a meat thermometer.
   7) Protect, purify and chlorinate public water supplies; chlorinate swimming pools. When the safety of drinking water is doubtful, boil it.
   8) Ensure adequate hygiene in childcare centers, and encourage frequent handwashing

   B. *Control of patient, contacts and the immediate environment:*

   1) Report to local health authority: Case report of STEC infection is obligatory in many countries, Class 2 (see Reporting). Recognition and reporting of outbreaks is especially important.
   2) Isolation: During acute illness, enteric precautions. Because of the small infective dose, infected patients should not be employed to handle food or provide child or patient care until 2 successive negative fecal samples or rectal swabs are obtained (collected 24 hours apart and not sooner than 48 hours after the last dose of antimicrobials).

3) Concurrent disinfection: Of feces and contaminated articles. In communities with a adequate sewage disposal system, feces can be discharged directly into sewers without preliminary disinfection. Terminal cleaning.

4) Quarantine: Not applicable.

5) Management of contacts: When feasible, contacts with diarrhea should be excluded from food handling and the care of children or patients until diarrhea ceases and 2 successive negative stool cultures are obtained. All contacts should be educated about thorough handwashing after defecation and before handling food or caring for children or patients.

6) Investigation of contacts and source of infection: Cultures in contacts should generally be confined to food handlers, attendants and children in child care centers and other situations where the spread of infection is particularly likely. Culture of suspected foods has rarely been productive in sporadic cases except when a specific ground beef item is strongly suspected.

7) Specific treatment: Reasonable concern exists that some antimicrobial agents increase the risk of HUS, although proof is lacking. Fluid replacement is the cornerstone of treatment for EHEC diarrhea; some clinicians choose to hospitalize all patients with *E. coli* O157:H7 infection for hydration to prevent the development of hemolytic uraemic syndrome.

C. *Epidemic measures:*

1) Report at once to the local health authority any group of acute bloody diarrhea cases or cases of hemolytic uraemic syndrome or thrombotic thrombocytopenic purpura, even in the absence of specific identification of the causal agent.

2) Search intensively for the specific vehicle (food or water) by which the infection was transmitted, evaluate potential for ongoing person-to-person transmission, and use the results of epidemiological investigations to guide specific control measures.

3) Exclude use of and trace the source of suspected food; in large common-source foodborne outbreaks, prompt recall may prevent many cases.

4) If a waterborne outbreak is suspected, issue an order to boil water and chlorinate suspected water supplies adequately under competent supervision or do not use them.

5) If a swimming-associated outbreak is suspected, close pools or beaches until chlorinated or shown to be free of fecal contamination and until adequate toilet facilities are provided to prevent further contamination of water by bathers.

6) If a milkborne outbreak is suspected, pasteurize or boil the milk.
7) Prophylactic administration of antibiotics is not recommended.
8) Publicize the importance of handwashing after defecation; provide soap and individual paper towels if otherwise not available.

D. Disaster implications: A potential problem where personal hygiene and environmental sanitation are deficient (see Typhoid fever, 9D).

E. International measures: WHO Collaborating Centres. *WHO Guide on Hygiene in Food Service and Mass Catering Establishments* http://whqlibdoc.who.int/hq/1994/WHO_FNU_FOS_94.5.pdf

II. DIARRHEA CAUSED BY ENTEROTOXIGENIC STRAINS (ETEC)   ICD-9 008.0; ICD-10 A04.1

1. Identification—A major cause of travellers' diarrhea in people from industrialized countries who visit developing countries, this disease is also an important cause of dehydrating diarrhea in infants and children in the latter countries. Enterotoxigenic strains may behave like *Vibrio cholerae* in producing a profuse watery diarrhea without blood or mucus. Abdominal cramping, vomiting, acidosis, prostration and dehydration can occur; low grade fever may or may not be present; symptoms usually last less than 5 days.

ETEC can be identified through demonstration of enterotoxin production, immunoassays, bioassays or DNA probe techniques that identify LT and ST genes (for heat labile and heat stable toxins) in colony blots. None of these assays are widely available in clinical laboratories, and ETEC infections are almost certainly underdiagnosed.

2. Infectious agent—ETEC elaborate a heat labile enterotoxin (LT), a heat stable toxin (ST) or both toxins (LT/ST). The most common O serogroups include O6, O8, O15, O20, O25, O27, O63, O78, O80, O114, O115, O128ac, O148, O153, O159 and O167. Recently, serogroup O169: H41 has emerged as the most common cause of ETEC outbreaks in the United States.

3. Occurrence—An infection primarily of developing countries. During the first 3 years of life, children in developing countries experience multiple ETEC infections that lead to the acquisition of immunity; consequently, illness in older children and adults occurs less frequently.

Infection occurs among travellers from industrialized countries that visit developing countries.

4. Reservoir—Humans. ETEC infections are largely species-specific; people constitute the reservoir for strains causing diarrhea in humans.

5. Mode of transmission—Contaminated food and, less often, contaminated water. Transmission via contaminated weaning foods may be particularly important in infection of infants. Direct contact transmission through fecally contaminated hands is believed to be rare.

6. Incubation period—Incubations as short as 10–12 hours have been observed in outbreaks and in volunteer studies with certain LT-only and ST-only strains. The incubation of LT/ST diarrhea in volunteer studies has usually been 24–72 hours.

7. Period of communicability—For the duration of excretion of the pathogenic ETEC, which may be prolonged.

8. Susceptibility—Epidemiological studies and rechallenge studies in volunteers demonstrate that ETEC infection is followed by serotype-specific immunity. Multiple infections with different serotypes are required to develop broad-spectrum immunity against ETEC.

9. Methods of control—

    A. Preventive measures:

      1) For general measures for prevention of fecal-oral spread of infection, see Typhoid fever, 9A.

      2) For adult travellers going for short periods of time to high-risk areas where it is not easy to obtain safe food or water, the use of prophylactic bismuth subsalicylate (2 tablets 4 times a day) or antibiotics (norfloxacin, 400 mg daily) may be considered; however each regimen is associated with health risks of its own. A much preferable approach is to initiate very early treatment, beginning with the onset of diarrhea, e.g. after the second or third loose stool (See section 9B7.)

    B. Control of patient, contacts and the immediate environment:

      1) Report to local health authority: Obligatory report of epidemics; no individual case report, Class 4 (see Reporting).

      2) Isolation: Enteric precautions for known and suspected cases.

      3) Concurrent disinfection: Of all fecal discharges and soiled articles. In communities with adequate sewage disposal system, feces can be discharged directly into sewers without preliminary disinfection. Thorough terminal cleaning.

      4) Quarantine: Not applicable.

    5) Immmunization of contacts: Not applicable.
    6) Investigation of contacts and source of infection: Not applicable.
    7) Specific treatment: Electrolyte-fluid therapy to prevent or treat dehydration is the most important measure (see Cholera, section 9B7). Most cases do not require any other treatment. For severe travellers' diarrhea in adults, early treatment with loperamide (not for children) and an antibiotic such as a fluoroquinolone (ciprofloxacin PO 500 mg twice daily) or norfloxacin (PO 400 mg daily) for 5 days. Fluoroquinolones are used as initial treatment because many ETEC strains worldwide are resistant to other antimicrobials. However, if local strains are known to be sensitive, trimethoprim-sulfoxazole (PO) (160 mg–800 mg) twice daily or doxycycline (PO) (100 mg) once daily, for 5 days are useful. Feeding should be continued according to the patient's appetite.

C. Epidemic measures: Epidemiological investigation may be indicated to determine how transmission is occurring.

D. Disaster implications: None.

E. International measures: WHO Collaborating Centres.

III. DIARRHEA CAUSED BY ENTEROINVASIVE STRAINS (EIEC)   ICD-9 008.0; ICD-10 A04.2

1. Identification—This inflammatory disease of the gut mucosa and submucosa caused by EIEC strains of *E. coli* closely resembles that produced by *Shigella*. The organisms possess the same plasmid-dependent ability to invade and multiply within epithelial cells. Clinically, the syndrome of watery diarrhea due to EIEC is much more common than dysentery. The O antigens of EIEC may cross-react with *Shigella* O antigens. Illness begins with severe abdominal cramps, malaise, watery stools, tenesmus and fever; in less than 10% of patients, it progresses to the passage of multiple, scanty, fluid stools containing blood and mucus.

    The presence of many fecal leukocytes visible in a stained smear of mucus, also seen in shigellosis, should raise the suspicion of EIEC. Tests available in reference laboratories include an immunoassay that detects the plasmid-encoded specific outer membrane proteins associated with epithelial cell invasiveness; a bioassay (guinea pig-keratoconjunctivitis test) detects epithelial cell invasiveness; DNA probes detect the enteroinvasiveness plasmid.

2. Infectious agent—Strains of *E. coli* shown to possess enteroinvasiveness dependent on the presence of a large virulence plasmid encoding invasion plasmid antigens. The main O serogroups in which EIEC fall include O28ac, O29, O112, O124, O136, O143, O144, O152, O164 and O167.

3. Occurrence—EIEC infections are endemic in developing countries, and cause about 1%-5% of diarrheal episodes among people visiting treatment centers. Rarely, infections and outbreaks of EIEC diarrhea have been reported in industrialized countries.

4. Reservoir—Humans.

5. Mode of transmission—The scant available evidence suggests that EIEC is transmitted by contaminated food.

6. Incubation period—Incubations as short as 10 and 18 hours have been observed in volunteer studies and outbreaks, respectively.

7. Period of communicability—Duration of excretion of EIEC strains.

8. Susceptibility—Little is known about susceptibility and immunity to EIEC.

9. Methods of control—Same as for ETEC. For the rare cases of severe diarrhea with enteroinvasive strains, as for shigellosis, treat using antimicrobials effective against local *Shigella* isolates.

IV. DIARRHEA CAUSED BY ENTEROPATHOGENIC STRAINS ICD-9 008.0; ICD-10 A04.0
(EPEC, Enteropathogenic *E. coli* enteritis)

1. Identification—The oldest recognized category of diarrhea-producing *E. coli*, implicated in 1940s and 1950s studies in which certain O:H serotypes were found to be associated with infant summer diarrhea, outbreaks of diarrhea in infant nurseries, and community epidemics of infant diarrhea. Diarrheal disease in this category is virtually confined to children under 1 in whom it causes watery diarrhea with mucus, fever and dehydration. EPEC cause dissolution of the microvilli of enterocytes and initiate attachment of the bacteria to enterocytes. The diarrhea in infants can be both severe and prolonged, and in developing countries may be associated with high case fatality.

EPEC can be tentatively identified through agglutination with antisera that detect EPEC O serogroups, but confirmation requires both O and H typing with high quality reagents. EPEC organisms exhibit localized adherence to HEp-2 cells in cell cultures, a property that postulates the presence of an EPEC virulence plasmid. The EPEC adherence factor (EAF) DNA probe detects the EPEC virulence plasmid; there is a 98% correlation between the detection of localized adherence and EAF probe positivity.

2. Infectious agent—The major EPEC O serogroups include O55, O86, O111, O119, O125, O126, O127, O128ab and O142.

3. Occurrence—Since the late 1960s, EPEC has largely disappeared as an important cause of infant diarrhea in North America and Europe. However, it remains a major agent of infant diarrhea in many developing areas, including South America, southern Africa and Asia.

4. Reservoir—Humans.

5. Mode of transmission—Through contaminated infant formula and weaning foods. In infant nurseries, transmission by fomites and by contaminated hands can occur if handwashing techniques are compromised.

6. Incubation period—As short as 9–12 hours in adult volunteer studies. It is not known whether the same incubation applies to infants who acquire infection through natural transmission.

7. Period of communicability—Limited to the duration of excretion of EPEC, which may be prolonged.

8. Susceptibility and resistance—Although susceptibility to clinical infection appears to be confined to infants in nature, it is not known whether this is because of immunity or of age-related, nonspecific host factors. Since diarrhea can be induced experimentally in some adult volunteers, specific immunity may be important in determining susceptibility. EPEC infection is uncommon in breastfed infants.

9. Methods of control—

  A. Preventive measures:

   1) Encourage mothers to practise exclusive breastfeeding from birth to 4–6 months. Provide adequate support for breastfeeding. Help the mother establish or re-establish breastfeeding.
      Where available, and only if a mother's breastmilk is unavailable or insufficient, give newborns pasteurized donor breastmilk until they go home. Infant formulas should be held at room temperature only for short periods. Cup feeding is preferred to bottle-feeding as early as possible.
   2) Practice rooming-in for mothers and infants in maternity facilities, unless there is a firm medical indication for separation. If mother or infant has a GI or respiratory infection, keep the pair together but isolate them from healthy pairs.
      In special care facilities, separate infected infants from those who are premature or ill in other ways.

3) Provide individual equipment for each infant; include a thermometer, kept at the bassinet. No common bathing or dressing tables should be used, and no bassinet stands should be used for holding or transporting more than one infant at a time.

4) Prevention of hospital outbreaks depends on washing hands between handling babies and maintaining high sanitary standards in the facilities in which babies are held.

B. *Control of patient, contacts and the immediate environment:*

1) Report to local health authority: Obligatory report of epidemics; no individual case report, Class 4 (see Reporting). Two or more concurrent cases of diarrhea requiring treatment for these symptoms in a nursery or among those recently discharged are to be interpreted as an outbreak requiring investigation.

2) Isolation: Enteric precautions for known and suspected cases.

3) Concurrent disinfection: Of all fecal discharges and soiled articles. In communities with adequate sewage disposal system, feces can be discharged directly into sewers without preliminary disinfection. Thorough terminal cleaning.

4) Quarantine: Use enteric precautions and cohort methods (see 9C).

5) Immmunization of contacts: Not applicable.

6) Investigation of contacts and source of infection: Families of discharged babies should be followed up for diarrheal status of the baby (see 9C).

7) Specific treatment: Electrolyte-fluid replacement (oral or IV) is the most important measure (see Cholera, 9B7). Most cases do not require any other treatment. For severe enteropathogenic infant diarrhea, oral trimethoprim-sufamethoxazole (10-50 mg/kg/day) has been shown to ameliorate the severity and duration of diarrheal illness; it should be administered in 3-4 divided doses for 5 days. Since many EPEC strains are resistant to a variety of antibiotics, selection should be based on the sensitivity of local isolated strains. Feeding, including breastfeeding, must continue.

C. *Epidemic measures:* For nursery epidemics (see section 9B1) the following:

1) All babies with diarrhea should be placed in one nursery under enteric precautions. Admit no more babies to the contaminated nursery. Suspend maternity service unless a clean nursery is available with separate personnel and facilities; promptly discharge infected infants when medically

possible. For babies exposed in the contaminated nursery, provide separate medical and nursing personnel skilled in the care of infants with communicable diseases. Observe contacts for at least 2 weeks after the last case leaves the nursery; promptly remove each new infected case to the single nursery ward used for these infants. Maternity service may be resumed after discharge of all contact babies and mothers, and thorough cleaning and terminal disinfection. Put into practice the recommendations of 9A, in so far as feasible, in the emergency.

2) Carry out a thorough epidemiological investigation into the distribution of cases by time, place, person and exposure to risk factors to determine how transmission is occurring.

D. Disaster implications: None.

E. International measures: WHO Collaborating Centres.

V. DIARRHEA CAUSED BY ENTEROAGGREGATIVE *E. COLI* (EAggEC) ICD-9 008.0; ICD-10 A04.4

This category of diarrhea-producing *E. coli* is increasingly recognized as an important cause of infant diarrhea in developing countries, where it may be the most common cause of persistent diarrhea in infants. In animal models, these *E. coli* organisms evoke a characteristic histopathology in which EAggEC adhere to enterocytes in a thick biofilm of aggregating bacteria and mucus. The most widely available method to identify EAggEC is the HEp-2 assay, wherein these strains produce a characteristic "stacked brick" aggregative pattern as they attach to one another and to the HEp-2 cells; this is a plasmid-dependent characteristic mediated by novel fimbriae. Most EAggEC encode one or more cytotoxin/enterotoxin that are believed to be responsible for the watery diarrhea with mucus seen in infants and children infected with this pathogen. A DNA probe has been described. The incubation period is estimated at 20−48 hours.

1. Identification—This category of diarrhea-producing *E. coli* was first associated with infant diarrhea in a study in Chile in the late 1980s. It was subsequently recognized in India as being associated with persistent diarrhea (continuing unabated for at least 14 days), an observation that has since been confirmed by reports from Bangladesh, Brazil and Mexico.

2. Infectious agent—EAggEC harbour a virulence plasmid required for expression of the unique fimbriae that encode aggregative adherence and many strains express a cytotoxin/enterotoxin. Among the most common EAggEC O serotypes are O3:H2 and O44:H18. Many EAggEC strains initially appear as rough strains lacking O antigens.

3. Occurrence—Reports associating EAggEC with infant diarrhea, and particularly persistent diarrhea, have come from many countries in Latin America and Asia and from the Democratic Republic of the Congo (formerly Zaire) in Africa. Reports from Germany and the United Kingdom suggest that EAggEC may also be responsible for a small proportion of diarrheal disease in industrialized countries. In the United States, EAggEC have been associated with diarrhea in HIV-infected adults.

VI. DIARRHEA CAUSED BY DIFFUSE-ADHERENCE *E. COLI* (DAEC)　　　　　　　　ICD-9 008.0; ICD-10 A04.4

A sixth category of diarrhea-producing *E. coli* now recognized is diffuse-adherence *E. coli* (DAEC). The name derives from the characteristic pattern of adherence of these bacteria to HEp-2 cells in tissue culture. DAEC is the least well-defined category of diarrhea-causing *E. coli*. Data from several epidemiological field studies of child diarrhea in developing countries have found DAEC to be significantly more common in children with diarrhea than in matched controls; other studies have failed to find such a difference. Preliminary evidence suggests that DAEC may be more pathogenic in children of preschool age than in infants and toddlers. Two DAEC strains failed to cause diarrhea when fed to volunteers and no outbreaks due to this category have yet been recognized. At present little is known about the reservoir, modes of transmission, host risk factors or period of communicability of DAEC.

[P. Braam]

DIPHTHERIA　　　　　　　　　　　ICD-9 032; ICD-10 A36

1. Identification—An acute bacterial disease primarily involving tonsils, pharynx, larynx, nose, occasionally other mucous membranes or skin and sometimes conjunctivae or vagina. The characteristic lesion, caused by liberation of a specific cytotoxin, is an asymmetrical adherent greyish white membrane with surrounding inflammation. The throat is moderately to severely sore in faucial or pharyngotonsillar diphtheria, with cervical lymph nodes somewhat enlarged and tender; in moderate to severe cases, there is marked swelling and oedema of the neck with extensive tracheal membranes that progress to airway obstruction.

Nasal diphtheria can be mild and chronic with one-sided nasal discharge and excoriations. Inapparent infections (colonization) outnumber clinical cases. The toxin can cause myocarditis, with heart block and progressive congestive failure beginning about 1 week after onset. Later effects include neuropathies that can mimic Guillain-Barré syndrome. The lesions of cutaneous diphtheria are variable and may be indistinguishable from, or a component of, impetigo; peripheral effects of the toxin are usually not evident. Case-fatality rates of 5%-10% for noncutaneous diphtheria have changed little in 50 years.

Diphtheria should be suspected in the differential diagnosis of bacterial (especially streptococcal) and viral pharyngitis, Vincent angina, infectious mononucleosis, oral syphilis and candidiasis.

Presumptive diagnosis is based on observation of an asymmetrical, greyish white membrane, especially if it extends to the uvula and soft palate and is associated with tonsillitis, pharyngitis or cervical lymphadenopathy, or a serosanguineous nasal discharge. Bacteriological examination of lesions confirms the diagnosis. If diphtheria is strongly suspected, specific treatment with antibiotics and antitoxin should be initiated while studies are pending and continued even in the face of a negative laboratory report.

2. **Infectious agent**—*Corynebacterium diphtheriae* of gravis, mitis or intermedius biotype. Toxin production results when bacteria are infected by corynebacteriophage containing the diphtheria toxin gene *tox*. Nontoxigenic strains rarely produce local lesions; however, they have been increasingly associated with infective endocarditis.

3. **Occurrence**—A disease of colder months in temperate zones, primarily involving nonimmunized children under 15; often found among adults in population groups whose immunization was neglected. In the tropics, seasonal trends are less distinct; inapparent, cutaneous and wound diphtheria cases are much more common.

A massive outbreak of diphtheria began in the Russian Federation in 1990 and spread to all countries of the former Soviet Union and Mongolia. Contributing factors included increased susceptibility among adults due to waning of vaccine-induced immunity, failure to fully immunize children due to unwarranted contraindications, antivaccine movements and declining socioeconomic conditions. This epidemic declined after reaching a peak in 1995; it was responsible for more than 150 000 reported cases and 5000 deaths (1990–1997). In Ecuador, an outbreak of about 200 cases, half of whom were 15 or older, occurred in 1993-94. In both epidemics, control was achieved through mass immunization activities.

4. **Reservoir**—Humans.

5. **Mode of transmission**—Contact with a patient or carrier; more rarely, contact with articles soiled with discharges from lesions of infected people. Raw milk has served as a vehicle.

6. **Incubation period**—Usually 2-5 days, occasionally longer.

7. **Period of communicability**—Variable, until virulent bacilli have disappeared from discharges and lesions; usually 2 weeks or less, seldom more than 4 weeks. Effective antibiotherapy promptly terminates shedding. The rare chronic carrier may shed organisms for 6 months or more.

8. **Susceptibility**—Infants born to immune mothers have passive protection, which is usually lost before the 6th month. Disease or inapparent infection usually, but not always, induces lifelong immunity. Immunization with toxoid produces prolonged but not lifelong immunity. Serosurveys in the USA indicate that more than 40% of adults lack protective levels of circulating antitoxin; decreasing immunity levels have also been found in Australia, Canada and several European countries. Many of these older adults may have immunological memory and would be protected against disease after exposure. Antitoxic immunity protects against systemic disease but not against colonization in the nasopharynx.

9. **Methods of control**—

   A. *Preventive measures:*

   1) Educational measures are important: inform the public, particularly parents of young children, of the hazards of diphtheria and the need for active immunization.

   2) The only effective control is widespread active immunization with diphtheria toxoid. Immunization should be initiated in infancy with a formulation containing diphtheria toxoid, tetanus toxoid and either acellular pertussis antigens (DTaP, preferred in the USA) or whole cell pertussis vaccine (DTP). Formulations that combine diphtheria and tetanus toxoid, whole cell pertussis, and *Haemophilus influenzae* type b vaccine (DTP-Hib) are also available.

   3) The schedule recommended in developing countries is at least 3 primary doses IM at 6, 10 and 14 weeks of age with a DTP booster at 18 months to 4.

      The following schedules are recommended for use in industrialized countries (some countries may recommend different ages or dosages):

      a) For children under 7—

         A primary series of diphtheria toxoid combined with other antigens, such as DTaP, or DTP-Hib. The first 3 doses are given at 4- to 8-week intervals beginning when the infant is 6−8 weeks; a fourth dose 6-12 months after the third dose. This schedule should not entail restarting immunizations because of delays in administering the scheduled doses. A fifth dose is given at 4-6 years prior to school entry; this dose is not necessary if the fourth dose was given after the fourth birthday. If the pertussis component of DTP is contraindicated, diphtheria and tetanus toxoids for children (DT) should be substituted.

b) For persons 7 and older—

Because adverse reactions may increase with age, a preparation with a reduced concentration of diphtheria toxoid (adult Td) is usually given after the seventh birthday for booster doses. For a previously unimmunized individual, a primary series of 3 doses of adsorbed tetanus and diphtheria toxoids (Td) is advised, 2 doses at 4- to 8-week intervals and the third 6 months to 1 year after the second dose. Limited data from Sweden suggest that this regimen may not induce protective antibody levels in most adults, and additional doses may be needed.

c) Active protection should be maintained by administering a dose of Td every 10 years thereafter.

4) Special efforts should be made to ensure that those who are at higher risk of patient exposure, such as health workers, are fully immunized and receive a booster dose of Td every 10 years.

5) For those who are severely immunocompromised or infected with HIV, diphtheria immunization is indicated, with the same schedule and dose as for immunocompetent persons, even though immune response may be suboptimal.

B. Control of patient, contacts and the immediate environment:

1) Report to local health authority: Case report obligatory in most countries, Class 2 (see Reporting).

2) Isolation: Strict isolation for pharyngeal diphtheria, contact isolation for cutaneous diphtheria, until 2 cultures from both throat and nose (and skin lesions in cutaneous diphtheria), not less than 24 hours apart, and not less than 24 hours after cessation of antibiotherapy, fail to show *C. diphtheriae*. Where culture is impractical, isolation may end after 14 days of appropriate antibiotherapy (see 9B7).

3) Concurrent disinfection: Of all articles in contact with patient and all articles soiled by discharges of patient. Terminal cleaning.

4) Quarantine: Adult contacts whose occupations involve handling food (especially milk) or close association with non-immunized children should be excluded from that work until treated as described below and bacteriological examination proves them not to be carriers.

5) Management of contacts: All close contacts should have cultures taken from nose and throat and be kept under

surveillance for 7 days. A single dose of benzathine penicillin (IM, see 9B7 for doses) or a 7–10 day course of erythromycin (PO, 40 mg/kg/day for children and 1 gram/day for adults) is recommended for all persons with household exposure to diphtheria, regardless of immunization status. Those who handle food or work with school children should be excluded from work or school until proven not to be carriers. Previously immunized contacts should receive a booster dose of diphtheria toxoid if more than 5 years have elapsed since their last dose, and a primary series should be initiated in nonimmunized contacts; use Td, DT, DTP, DTaP or DTP-Hib vaccine, depending on the contact's age.

6) Investigation of contacts and source of infection: Searching for carriers by use of nose and throat cultures, other than among close contacts, is neither useful nor indicated if provisions of 9B5 are carried out.

7) Specific treatment: Sensitivity testing (skin or eye testing) should be undertaken before giving antitoxin—only antitoxin of equine origin is available. After completion of tests to rule out hypersensitivity, if diphtheria is strongly suspected on the basis of clinical findings, a single dose of antitoxin (in the range of 20 000 units for anterior nasal diphtheria to 100 000 units for extensive disease of >3days' duration) given daily intramuscularly for 14 days immediately after bacteriological specimens are taken, without waiting for results (in the USA: 404-639-8255 or 404-639-2888). Antibiotics are not a substitute for antitoxin. Procaine penicillin G (IM) (25 000 to 50 000 units/kg/day for children and 1.2 million units/kg/day for adults, in 2 divided doses) or parenteral erythromycin (40–50 mg/kg/day, with a maximum of 2 grams/day) has been recommended until the patient can swallow comfortably, at which point erythromycin PO in 4 divided doses or penicillin V PO (125–250 mg 4 times daily) may be substituted for a recommended total treatment period of 14 days. Some erythromycin-resistant strains have been identified, but they are uncommon and not a public health problem. Newer macrolide antibiotics, including azithromycin and clarithromycin, do not offer any substantial advantage over erythromycin.

Prophylactic treatment of carriers: A single dose of benzathine penicillin G (IM) (600 000 units for persons under 6 years and 1.2 million units for persons 6 or older) or a 7–10 day course of erythromycin (PO, 40 mg/kg/day for children and 1 gram/day for adults) has been recommended. If culture is positive, treat as patients.

C. Epidemic measures:

1) Immunize the largest possible proportion of the population group involved, especially infants and preschool children. In an epidemic involving adults, immunize groups that are most affected or at high risk. Repeat immunization procedures 1 month later to provide at least 2 doses to recipients.

2) Identify close contacts and define population groups at special risk. In areas with appropriate facilities, carry out a prompt field investigation of reported cases to verify the diagnosis and to determine the biotype and toxigenicity of *C. diphtheriae.*

D. Disaster implications:
Outbreaks can occur when social or natural conditions lead to crowding of susceptible groups, especially infants and children. This frequently occurs when there are large-scale movements of susceptible populations.

E. International measures:
People travelling to or through countries where either faucial or cutaneous diphtheria is common should receive primary immunization if necessary, or a booster dose of Td for those previously immunized.

[J. Clements]

DIPHYLLOBOTHRIASIS ICD-9 123.4; ICD-10 B70.0
(Dibothriocephaliasis, Broad or fish tapeworm infection)

1. Identification—An intestinal tapeworm infection of long duration; symptoms commonly are trivial or absent. A few patients in whom the worms are attached to the jejunum rather than to the ileum develop vitamin B12 deficiency anaemia. Massive infections may be associated with diarrhea, obstruction of the bile duct or intestine, and toxic symptoms.

Identification of eggs or segments (proglottids) of the worm in feces confirms the diagnosis.

2. Infectious agents—*Diphyllobothrium latum* (*Dibothriocephalus latus*), *D. pacificum, D. dendriticum, D. ursi, D. dalliae* and *D. klebanovskii,* all cestodes.

3. Occurrence—The disease occurs in lake regions in the northern hemisphere, and subarctic, temperate and tropical zones where eating raw or partly cooked freshwater fish is popular. Prevalence increases with age. In North America, endemic foci have been found among Eskimos in Alaska and Canada. Infections in the USA are sporadic and usually come from eating uncooked fish from Alaska or, less commonly, from midwestern or Canadian lakes. Japan and Peru report cases of *D. pacificum* infection among consumers of marine (but not freshwater) fish.

4. Reservoir—Humans; mainly infected hosts discharging eggs in feces; reservoir hosts other than people include dogs, bears and other fish eating mammals.

5. Mode of transmission—Humans acquire the infection by eating raw or inadequately cooked fish. Eggs in mature segments of the worm are discharged in feces into bodies of fresh water, where they mature and hatch; ciliated embryos (coracidium) infect the first intermediate host (copepods of the genera *Cyclops* and *Diaptomus*) and become procercoid larvae. Susceptible species of freshwater fish (pike, perch, turbot, salmon) ingest infected copepods and become second intermediate hosts, in which the worms transform into the plerocercoid (larval) stage, which is infective for people and fish eating mammals, e.g. fox, mink, bear, cat, dog, pig, walrus and seal. The egg-to-egg cycle takes at least 11 weeks.

6. Incubation period—From 3 to 6 weeks between ingestion and passage of eggs in the stool.

7. Period of communicability—No direct person-to-person transmission. Humans and other definitive hosts disseminate eggs into the environment as long as worms remain in the intestine, sometimes for many years.

8. Susceptibility—People are universally susceptible. No apparent resistance follows infection.

9. Methods of control—

   A. Preventive measures: Thorough heating of freshwater fish (56°C/133°F for 5 minutes), freezing for 24 hours at −18°C (0°F), or irradiation.

   B. Control of patient, contacts and the immediate environment:

     1) Report to local health authority: Official report not ordinarily justifiable, Class 5 (see Reporting). Report indicated if a commercial source is implicated.
     2) Isolation: Not applicable.
     3) Concurrent disinfection: Sanitary disposal of feces.
     4) Quarantine: Not applicable.
     5) Immmunization of contacts: Not applicable.
     6) Investigation of contacts and source of infection: Not usually justified.
     7) Specific treatment: Praziquantel or niclosamide are the drugs of choice.

C. Epidemic measures: None.

D. Disaster implications: None.

E. International measures: None.

[L. Savioli]

DRACUNCULIASIS   ICD-9 125.7; ICD-10 B72
(Guinea worm disease, Dracontiasis)

1. Identification—An infection of the subcutaneous and deeper tissues by a large nematode. A blister appears, usually on a lower extremity (especially the foot) when the gravid 60–100 cm long adult female worm is ready to discharge its larvae. Burning and itching of the skin in the area of the lesion and frequently fever, nausea, vomiting, diarrhea, dyspnoea, generalized urticaria and eosinophilia may accompany or precede vesicle formation. After the vesicle ruptures, the worm discharges larvae whenever the infected part is immersed in fresh water. The prognosis is good unless bacterial infection of the lesion occurs; such secondary infections may produce arthritis, synovitis, ankylosis and contractures of the involved limb and may be life-threatening. Tetanus infections may occur via the site of the lesion.

Diagnosis is made by visual recognition of the adult worm protruding from a skin lesion or by microscopic identification of larvae.

2. Infectious agent—*Dracunculus medinensis*, a nematode.

3. Occurrence—In Africa (13 countries south of the Sahara). Local prevalence varies greatly. In some locales, nearly all inhabitants are infected, in others, few, mainly young adults.

4. Reservoir—Humans; there are no other known animal reservoirs.

5. Mode of transmission—Larvae discharged by the female worm into stagnant fresh water are ingested by minute crustacean copepods (*Cyclops* spp). In about 2 weeks, the larvae develop into the infective stage. People swallow the infected copepods in drinking water from infested step wells and ponds. The larvae are liberated in the stomach, cross the duodenal wall, migrate through the viscera and become adults. The female, after mating, grows and develops to full maturity, then migrates to the subcutaneous tissues (most frequently of the legs).

6. Incubation period—About 12 months.

7. Period of communicability—From rupture of vesicle until larvae have been completely evacuated from the uterus of the gravid worm, usually 2–3 weeks. In water, the larvae are infective for the copepods for about 5 days. After ingestion by copepods, the larvae become infective for people after 12–14 days at temperatures above 25°C (77°F), and remain infective in the copepods for about 3 weeks, the life span of an infected copepod. No direct person-to-person transmision.

8. Susceptibility—Susceptibility is universal. No acquired immunity; multiple and repeated infections may occur in the same person.

9. Methods of control/eradication—The provision of safe, filtered drinking water and health education of the populations at risk could lead to eradication of the disease. Foci of disease formerly present in some parts of the Middle East and the Indian subcontinent have been eliminated in this manner.

A. Preventive measures:

1) Provide health education programs in endemic communities to convey 3 messages: 1) that guinea worm infection comes from their drinking unsafe water; 2) that villagers with blisters or ulcers should not enter any source of drinking water; and 3) that drinking water should be filtered through fine mesh cloth (such as nylon gauze with a mesh size of 100 micrometers) to remove copepods.
2) Provide potable water. Abolish step wells or convert them to draw wells. Construction of protected wells or rainwater catchments can provide noninfected water.
3) Control copepod populations in ponds, tanks, reservoirs and step wells by use of the insecticide temephos, which is effective and safe.
4) Immunize high-risk populations against tetanus.

B. Control of patient, contacts and the immediate environment:

1) Report to local health authority: Case report required wherever the disease occurs, as part of the WHO eradication program, Class 2 (see Reporting).
2) Isolation: Cases are contained and advised not to enter drinking water sources while worm is emerged.
3) Concurrent disinfection: Not applicable.
4) Quarantine: Not applicable.
5) Immmunization of contacts: Not applicable.
6) Investigation of contacts and source of infection: Obtain information as to source of drinking water at probable time of infection (about 1 year previously). Search for other cases.
7) Specific treatment: Tetanus toxoid and local treatment with antibiotic ointment and occlusive bandage. Aseptic surgical extraction just prior to worm emergence is only possible on an individual basis but not applicable as a public health

measure of eradication. Drugs, such as thiabendazole, albendazole, ivermectin and metronidazole have no therapeutic value.

C. *Epidemic measures:* In hyperendemic situations, field survey to determine prevalence, discover sources of infection and guide control/eradication measures as described under 9A.

D. *Disaster implications:* None.

E. *International measures:* The World Health Assembly adopted a resolution (WHA 44.5, May 1991) to eradicate dracunculiasis by 1995. As of mid-2003, the disease remains endemic in 13 sub-Saharan countries only.

[M. Karam]

EBOLA-MARBURG VIRAL DISEASES   ICD-9 078.8; ICD-10 A98.4, A98.3
(African hemorrhagic fever, Ebola virus hemorrhagic fever, Marburg virus hemorrhagic fever)

1. Identification—Severe acute viral illnesses, usually with sudden onset of fever, malaise, myalgia and headache, followed by pharyngitis, vomiting, diarrhea and maculopapular rash. In severe and fatal forms, the hemorrhagic diathesis is often accompanied by hepatic damage, renal failure, CNS involvement and terminal shock with multiorgan dysfunction. Laboratory findings usually show lymphopenia, severe thrombocytopenia and transaminase elevation (AST greater than ALT), sometimes with hyperamylasaemia, elevated creatinine and blood urea nitrogen levels during the final renal failure phase. Case-fatality rates for Ebola infections in Africa have ranged from 50% to nearly 90%; 25%–80% of reported cases of Marburg virus infection have been fatal.

Diagnosis is usually through a combination of assays detecting antigen or RNA and antibody IgM or IgG. RT-PCR or ELISA antigen detection can be used on blood, serum or organ homogenates (the presence of IgM antibody suggests recent infection). Virus isolation attempts in cell culture or suckling mice must be undertaken in a BSL-4 laboratory. ELISA is used for specific IgM and IgG antibody detection in serum (the presence of IgM antibody suggesting recent infection). Virus may sometimes be visualized in liver, spleen, skin and other tissue sections by EM. Postmortem diagnosis through immunohistochemical examination of formalin-fixed skin biopsy or autopsy specimens is possible. IFA tests for antibodies have often been misleading, particularly in serological surveys for past infection. Laboratory studies represent an extreme biohazard and should be carried out only where protection against infection of the staff and community is available (BSL-4 containment).

2. Infectious agents—Virions are 80 nanometers in diameter and 970 (Ebola) or 790 nanometers (Marburg) in length, and are respectively members of *Ebolavirus* and *Marburgvirus* genus in the family Filoviridae. Pleomorphic virions with branched, circular or coiled shapes are frequent on electron microscopy preparation and may reach micrometers in length. The Ebola and Marburg viruses are antigenically distinct. In the Republic of Congo, Côte d'Ivoire, the Democratic Republic of the Congo (formerly Zaire), Gabon, Sudan and Uganda, 3 different subtypes of *Ebolavirus* (Côte d'Ivoire, Sudan and Zaire) have been associated with human disease. A 4th Ebola subtype, Reston, causes fatal hemorrhagic disease in nonhuman primates originated from the Philippines in Asia; few human infections have been documented and those were clinically asymptomatic.

3. Occurrence—Ebola disease was first recognized in 1976 in the western Equatoria province of the Sudan and 800 kilometers away in Zaire (now Democratic Republic of the Congo); more than 600 cases were identified in rural hospitals and villages; the case-fatality rate for these nearly simultaneous outbreaks was respectively about 55% and about 90%. A second outbreak occurred in the same area in Sudan in 1979. A new subtype of Ebola virus was recovered from one person probably infected while dissecting an infected chimpanzee in Côte-d'Ivoire in 1994. In 1995, a major Ebola outbreak with 315 cases and 244 deaths was centered on Kikwit (Democratic Republic of the Congo, formerly Zaire). Between the end of 1994 and the third trimester of 1996 three outbreaks reported in Gabon resulted in 150 cases and 98 deaths. A fatal secondary infection occurred in a nurse in South Africa.

Between August 2000 and January 2001 an epidemic (425 cases, 224 deaths) occurred in northern Uganda. From October 2001 to April 2003, several outbreaks were reported in Gabon and the Republic of Congo with a total of 278 cases and 235 deaths; high numbers of deaths were reported among wild animals in the region, particularly non-human primates. Antibodies have been found in residents of other areas of sub-Saharan Africa; their relation to the Ebola virus is unknown. End 2003, an outbreak in the Republic of Congo, with high case-fatality and thought to be related to contact with non-human primates, was rapidly controlled. In 2004 the Russian Federation and the USA reported 2 laboratory infections (1 fatal).

Ebolavirus, Reston subtype, have been isolated from cynomolgus monkeys (*Macaca fascicularis*) imported in 1989, 1990 and 1996 to the USA and in 1992 to Italy from the same export facility Philippines; many of these monkeys died. In Reston, 4 animal handlers with daily exposure to these monkeys in 1989 developed specific antibodies.

Marburg disease has been recognized on 5 occasions: in 1967, in Germany and what was then the Federal Republic of Yugoslavia, 31 humans (7 fatalities) were infected following exposure to African green monkeys (*Cercopithecus aethiops*) imported from Uganda; in 1975, the fatal index case of 3 cases diagnosed in South Africa had been infected in Zimbabwe; in 1980, 2 linked cases, 1 of which fatal, were confirmed in Kenya; in 1987, a fatal case occurred in Kenya. From 1998 to 2000, in the Democratic Republic of the Congo, at least 12 cases were confirmed among more than 145 suspected cases (case-fatality rate 80%) of Marburg viral hemorrhagic fever.

4. Reservoir—Unknown despite extensive studies. In Africa, Ebola infections of human index cases were linked to contact with gorillas, chimpanzees, monkeys, forest duikers and porcupines found dead or killed in the rainforest. So far, Ebola virus has been detected in the wild in carcases of chimpanzees (in Côte-d'Ivoire and Republic of Congo), gorillas (Gabon and Republic of Congo) and duikers (Republic of Congo), found dead in the rainforest.

5. Mode of transmission—Ebola infection of index cases seems to occur (i) in Africa, while manipulating infected wild mammals found dead in the rainforest; (ii) for Ebola Reston, while handling infected cynomolgus monkeys through direct contact with their infected blood or fresh organs. Person-to-person transmission occurs through direct contact with infected blood, secretions, organs or semen. Risk is highest during the late stages of illness when the patient is vomiting, having diarrhea or hemorrhaging, and during funerals with unprotected body preparation. Risk during the incubation period is low. Under natural conditions, airborne transmission among humans has not been documented. Nosocomial infections have been frequent; virtually all patients who acquired infection from contaminated syringes and needles died. Transmission through semen has occurred 7 weeks after clinical recovery.

6. Incubation period—Probably 2 to 21 days for both Ebola and Marburg virus disease.

7. Period of communicability—Not before the febrile phase and increasing with stages of illness, as long as blood and secretions contain virus. Ebola virus was isolated from the seminal fluid on the 61st, but not on the 76th, day after onset of illness in a laboratory acquired case.

8. Susceptibility—All ages are susceptible.

9. Methods of control—No vaccine and no specific treatment available as yet for either Ebola or Marburg. See control measures for Lassa fever: 9B, C, D and E; plus protection of sexual intercourse for 3 months or until semen can be shown to be free of virus.

[P. Formenty]

ECHINOCOCCOSIS ICD-9 122; ICD-10 B67

The larval stage (hydatid or cystic) of species of *Echinococcus* produces disease in humans and other animals; disease characteristics depend upon the infecting species. Cysts usually develop in the liver but also in other viscera, nervous tissue or bone. They can be: a) unilocular or cystic, b) multilocular or alveolar, c) polycystic.

I. ECHINOCOCCOSIS DUE TO *ECHINOCOCCUS GRANULOSUS* ICD-9 122.4; ICD-10 B67.0-B67.4
(Cystic or unilocular echinococcosis, Cystic hydatid disease)

1. Identification—Larval stages of the tapeworm *Echinococcus granulosus*, the most common *Echinococcus*, cause cystic echinococcosis or hydatid disease. Hydatid cysts enlarge slowly and require several years for development. Developed cysts range from 1–15 cm in diameter, but may be larger. Infections may be asymptomatic until cysts cause noticeable mass effect; signs and symptoms will vary according to location, cyst size, cyst type and numbers. Ruptured or leaking cysts can cause severe anaphylactoid reactions and may release protoscolices that can produce secondary echinococcosis. Cysts are typically spherical, thick-walled and unilocular, most frequently found in the liver and lungs, although they may occur in other organs.

Clinical diagnosis is based on signs and symptoms compatible with a slowly growing tumour, a history of residence in an endemic area, along with association with canines. Differential diagnoses include malignancies, amoebic abscesses, congenital cysts and tuberculosis. Radiography, computerized tomography and sonography along with serological testing are useful for laboratory diagnosis. WHO has developed a classification of ultrasound images on cystic echinococcosis for diagnostic and prognostic purposes and determination of the type of intervention required (see Treatment 9B7). Definitive diagnosis in seronegative patients, however, requires microscopic identification from specimens obtained at surgery or by percutaneous aspiration; the potential risks of this (anaphylaxis, spillage) can be avoided by ultrasound guidance and anthelmintic coverage. Species identification is based on finding thick laminated cyst walls and protoscolices as well as on the structure and measurements of protoscolex hooks.

2. Infectious agent—*Echinococcus granulosus*, a small tapeworm of dogs and other canids.

3. Occurrence—All continents except Antarctica; depends on close association of humans and infected dogs. Especially common in grazing countries where dogs consume viscera containing cysts. Transmission has been eliminated in Iceland and greatly reduced in Tasmania (Australia), Cyprus and New Zealand. Control programs exist in Argentina, Brazil, China, Kenya (Turkana district), Spain, Uruguay and other countries, including those of the Mediterranean basin.

4. **Reservoir**—The domestic dog and other canids, definitive hosts for *E. granulosus*, may harbour thousands of adult tapeworms in their intestines without signs of infection. Felines and most other carnivores are normally not suitable hosts for the parasite. Intermediate hosts include herbivores, primarily sheep, cattle, goats, pigs, horses, camels and other animals.

5. **Mode of transmission**—Human infection often takes place during childhood, directly with hand-to-mouth transfer of eggs after association with infected dogs or indirectly through contaminated food, water, soil or fomites. In some instances, flies have dispersed eggs after feeding on infected feces.

Adult worms in the small intestines of canines produce eggs containing infective embryos (oncospheres); these are passed in feces and may survive for several months in pastures or gardens. When ingested by susceptible intermediate hosts, including humans, eggs hatch, releasing oncospheres that migrate through the mucosa and are bloodborne to organs, primarily the liver (first filter), then the lungs (second filter), where they form cysts. Strains of *E. granulosus* vary in their ability to adapt to various hosts as well as their infectivity to humans.

Canines become infected by eating animal viscera containing hydatid cysts. Sheep and other intermediate hosts are infected while grazing in areas contaminated with dog feces containing parasite eggs.

6. **Incubation period**—12 months to years, depending on number and location of cysts and how rapidly they grow.

7. **Period of communicability**—Not directly transmitted from person to person or from one intermediate host to another. Infected dogs begin to pass eggs 5 to 7 weeks after infection. Most canine infections resolve spontaneously by 6 months; adult worms may survive up to 2−3 years. Dogs may become infected repeatedly.

8. **Susceptibility**—Children, who are more likely to have close contact with infected dogs and less likely to have adequate hygienic habits, are at greater risk of infection, especially in rural areas. There is no evidence that they are more susceptible to infection than are adults.

9. Methods of control—

A. Preventive measures:

1) Educate those at risk on avoidance of exposure to dog feces. Emphasize basic hygiene practices such as handwashing, washing fruits and vegetables and control of contacts with infected dogs.
2) Interrupt transmission from intermediate to definitive hosts by preventing access of dogs to potentially contaminated (uncooked) viscera through supervision of livestock slaughtering and safe disposal of infected viscera.
3) Incinerate or deeply bury infected organs from intermediate hosts.
4) Periodically treat high-risk dogs; reduce dog populations to the occupational need for them. Eliminate ownerless dogs whenever possible and encourage responsible dog ownership.
5) Field and laboratory personnel must observe strict safety precautions to avoid ingestion of tapeworm eggs.

B. Control of patient, contacts and the immediate environment:

1) Report to the local health authority: Not normally a reportable disease, Class 3 (see Reporting).
2) Isolation: Not applicable.
3) Concurrent disinfection. Not applicable.
4) Quarantine: Not applicable.
5) Immmunization of contacts: Not applicable.
6) Investigation of contacts and source of infection: Examine families and associates for suspicious tumours. Check dogs kept in and about houses for infection. Determine practices leading to infection.
7) Specific treatment: Surgical resection of isolated cysts is the most common treatment; PAIR (Puncture, Aspiration, Injection, Re-aspiration—percutaneous drainage of echinococcal cysts located in the abdomen with a fine needle or a catheter, followed by the killing of remaining protoscolices with a protoscolicide and by the re-aspiration of protoscolicide solution) is a minimally invasive technique of lesser risk than surgery; WHO recommends it for certain cysts (see *Puncture, Aspiration, Injection, Re-aspiration: an option for the treatment of cystic echinococcosis* http://whqlibdoc.who.int/hq/2001/WHO_CDS_CSR_APH_2001.6.pdf). Chemotherapy with mebendazole and albendazole has proved successful and may be the preferred treatment in many cases. If a primary cyst ruptures, praziquantel, a protoscolicidal agent, reduces the probability of secondary cysts.

C. *Epidemic measures:* In hyperendemic areas, control populations of wild and ownerless dogs. Periodical treatment of owned and community dogs with praziquantel. Strict control of livestock slaughtering; mandatory condemnation and destruction of infested organs. Improvement of infrastructure and inspection in rural abattoirs.

D. *Disaster implications:* None.

E. *International measures:* Control the movement of dogs from known enzootic areas.

II. ECHINOCOCCOSIS DUE TO *ECHINOCOCCUS MULTILOCULARIS*   ICD-9 122.7; ICD-10 B67.5-B67.7
(Alveolar echinococcosis or hydatidosis; Multilocular echinococcosis)

1. **Identification**—A highly invasive, destructive disease caused by the larval stage of *E. multilocularis*. Cysts are usually found in the liver; because their growth is not restricted by a thick laminated cyst wall, they expand at the periphery to produce solid, tumour-like masses. Metastases can result in secondary cysts in other organs. Clinical manifestations depend on the size and location of cysts but are often confused with hepatic cirrhosis or carcinoma. The disease is often fatal, although spontaneous cure through calcification has been observed.

Diagnosis is often based on histopathology, i.e. evidence of the thin host pericyst and multiple microvesicles formed by external proliferation. Humans are an abnormal host, and the cysts rarely produce brood capsules, protoscolices or calcareous corpuscles. Serodiagnosis using purified *E. multilocularis* antigen is highly sensitive and specific. A recently proposed staging and classification system (PNM) is based on a) Hepatic localisation of the parasite (P); b) extrahepatic involvement of neighboring organs (N); c) metastases (M).

2. **Infectious agent**—*Echinococcus multilocularis*.

3. **Occurrence**—Distribution is limited to areas of the northern hemisphere: Canada, central Europe, former Soviet Union, northern Japan, Alaska and rarely the north central USA. The disease is usually diagnosed in adults.

4. **Reservoir**—Adult tapeworms are largely restricted to wild animals such as foxes, and *E. multilocularis* is commonly maintained in nature in fox-rodent cycles. Dogs and cats can be sources of human infection if hunting wild (and rarely domestic) intermediate hosts such as rodents, including voles, lemmings and mice.

5. **Mode of transmission**—Ingestion of eggs passed in the feces of

Canidae and Felidae that have fed on infected rodents. Fecally soiled dog hair, harnesses and environmental fomites also serve as vehicles of infection.

6., 7., 8. and **9. Incubation period, Period of communicability, Susceptibility, Methods of control**—As in section I, *Echinococcus granulosus*; radical surgical excision is less often successful and must be followed by chemotherapy. Mebendazole or albendazole for a limited period after surgery, or long-term (several years) for inoperable patients may prevent progression of the disease; presurgery chemotherapy is indicated in rare cases. Liver transplantation has been carried out with limited success.

III. ECHINOCOCCOSIS DUE TO ECHINOCOCCUS VOGELI AND E. OLIGARTHRUS ICD-9 122.9; ICD-10 B67.9
(Polycystic hydatid disease)

This disease occurs in the liver, lungs and other viscera. Symptoms vary depending on cyst size and location. This species is distinguished by its rostellar hooks. The polycystic hydatid is unique in that the germinal membrane proliferates externally to form new cysts and internally to form septae that divide the cavity into numerous microcysts. Brood capsules containing many protoscolices develop in the microcysts. The causal agents are *Echinococcus vogeli* (over 100 cases) and *E. oligarthrus* (a few cases), encountered in Latin America. Immunodiagnosis using a purified antigen of *E. vogeli* does not always allow differentiation from alveolar echinococcosis. Albendazole has been used for chemotherapy.

[F. Meslin]

EHRLICHIOSES ICD-9 083.8; ICD-10 A79.8
(Human monocytotropic ehrlichiosis, Ehrlichiosis ewingii, Human granulocytotropic anaplasmosis, Sennetsu fever)

1. Identification—Ehrlichioses, or *Anaplasmataceae* infections, are acute, febrile, bacterial illnesses caused by a group of small, obligate intracellular, pleomorphic bacteria that survive and reproduce in the phagosomes of mononuclear or polymorphonuclear leukocytes of the infected host. The organisms are sometimes observed within these cells in the peripheral blood.

Human ehrlichioses in the USA, Asia and Europe are caused by 3 similar but distinct organisms. *Ehrlichia chaffeensis* affects primarily mononuclear phagocytes; the disease is known as human monocytotropic ehrli chiosis. *Ehrlichia ewingii* infects neutrophils of immunocompromised patients, the disease is ehrlichiosis ewingii. *Ehrlichia muris* detected in ticks in Japan and the Russian Federation appears to be an agent of human monocytotropic ehrlichiosis in the Russian Federation. The clinical spectrum ranges from mild illness to severe, life threatening or fatal disease. Ehrlichiosis ewingii and *E. muris* infection have not been associated with fatalities. Symptoms are usually nonspecific; commonly fever, headache, anorexia, nausea, myalgia and vomiting. About 20% of patients have meningoencephalitis. Human monocytotropic ehrlichiosis may be confused clinically with Rocky Mountain spotted fever, although rash occurs less often in the former. Laboratory findings include leukopenia, thrombocytopenia and elevation of one or more hepatocellular enzymes.

Anaplasma phagocytophilum, which infects neutrophils, causes human granulocytotropic anaplasmosis, an emerging infectious disease in Asia, Europe and North America, characterized by acute and usually self-limited fever, headache, malaise, myalgia, thrombocytopenia, leukopenia, and increased hepatic transaminases. Meningoencephalitis is rare. The illness ranges from mild to severe, with less than 1% case-fatality. Co-infections with *Borrelia burgdorferi*, *Babesia* spp., and tick-borne encephalitis viruses can occur (transmission from *Ixodes* ticks). There is no current evidence for persistent infection in humans.

Sennetsu fever caused by *Neorickettsia sennetsu* is characterized by sudden onset of fever, chills, malaise, headache, muscle and joint pain, sore throat and sleeplessness. Generalized lymphadenopathy with tenderness of the enlarged nodes is common. Atypical lymphocytosis with postauricular and posterior cervical lymphadenopathy is similar to that seen in infectious mononucleosis. The course is usually benign; fatal cases have not been reported.

Differential diagnosis includes various viral syndromes, Rocky Mountain Spotted Fever, sepsis, toxic shock syndrome, gastroenteritis, meningoencephalitis, tularaemia, Colorado tick fever, tick-borne encephalitis, babesiosis, Lyme borreliosis, leptospirosis, hepatitis, typhoid fever, murine typhus and blood malignancies. Diagnosis is based on clinical and laboratory findings and antibody detection using organism-specific antigens or *E. chaffeensis* as surrogate antigen for the uncultivated agent, *E. ewingii* (4-fold rise or fall in titre). Blood smears or buffy coat smears should be examined for the characteristic inclusions (morulae). Other diagnostic techniques include DNA amplification methods (e.g. PCR), culture, and immunohistochemistry.

2. Infectious agents—The agent of human monocytotropic ehrlichiosis, *E. chaffeensis*, is named after Fort Chaffee AK, USA, where the first patient from whom an isolate was obtained was infected. Human granulocytotropic anaplasmosis is caused by *A. phagocytophilum*, described in animals in 1932 and in humans in 1994. *E. ewingii*, which like *E. chaffeensis* is commonly found in deer and dogs, was identified in 1999 as another cause of human granulocytotropic ehrlichiosis. *Neorickettsia* *sennetsu* is the causal agent of sennetsu fever. These organisms are members of the family *Anaplasmataceae*. They were classified as members of the family *Rickettsiaceae* until 1984. The sennetsu agent was reclassified as *Ehrlichia* until 2001 when it was moved to the genus *Neorickettsia*.

3. **Occurrence**—In the USA, active prospective surveillance for human monocytotropic ehrlichiosis detects 10 cases per 100 000 population in rural and suburban areas south of New Jersey to Kansas as well as in California. Human granulocytotropic anaplasmosis occurs in areas of the USA endemic for Lyme disease as well as in Asia and Europe. Sennetsu fever appears confined to western Japan and perhaps Malaysia.

4. **Reservoirs**—The major reservoirs of *E. chaffeensis* and *E. ewingii* are white-tailed deer and dogs and for *A. phagocytophilum,* ruminants, cervids, and field rodents. *Neorickettsia* generally parasitize trematodes that live in aquatic hosts such as snails, insects, and fish. The trematode and aquatic hosts of *N. sennetsu* have not been identified.

5. **Mode of transmission**—Feeding ticks, particularly *Amblyomma americanum*, transmit *E. chaffeensis* and *E. ewingii*. *E. muris* has been identified in *Ixodes persulcatus* and *Haemaphysalis flava* ticks. The vectors of *A. phagocytophilum* are *Ixodes* spp., including *I. scapularis, I. ricinus, I. pacificus, I. trianguliceps, I. spinipalpis* and *I. persulcatus* ticks. The means of transmission is not known for sennetsu fever, although ingestion of an uncooked trematode-parasitized aquatic host by patients is suspected.

6. **Incubation period**—For sennetsu fever 14 days; 7–10 days for American ehrlichioses and 7–14 days for human granulocytotropic anaplasmosis.

7. **Period of communicability**—No evidence of person-to-person transmission.

8. **Susceptibility**—Susceptibility is believed to be general; older or immunocompromised individuals are likely to suffer a more serious illness. No data are available on protective immunity in humans due to infections caused by these organisms; reinfection is rare, but has been reported.

9. **Methods of control**—

    A. *Preventive measures:*

        1) None established for sennetsu fever.
        2) Measures against ticks should be employed (see Lyme disease, 9A) to prevent other ehrlichioses and human granulocytotropic anaplasmosis.

B. Control of patient, contacts and the immediate environment:

1) Report to local health authority: Case report required in most countries, Class 2 (see Reporting).
2) Isolation: Not applicable.
3) Concurrent disinfection: Remove any ticks.
4), 5) and 6) Quarantine, Immunization of contacts and Investigation of contacts and source of infection: Not applicable.
7) Specific treatment: Doxycycline is the drug of choice for adults and children. Rifampicin has been used for human granulocytotropic anaplasmosis in pregnant and pediatric patients. There is no established alternative drug for human monocytotropic ehrlichiosis. *E. chaffeensis* and *A. phagocytophilum* have shown resistance to chloramphenicol.

C. Epidemic measures: Not applicable.

D. Disaster implications: Not applicable.

E. International measures: Not applicable.

[D. H. Walker, J. S. Dumler]

ENCEPHALOPATHY, SUBACUTE SPONGIFORM ICD-9 046; ICD-10 A81
(Slow virus infections of the CNS)

A group of subacute degenerative diseases of the brain caused by unconventional filterable infectious agents, with very long incubation periods and no demonstrable inflammatory or immune response. The infectious agents are thought to be unique proteins replicating by an as yet unknown mechanism; the term prion may be an appropriate name and is generally accepted. Humans evidence 4 prion diseases: Creutzfeldt-Jakob disease (CJD), Gerstmann-Staussler-Scheinker syndrome (GSS), kuru, fatal familial insomnia; and animals 5: scrapie in sheep and goats, transmissible mink encephalopathy, chronic wasting disease of North American mule deer and elk, feline spongiform encephalopathy affecting domestic cats and bovine spongiform encephalopathy (BSE or "mad cow disease"). During the late 1990s, a new form of Creutzfeldt-Jakob disease, variant CJD (vCJD) emerged and has been linked causally to bovine spongiform encephalopathy.

I. CREUTZFELDT-JAKOB
DISEASE   ICD-9 046; ICD-10 A81.0
(Jakob-Creutzfeldt syndrome, Subacute spongiform
encephalopathy)

1. Identification—CJD has 4 different categories: sporadic (sCJD) accounting for 80%–90% of cases, iatrogenic CJD associated with medical use of infected pituitary-derived hormones and dura mater, familial CJD and the recently described vCJD. Subacute onset with confusion, progressive dementia and variable ataxia in patients aged 14 to over 80, almost all (more than 95%) 35 or older. Myoclonic jerks appear later, together with a variable spectrum of other neurological signs. Characteristically, routine laboratory studies and the CSF cell count are normal and there is no fever. Typical periodic high-voltage complexes are present in the electroencephalogram (EEG) in about 70% of cases and the CSF 14-3-3 protein is elevated in about 90%. The EEG is non-specific and the CSF 14-3-3 is not elevated in vCJD. Disease progresses rapidly; death usually occurs within 3–12 months (median 4 months, mean 7 months). Pathological changes are restricted to the CNS. About 10% of cases are associated with one of several mutations in the gene on chromosome 20 that encodes for prion protein (PrP), but only about one-third have a family history of CJD. One familial form of human prion disease, GSS, is characterised neuropathologically by many multicentric plaques and differs from CJD by an extended duration of illness and early ataxia.

CJD must be differentiated from other forms of dementia (especially Alzheimer disease), other infections (including encephalitis), toxic and metabolic encephalopathies and, occasionally, tumours.

Reports from the United Kingdom over the past 15 years have described over 130 000 BSE cases in domestic cattle. Concern that BSE might transmit to humans through consumption of beef products led to large-scale epidemiological and laboratory studies of BSE and CJD. In 1996 these studies suggested that a new form of CJD, designated variant CJD (vCJD), had occurred in the United Kingdom. This condition differs in several ways from conventional or sporadic CJD (sCJD). vCJD occurs in a younger age group (mean age at death 29, range 15–73) than sCJD and its clinical course is longer (mean 14 months vs. 7 months). The typical EEG changes of sCJD are not seen in vCJD, but the MRI scan in vCJD shows high signal in the posterior thalamus in about 90% of cases. By 2003 over 130 cases of vCJD had been identified in the United Kingdom and a few cases have been identified in other countries including Canada (1), France (6), Ireland (1), Italy (1) and the USA (1). The cases in Canada, Italy and the USA had a history of residence in the United Kingdom, where they may have been exposed to BSE. All tested cases of vCJD to date have been homozygous for methionine at codon 129 of the PrP gene. Laboratory transmission studies show that the infectious agent in vCJD is likely to be that of BSE.

Diagnosis of all forms of CJD is based on clinical features together with investigations, including EEG, CSF 14-3-3 assay and neuro-imaging. Brain biopsy and, in vCJD, tonsil biopsy can provide antemortem diagnosis, but these are invasive procedures and a definite diagnosis depends on postmortem examination of brain tissue.

2. Infectious agent—CJD is believed to be caused by a self-replicating host-encoded protein or prion protein. This is transmissible in the laboratory to many species, including wild and transgenic mice and non-human primates.

3. Occurrence—sCJD has been reported worldwide. The annual mortality rate for sCJD approaches or exceeds 1 per million, with familial clusters reported from Chile, Israel and Slovakia. The highest age-specific average mortality rate (more than 5 cases/million) occurs in the 65-79 age group. Over 130 cases of vCJD have been reported, mainly from the United Kingdom.

4. Reservoir—Human cases constitute the only known reservoir for sCJD. The reservoir for vCJD is believed to be BSE-infected cattle.

5. Mode of transmission—The mode of transmission for conventional or sporadic CJD (sCJD) is unknown; de novo spontaneous generation of the self-replicating protein has been hypothesized. Iatrogenic cases include 170 cases following human pituitary hormone therapy, 136 following human dura mater grafts, 3 linked to corneal grafts, and 6 linked to neurosurgical instruments. In all these cases it is presumed that infection from a case or cases of sCJD was inadvertently transmitted to another person in the course of medical/surgical treatment. The mechanism of transmission of BSE to humans has not been established, but the favored hypothesis is that humans are infected through dietary consumption of the BSE agent, probably beginning in the 1980s and now thought to have ended because of changes in animal feeding and slaughtering practices.

6. Incubation period—Iatrogenic cases: 15 months to over 30 years; the route of exposure influences incubation period: 15-120 months with direct CNS exposure, 4.5->30 years with peripheral exposure (human pituitary hormones given by injection). Incubation period unknown in naturally occurring sCJD and vCJD.

7. Period of communicability—Infection present in lymphoid tissues from early in the incubation period. The level of infectivity in the CNS rises late in the incubation period and high levels of infectivity occur in the CNS throughout symptomatic illness. In vCJD higher levels of infectivity are present in lymphoid tissues during clinical illness (and probably during incubation) than in sCJD. There is evidence that blood may be infective in some forms of experimental prion disease.

8. Susceptibility—Mutations of the PrP gene are associated with familial forms of human prion disease, with an autosomal pattern of inheritance. Polymorphic regions of the PrP gene influence susceptibility to infection and incubation period in animal species, including sheep and mice. In human disease, the genotype at codon 129 of the PrP gene influences susceptibility to sCJD (>70% methionine homozygous), vCJD (100% methionine homozygous) and iatrogenic CJD (an excess of homozygotes for either valine or methionine).

9. **Methods of control—**

    A. *Preventive measures:* Absolute avoidance of organ or tissue transplants from infected patients, and of reuse for potentially contaminated surgical instruments. WHO guidelines to minimize the risk of transmission of CJD (WHO/CDS/CSR/APH/2000.3 http://whqlibdoc.who.int/hq/2000/WHO_CDS_CSR_APH_2000.3.pdf) identify categories of individuals at higher risk of human prion diseases (family history of CJD, prior treatment with human pituitary hormones, prior neurosurgery). Blood transfusion has not been shown to have resulted in the transmission of CJD, but patients in higher risk groups should not act as blood donors.

    In relation to vCJD, the United Kingdom has introduced universal leukodepletion of blood donations; plasma products are now produced from blood sourced outside the United Kingdom. As a precautionary measure to reduce the theoretical risk of transmission of vCJD through blood or blood products some countries, including Canada and the USA, have requested blood centers to exclude potential blood donors who have resided for a specified period in the United Kingdom (and in some continental European countries).

    B. *Control of patient, contacts and the immediate environment:*

        1) Report to local health authority: official case report not ordinarily justifiable, Class 5 (see Reporting). The United Kingdom advises reporting to the local Consultant in Communicable Disease Control. Many countries have made CJD (including vCJD) a notifiable disease.

        2) Isolation: Universal precautions.

        3) Concurrent disinfection: the preferred policy for neurosurgical and ophthalmic instruments used in a patient with suspect CJD is their quarantine, with later destruction if the diagnosis of CJD is confirmed. Prions are remarkably resistant to disinfection and sterilisation, but sodium hydroxide (2M for 1 hour), sodium hypochlorite (20 000 ppm for 1 hour) and porous load autoclaving (134–137°C (273.2–278.6°F) for 18 minutes or 6 cycles at the same temperature for 3 minutes per cycle) all significantly decrease levels of infectivity.

        4) Quarantine: Not applicable

5) Immunisation of contacts: None
6) Investigation of contacts and source of infection: Obtain detailed history of past surgical procedures, exposure to human pituitary hormones or human dura mater grafts, as well as a family history.
7) Specific treatment: None.

C., D. and *E. Epidemic measures, Disaster Implications* and *International measures:* None, except for control of transborder passage of cattle and bovine meat.

II. KURU   ICD-9 046.0; ICD-10 A81.8

A fatal disease of the CNS presenting with cerebellar ataxia, incoordination, tremor and rigidity in patients aged 4 years or older. The disease occurs exclusively in the Fore language group in the highlands of Papua New Guinea and is caused by a self-replicating protein or prion. Kuru was transmitted by traditional burial practices involving consumption or smearing on the skin of infected tissues, including the brain. Formerly very common, the annual incidence of kuru has declined and only occasional cases now occur.

[F. Meslin]

ENTEROBIASIS   ICD-9 127.4; ICD-10 B80
(Pinworm infection, Oxyuriasis)

1. **Identification**—A common intestinal helminthic infection that is often asymptomatic. There may be perianal itching, disturbed sleep, irritability and sometimes secondary infection of the scratched skin. Other clinical manifestations include vulvovaginitis, salpingitis, and pelvic and liver granulomata. Appendicitis and enuresis have rarely been reported as possible associated conditions.

Diagnosis is made by applying transparent adhesive tape (tape swab or pinworm paddle) to the perianal region and examining the tape or paddle microscopically for eggs; the material is best obtained in the morning before bathing or passage of stools. Examination should be repeated 3 or more times before accepting a negative result. Eggs are sometimes found on microscopic stool and urine examination. Female worms may be found in feces and in the perianal region during rectal or vaginal examinations.

2. **Infectious agent**—*Enterobius vermicularis*, an intestinal nematode.

3. Occurrence—Worldwide, affecting all socioeconomic classes, with high rates in some areas. It is the most common worm infection in North America and other countries of temperate climate; prevalence is highest in school-age children (in some groups near 50%), followed by preschoolers, and is lowest in adults except for mothers of infected children. Infection often occurs in more than one family member. Prevalence is often high in domiciliary institutions.

4. Reservoir—Humans. Pinworms of other animals are not transmissible to people.

5. Mode of transmission—Direct transfer of infective eggs by hand from anus to mouth of the same or another person, or indirectly through clothing, bedding, food or other articles contaminated with parasite eggs. Dustborne infection is possible in heavily contaminated households and institutions. Eggs become infective within a few hours after being deposited at the anus by migrating gravid females; eggs survive less than 2 weeks outside the host. Larvae from ingested eggs hatch in the small intestine; young worms mature in the caecum and upper portions of the colon. Gravid worms usually migrate actively from the rectum and may enter adjacent orifices.

6. Incubation period—The life cycle requires 2–6 weeks. Symptomatic disease with high worm burdens results from successive reinfections occurring within months after initial exposure.

7. Period of communicability—As long as gravid females discharge eggs on perianal skin. Eggs remain infective in an indoor environment for about 2 weeks.

8. Susceptibility—Universal. Differences in frequency and intensity of infection are due primarily to differences in exposure.

9. Methods of control—

   A. Preventive measures:

1) Educate the public in personal hygiene, particularly the need to wash hands before eating or preparing food. Keep nails short; discourage nail biting and scratching anal area.
2) Remove sources of infection through treatment of cases.
3) Daily morning bathing, with showers (or stand-up baths) preferred to tub baths.
4) Change to clean underclothing, nightclothes and bedsheets frequently, preferably after bathing.
5) Clean and vacuum house daily for several days after treatment of cases.
6) Reduce overcrowding in living accommodations.
7) Provide adequate toilets; maintain cleanliness in these facilities.

B. *Control of patient, contacts and the immediate environment:*

1) Report to local health authority: Official report not ordinarily justifiable, Class 5 (see Reporting).
2) Isolation: Not applicable.
3) Concurrent disinfection: Change bed linen and underwear of infected person daily for several days after treatment, avoiding aerial dispersal of eggs. Use closed sleeping garments. Eggs on discarded linen are killed by exposure to temperatures of 55°C (131°F) for a few seconds; either boil bed clothing or use a washing machine on the "hot" cycle. Clean and vacuum sleeping and living areas daily for several days after treatment.
4) Quarantine: Not applicable.
5) Immunization of contacts: Not applicable
6) Investigation of contacts and source of infection: Examine all members of an affected family or institution.
7) Specific treatment: Pyrantel pamoate, mebendazole or albendazole. Treatment to be repeated after 2 weeks; concurrent treatment of the whole family may be advisable if several members are infected.

C. *Epidemic measures:* Multiple cases in schools and institutions can best be controlled through systematic treatment of all infected individuals and household contacts.

D. *Disaster implications:* None.

E. *International measures:* None.

[L. Savioli]

ERYTHEMA INFECTIOSUM HUMAN PARVOVIRUS INFECTION ICD-9 057.0; ICD-10 B08.3
(Fifth Disease)

1. Identification—Erythema infectiosum is a mild, usually nonfebrile, viral disease with an erythematous eruption that occurs sporadically or in epidemics, especially among children. Characteristic is a striking erythema of the cheeks (slapped face appearance) frequently associated with a lace-like rash on the trunk and extremities that fades but may recur for 1–3 weeks or longer on exposure to sunlight or heat (e.g. bathing). Mild constitutional symptoms may precede onset of rash. In adults, the rash is often atypical or absent, but arthralgias or arthritis lasting days to months or even years may occur; 25% or more of infections may be asymptomatic. Differentiation from rubella, scarlet fever and erythema multiforme often necessary.

Severe complications of infection with the causal virus are unusual, but persons with anaemia that requires increased red cell production (e.g. sickle cell disease) may develop transient aplastic crisis, often in the absence of a preceding rash. Intrauterine infection in the first half of pregnancy has resulted in fetal anaemia with hydrops fetalis and fetal death in less than 10% of such infections. Immunosuppressed people may develop severe, chronic anaemia. Several diseases (e.g. rheumatoid arthritis, systemic vasculitis, fulminant hepatitis and myocarditis) have been reported to occur in association with erythema infectiosum, but no causal link has been established.

Diagnosis, usually on clinical and epidemiological grounds; can be confirmed by detection of specific IgM antibodies against parvovirus B19 (B19), or by a rise in B19 IgG antibodies. IgM titres begin to decline 30-60 days after the onset of symptoms. Diagnosis of B19 infection can also be made by detecting viral antigens of DNA. PCR for B19 DNA is the most sensitive of these tests and will often be positive during the first month of an acute infection and in some persons for prolonged periods.

2. Infectious agent—Human parvovirus B19, a 20-25-nanometer DNA virus belonging to the family Parvoviridae. The virus replicates primarily in erythroid precursor cells.

3. Occurrence—Worldwide. Common in children; both sporadic and epidemic. In temperate zones, epidemics tend to occur in winter and spring, with a periodicity of 3-7 years in a given community.

4. Reservoir—Humans.

5. Mode of transmission—Primarily through contact with infected respiratory secretions; also, from mother to fetus, and parenterally through transfusion of blood and blood products. B19 is resistant to inactivation by various methods, including heating to 80°C (176°F) for 72 hours.

6. Incubation period—Variable; 4-20 days to development of rash or symptoms of aplastic crisis.

7. Period of communicability—In people with rash illness alone, greatest before onset of rash and probably not communicable thereafter. People with aplastic crisis are infectious up to 1 week after onset of symptoms, immunosuppressed people with chronic infection and severe anaemia for months to years.

8. Susceptibility—Universal susceptibility in persons with blood group P antigen, the receptor for B19 erythroid cells; protection appears to be conferred with development of B19 antibodies. Attack rates among susceptibles can be high: 50% in household contacts, and 10%–60% in the day care or school setting over a 2–6 month outbreak period. In the USA, 50%–80% of adults have serological evidence of past infection depending on age and location.

9. **Methods of control—**

  A. *Preventive measures:*

  1) Since the disease is generally benign, prevention should focus on those most likely to develop complications (e.g. underlying anaemia, immunodeficiency and pregnant women not immune to B19), who should avoid exposure to potentially infectious people in hospital or outbreak settings. Immunoglobulin (IG) has not yet had a trial for efficacy.
  2) Susceptible women who are pregnant or who might become pregnant, and have continued close contact to people with B19 infection (e.g. at school, at home, in health care facilities) should be advised of the potential for acquiring infection and of the potential risk of complications to the fetus. Pregnant women with sick children at home are advised to wash hands frequently and to avoid sharing eating utensils.
  3) Health care workers should be advised of the importance of following good infection control measures. Rare nosocomial outbreaks have been reported.

  B. *Control of patient, contacts and the immediate environment:*

  1) Report to local health authority: Community-wide outbreaks, Class 4 (see Reporting).
  2) Isolation: Impractical in the community at large. Cases of transient aplastic crisis in the hospital setting should be placed on droplet precautions. Although children with B19 infection are most infectious before onset of illness, it may be prudent to exclude them from school or day care attendance while fever is present.
  3) Concurrent disinfection: Strict handwashing after patient contact.
  4) Quarantine: Not applicable.
  5) Immunization of contacts: A recombinant B19 capsid vaccine is in the early stages of development.
  6) Investigation of contacts and source of infection: Exposed pregnant women should be offered B19 IgG and IgM antibody testing to determine susceptibility and to assist with counselling regarding risks to their fetuses.
  7) Specific treatment: Intravenous immunoglobulin (IGIV) has been successfully used to treat chronic anaemia in persistent

infections, but relapses can occur and require additional IGIV therapy.

C. *Epidemic measures:* During outbreaks in school or day care settings, those with anaemia or immunodeficiencies and pregnant women should be informed of the possible risk of acquiring and transmitting infection.

D. *Disaster implications:* None.

E. *International measures:* None.

EXANTHEMA SUBITUM ICD-9 057.8; ICD-10 B08.2
(Sixth disease, Roseola infantum)

1. Identification—Exanthema subitum is an acute, febrile rash illness of viral etiology, that occurs usually in children under 4 but is most common before 2. It is one manifestation of illnesses caused by human herpesvirus-6B (HHV-6B). A fever, sometimes as high as 41°C (106°F), appears suddenly and lasts 3–5 days. A maculopapular rash on the trunk and later on the remainder of the body ordinarily follows lysis of the fever, and the rash usually fades rapidly. Symptoms are generally mild, but febrile seizures have been reported.

The spectrum of clinical illness in children includes high fever without rash, inflamed tympanic membranes and, rarely, meningoencephalitis, recurrent seizures or fulminant hepatitis. In immunocompetent adults, a mononucleosis-like syndrome has been described, and in immunocompromised hosts, pneumonitis has been noted. HHV-6 also causes asymptomatic and latent infection. Differentiation from similar vaccine-preventable exanthems (e.g. measles, rubella) is often necessary.

Diagnosis can be confirmed by testing of paired sera for antibodies to HHV-6 by IFA or by isolation of HHV-6. Practical IgM tests are not available; an IgM response is usually not detectable until at least 5 days following the onset of symptoms. Detection of HHV-6 DNA in blood by PCR in the absence of concurrent IgG antibody shows promise as a future practical method for rapid diagnosis.

2. Infectious agent—Human herpesvirus-6 (subfamily, betaherpesvirus, genus Roseolovirus) is the most common cause of exanthema subitum. HHV-6 can be divided into HHV-6A and HHV-6B by using monoclonal techniques. Most HHV-6 infections in humans are now known to be caused by HHV-6B. Cases of exanthema subitum due to human herpesvirus 7 also occur.

3. Occurrence—Worldwide. In Hong Kong (China), Japan, the United

Kingdom and USA, where the seroepidemiology of HHV-6 has been best described, incidence peaks in 6-12 month olds, with 65%-100% sero-prevalence by age 2 years. Seroprevalence in childbearing women ranges from 80%-100% in most of the world, although rates as low as 20% have been observed in Morocco and 49% in Malaysia. Distinct outbreaks of exanthema subitum or HHV-6 are rarely recognized; a seasonal predilection (late winter, early spring) has been described only in Japan.

4. **Reservoir**—Humans appear to be the main reservoir of infection.

5. **Mode of transmission**—In children, the rapid acquisition of early childhood infection that follows the waning of maternal antibodies and the high prevalence of HHV-6 viral DNA in salivary glands of adults suggest that salivary contact with caregivers and parents is the most likely mode of infection. However, in one USA study, the age specific infection rate increased when there was more than one sibling in the household, which suggests that children may also be important reservoirs for transmission. Renal and hepatic transplants from HHV-6-infected donors can cause primary infection in seronegative transplant recipients.

6. **Incubation period**—Ten days, with a usual range of 5-15 days. Onset of illness is usually 2-4 weeks after transplantation in susceptible transplant recipients.

7. **Period of communicability**—In acute infection, unknown. Following acute infection, the virus may establish latency in lymph nodes, kidney, liver, salivary glands and in monocytes. The duration of potential communicability from these latent infections is unknown but may be lifelong.

8. **Susceptibility**—Susceptibility is general. Infection rates in infants under 6 months are low but increase rapidly thereafter, which suggests that temporary protection is conferred by transplacentally acquired maternal antibodies. Second cases of exanthema subitum are rare. Latent infection appears to be established in most persons but is of uncertain clinical significance, notably in persons who are immunosuppressed, among whom primary disease may be more severe and symptoms last longer.

9. **Methods of control**—Effective measures are not available.

   A. *Preventive measures:*

   1. Transplantation of organ tissues from HHV-6 seropositive donors to seronegative recipients is better avoided.

   B. *Control of patient, contacts and the immediate environment:*

   1. Report to local health authority: Official report not ordinarily justifiable, Class 5 (see Reporting).

2. Isolation: In hospitals and institutions, patients suspected of having exanthema subitum should preferably be managed under contact isolation precautions.
3. Concurrent disinfection: Not applicable.
4. Quarantine: Not applicable.
5. Immunization of contacts: Not applicable. Sustained immunity against reinfection following primary infections appears to occur and there is potential for a vaccine.
6. Investigation of contacts and source of infection: None, because of the high prevalence of asymptomatic shedders in the population.
7. Specific treatment: None

C. Epidemic measures: None.

D. Disaster implications: None.

E. International measures: None.

FASCIOLIASIS   ICD-9 121.3; ICD-10 B66.3

1. Identification—A disease of the liver caused by a large trematode that is a natural parasite of sheep, cattle and related animals worldwide. Flukes measuring up to about 3 cm live in the bile ducts; the young stages live in the liver parenchyma and cause tissue damage and enlargement of the liver. During the early period of parenchymal invasion, there may be right upper quadrant pain, liver function abnormalities and eosinophilia. After migration to the biliary ducts, the flukes may cause biliary colic or obstructive jaundice. Ectopic infection, especially by *Fasciola gigantica*, may produce transient or migrating areas of inflammation in the skin over the trunk or other areas of the body.

Diagnosis is based on finding eggs in feces or in bile aspirated from the duodenum. Serodiagnostic tests, available in some centers, suggest the diagnosis when positive. "Spurious infection" may be diagnosed when nonviable eggs appear in the feces after consumption of liver from infected animals.

2. Infectious agents—*Fasciola hepatica* and *F. gigantica*.

3. Occurrence—Human infection has been reported from 61 countries, mainly in sheep- and cattle-raising areas. Sporadic cases are reported in the USA. The infection is a public health problem in countries such as Bolivia, Ecuador, Egypt, Georgia, Peru, the Russian Federation and Viet Nam. Outbreaks have occurred in Cuba, the Islamic Republic of Iran, and to a lesser extent in Bolivia.

4. Reservoir—Traditionally humans are considered as an accidental host. The infection in nature is known to be maintained in a cycle between other animal species, mainly sheep, cattle, water buffalo and other large herbivorous mammals and snails of the family Lymnaeidae. In certain areas humans may also act as reservoir.

5. Mode of transmission—Eggs passed in the feces develop in water; in about 2 weeks a motile ciliated larva (miracidium) hatches. On entering a snail (lymnaeid), larvae develop to produce large numbers of free-swimming cercariae that attach to aquatic plants and encyst; these encysted forms (metacercariae) resist to drying. Infection is acquired by eating uncooked aquatic plants (such as watercress) bearing metacercariae. Free-floating metacercariae in drinking water can also transmit the disease. On reaching the intestine, the larvae migrate through the wall into the peritoneal cavity, enter the liver and, after development, enter the bile ducts to lay eggs 3–4 months after initial exposure.

6. Incubation period—Variable.

7. Period of communicability—Infection is not transmitted directly from person to person.

8. Susceptibility—People of all ages are susceptible; infection persists indefinitely.

9. Methods of control—

    A. Preventive measures:

        1) Educate the public in endemic areas to abstain from eating watercress or other aquatic plants of wild or unknown origin, especially from grazing areas or places where the disease is known to be endemic.
        2) Avoid using livestock feces to fertilize water plants.
        3) Drain the land or use chemical molluscicides to eliminate molluscs where this is technically and economically feasible.

    B. Control of patient, contacts and the immediate environment:

        1) Report to local health authority: Official report not ordinarily justifiable, Class 5 (see Reporting).
        2) Isolation: Not applicable.
        3) Concurrent disinfection: Not applicable.
        4) Quarantine: Not applicable.
        5) Immmunization of contacts: Not applicable.
        6) Investigation of contacts and source of infection: Identification of the source of infection may be useful in preventing additional infections in the patient or others.

7) Specific treatment: Bithionol was formerly the drug of choice but cure rates with this or praziquantel are not dependable. As of late 1999, the treatment of choice is triclabendazole. During the migratory phase, symptomatic relief may be provided by dehydroemetine, chloroquine or metronidazole. Nitrazoxinide is under investigation.

C. *Epidemic measures:* Determine source of infection and identify plants and snails involved in transmission. Prevent the consumption of aquatic plants from contaminated areas.

D. *Disaster implications:* None.

E. *International measures:* None.

[D. Engels]

FASCIOLOPSIASIS ICD-9 121.4; ICD-10 B66.5

1. Identification—A trematode infection of the small intestine, particularly the duodenum. Symptoms result from local inflammation, ulceration of intestinal wall and systemic toxic effects. Diarrhea usually alternates with constipation; vomiting and anorexia are frequent. Large numbers of flukes may produce acute intestinal obstruction. Patients may show oedema of the face, abdominal wall and legs within 20 days after massive infection; ascites is common. Eosinophilia is usual; secondary anaemia may occur. Death is rare; light infections are usually asymptomatic.

Diagnosis is made by finding the large flukes or characteristic eggs in feces; worms are occasionally vomited.

2. Infectious agent—*Fasciolopsis buski*, a large trematode reaching lengths up to 7 cm.

3. Occurrence—Widely distributed in rural southeastern Asia, especially central and south China, parts of India, and Thailand. Prevalence is often high in pig rearing areas.

4. Reservoir—Swine and humans are definitive hosts of adult flukes; dogs less commonly.

5. Mode of transmission—Eggs passed in feces, most often of swine, develop in water within 3–7 weeks under favorable conditions; miracidia hatch and penetrate planorbid snails as intermediate hosts; cercariae develop, are liberated and encyst on aquatic plants to become infective metacercariae. Human infections result from eating these plants uncooked. In China, the chief sources of infection are the nuts of the red water caltrop (*Tapa bicornis, T. natans*), grown in enclosed ponds, and tubers of the so-called water chestnut (*Eliocharis tuberosa*) and water bamboo (*Zizania aquatica*); infection frequently results when the hull or skin is peeled off with teeth and lips; less often from metacercaria in pond water.

6. **Incubation period**—Eggs appear in feces about 3 months after infection.

7. **Period of communicability**—As long as viable eggs are discharged in feces; without treatment, probably for 1 year. No direct person-to-person transmission.

8. **Susceptibility**—Susceptibility is universal. In malnourished individuals, ill effects are pronounced; the number of worms influences severity of disease.

9. **Methods of control**—

A. *Preventive measures:*

1) Educate the population at risk in endemic areas on the mode of transmission and life cycle of the parasite.
2) Treat night soil to destroy eggs.
3) Bar swine from contaminating areas where water plants are growing; do not feed water plants to pigs.
4) Dry suspected plants, or if plants are to be eaten fresh, dip them in boiling water for a few seconds; both methods kill metacercariae.

B. *Control of patient, contacts and the immediate environment:*

1) Report to local health authority: In selected endemic areas; in most countries, not a reportable disease, Class 3 (see Reporting).
2) Isolation: Not applicable.
3) Concurrent disinfection: Safe disposal of feces.
4) Quarantine: Not applicable.
5) Immmunization of contacts: Not applicable.
6) Investigation of contacts and source of infection: In the individual case, of little value. A community problem (see 9C).
7) Specific treatment: Praziquantel is the drug of choice.

C. *Epidemic measures:* Identify aquatic plants that harbour encysted metacercariae and are eaten fresh, identify infected snail species living in water with such plants and prevent contamination of water with human and pig feces.

D. Disaster implications: None.

E. International measures: None.

[D. Engels]

FILARIASIS   ICD-9 125; ICD-10 B74

The term filariasis denotes infection with any of several nematodes belonging to the family Filarioidea. However, as used here, the term refers only to the lymphatic-dwelling filariae listed below. For others, refer to the specific disease.

FILARIASIS DUE TO WUCHERERIA BANCROFTI   ICD-9 125.0; ICD-10 B74.0
(Bancroftian filariasis)
FILARIASIS DUE TO BRUGIA MALAYI   ICD-9 125.1; ICD-10 B74.1
(Malayan filariasis, Brugian filariasis)
FILARIASIS DUE TO BRUGIA TIMORI   ICD-9 125.6; ICD-10 B74.2
(Timorean filariasis)

1. Identification—Bancroftian filariasis is an infection with the nematode *Wuchereria bancrofti*, which normally resides in the lymphatics in infected people. Female worms produce microfilariae that reach the bloodstream 6–12 months after infection. Two biologically different forms occur: in one, the microfilariae circulate in the peripheral blood at night (nocturnal periodicity) with greatest concentrations between 10 pm and 2 am; in the other, microfilariae circulate continuously in the peripheral blood, but occur in greater concentration in the daytime (diurnal). The latter form is endemic in the South Pacific and in small rural foci in southeastern Asia where the principal vectors are day-biting *Aedes* mosquitoes.

Clinical manifestations in regions of endemic filariasis include: a) asymptomatic and parasitologically negative form; b) asymptomatic microfilaraemia; c) filarial fevers manifested by high fever, acute recurrent lymphadenitis and retrograde lymphangitis with or without microfilaraemia; d) lymphostasis associated with chronic signs, including hydrocoele, chyluria, lymphoedema and elephantiasis of the limbs, breasts and genitalia, with low-level or undetectable microfilaraemia; and e) tropical pulmonary eosinophilic syndrome, manifested by paroxysmal nocturnal asthma, chronic interstitial lung disease, recurrent low-grade fever, profound eosinophilia and degenerating microfilariae in lung tissues but not in the bloodstream (occult filariasis).

Brugian and Timorean filariasis are caused by the nematodes *Brugia malayi* and *B. timori* respectively. The nocturnally periodic form of *B. malayi* occurs in rural populations living in open rice-growing areas throughout much of southeastern Asia. The subperiodic form infects humans, monkeys and wild and domestic carnivores in the forests of Malaysia and Indonesia. Clinical manifestations are similar to those of Bancroftian filariasis, except that the recurrent acute attacks of adenitis and retrograde lymphangitis associated with fever are more severe, while chyluria is uncommon and elephantiasis is usually confined to the distal extremities, most frequently to the legs below the knees. Hydrocele and breast lymphoedema are rarely if ever seen.

Brugia timori infections have been described on Timor (now Timor-Leste) and on southeastern islands of Indonesia. Clinical manifestations are comparable to those seen in *B. malayi* infections.

Microfilariae are best detected during periods of maximal microfilaraemia. Live microfilariae can be seen under low power in a drop of peripheral blood (finger prick) on a slide or in hemolysed blood in a counting chamber. Giemsa-stained thick and thin smears permit species identification. Microfilariae may be concentrated by filtration of anticoagulated blood through a Nuclepore® filter (2-5 micrometer pore size), in a Swinnex® adapter, by the Knott technique (centrifugal sedimentation of 2 ml of anticoagulated blood mixed with 10 ml of 2% formalin), or by the Quantitative Buffy Coat (QBC) acridine orange/microhematocrit tube technique. More sensitive techniques to detect circulating filarial antigen of *W. bancrofti* by ELISA or immunochromatic test cards have recently become available commercially. The adult worms in nests can be diagnosed on ultrasound by the "filarial dance sign".

2. Infectious agents—*Wuchereria bancrofti*, *Brugia malayi* and *B. timori*; long threadlike worms.

3. Occurrence—*W. bancrofti*, the most commonly prevalent of the 3 parasites responsible for 90% of the lymphatic filariases, is endemic in most of the warm humid regions of the world, including Latin America (scattered foci in Brazil, Costa Rica, the Dominican Republic, French Guyana, Guyana, Haiti, and Suriname), Africa, Asia and the Pacific islands. It is common in those urban areas where conditions favor breeding of vector mosquitoes. In general, nocturnal subperiodicity in *Wuchereria*-infected areas of the Pacific is found West of 140°E longitude, and diurnal subperiodicity East of 180°E longitude. *B. malayi* is endemic in rural southwestern India, southeastern Asia, central and northern coastal areas of China and the Republic of Korea. *B. timori* occurs in Timor-Leste and on the rural islands of Flores, Alor and Roti in southeastern Indonesia.

4. Reservoir—Humans with microfilariae in the blood for *W. bancrofti*, periodic *B. malayi* and *B. timori*. In Malaysia, southern Thailand, the Philippines and Indonesia, cats, civets (*Viverra tangalunga*) and nonhuman primates serve as reservoirs for subperiodic *B. malayi* but zoonotic transmission is not of much significance.

5. Mode of transmission—Bite of a mosquito harbouring infective larvae. *W. bancrofti* is transmitted by many species, the most important being *Culex quinquefasciatus*, *Anopheles gambiae*, *An. funestus*, *Aedes polynesiensis*, *Ae. scapularis* and *Ae. pseudoscutellaris*. *B. malayi* is transmitted by various species of Mansonia, Anopheles and Aedes. *B. timori* is transmitted by *An. barbirostris*. In the female mosquito, ingested microfilariae penetrate the stomach wall and develop in the thoracic muscles into elongated, infective filariform larvae that migrate to the proboscis. When the mosquito feeds, the larvae emerge and enter the punctured skin following the mosquito bite. They travel via the lymphatics, where they moult twice before becoming adults.

6. Incubation period—Microfilariae may not appear in the blood until 3–6 months in *B. malayi* or 6–12 months in *W. bancrofti* infections described as the prepatent period.

7. Period of communicability—Not directly transmitted from person to person. Humans may infect mosquitoes when microfilariae are present in the peripheral blood; microfilaraemia may persist for 5–10 years or longer after initial infection. The mosquito becomes infective about 12–14 days after an infective blood meal. A large number of infected mosquito bites are required to initiate infection in the host.

8. Susceptibility—Universal susceptibility to infection is probable; there is considerable geographic difference in the type and severity of disease. Repeated infections may occur in endemic regions.

9. Methods of control—

   A. Preventive measures:

   1) Educate the inhabitants of endemic areas on the mode of transmission and methods of mosquito control.
   2) Identify the vectors by detecting infective larvae in mosquitoes caught; identify times and places of mosquito biting and locate breeding places. If indoor night biters are responsible, screen houses or use bednets (preferably impregnated with synthetic pyrethroid) and insect repellents. Eliminate breeding places (e.g. open latrines, tires, coconut husks) and treat with polystyrene beads or larvicides. Where *Mansonia* species are vectors, clear ponds of vegetation (*Pistia*) that serve as sources of oxygen for the larvae.
   3) Long-term vector control may involve changes in housing construction to include screening, and environmental control in order to eliminate mosquito breeding sites.

4) Mass treatment with diethylcarbamazine citrate (DEC), especially when followed by monthly treatment with a low dose (25–50 mg/kg body weight) of DEC for 1–2 years or the use of DEC-medicated cooking salt (0.2–0.4% w/w of salt) for 6 months to 2 years, has proven efficacious. However, DEC cannot be used in areas where onchocerciasis is co-endemic due to possible adverse reactions (see also Onchocerciasis, Mazzotti reaction). In areas co-endemic for onchocerciasis, ivermectin is used; albendazole in multiple and single doses also has anti-filarial properties. In lymphatic filariasis where onchocerciasis is not endemic, WHO currently recommends mass drug administration, as an annual single dose, of combinations of DEC 6 mg/kg body weight with 400 mg of albendazole for 4–6 years, or the regular use of DEC⁻ fortified salt for 1–2 years. In areas where onchocerciasis is co-endemic, the use of ivermectin and albendazole (400mg) is recommended. Certain groups of individuals such as pregnant women and children below 2 years (DEC and albendazole co-administration) or children under 90cm height and lactating women in the first week (ivermectin and albendazole co-administration), as well as severely ill persons, should not receive the drugs. Mass drug administration is contraindicated for the time being in areas with concurrent loiasis due to the risk of severe adverse reactions in patients with high density *Loa loa* infections.

B. *Control of patient, contacts and the immediate environment:*

1) Report to local health authority: In selected endemic regions; in most countries, not a reportable disease, Class 3 (see Reporting). Reporting of cases with demonstrated microfilariae or circulating filarial antigen provides information on areas of transmission.
2) Isolation: Not practicable. As far as possible, patients with microfilaraemia treated with anti-filarial drugs and should be protected from mosquitoes to reduce transmission.
3) Concurrent disinfection: Not applicable.
4) Quarantine: Not applicable.
5) Immmunization of contacts: Not applicable.
6) Investigation of contacts and source of infection: Only as part of a general community effort (see 9A and 9C).
7) Specific treatment: Diethylcarbamazine citrate (DEC) and ivermectin in combination with albendazole result in rapid and sustained suppression of most or all microfilariae from the blood, but may not destroy all the adult worms. Low level microfilaraemia may reappear after treatment. Therefore, treatment must usually be repeated at yearly intervals. Low

level microfilaraemia can be detected only by concentration techniques. DEC may cause acute generalized reactions during the first 24 hours of treatment because of death and degeneration of microfilariae; these reactions are mostly self-limiting and often controlled by paracetamol and antihistamines. Localized lymphadenitis and lymphangitis may follow the death of the adult worms and usually occurs 5–7 days after taking the drugs. Parasites primarily result in lymphatic damage, the subsequent lymphoedema and its progression are due to secondary bacterial infections.

Care of the skin to prevent entry lesions, exercise, elevation of affected limbs and use of topical anti-fungal or antibiotics when infected prevent acute dermato-adenolymphangitis and subsequent progression to lymphoedema. Management of lymphoedema includes local limb care; surgical decompression may be required. Hydrocoeles can be surgically repaired.

C. *Epidemic measures:* Because of low infectivity and long incubation period, epidemics of filariasis are almost unlikely.

D. *Disaster implications:* None.

E. *International measures:* WHO has launched a global program subsequent to the Resolution of the 1997 World Health Assembly calling for the elimination of lymphatic filariasis as a public health problem, through an alliance of endemic countries and partners from the public and private sectors. WHO Collaborating Centres. Further information on http://www.filariasis.org and http://www.who.int/tdr/diseases/lymphfil/default.htm

DIROFILARIASIS
(Zoonotic filariasis)

ICD-9 125.6; ICD-10 B74.8

Certain species of filariae commonly seen in wild or domestic animals occasionally infect humans, but microfilaraemia occurs rarely. The genus Dirofilaria causes pulmonary and cutaneous disease in humans. *D. immitis*, the dog heartworm, has caused a few reported infections in Australia, Japan, the USA and Asia. Transmission to humans is by mosquito bite. The worm lodges in a pulmonary artery, where it may form the nidus of a thrombus; this can then lead to vascular occlusion, coagulation, necrosis and fibrosis. Symptoms are chest pain, cough and hemoptysis. Eosinophilia is infrequent. A fibrotic nodule, 1–3 cm in diameter, which most commonly is asymptomatic, is recognizable by X-ray as a "coin lesion."

Various species, including *D. tenuis*, a parasite of the racoon in the

USA; *D. ursi*, a parasite of bears in Canada; and adult *D. repens*, a parasite of dogs and cats in Europe, Africa and Asia cause cutaneous lesions. The worms develop in or migrate to the conjunctivae and the subcutaneous tissues of the scrotum, breasts, arms and legs, but microfilaraemia is rare. Others (*Brugia*) localize in lymph nodes. Diagnosis is usually made by the finding of worms in tissue sections of surgically excised lesions.

OTHER NEMATODES PRODUCING MICROFILARIAE IN HUMANS

Several other nematodes may infect humans and produce microfilariae. These include *Onchocerca volvulus* and *Loa loa*, which cause onchocerciasis and loiasis, respectively (see under each disease listing). Other infections are forms of mansonellosis (ICD-9 125.4 and 125.5; ICD-10 B74.4): *Mansonella perstans* is widely distributed in western Africa and northeastern South America; the adult is found in the body cavities, and the unsheathed microfilariae circulate with no regular periodicity. Infection is usually asymptomatic, but eye infection from immature stages has been reported.

In some countries of western and central Africa, infection with *M. streptocerca* (ICD-9 125.4-125.6; ICD-10 B74.4) is common and is suspected of causing cutaneous oedema and thickening of the skin, hypopigmented macules, pruritus and papules. Adult worms and unsheathed microfilariae occur in the skin as in onchocerciasis. *M. ozzardi* (ICD-9 125.5; ICD-10 B74.4) occurs from the Yucatan Peninsula in Mexico to northern Argentina and in the West Indies; diagnosis is based on demonstration of the circulating unsheathed nonperiodic microfilariae. Infection is generally asymptomatic but may be associated with allergic manifestations such as arthralgia, pruritus, headaches and lymphadenopathy.

Culicoides midges are the main vectors for *M. streptocerca*, *M. ozzardi* and *M. perstans*; in the Caribbean area, blackflies also transmit *M. ozzardi*. *M. rodhaini*, a parasite of chimpanzees, was found in 1.7% of skin snips taken in Gabon.

Diethyl carbamazine is effective against *M. streptocerca* and occasionally against *M. perstans* and *M. ozzardi*. Ivermectin is effective against *M. ozzardi*.

[G. Biswas]

FOODBORNE INTOXICATIONS
(Food poisoning)

Foodborne diseases, including foodborne intoxications and foodborne infections, are terms applied to illnesses acquired through consumption of contaminated food; they are frequently and inaccurately referred to as food poisoning. These diseases include those caused by chemical contaminants such as heavy metals and many organic compounds; the more frequent causes of foodborne illnesses are: 1) toxins elaborated by bacterial growth in the food before consumption (*Clostridium botulinum*, *Staphylococcus aureus* and *Bacillus cereus*; scombroid fish poisoning—associated not with a specific toxin but with elevated histamine levels) or in the intestines (*Clostridium perfringens*); 2) bacterial, viral, or parasitic infections (brucellosis, *Campylobacter* enteritis, diarrhea caused by *Escherichia coli*, hepatitis A, listeriosis, salmonellosis, shigellosis, toxoplasmosis, viral gastroenteritis, taeniasis, trichinosis, and infection with vibrios); 3) toxins produced by harmful algal species (ciguatera fish poisoning, paralytic, neurotoxic, diarrhoeic or amnesic shellfish poisoning) or present in specific species (puffer fish poisoning, AZP).

This chapter deals specifically with toxin-related foodborne illnesses (with the exception of botulism). Foodborne illnesses associated with infection by specific agents are covered in chapters dealing with these agents.

Foodborne disease outbreaks are recognized by the occurrence of illness within a variable but usually short time period (a few hours to a few weeks) after a meal, among individuals who have consumed foods in common. Prompt and thorough laboratory evaluation of cases and implicated foods is essential. Single cases of foodborne disease are difficult to identify unless, as in botulism, there is a distinctive clinical syndrome. Foodborne disease may be one of the most common causes of acute illness; many cases and outbreaks are unrecognized and unreported.

Prevention and control of these diseases, regardless of specific cause, are based on the same principles: avoiding food contamination, destroying or denaturing contaminants, preventing further spread or multiplication of these contaminants. Specific problems and appropriate modes of intervention may vary from one country to another and depend on environmental, economic, political, technological and sociocultural factors. Ultimately, prevention depends on educating food handlers about proper practices in cooking and storage of food and personal hygiene. Toward this end, WHO has developed a document (http://www.who.int/fsf/Documents/5keys-ID-eng.pdf) called "Five Keys to Safer Food, as follows:

1. Keep Clean.
2. Separate raw and cooked.
3. Cook thoroughly.
4. Keep food at safe temperatures.
5. Use safe water and raw materials.

I. STAPHYLOCOCCAL FOOD INTOXICATION ICD-9 005.0; ICD-10 A05.0

1. Identification—An intoxication (not an infection) of abrupt and sometimes violent onset, with severe nausea, cramps, vomiting and prostration, often accompanied by diarrhea and sometimes with subnormal temperature and lowered blood pressure. Deaths are rare; illness commonly lasts only a day or two, but can take longer in severe cases; in rare cases, the intensity of symptoms may require hospitalization and surgical exploration. Diagnosis is easier when a group of cases presents the characteristic acute, predominantly upper GI symptoms and the short interval between eating a common food item and the onset of symptoms (usually within 4 hours).

Differential diagnosis includes other recognized forms of food poisoning as well as chemical poisons.

In the outbreak setting, recovery of large numbers of staphylococci (10^5 organisms or more/gram of food) on routine culture media, or detection of enterotoxin from an epidemiologically implicated food item confirms the diagnosis. Absence of staphylococci on culture from heated food does not rule out the diagnosis; a Gram stain of the food may disclose the organisms that have been heat killed. It may be possible to identify enterotoxin or thermonuclease in the food in the absence of viable organisms. Isolation of organisms of the same phage type from stools or vomitus of 2 or more ill persons confirms the diagnosis. Recovery of large numbers of enterotoxin-producing staphylococci from stool or vomitus from a single person supports the diagnosis. Phage typing and enterotoxin tests may help epidemiological investigations but are not routinely available or indicated; in outbreak settings, pulsed field gel electrophoresis may be more useful in subtyping strains.

2. Toxic agent—Several enterotoxins of *Staphylococcus aureus*, stable at boiling temperature, even by thermal process. Staphylococci multiply in food and produce the toxins at levels of water activity too low for the growth of many competing bacteria.

3. Occurrence—Widespread and relatively frequent; one of the principal acute food intoxications worldwide. About 25% of people are carriers of this pathogen.

4. Reservoir—Humans in most instances; occasionally cows with infected udders, as well as dogs and fowl.

5. Mode of transmission—Ingestion of a food product containing staphylococcal enterotoxin, particularly those foods that come in contact with food handlers' hands, either without subsequent cooking or with inadequate heating or refrigeration, such as pastries, custards, salad dressings, sandwiches, sliced meat and meat products. Toxin has also developed in inadequately cured ham and salami, and in unprocessed or inadequately processed cheese. When these foods remain at room temperature for several hours before being eaten, toxin-producing staphylococci multiply and elaborate the heat-stable toxin.

Organisms may be of human origin from purulent discharges of an infected finger or eye, abscesses, acneiform facial eruptions, nasopharyngeal secretions or apparently normal skin; or of bovine origin, such as contaminated milk or milk products, especially cheese.

6. Incubation period—Interval between eating food and onset of symptoms is 30 minutes to 8 hours, usually 2–4 hours.

7. Period of communicability—Not applicable.

8. Susceptibility—Most people are susceptible.

9. Methods of control

    A. Preventive measures:

        1) Educate food handlers about: (a) strict food hygiene, sanitation and cleanliness of kitchens, proper temperature control, handwashing, cleaning of fingernails; (b) the danger of working with exposed skin, nose or eye infections and uncovered wounds.

        2) Reduce food-handling time (from initial preparation to service) to a minimum, no more than 4 hours at ambient temperature. If they are to be stored for more than 2 hours, keep perishable foods hot (above 60°C/140°F) or cold (below 7°C/45°F; best is below 4°C/39°F) in shallow containers and covered.

        3) Temporarily exclude people with boils, abscesses and other purulent lesions of hands, face or nose from food handling.

    B. Control of patient, contacts and the immediate environment:

        1) Report to local health authority: Obligatory report of outbreaks of suspected or confirmed cases in some countries, Class 4 (see Reporting).

        2), 3), 4), 5) and 6) Isolation, Concurrent disinfection, Quarantine, Immunization of contacts and Investigation of contacts and source of infection: Not pertinent. Control is of outbreaks; single cases are rarely identified.

        7) Specific treatment: Fluid replacement when indicated.

C. Epidemic measures:

1) Through quick review of reported cases, determine time and place of exposure and population at risk; obtain a complete listing of the foods served and embargo, under refrigeration, all foods still available. The prominent clinical features, coupled with an estimate of the incubation period, provide useful leads to the most probable causal agent. Collect specimens of feces and vomitus for laboratory examination; alert the laboratory to suspected causal agents. Conduct an epidemiological investigation including interviews of ill and well persons to determine the association of illness with consumption of a given food. Compare attack rates for specific food items eaten and not eaten; the implicated food item(s) will usually have the greatest difference in attack rates and most of the sick will remember having eaten the contaminated food.

2) Inquire about the origin of incriminated food and the manner of its preparation and storage before serving. Look for possible sources of contamination and periods of inadequate refrigeration and heating that would permit growth of staphylococci. Submit leftover suspected foods promptly for laboratory examination; failure to isolate staphylococci does not exclude the presence of the heat-resistant enterotoxin if the food has been heated.

3) Search for food handlers with skin infections, particularly of the hands. Culture all purulent lesions and collect nasal swabs from all foodhandlers. Antibiograms and/or phage typing of representative strains of enterotoxin producing staphylococci isolated from foods and food handlers and from patient vomitus or feces may be helpful.

D. Disaster implications: A potential hazard in situations involving mass feeding and lack of refrigeration facilities, including feeding during air travel.

E. International measures: WHO Collaborating Centres.

II. CLOSTRIDIUM PERFRINGENS
FOOD INTOXICATION   ICD-9 005.2; ICD-10 A05.2
(C. welchii food poisoning, Enteritis necroticans, Pigbel)

1. Identification—An intestinal disorder characterized by sudden onset of colic followed by diarrhea; nausea is common, vomiting and fever are usually absent. Generally a mild disease of short duration, 1 day or less, rarely fatal in healthy people. Outbreaks of severe disease with high case-fatality rates associated with a necrotizing enteritis have been documented in postwar Germany and in Papua New Guinea (pigbel).

In the outbreak setting, diagnosis is confirmed by demonstration of *Clostridium perfringens* in semiquantitative anaerobic cultures of food (10^5/g or more) or patients' stool (10^6/g or more) in addition to clinical and epidemiological evidence. Detection of enterotoxin in patients' stool also confirms the diagnosis. When serotyping is possible, the same serotype is usually demonstrated in different specimens; serotyping is done routinely only in Japan and the United Kingdom.

2. Infectious agent—Type A strains of *C. perfringens* (*C. welchii*) cause typical food poisoning outbreaks (they also cause gas-gangrene); type C strains cause necrotizing enteritis. Disease is produced by toxins elaborated by the organisms.

3. Occurrence—Widespread and relatively frequent in countries with cooking practices that favor multiplication of clostridia to high levels.

4. Reservoir—GI tract of healthy people and animals (cattle, fish, pigs and poultry).

5. Mode of transmission—Ingestion of food containing soil or feces and then held under conditions that permit multiplication of the organism. Almost all outbreaks are associated with inadequately heated or reheated meats, usually stews, meat pies, and gravies made of beef, turkey or chicken. Spores survive normal cooking temperatures, germinate and multiply during slow cooling, storage at ambient temperature, and/or inadequate rewarming. Outbreaks are usually traced to catering firms, restaurants, cafeterias and schools with inadequate cooling and refrigeration facilities for large-scale service. Illness results from the release of toxin by cells undergoing sporulation in the lower intestinal tract. Heavy bacterial contamination (more than 10^5 organisms/gram of food) is usually required to produce toxin in the human intestine for clinical disease.

6. Incubation period—From 6 to 24 hours, usually 10–12 hours.

7. Period of communicability—Not applicable.

8. Susceptibility—Most people are probably susceptible. In volunteer studies, no resistance was observed after repeated exposures.

9. Methods of control—

A. Preventive measures:

1) Educate food handlers about the risks inherent in large-scale cooking, especially of meat dishes. Where possible, encourage serving hot dishes (above 60°C/140°F) while still hot from initial cooking.

2) Serve meat dishes hot, as soon as cooked, or cool them rapidly in a properly designed chiller and refrigerate until serving time; reheating, if necessary, should be thorough (internal temperature of at least 70°C/158°F, preferably 75°C/167°F or higher) and rapid. Do not partially cook meat and poultry one day and reheat the next, unless it can be stored at a safe temperature. Large cuts of meat must be thoroughly cooked; for more rapid cooling of cooked foods, divide stews and similar dishes prepared in bulk into many shallow containers and place in a rapid chiller.

B., C. and **D.** **Control of patient, contacts and the immediate environment, Epidemic measures** and **Disaster implications:** See Staphylococcal food intoxication (I, 9B, 9C and 9D).

E. **International measures:** None.

III. *BACILLUS CEREUS* FOOD INTOXICATION   ICD-9 005.8; ICD-10 A05.4

1. Identification—An intoxication characterized in some cases by sudden onset of nausea and vomiting, and in others by colic and diarrhea. Illness generally persists no longer than 24 hours and is rarely fatal.

In outbreak settings, diagnosis is confirmed through quantitative cultures on selective media to estimate the number of organisms present in the suspected food (generally more than 10^5 to 10^6 organisms per gram of the incriminated food are required). Isolation of organisms from the stool of 2 or more ill persons and not from stools of controls also confirms the diagnosis. Enterotoxin testing is valuable but may not be widely available.

2. Toxic agent—*Bacillus cereus*, an aerobic spore former. Two enterotoxins have been identified: one (heat stable) causing vomiting, is produced in food when *B. cereus* levels reach 10^5 colony-forming units/gram of food and one (heat labile) causing diarrhea, formed in the small intestine of the human host.

3. Occurrence—A well recognized cause of foodborne disease in the world.

4. Reservoir—A ubiquitous organism in soil and environment, commonly found at low levels in raw, dried and processed foods.

5. Mode of transmission—Ingestion of food kept at ambient temperatures after cooking, with multiplication of the organisms. Outbreaks associated with vomiting have been most commonly associated with cooked rice held at ambient room temperatures before reheating. Various mishandled foods have been implicated in outbreaks associated with diarrhea.

6. Incubation period—From 0.5 to 6 hours in cases where vomiting is the predominant symptom; from 6 to 24 hours where diarrhea predominates.

7. Period of communicability—Not communicable from person to person.

8. Susceptibility—Unknown.

9. Methods of control—

A. *Preventive measures:* Foods should not remain at ambient temperature after cooking, since the ubiquitous *B. cereus* spores can survive boiling, germinate, and multiply rapidly at room temperature. The emetic toxin is also heat-resistant. Refrigerate leftover food promptly (toxin formation is unlikely at temperatures below 10°C/50°F); reheat thoroughly and rapidly to avoid multiplication of microorganisms.

B, C. and D. *Control of patient, contacts and the immediate environment, Epidemic measures* and *Disaster implications:* See Staphylococcal food intoxication (I, 9B, 9C and 9D).

E. *International measures:* None.

IV. SCOMBROID FISH
  POISONING   ICD-9 988.0; ICD-10 T61.1
(Histamine poisoning)

A syndrome of tingling and burning sensations around the mouth, facial flushing and sweating, nausea and vomiting, headache, palpitations, dizziness and rash occurring within a few hours after eating fish containing high levels of free histamine (more than 20 mg/100 grams of fish); this occurs when the fish undergoes bacterial decomposition after capture. Symptoms resolve spontaneously within 12 hours and there are no long-term sequelae.

Occurrence is worldwide; the syndrome was initially associated with fish in the families Scombroidea and Scomberesocidae (tuna, mackerel, skipjack and bonito) containing high levels of histidine that can be decarboxylated to form histamine by histidine-decarboxylase-producing bacteria in the fish. Nonscombroid fish, such as mahi-mahi (*Coryphaena hippurus*), and bluefish (*Pomatomus saltatrix*), are also associated with illness. Risks appear to be greatest for fish imported from tropical or semitropical areas and fish caught by recreational or artisanal fishermen, who may lack appropriate storage facilities for large fish. Detection of histamine in epidemiologically implicated fish confirms the diagnosis,

Adequate and rapid refrigeration, with evisceration and removal of the gills in a sanitary manner prevents this spoilage. Symptoms usually resolve spontaneously. In severe cases, antihistamines may be effective in relieving symptoms.

While this is most often associated with fish, any food (such as certain cheeses) that contains the appropriate amino acids and is subjected to certain bacterial contamination and growth may lead to scombroid poisoning when ingested, especially in patients taking isoniazid or other drugs interfering with histamine metabolism.

V. CIGUATERA FISH
   POISONING   ICD-9 988.0; ICD-10 T61.0

A characteristic GI and neurological syndrome may occur within 1 hour after eating tropical reef fish. GI symptoms (diarrhea, vomiting, abdominal pain) occur first, usually within 24 hours of consumption. In severe cases, patients may also become hypotensive, with a paradoxical bradycardia. Neurological symptoms, including pain and weakness in the lower extremities and circumoral and peripheral paresthaesias, may occur at the same time as the acute symptoms or follow 1–2 days later; they may persist for weeks or months.

Symptoms such as temperature reversal (ice cream tastes hot, hot coffee seems cold) and "aching teeth" are frequently reported. In very severe cases neurological symptoms may progress to coma and respiratory arrest within the first 24 hours of illness. Most patients recover completely within a few weeks; intermittent recrudescence of symptoms can occur over a period of months to years.

This syndrome is caused by the presence in the fish of toxins elaborated by the dinoflagellate *Gambierdiscus toxicus* and algae growing on underwater reefs. Fish eating the algae become toxic, and the effect is magnified through the food chain so that large predatory fish become the most toxic; this occurs worldwide in tropical areas.

Ciguatera is a significant cause of morbidity where consumption of reef fish is common—Australia, the Caribbean, southern Florida, Hawaii and the South Pacific. Incidence has been estimated at 500-odd cases/100 000 population/year in the South Pacific, with rates 50 times higher reported for some island groups. More than 400 fish species may have the potential for becoming toxic. Worldwide, 50 000 cases of ciguatera occur per year. Evidence of ciguatoxin in epidemiologically implicated fish confirms the diagnosis.

The consumption of large predatory fish should be avoided, especially in the reef area, particularly the barracuda. Where assays for toxic fish are available, screening all large "high-risk" fish before consumption can reduce risk. The occurrence of toxic fish is sporadic and not all fish of a given species or from a given locale will be toxic. Intravenous infusion of mannitol (1 gram/kg of a 20% solution over 45 minutes) may have a dramatic effect on acute symptoms of ciguatera fish poisoning, particularly in severe cases, and may be lifesaving in severe cases that have progressed to coma.

VI. PARALYTIC SHELLFISH POISONING (PSP)   ICD-9 988.0; ICD-10 T61.2

Classic PSP is a characteristic syndrome (predominantly neurological) starting within minutes to several hours after eating bivalve molluscs. Initial symptoms include paresthaesias of the mouth and extremities, accompanied by GI symptoms, and usually resolving within a few days. In severe cases, ataxia, dysphonia, dysphagia and muscle paralysis with respiratory arrest and death may occur within 12 hours. Symptoms usually resolve completely within hours to days after shellfish ingestion.

This syndrome is caused by the presence in shellfish of saxitoxins and gonyautoxins produced by *Alexandrium* species and other dinoflagellates. Concentration of these toxins occurs during massive algal blooms known as "red tides" but also in the absence of recognizable algal bloom. PSP is common in shellfish harvested from colder waters above 30°N and below 30°S latitude, but may also occur in tropical waters. In the USA, PSP is primarily a problem in the New England states, Alaska, California and Washington. Blooms of the causative *Alexandrium* species occur several times each year, primarily from April through October. Shellfish remain toxic for several weeks after the bloom subsides; some shellfish species remain toxic constantly. Most cases occur in individuals or small groups who gather shellfish for personal consumption. Detection of toxin in epidemiologically implicated food confirms the diagnosis. On an experimental basis, saxitoxins have been demonstrated in serum during acute illness and in urine after acute symptoms resolve.

PSP neurotoxins are heat-stable. Surveillance of high-risk harvest areas is routine in Canada, the European Union; Japan and the USA use a standard mouse bioassay; when toxin levels in shellfish exceed 80 micrograms of saxitoxin equivalent/100 grams, areas are closed to harvesting and warnings posted in shellfish-growing areas, on beaches and in the media.

VII. NEUROTOXIC SHELLFISH POISONING   ICD-9 988.0; ICD-10 T61.2

Neurotoxic shellfish poisoning is associated with algal blooms of *Gymnodinium breve*, which produce brevetoxin. Red tides caused by *G. breve* have long occurred along the Florida coast, with associated mortality in fish, seabirds and marine mammals. Symptoms after eating toxic shellfish, including circumoral paresthaesias and paresthaesias of the extremities, dizziness and ataxia, myalgia and GI symptoms, tend to be mild and resolve quickly and completely. Respiratory and eye irritation also occur in association with *G. breve* blooms, apparently through aerosolization of the toxin through wind and wave action.

VIII. DIARRHETIC SHELLFISH
POISONING   ICD-9 988.0; ICD-10 T61.2

This was first reported in Japan in 1978, and thereafter worldwide. The causative toxins, dinophysistoxin-1 (DTX1), dinophysistoxin-2 (DTX2), dinophysistoxin-3 (DTX3), okadaic acid (OA), 7-*O*-acylDTX2 (acylDTX2), and 7-*O*-acylOA (acylOA) have been isolated. Illness results from eating mussels, scallops, or clams that have fed on *Dinophysis fortii* or *Dinophysis acuminata*. Symptoms include diarrhea, nausea, vomiting, and abdominal pain.

In scallops, the distribution of toxins was localized in the hepatopancreas (midgut gland), the elimination of which renders scallops safe to eat. Ordinary cooking such as boiling in water or steaming cannot reduce OAs in this gland because of their chemical stability and lipophilic properties. Methods of detection of PSP in shellfish include mouse bioassay, ELISA and liquid chromatography-mass spectrometry. The USA has established action level for DSP at 0.2 ppm okadaic acid (OA) plus 35-methyl okadaic acid (DXT1).

IX. AMNESIC SHELLFISH
POISONING   ICD-9 988.0; ICD-10 T61.2

Amnesic shellfish poisoning results from ingestion of shellfish containing domoic acid, produced by the diatom *Pseudonitzschia pungens*. Cases were reported in the Atlantic provinces of Canada in 1987, with vomiting, abdominal cramps, diarrhea, headache and loss of short term memory. When tested several months after acute intoxication, patients show antegrade memory deficits with relative preservation of other cognitive functions, together with clinical and electromyographical evidence of pure motor or sensorimotor neuropathy and axonopathy. Canadian authorities now analyse mussels and clams for domoic acid, and close shellfish beds to harvesting when levels exceed 20 ppm domoic acid.

In 1991, domoic acid was also identified in razor clams and Dungeness crabs on the Oregon and Washington coast (USA), and in the marine food web along the Texas coast. The clinical significance of ingestion of low levels of domoic acid (in persons eating shellfish and anchovies harvested from areas where *Pseudonitzschia* species are present) is unknown.

EC-directive 91/492/EEC and amendments for the safety of shellfish (Amendment 97/61/EC) state that: "total Amnesic Shellfish Poison (ASP) content in the edible part of molluscs (the entire body or any part edible separately) must not exceed 20 micrograms of domoic acid per gram using HPLC [high pressure liquid chromatography]."

X. PUFFER FISH POISONING
(TETRODOTOXIN)   ICD-9 988.0; ICD-10 T61.2

Puffer fish poisoning is characterized by onset of paresthaesias, dizziness, GI symptoms and ataxia, often progressing to paralysis and death within several hours after eating. The case-fatality rate approaches 60%. The causative toxin is tetrodotoxin, a heat-stable, nonprotein neurotoxin concentrated in the skin and viscera of puffer fish, porcupine fish, ocean sunfish, and species of newts and salamanders. More than 6000 cases have been documented, mostly in Japan. Toxicity can be avoided by not consuming any of the tetrodotoxin-producing species of fish or amphibians. Some fish species contain no or little tetrodotoxin in the muscle. Japan implements control measures such as species identification and adequate removal of toxic parts (e.g. ova, intestine) by qualified cooks.

XI. AZASPIRACID POISONING
(AZP)   ICD-9 988.0; ICD-10 T61.2

Occurrence of AZP was first reported when mussels harvested in Ireland caused diarrhea in humans in the Netherlands in 1995. Since 1996 several AZP incidents have been identified in several European countries, mainly through mussels. Symptoms occur 12 to 24 hours after consumption and persist for up to 5 days: they include severe diarrhea and vomiting with abdominal pain and occasional nausea, chills, headaches, vomiting, stomach cramps. Azaspiracid can cause necrosis in the intestine, thymus, and liver.

[H. Toyofuku]

GASTRITIS CAUSED BY
HELICOBACTER PYLORI   ICD-9 535; ICD-10 B96.8

1. Identification—A bacterial infection causing chronic gastritis, primarily in the antrum of the stomach, and duodenal ulcer disease. Infection with *Helicobacter pylori* is epidemiologically associated with gastric adenocarcinoma. The key pathophysiological event in *H. pylori* infection is initiation and continuance of an inflammatory response. Development of atrophy and metaplasia of the gastric mucosa are strongly associated with *H. pylori* infection. Oxidative and nitrosative stress in combination with inflamation plays an important role in gastric carcinogenesis.

Diagnosis may be made from a gastric biopsy specimen through the use of culture, histology or the detection of *H. pylori* urease using commercially available kits. The organism requires nutrient media for growth, such as Brain-Heart Infusion Agar with added horse blood. Selective media have been developed to prevent contaminating growth when culturing gastric biopsy material. Cultures should be incubated at 37°C (98.6°F) in microaerophilic conditions for 48–72 hours. Specific urea-based breath tests may also be used and are based on the organism's extremely high urease activity. The presence of specific serum antibodies can also be measured, most commonly by ELISA.

2. Infectious agent—*Helicobacter pylori* is a Gram-negative, "S" and "U" spirally shaped bacillus, catalase-, oxidase- and urease-positive. Many different *Helicobacter* species have been identified in other animals; *H. cinaedi* and *H. fennelliae* have been associated with diarrhea in men who have sex with men.

3. Occurrence—*H. pylori* has an estimated rate of infection of over one-half of the world population. It could reach up to 70% in developing countries and up to 20%–30% in industrialized countries. Only a minority of those infected develop duodenal ulcer disease. Although individuals infected with the organism often have histological evidence of gastritis, the vast majority are asymptomatic. Most *H. pylori* infections occur in children and atrophy of the gastric mucosa progresses during ageing. Cross-sectional serological studies demonstrate increasing prevalence with increasing age. Low socioeconomic status, especially in childhood, is associated with infection.

4. Reservoir—Mainly humans, though recently *H. pylori* has been found in other primates. Most infected persons are asymptomatic, and without treatment infection is often lifelong. Isolation of *H. pylori* from nongastric sites such as oral secretions and stool has been reported but is infrequent.

5. Mode of transmission—Not clearly established, but infection is almost certainly a result of ingesting organisms. Transmission is presumed to be either oral-oral and/or fecal-oral. *H. pylori* has been transmitted through incompletely decontaminated gastroscopes and pH electrodes.

6. Incubation period—Data collected from two volunteers who ingested 10^6–10^9 organisms indicate that the onset of gastritis occurred within 5–10 days. No other information about inoculum size or incubation period is available.

7. Period of communicability—Not known. Since infection may be lifelong, those infected are potentially infectious for life. It is not known whether acutely infected patients are more infectious than those with long-standing infection. There is some evidence that persons with low stomach acidity may be more infectious.

8. Susceptibility—All individuals are presumed to be susceptible to infection. Although poor socioeconomic conditions are an important risk factor for infection, there are scant data on individual susceptibility. A variety of cofactors may be required for the development of disease. No protective immunity apparent after infection.

9. **Methods of control—**

   A. *Preventive measures:*

      1) Persons living in uncrowded and clean environments are less likely to acquire *H. pylori*.
      2) Complete disinfection of gastroscopes, pH electrodes and other instruments entering the stomach.

   B. *Control of patient, contacts and the immediate environment:*

      1) Report to local health authority: Official report not ordinarily justifiable, Class 5 (see Reporting).
      2) Isolation: Not applicable.
      3) Concurrent disinfection: Of intragastric instruments.
      4) Quarantine: Patients infected with *H. pylori* need not be placed in quarantine restrictions.
      5) Immunization of contacts: Prototype protein-based vaccines have shown promising results, but have not cleared infection and/or prevented reinfection.
      6) Investigation of contacts and source of infection: Testing is recommended only if the intention is to treat. Patients with asymptomatic infection should not undergo testing.
      7) Specific treatment: Treatment for asymptomatic infection remains controversial. There is a wide variety of treatment regimens available for eradicating infections in individuals with symptoms of disease attributable to *H. pylori*. Regimens for first and second line treatment include: a) combinations of proton-pump inhibitor (PPI) drugs with clarithromycin and amoxicillin; or b) bismuth subsalicylate with tetracycline and metronidazole, each for one week. Cure rates of up to 90% have been reported with these regimens. If infection persists, the isolates should be checked for resistance to the antibiotics. Ulcers relapse in those patients in whom cure was not achieved. In industrialized countries, reinfection following cure is infrequent. There are no data on reinfection rates in developing countries.

   C. *Epidemic measures:* None.

   D. *Disaster implications:* None

   E. *International measures:* None.

[I. Lcjncv]

GASTROENTERITIS, ACUTE
VIRAL   ICD-9 008.6; ICD-10 A08

Viral gastroenteritis presents as an endemic or epidemic illness in infants, children and adults. Several viruses (rotaviruses, enteric adenoviruses, astroviruses and caliciviruses including Norwalk-like viruses) infect children in their early years and cause a diarrheal illness that may be severe enough to produce dehydration. Viral agents such as Norwalk-like viruses are also common causes of epidemics of gastroenteritis among children and adults. The epidemiology, natural history and clinical expression of enteric viral infections are best understood for type A rotavirus in infants and Norwalk agent in adults.

I. ROTAVIRAL ENTERITIS   ICD-9 008.61; ICD-10 A08.0
(Sporadic viral gastroenteritis, Severe viral gastroenteritis of infants and children)

1. Identification—A sporadic, seasonal, often severe gastroenteritis of infants and young children, characterized by vomiting, fever and watery diarrhea. Rotaviral enteritis is occasionally associated with severe dehydration and death in young children. Secondary symptomatic cases among adult family contacts can occur, although subclinical infections are more common. Rotavirus infection has occasionally been found in pediatric patients with a variety of other clinical manifestations, but the virus is probably coincidental rather than causative in these conditions. Rotavirus is a major cause of nosocomial diarrhea of newborns and infants. Although rotaviral diarrhea is generally more severe than acute diarrhea due to other agents, illness caused by rotavirus is not distinguishable from that caused by other enteric viruses for any individual patient.

EM, ELISA, LA and other immunological techniques for which commercial kits are available can identify rotavirus in stool specimens or rectal swabs. Evidence of rotavirus infection can be demonstrated by serological techniques, but diagnosis is usually based on the demonstration of rotavirus antigen in stools. False-positive ELISA reactions are common in newborns; positive reactions require confirmation by an alternative test.

2. Infectious agent—The 70-nanometer rotavirus belongs to the Reoviridae family. Group A is common, group B is uncommon in infants but has caused large epidemics in adults in China, while group C appears to be uncommon in humans. Groups A, B, C, D, E and F occur in animals. There are 4 major and at least 10 minor serotypes of group A human rotavirus, based on antigenic differences in the viral protein 7 (VP7) outer capsid surface protein, the major neutralization antigen. Another outer capsid protein called VP4, is associated with virulence and also plays a role in virus neutralization.

3. Occurrence—In both industrialized and developing countries, rotavirus is associated with about one-third of hospitalized cases of diarrheal illness in infants and young children under 5. Neonatal rotaviral infections are frequent in certain settings but are usually asymptomatic. Essentially all children are infected by rotavirus in their first 2–3 years of life, with peak incidence of clinical disease in the 6- to 24-month age group. Outbreaks occur among children in day care settings. Rotavirus is more frequently associated with severe diarrhea than other enteric pathogens; in developing countries, it is responsible for an estimated 600 000-870 000 diarrheal deaths each year.

In temperate climates, rotavirus diarrhea occurs in seasonal peaks during cooler months; in tropical climates, cases occur throughout the year, often with a moderate peak in the cooler dry months. Infection of adults is usually subclinical, but outbreaks of clinical disease occur in geriatric units. Rotavirus occasionally causes travellers' diarrhea in adults and diarrhea in immunocompromised persons (including those with HIV infection), parents of children with rotavirus diarrhea and the elderly.

4. Reservoir—Probably humans. The animal viruses do not produce disease in humans; group B and group C rotaviruses identified in humans appear to be quite distinct from those found in animals.

5. Mode of transmission—Probably fecal-oral with possible contact or respiratory spread. Although rotaviruses do not effectively multiply in the respiratory tract, they may be encountered in respiratory secretions. There is some evidence that rotavirus may be present in contaminated water.

6. Incubation period—Approximately 24–72 hours.

7. Period of communicability—During the acute stage, and later while virus shedding continues. Rotavirus is not usually detectable after about the eighth day of infection, although excretion of virus for 30 days or more has been reported in immunocompromised patients. Symptoms last for an average of 4–6 days.

8. Susceptibility—Susceptibility is greatest between 6 and 24 months of age. By age 3, most individuals have acquired rotavirus antibodies. Diarrhea is uncommon in infected infants under 3 months. Immunocompromised individuals are at particular risk for prolonged rotavirus antigen excretion and intermittent rotavirus diarrhea.

9. **Methods of control—**

   A. *Preventive measures*

   1) In August 1998, an oral, live, tetravalent, rhesus-based rotavirus vaccine (RRV-TV) was licensed for use among infants in the USA. This was recommended for administration to infants between the ages of 6 weeks and 1 year as a 3-dose series at ages 2, 4 and 6 months; the first dose to be administered at ages 6 weeks to 6 months; subsequent doses to be administered with a minimum interval of 3 weeks between any two doses. Routine use of this vaccine was intended to reduce numbers of physician visits for rotavirus gastroenteritis and to prevent at least 2/3 of hospitalizations and deaths related to rotavirus.

   Intussusception (a bowel obstruction in which one segment of bowel becomes enfolded within another segment) was identified in prelicensure trials as a potential problem associated with RRV-TV. Because of continued reports of an association between administration of the vaccine and the development of intussusception, the Advisory Committee on Immunization Practices (ACIP) withdrew this vaccine. New rotavirus vaccines are now under development and testing in several countries.

   2) The effectiveness of other preventive measures is undetermined. Hygienic measures applicable to diseases transmitted via the fecal-oral route may not be effective in preventing transmission. The virus survives for long periods on hard surfaces, in contaminated water and on hands. It is relatively resistant to commonly used disinfectants but is inactivated by chlorine.

   3) In day care, dressing infants with overalls to cover diapers has been demonstrated to decrease transmission of the infection.

   4) Prevent exposure of infants and young children to individuals with acute gastroenteritis in family and institutional (day care or hospital) settings by maintaining a high level of sanitary practices; exclusion from day care centers is not necessary.

   5) Passive immunization by oral administration of IG has been shown to protect low birthweight neonates and immunocompromised children. Breastfeeding does not affect infection rates, but may reduce the severity of the gastroenteritis.

   B. *Control of patient, contacts and the immediate environment:*

   1) Report to local health authority: Obligatory report of epidemics in some countries; no individual case report, Class 4 (see Reporting).

2) Isolation: Enteric precautions, with frequent handwashing by caretakers of infants.

3) Concurrent disinfection: Sanitary disposal of diapers; place overalls over diapers to prevent leakage.

4) Quarantine: Not applicable.

5) Immmunization of contacts: Not applicable.

6) Investigation of contacts and source of infection: Sources of infection should be sought in certain high-risk populations and antigen excretors.

7) Specific treatment: None. Oral rehydration therapy with oral glucose-electrolyte solution is adequate in most cases. Parenteral fluids are needed in cases with vascular collapse or uncontrolled vomiting (see Cholera, 9B7). Antibiotics and antimotility drugs are contraindicated.

C. *Epidemic measures:* Search for vehicles of transmission and source on epidemiological bases.

D. *Disaster implications:* A potential problem with dislocated populations.

E. *International measures:* WHO Collaborating Centres.

II. EPIDEMIC VIRAL GASTROENTEROPATHY   ICD-9 008.6, 008.8; ICD-10 A08.1

(Norwalk agent disease, Norwalk-like disease, Viral gastroenteritis in adults, Epidemic viral gastroenteritis, Acute infectious nonbacterial gastroenteritis, Viral diarrhea, Epidemic diarrhea and vomiting, Winter vomiting disease, Epidemic nausea and vomiting)

1. Identification—Usually a self-limited, mild to moderate disease that often occurs in outbreaks, with clinical symptoms of nausea, vomiting, diarrhea, abdominal pain, myalgia, headache, malaise, low grade fever or a combination of these symptoms. GI symptoms characteristically last 24–48 hours.

The virus may be identified in stools through direct or immune EM or, for the Norwalk virus, through RIA or reverse transcription polymerase chain reaction (RT-PCR). Serological evidence of infection may be demonstrated by IEM or, for the Norwalk virus, by RIA. Diagnosis requires collection of a large volume of stools, with aliquots stored at 4°C (39°F) for EM, and at −20°C (−4°F) for antigen assays. Acute and convalescent sera (3–4-week interval) are essential to link particles observed by EM with disease etiology. RT-PCR seems to be more sensitive than IEM and can be used to examine links among widely scattered clusters of disease.

2. Infectious agents—Norwalk-like viruses are small (27–32-nanometers), structured RNA viruses classified as caliciviruses; they have been implicated as the most common causal agent of nonbacterial gastroenteritis outbreaks. Several morphologically similar but antigenically distinct viruses have been associated with gastroenteritis outbreaks; these include Hawaii, Taunton, Ditchling or W, Cockle, Parramatta, Oklahoma and Snow Mountain agents.

3. Occurrence—Worldwide and common; most often in outbreaks but also sporadically; all age groups are affected. Outbreaks in the USA and other industrialized countries are usually associated with consumption of raw shellfish. In one study in the USA, antibodies to Norwalk agent were acquired slowly; by the fifth decade of life, more than 60% of the population had antibodies. In most developing countries studied, antibodies are acquired much earlier. Seroresponse to Norwalk virus has been widely detected in infants and young children from Bangladesh and Finland.

4. Reservoir—Humans are the only known reservoir.

5. Mode of transmission—Probably by the fecal-oral route, although contact or airborne transmission from fomites has been suggested to explain the rapid spread in hospital settings. Several recent outbreaks have strongly suggested primary community foodborne, waterborne and shellfish transmission, with secondary transmission to family members.

6. Incubation period—Usually 24–48 hours; in volunteer studies with Norwalk agent, the range was 10–50 hours.

7. Period of communicability—During acute stage of disease and up to 48 hours after Norwalk diarrhea stops.

8. Susceptibility and resistance—Susceptibility is widespread. Short-term immunity lasting up to 14 weeks has been demonstrated in volunteers after induced Norwalk illness, but long-term immunity was variable; some individuals became ill on rechallenge 27–42 months later. Levels of pre-existing serum antibody to Norwalk virus did not correlate with susceptibility or resistance.

9. Methods of control—

    A. *Preventive measures:* Use hygienic measures applicable to diseases transmitted via fecal-oral route (see Typhoid fever, 9A). In particular, cooking shellfish and surveillance of shellfish breeding waters can prevent infection from that source.

B. *Control of patient, contacts and the immediate environment:*

1) Report to local health authority: Obligatory report of epidemics in some countries; no individual case report, Class 4 (see Reporting).
2) Isolation: Enteric precautions.
3) Concurrent disinfection: Not applicable.
4) Quarantine: Not applicable.
5) Immmunization of contacts: Not applicable.
6) Investigation of contacts and source of infection: Search for means of spread of infection in outbreak situations.
7) Specific treatment: Fluid and electrolyte replacement in severe cases (see Cholera, 9B7).

C. *Epidemic measures:* Search for vehicles of transmission and source; determine course of outbreak to define epidemiology.

D. *Disaster implications:* A potential problem.

E. *International measures:* None.

[O. Fontaine]

GIARDIASIS
(*Giardia* enteritis)

ICD-9 007.1; ICD-10 A07.1

1. Identification—A protozoan infection principally of the upper small intestine; it can a) remain asymptomatic; b) bring on acute, self-limited diarrhea; c) lead to intestinal symptoms such as chronic diarrhea, steatorrhea, abdominal cramps, bloating, frequent loose and pale greasy stools, fatigue, malabsorption (of fats and fat-soluble vitamins) and weight loss. There is usually no extraintestinal invasion, but reactive arthritis and, in severe giardiasis, damage to duodenal and jejunal mucosal cells may occur.

Diagnosis is traditionally made through identification of cysts or trophozoites in feces (to rule out the diagnosis at least 3 negative results are needed). Because *Giardia* infection is usually asymptomatic, the presence of *G. lamblia* (in stool or duodenum) does not necessarily indicate that *Giardia* is the cause of illness. Tests using ELISA or direct fluorescent antibody methods to detect antigens in the stool, generally more sensitive than direct microscopy, are commercially available. Where results of stool examination and antigen assays are questionable, it may be useful to examine for trophozoites from duodenal fluid (aspiration or string test) or mucosa obtained by small intestine biopsy.

2. Infectious agent—*Giardia lamblia* (*G. intestinalis*, *G. duodenalis*), a flagellate protozoan.

3. Occurrence—Worldwide. Children are infected more frequently than adults. Prevalence is higher in areas of poor sanitation and in institutions with children not toilet trained, including day care centers. The prevalence of stool positivity in different areas may range between 1% and 30%, depending on the community and age group surveyed. Endemic infection in Mexico, the United Kingdom and the USA most commonly occurs in July-October among children under 5 and adults 25–39. It is associated with drinking-water from unfiltered surface water sources or shallow wells, swimming in bodies of freshwater and having a young family member in day care. Large community outbreaks have occurred from drinking treated but unfiltered water. Smaller outbreaks have resulted from contaminated food, person-to-person transmission in day care centers and contaminated recreational waters (including swimming and wading pools).

4. Reservoir—Humans; possibly beaver and other wild and domestic animals.

5. Mode of transmission—Person-to-person transmission occurs by hand-to-mouth transfer of cysts from the feces of an infected individual, especially in institutions and day care centers; this is probably the principal mode of spread. Anal intercourse also facilitates transmission. Localized outbreaks may occur from ingestion of cysts in fecally contaminated drinking and recreational water less often than from fecally contaminated food. Concentrations of chlorine used in routine water treatment do not kill *Giardia* cysts, especially when the water is cold; unfiltered stream and lake waters open to contamination by human and animal feces are a source of infection.

6. Incubation period—Usually 3–25 days or longer; median 7–10 days.

7. Period of communicability—Entire period of infection, often months.

8. Susceptibility—Asymptomatic carrier rate is high; infection is frequently self-limited. Pathogenicity of *G. lamblia* for humans has been established by clinical studies. Persons with HIV infection may have more serious and prolonged giardiasis.

9. Methods of control—

   A. Preventive measures:

   1) Educate families, personnel and inmates of institutions, and especially adult personnel of day care centers, in personal

hygiene and the need for washing hands before handling food, before eating and after toilet use.
2) Filter public water supplies exposed to human or animal fecal contamination.
3) Protect public water supplies against contamination with human and animal feces.
4) Dispose of feces in a sanitary manner.
5) Boil emergency water supplies. Chemical treatment with hypochlorite or iodine less reliable; use 0.1 to 0.2 ml (2 to 4 drops) of household bleach or 0.5 ml of 2% tincture of iodine per liter for 20 minutes (longer if water is cold or turbid).

B. *Control of patient, contacts and the immediate environment:*

1) Report to local health authority: Case report in selected areas, Class 3 (see Reporting).
2) Isolation: Enteric precautions.
3) Concurrent disinfection: Of feces and articles soiled therewith. In communities with a modern and adequate sewage disposal system, feces can be discharged directly into sewers without preliminary disinfection. Terminal cleaning.
4) Quarantine: Not applicable.
5) Immmunization of contacts: Not applicable.
6) Investigation of contacts and source of infection: Microscopic examination of feces of household members and other suspected contacts, especially if symptomatic.
7) Specific treatment: 5-nitroimidazoles: one daily dose of 2 grams metronidazole (children 15 mg/kg) for 3 days, or tinidazole 2 grams in a single dose (children 50–75 mg/kg) are the drugs of choice. Furazolidone is available in pediatric suspension for young children and infants (2 mg/kg thrice daily for 7–10 days). Paromomycin can be used during pregnancy, but when disease is mild, delay of treatment till after delivery is recommended. Drug resistance and relapses may occur with any drug.

C. *Epidemic measures:* Institute an epidemiological investigation of clustered cases in an area or institution to determine source of infection and mode of transmission. A common vehicle, such as water, food or association with a day care center or recreational area must be sought; institute applicable preventive or control measures. Control of person-to-person transmission requires special emphasis on personal cleanliness and sanitary disposal of feces.

D. *Disaster implications:* None.

E. *International measures:* None.

[A. Montresor]

GONOCOCCAL INFECTIONS   ICD-9 098; ICD-10 A54

Urethritis, epididymitis, proctitis, cervicitis, Bartholinitis, pelvic inflammatory disease (salpingitis and/or endometritis) and pharyngitis of adults; vulvovaginitis of children; and conjunctivitis of the newborn and adults are localized inflammatory conditions caused by *Neisseria gonorrhoeae*. Gonococcal bacteraemia results in the arthritis-dermatitis syndrome, occasionally associated with endocarditis or meningitis. Other complications include perihepatitis and the neonatal amniotic infection syndrome.

Clinically similar infections of the same genital structures may be caused by *Chlamydia trachomatis* and other infectious agents. Simultaneous infections are not uncommon.

I. GONOCOCCAL INFECTION   ICD-9 098.0-098.3;
ICD-10 A54.0-A54.2
(Gonorrhea, Gonococcal urethritis, Gonococcal vulvovaginitis, Gonococcal cervicitis, Gonococcal Bartholinitis, Clap, Strain, Gleet, Dose, GC)

1. Identification—A sexually transmitted bacterial disease limited to columnar and transitional epithelium, which differs in males and females in course, severity and ease of recognition. In males, gonococcal infection presents as an acute purulent discharge from the anterior urethra with dysuria within 2–7 days after exposure. Urethritis can be documented by: a) the presence of mucopurulent or purulent discharge; b) Gram stain of urethral discharge showing 5 or more WBC per oil immersion field. The Gram stain is highly sensitive and specific for documenting urethritis and the presence of gonococcal infection in symptomatic males. A small percentage of gonococcal infections in males are asymptomatic.

In females infection is followed by the development of mucopurulent cervicitis, often asymptomatic, although some women have abnormal vaginal discharge and vaginal bleeding after intercourse. In about 20% there is also uterine invasion, often at the first, second or later menstrual period, with symptoms of endometritis, salpingitis or pelvic peritonitis and subsequent risk of infertility and ectopic pregnancy. Prepubescent girls may develop gonococcal vulvovaginitis through direct genital contact with exudate from infected people during sexual abuse.

In females and homosexual males, pharyngeal and anorectal infections are common and, while usually asymptomatic, may cause pruritus, tenesmus and discharge. Conjunctivitis occurs in newborns and rarely in adults, with resultant blindness if not rapidly and adequately treated. Septicaemia may occur in 0.5%–1% of all gonococcal infections, with arthritis, skin lesions and (rarely) endocarditis and meningitis. Arthritis can produce permanent joint damage if appropriate antibiotherapy is delayed. Death is rare except among persons with endocarditis.

Nongonococcal urethritis (NGU) and nongonococcal mucopurulent cervicitis (MPC) are also caused by other sexually transmitted agents and seriously complicate the clinical diagnosis of gonorrhoea; the organisms that cause these diseases often coexist with gonococcal infections. In many populations, the incidence of NGU exceeds that of gonorrhoea. *Chlamydia trachomatis* (see Chlamydial infections) causes about 30%–40% of NGU in the USA and other industrialized countries.

Diagnosis is made by Gram stain of discharges, bacteriological culture on selective media (e.g. modified Thayer-Martin agar) or tests that detect gonococcal nucleic acid. Typical Gram-negative intracellular diplococci can be considered diagnostic in male urethral smears; they are nearly diagnostic when seen in cervical smears (specificity 90%–97%). Cultures on selective media, plus presumptive identification based on both macroscopic and microscopic examination and biochemical testing, are sensitive and specific, as are nucleic acid detection tests. In cases with potential legal implications, specimens should be cultured and isolates confirmed as *N. gonorrhoeae* by 2 different methods.

2. Infectious agent—*Neisseria gonorrhoeae*, the gonococcus.

3. Occurrence—Worldwide, the disease affects both men and women, especially sexually active adolescents and younger adults. Prevalence is highest in communities of lower socioeconomic status. In most industrialized countries, incidence has decreased during the past 20-odd years, although it appears to have increased again since 1995; the rise has been greatest in the younger age groups. New infections tend to be concentrated in population subgroups at increased risk, such as men who have sex with men and ethnic minorities. Resistance to penicillin and tetracycline is widespread. Quinolone-resistant *N. gonorrhoeae* (QRNG) continues to spread; it is common in parts of Asia and the Pacific and becoming increasingly common on the West Coast of the USA. Resistance to recommended cephalosporins has not been documented.

4. Reservoir—Strictly a human disease.

5. Mode of transmission—Contact with exudates from mucous membranes of infected people, almost always as a result of sexual activity. In children over 1 year, it is considered an indicator of sexual abuse.

6. Incubation period—Usually 2–7 days, sometimes longer when symptoms occur.

7. Period of communicability—May extend for months in untreated individuals. Effective treatment ends communicability within hours.

8. Susceptibility—Susceptibility is general. Humoral and secretory antibodies have been demonstrated, but gonococcal strains are antigenically heterogeneous and reinfection is common. Women using an intra-uterine contraceptive device have higher risks of gonococcal salpingitis during the first 3 months after insertion; some people deficient in complement components are uniquely susceptible to bacteraemia. Since only columnar and transitional epithelium can be infected by the gono-coccus, the vaginal epithelium of adult women (which is covered by stratified squamous epithelium) is resistant to infection, whereas the prepubertal columnar or transitional vaginal epithelium is susceptible.

9. **Methods of control—**

A. *Preventive measures:*

1) Same as for syphilis (see Syphilis, 9A), except for measures that apply specifically to gonorrhoea, i.e. the use of prophy-lactic agents in the eyes of the newborn (see section II, 9A2) and special attention (presumptive treatment) to contacts of infected patients (see 9B6).
2) Prevention is based primarily on safer sexual practices; i.e. consistent and correct use of condoms with all partners not known to be infection-free, avoiding multiple sexual encoun-ters or anonymous/casual sex, mutual monogamy with a noninfected partner

B. *Control of patient, contacts and the immediate environment:*

1) Report to local health authority: Case report is required in many countries, Class 2 (see Reporting).
2) Isolation: Contact isolation for all newborn infants and pre-pubertal children with gonococcal infection until effective parenteral antimicrobial therapy has been administered for 24 hours. Effective antibiotics in adequate dosage promptly render discharges noninfectious. Patients should refrain from sexual intercourse until antimicrobial therapy is completed, and, to avoid reinfection, abstain from sex with previous sexual partners until these have been treated.
3) Concurrent disinfection: Care in disposal of discharges from lesions and contaminated articles.
4) Quarantine: Not applicable.
5) Immmunization of contacts: Not applicable.
6) Investigation of contacts and source of infection: Interview patients and notify sexual partners. With uncooperative patients, trained interviewers obtain the best results, but clinicians can motivate most patients to help arrange treat-ment for their partners. Sexual contacts of cases should be examined, tested and treated if their last sexual contact with the case was within 60 days before the onset of symptoms or diagnosis in the case. Even outside these time-limits the most

recent sexual partner should be examined, tested and treated. All infants born to infected mothers must receive prophylactic treatment.

7) Specific treatment: On clinical, laboratory or epidemiological grounds (contacts of a diagnosed case), adequate treatment must be given as follows:

For uncomplicated gonococcal infections of the cervix, rectum and urethra in adults, recommended treatments include ceftriaxone IM (125 mg single dose), cefixime PO (400 mg single dose), ciprofloxacin PO (500 mg single dose), floxacin PO (400 mg single dose) or levofloxacin PO (250 mg single dose). Patients who can take neither cephalosporins nor quinolones may be treated with spectinomycin 2 grams IM (single dose). If chlamydial infection is not ruled out patients infected with *N. gonorrhoeae* must also be treated orally with azithromycin (1 gram single dose) or doxycyline (100 mg twice daily for 7 days).

Providing patients under treatment for gonorrhoea with a treatment effective against genital chlamydial infection is recommended routinely because chlamydial infection is common among patients diagnosed with gonorrhoea. This will also cure incubating syphilis and may inhibit emergence of antimicrobial-resistant gonococci.

Gonococcal infections of the pharynx are more difficult to eliminate than infections of the urethra, cervix or rectum. Recommended regimens for this infection include ceftriaxone 125 mg IM in a single dose or ciprofloxacin 500 mg orally in a single dose.

Resistance of the gonococcus to common antimicrobials is due to the widespread presence of plasmids that carry genes for resistance. Thus, strains of gonococcus are resistant to penicillin (PPNG), tetracycline (TRNG), and the fluoroquinolones (QRNG). Resistance to third-generation and extended spectrum cephalosporins (e.g. ceftriaxone and cefixime) is unknown; resistance to spectinomycin is rare. Cases of gonorrhoea resistant to fluoroquinolones (e.g. ciprofloxacin and ofloxacin) are becoming widespread in Asia and have been reported sporadically from many parts of the world, including North America. In 2000, fluoroquinolone resistance was present in up to 0.2% of infections in the USA.

Treatment failure following any of the antigonococcal regimens listed above is rare, and routine culture as a test of cure is unnecessary. If symptoms persist, reinfection is most likely, but specimens should be obtained for culture and antimicrobial susceptibility testing. Retesting of high-risk patients after 1–2 months is advisable to detect late asymptomatic reinfections. Patients with gonococcal infections are at increased risk of HIV infection and should be offered confidential counselling and testing.

C. Epidemic measures: Intensify routine procedures, especially treatment of contacts on epidemiological grounds.

D. Disaster implications: None.

E. International measures: See Syphilis, 9E.

[F. Ndowa]

II. GONOCOCCAL
CONJUNCTIVITIS
(NEONATORUM)   ICD-9 098.4; ICD-10 A54.3
(Gonorrhoeal ophthalmia neonatorum)

1. Identification—Acute redness and swelling of conjunctiva in one or both eyes, with mucopurulent or purulent discharge in which gonococci are identifiable by microscopic and culture methods. Corneal ulcer, perforation and blindness may occur if specific treatment is not given promptly.

Gonococcal ophthalmia neonatorum is only one of several acute inflammatory conditions of the eye or the conjunctiva occurring within the first 3 weeks of life, collectively known as ophthalmia neonatorum. The gonococcus is the most serious but not the most frequent infectious agent. The commonest infectious cause is *Chlamydia trachomatis*, which produces inclusion conjunctivitis that tends to be less acute than gonococcal conjunctivitis and usually appears 5–14 days after birth (see Conjunctivitis, chlamydial). Any purulent neonatal conjunctivitis should be considered gonococcal until proven otherwise.

2. Infectious agent—*Neisseria gonorrhoeae*, the gonococcus.

3. Occurrence—Varies widely according to prevalence of maternal infections and availability of measures to prevent eye infections in the newborn at delivery; it is infrequent where infant eye prophylaxis is adequate. The disease continues to be an important cause of blindness throughout the world.

4. Reservoir—Infection of the maternal cervix.

5. Mode of transmission—Contact with the infected birth canal during childbirth.

6. Incubation period—Usually 1–5 days.

7. Period of communicability—While discharge persists if untreated; for 24 hours following initiation of specific treatment.

8. Susceptibility and resistance—Susceptibility is general.

9. Methods of control—

A. Preventive measures:

1) Prevent maternal infection (see section I, 9A and Syphilis, 9A). Diagnose gonorrhoea in pregnant women and treat the woman and her sexual partners. Routine culture of the cervix and rectum for gonococci should be considered prenatally, especially in the third trimester where infection is prevalent.

2) Use an established effective preparation for protection of babies' eyes at birth; instillation of 1% silver nitrate aqueous solution stored in individual wax capsules remains the agent most widely used. Erythromycin (0.5%) and tetracycline (1%) ophthalmic ointments are also effective. A study carried out in Kenya found that the incidence of ophthalmia neonatorum in infants treated with a 2.5% ophthalmic solution of povidone-iodine was significantly lower than in those treated with 1% silver nitrate or with 0.5% erythromycin ointment.

B. Control of patient, contacts and the immediate environment:

1) Report to local health authority: Case report is required in many countries, Class 2 (see Reporting).

2) Isolation: Contact isolation for the first 24 hours after administration of effective therapy. Hospitalize patients if possible. Bacterial cure after therapy should be confirmed by culture.

3) Concurrent disinfection: Care in disposal of conjunctival discharges and contaminated articles.

4) Quarantine: Not applicable.

5) Immunization of contacts: Not applicable; prompt treatment on diagnosis or clinical suspicion of infection.

6) Investigation of contacts and source of infection: Examination and treatment of mothers and their sexual partners.

7) Specific treatment: For gonococcal infections when antibiotic susceptibility is not known, or for penicillin-resistant organisms, a single dose of ceftriaxone, 25–50 mg/kg (not to exceed 125 mg) IV or IM, is recommended. Mother and infant should also be treated for chlamydial infection.

C. Epidemic measures: None.

D. Disaster implications: None.

E. International measures: None.

[S Pernikoff]

GRANULOMA INGUINALE ICD-9 099.2; ICD-10 A.58
(Donovanosis)

1. Identification—A chronic and progressively destructive, but poorly communicable bacterial disease of the skin and mucous membranes of the external genitalia, inguinal and anal regions. One or more indurated nodules or papules lead to a slowly spreading, nontender, exuberant, granulomatous, ulcerative or cicatricial lesions. The lesions are characteristically nonfriable beefy red granulomas that extend peripherally with characteristic rolled edges and eventually form fibrous tissue. Lesions occur most commonly in warm, moist surfaces such as the folds between the thighs, the perianal area, the scrotum, or the vulvar labia and vagina. The genitalia are involved in close to 90% of cases, the inguinal region in close to 10%, the anal region in 5%–10% and distant sites in 1%–5%. If neglected, the process may result in extensive destruction of genital organs and spread by autoinoculation to other parts of the body.

Laboratory diagnosis is based on demonstration of intracytoplasmic rod shaped organisms (Donovan bodies) in Wright- or Giemsa-stained smears of granulation tissue or on histological examination of biopsy specimens; the presence of large infected mononuclear cells filled with deeply staining Donovan bodies is pathognomonic. Culture is difficult and unreliable. PCR and serology are available on a research basis. *Haemophilus ducreyi* should be excluded by culture on appropriate selective media.

2. Infectious agent—*Klebsiella granulomatis* (*Donovania granulomatis*, *Calymmatobacterium granulomatis*), a Gram-negative bacillus, is the presumed causal agent; this is not certain.

3. Occurrence—Rare in industrialized countries, but cluster outbreaks occasionally occur. Endemic in tropical and subtropical areas, such as central and northern Australia, southern India, Papua New Guinea, Viet Nam; occasionally in Latin America, the Caribbean islands and central, eastern and southern Africa. It is more frequently seen among males than females and among people of lower socioeconomic status; it may occur in children aged 1–4 years but is predominantly seen at ages 20–40.

4. Reservoir—Humans.

5. Mode of transmission—Presumably by direct contact with lesions during sexual activity, but in various studies only 20%–65% of sexual partners were infected, thus not quite fulfilling the criteria for sexual transmission. Donovanosis occurs in sexually inactive individuals and the very young, suggesting that some cases are transmitted nonsexually.

6. Incubation period—Unknown; probably between 1 and 16 weeks.

7. Period of communicability—Unknown; probably for the duration of open lesions on the skin or mucous membranes.

8. Susceptibility and resistance—Susceptibility is variable; immunity apparently does not follow attack.

9. Methods of control—

A. *Preventive measures:* Except for those measures applicable only to syphilis, preventive measures are those for Syphilis, 9A. Educational programs in endemic areas should stress the importance of early diagnosis and treatment.

B. *Control of patient, contacts and the immediate environment:*

   1) Report to local health authority: A reportable disease in most states and countries, Class 3 (see Reporting).
   2) Isolation: Avoid close personal contact until lesions are healed.
   3) Concurrent disinfection: Care in disposal of discharges from lesions and articles soiled therewith.
   4) Quarantine: Not applicable.
   5) Immunization of contacts: Not applicable; prompt treatment upon recognition or clinical suspicion of infection.
   6) Investigation of contacts and source of infection: Examination of sexual contacts.
   7) Specific treatment: Azithromycin is effective and its long tissue half-life allows a flexible dosing regimen and short course treatment. Erythromycin, trimethoprim-sufamethoxazole and doxycycline have been reported to be effective but drug-resistant strains of the organism occur. Treatment is continued for 3 weeks or until the lesions have resolved; recurrence is not rare but usually responds to a repeat course unless malignancy is present. Single dose treatment with ceftriaxone IM or ciprofloxacin PO are anecdotally reported to be effective.

C. *Epidemic measures:* Not applicable.

D. *Disaster implications:* None.

E. *International measures:* See Syphilis, 9E.

[F. Ndowa]

HANTAVIRAL DISEASES

Hantaviruses infect rodents worldwide; several species are known to infect humans with varying severity, with primary impact effect on the vascular endothelium, resulting in increased vascular permeability, hypotensive shock and hemorrhagic manifestations. Many of these agents have been isolated from rodents but are not associated with human cases. In 1993, an outbreak of disease caused by a previously unrecognized hantavirus occurred in the USA; the principal target organ was not the kidney (the usual target organ in human hantaviral infections) but the lung. Because they are caused by related causal organisms and have similar features of epidemiology and pathology (febrile prodrome, thrombocytopenia, leukocytosis and capillary leakage), both the renal and the pulmonary syndrome are presented under Hantaviral diseases.

I. HEMORRHAGIC FEVER WITH
RENAL SYNDROME   ICD-9 078.6; ICD-10 A98.5
(Epidemic hemorrhagic fever, Korean hemorrhagic fever,
Nephropathia epidemica, Hemorrhagic nephrosonephritis, HFRS)

1. Identification—Acute zoonotic viral disease with abrupt onset of fever, lower back pain, varying degrees of hemorrhagic manifestations and renal involvement. Severe illness is associated with Hantaan (primarily in Asia) and Dobrava viruses (in the Balkans). Disease is characterized by 5 clinical phases which frequently overlap: febrile, hypotensive, oliguric, diuretic and convalescent. High fever, headache, malaise and anorexia, followed by severe abdominal or lower back pain, often accompanied by nausea and vomiting, facial flushing, petechiae and conjunctival injection characterize the febrile phase, which lasts 3-7 days. The hypotensive phase lasts from several hours to 3 days and is characterized by defervescence and abrupt onset of hypotension, which may progress to shock and more apparent hemorrhagic manifestations. Blood pressure returns to normal or is high in the oliguric phase (3-7 days); nausea and vomiting may persist, severe hemorrhage may occur and urinary output falls dramatically.

The majority of deaths (the case-fatality rate ranges from 5% to 15%) occur during the hypotensive and oliguric phases. Diuresis heralds the onset of recovery in most cases, with polyuria of 3-6 liters per day. Convalescence takes weeks to months.

A less severe illness (case-fatality rate <1%) caused by Puumala virus and referred to as nephropathia epidemica is predominant in Europe. Infections caused by Seoul virus, carried by brown or Norway rats, are clinically milder, although severe disease may occur with this strain. They show less clear distinction between clinical phases.

Diagnosis is through demonstration of specific antibodies using ELISA or IFA; most patients have IgM antibodies at the time of hospitalization. The presence of proteinuria, leukocytosis, hemoconcentration, thrombocytopenia and elevated blood urea nitrogen supports the diagnosis. Hantaviruses can be propagated in a limited range of cell cultures and laboratory rats and mice, mainly for research purposes. Leptospirosis and rickettsioses must be considered in the differential diagnosis.

2. Infectious agent—Hantaviruses (a genus of the family Bunyaviridae, the only genus without an arthropod vector); 3-segmented RNA viruses with spherical to oval particles, 95–110 nanometers in diameter. More than 25 antigenically distinguishable viral species exist, each associated primarily with a single rodent species. Seoul virus is found worldwide, Puumala virus in Europe, Hantaan virus principally in Asia, less often in Europe, Dobrava (Belgrade) virus in Serbia and Montenegro (formerly the Federal Republic of Yugoslavia).

3. Occurrence—Prior to World War II, Japanese and Soviet authors described the disease in Manchuria along the Amur River. In 1951, it was recognized among United Nations troops in Asia and later in both military personnel and civilians—the virus was first isolated from a field rodent (*Apodemus agrarius*) in 1977 near the Hantaan river. The disease is considered a major public health problem in China and the Republic of Korea. Occurrence is seasonal, most cases occurring in late autumn and early winter, primarily among rural populations. In the Balkans, a severe form of the disease due to Dobrava virus affects a few hundred people annually, with fatality rates at least as high as those in Asia (5%–15%). Most cases there are seen during spring and early summer.

Nephropathia epidemica, due to Puumala virus, is found in most of Europe, including the Balkans and the Russian Federation West of the Ural mountains. It is often seen in summer and in the autumn and early winter. Seasonal occupational and recreational activities probably influence the risk of exposure, as do climate and other ecological factors of rodent population densities. Among medical research personnel and animal handlers in Asia and Europe, the disease has been traced to laboratory rats infected with Seoul virus, which has been identified in captured urban rats worldwide, including Argentina, Brazil, Thailand and USA; only in Asia has it been regularly associated with human disease. The availability of newer diagnostic techniques has led to increasing recognition of hantaviruses and hantaviral infections.

4. Reservoir—Field rodents (*Apodemus* spp. for Hantaan and Dobrava-Belgrade viruses in Asia and the Balkans; *Clethrionomys* spp. for Puumala in Europe; *Rattus* spp. for Seoul virus worldwide). Humans are accidental hosts.

5. Mode of transmission—Presumed aerosol transmission from rodent excreta (aerosol infectivity has been demonstrated experimentally), though this may not explain all human cases or all forms of inter-rodent transmission. Virus occurs in urine, feces and saliva of persistently infected asymptomatic rodents, with maximal virus concentration in the lungs. Nosocomial transmission of hantaviruses has been documented but is believed rare.

6. Incubation period—From a few days to nearly 2 months, usually 2–4 weeks.

7. Period of communicability—Not well defined. Person-to-person transmission is rare.

8. Susceptibility—Persons without serological evidence of past infection appear to be uniformly susceptible. Inapparent infections occur; second attacks have not been documented.

9. Methods of control—

A. *Preventive measures:*

1) Exclude and prevent rodent access to houses and other buildings.
2) Store human and animal food under rodent-proof conditions.
3) Disinfect rodent-contaminated areas by spraying a disinfectant solution (e.g. diluted bleach) prior to cleaning. Do not sweep or vacuum rat-contaminated areas; use a wet mop or towels moistened with disinfectant. In so far as possible, avoid inhalation of dust by using approved respirators when cleaning previously unoccupied areas.
4) Trap rodents and dispose using suitable precautions. Live trapping is not recommended.
5) In enzootic areas, minimize exposure to wild rodents and their excreta.
6) Laboratory rodent colonies, particularly *Rattus norvegicus*, must be tested to ensure freedom from asymptomatic hantavirus infection.

B. *Control of patient, contacts and the immediate environment:*

1) Report to local health authority: In endemic countries where reporting is required, Class 3 (see Reporting).
2) Isolation: Not applicable.
3) Concurrent disinfection: Not applicable.
4) Quarantine: Not applicable.
5) Immmunization of contacts: Not applicable.
6) Investigate contacts and source of infection: Exterminate rodents in and around households if feasible.
7) Specific treatment: Bed rest and early hospitalization are critical. Jostling and the effect of lowered atmospheric

pressures during airborne evacuation of cases can be deleterious to patients critically ill with hantavirus. Careful attention to fluid management is important to avoid overload and minimize the effects of shock and renal failure. Dialysis is often required. Ribavirin IV as early as possible during the first few days of illness has shown benefit.

C. *Epidemic measures:* Rodent control; surveillance for hantavirus infections in wild rodents. Laboratory-associated outbreaks call for evaluation of the associated rodents and, if positive, elimination of the rodents and thorough disinfection.

D. *Disaster implications:* Natural disasters and wars often result in increased numbers of rodents and rodent contact with humans.

E. *International measures:* Control transport of exotic reservoir rodents.

II. HANTAVIRUS PULMONARY SYNDROME ICD-9 480.8; ICD-10 B33.4
(Hantavirus adult respiratory distress syndrome, Hantavirus cardiopulmonary syndrome)

1. **Identification**—An acute zoonotic viral disease characterized by fever, myalgias and GI complaints followed by the abrupt onset of respiratory distress and hypotension. The illness progresses rapidly to severe respiratory failure and shock. Most cases show an elevated hematocrit, hypoalbuminaemia and thrombocytopenia. The crude fatality rate is approximately 40%–50%. In survivors, recovery from acute illness is rapid, but full convalescence may require weeks to months. Restoration of normal lung function generally occurs, but pulmonary function abnormalities may persist in some individuals. Renal and hemorrhagic manifestations are usually absent except in some severe cases.

Diagnosis is through demonstration of specific IgM antibodies using ELISA, Western blot or strip immunoblot techniques. Most patients have IgM antibodies at the time of hospitalization. PCR analysis of autopsy or biopsy tissues and immunohistochemistry in specialized laboratories are also established diagnostic techniques.

2. **Infectious agents**—Many hantaviruses have been identified in the Americas: Andes virus (Argentina, Chile), Laguna Negra virus (Bolivia, Paraguay), Juquitiba virus (Brazil), Black Creek Canal and Bayou viruses (southeastern USA), New York-1 and Monongahela viruses (eastern USA). Sin Nombre virus was responsible for the 1993 epidemic in southwestern USA and many other cases in North America.

3. **Occurrence**—The disease was first recognized in the spring and

summer of 1993 among resident Native American populations; cases have been confirmed in Canada and in many eastern and western regions of the USA. Sporadic cases and several outbreaks have been reported in South America (Argentina, Bolivia, Brazil, Chile, Paraguay). The disease is not restricted to any ethnic group. Incidence appears to coincide with the geographic distribution and population density of infected carrier rodents and their infection levels.

4. **Reservoir**—The major reservoir of Sin Nombre virus appears to be the deer mouse, *Peromyscus maniculatus*. Antibodies have also been found in other *Peromyscus* species, pack rats, the chipmunk and other rodents. Other hantavirus strains have been associated mainly with other rodent species of the subfamily Sigmodontinae.

5. **Mode of transmission**—As with hantaviral hemorrhagic fever with renal syndrome, aerosol transmission from rodent excreta is presumed. The natural history of viral infections of host rodents has not been characterized. Indoor exposure in closed, poorly ventilated homes, vehicles and outbuildings with visible rodent infestation is especially important.

6. **Incubation period**—Incompletely defined but thought to be approximately 2 weeks with a range of a few days to 6 weeks.

7. **Period of communicability**—Person-to-person spread of hantaviruses has been reported during an outbreak in Argentina.

8. **Susceptibility**—All persons without prior infection are presumed to be susceptible. No inapparent infections have been documented to date, but milder infections without frank pulmonary oedema have occurred. No second cases have been identified, but the protection and duration of immunity conferred by previous infection is unknown.

9. **Methods of control**—

   A. *Preventive measures:* See section I, 9A.

   B. *Control of patient, contacts and the immediate environment:*

      1), 2), 3), 4), 5) and 6) Report to local health authority, Isolation, Concurrent disinfection, Quarantine, Immunization of contacts and Investigation of contacts and source of infection–See section I, 9B1 through 9B6.

      7) Specific treatment: Provide respiratory intensive care management, carefully avoid overhydration that might lead to exacerbation of pulmonary oedema. Cardiotonic drugs and pressors given early under careful monitoring help prevent shock. Strictly avoid hypoxia, particularly if transfer is contemplated. Ribavirin is under investigation and as yet of no

proven benefit. Extracorporeal membrane oxygenation has been used with some success.

C. **Epidemic measures:** Public education regarding rodent avoidance and rodent control in homes is desirable in endemic situations and should be intensified during epidemics. Monitoring of rodent numbers and infection rates is desirable but as yet of unproven value. See section I, 9C.

D. **Disaster implications:** See section I, 9D.

E. **International measures:** Control transport of exotic reservoir rodents.

[J. Mackenzie/A. Plant]

HENDRA AND NIPAH VIRAL
DISEASES   ICD-9 078.8; ICD-10 B33.8

1. Identification—These are newly recognized zoonotic viral diseases named for the locations in Australia and Malaysia where the first human isolates were confirmed in 1994 and 1999, respectively. Nipah virus manifests mainly as encephalitis; Hendra virus as a respiratory illness (2 cases) and as a prolonged and initially mild meningoencephalitis (1 case). The full course and spectrum of these diseases is still unknown; symptoms range in severity from mild to coma and death and include fever and headaches, sore throat, dizziness, drowsiness and disorientation. Pneumonitis was prominent in the initial Hendra cases, one of which was fatal. Coma usually leads to death in 3–30 days. The case-fatality rate for clinical cases is about 50%; subclinical infections occur.

Serological diagnosis is available through detection of IgM and IgG with an antibody capture ELISA or serum neutralization. Virus isolation from infected tissues confirms the diagnosis.

2. Infectious agent—Hendra (formerly called equine morbillivirus) and Nipah viruses are members of a new genus, *Henipaviruses*, of the Paramyxoviridae family.

3. Occurrence—Hendra virus caused disease in horses in Queensland, Australia. In 1994, 3 human cases followed close contact with sick horses, the first 2 during the initial outbreak in Hendra, the 3rd occurring 13 months after an initially mild meningitic illness when the virus reactivated to cause a fatal encephalitis. Nipah virus affected swine in the pig-farming provinces of Perak, Negeri Sembilan, and Selangor in Malaysia. The first human case is believed to have occurred in 1996; although the disease became apparent in late 1998, most cases were identified in the first months of 1999, with over 100 confirmed deaths as of mid-1999. During 1999 11 abattoir workers in Singapore developed Nipah virus infection following contact with pigs imported from Malaysia.

4. Reservoir—Fruit bats for Hendra virus; virus isolation and serological data suggest that Nipah virus may have a similar reservoir. Hendra virus (in horses) and Nipah virus (domestic swine) cause an acute febrile illness, which may lead to severe respiratory and CNS involvement and death. Dogs infected with Nipah virus show a distemper-like manifestation but their epidemiological role has not been defined. Nipah-seropositive horses have been identified, but their role is also undetermined. Testing of other animals is under way; susceptibility testing suggests that cats and guineapigs can be infected, sometimes with fatal outcomes, mice, rabbits and rats appear refractory to infection.

5. Mode of transmission—Primarily through direct contact with infected horses (Hendra) or swine (Nipah) or contaminated tissues. Oral and nasal routes are suspected in most cases. There is no evidence for person-to-person transmission.

6. Incubation period—From 4 to 18 days, occasionally up to several months.

7. Period of communicability— unknown

8. Susceptibility— undetermined—recurrent infection appear to occur

9. Methods of control

> **A. Preventive measures:** Health education about measures to be taken and the need to avoid fruit bats.
>
> **B. Control of patient, contacts, and the immediate environment:**
>
> 1. Report to local authority: Case report should be obligatory wherever these diseases occur; Class 2 (see Reporting).
> 2. Isolation: Of infected horses or swine; no evidence for person-to-person transmission.
> 3. Concurrent disinfection: Slaughter of infected horses or swine with burial or incineration of carcases under government supervision.
> 4. Quarantine: Restrict movement of horses or pigs from infected farms to other areas.
> 5. Immmunization of contacts: Not applicable.
> 6. Investigation of contacts and source of infection: Search for missed cases.

7. Specific treatment: None at present, although there is some research evidence that ribavirin may decrease mortality from Nipah virus.

C. Epidemic measures:

1. Precautions by animal handlers: protective clothing, boots, gloves, gowns, goggles and face shields; washing of hands and body parts with soap before leaving pig farms.
2. Slaughter of infected horses or swine with burial or incineration of carcases under government supervision.
3. Restrict movement of horses or pigs from infected farms to other areas.

D. Disaster implications: None

E. International measures: Prohibit exportation of horses or pigs and horse/pig products from infected areas.

[A. Plant]

HEPATITIS, VIRAL   ICD-9 070; ICD-10 B15-B19

Several distinct infections are grouped as the viral hepatitides; they are primarily hepatotrophic and have similar clinical presentations, but differ in etiology and in some epidemiological, immunological, clinical and pathological characteristics. Their prevention and control vary greatly. Each will be presented in a separate section.

I. VIRAL HEPATITIS A   ICD-9 070.1; ICD-10 B15
(Infectious hepatitis, Epidemic hepatitis, Epidemic jaundice, Catarrhal jaundice, Type A hepatitis, HA)

1. Identification—In most of the industrialized countries, infection occurs in childhood asymptomatically or with a mild illness. The latter infections may be detectable only through laboratory tests of liver function. Onset of illness in adults in nonendemic areas is usually abrupt with fever, malaise, anorexia, nausea and abdominal discomfort, followed within a few days by jaundice. The disease varies in clinical severity from a mild illness lasting 1–2 weeks to a severely disabling disease lasting several months. Prolonged, relapsing hepatitis for up to 1 year occurs in 15% of cases; no chronic infection is known to occur. Convalescence is often prolonged. In general, severity increases with age, but complete recovery without sequelae or recurrences is the rule. Reported case-fatality is normally low, 0.1%–0.3%; it can reach 1.8% for adults over 50;

persons with chronic liver disease have an elevated risk of death from fulminant hepatitis A.

Demonstration of IgM antibodies against hepatitis A virus (IgM anti-HAV) in the serum of acutely or recently ill patients establishes the diagnosis. IgM anti-HAV becomes detectable 5–10 days after exposure. A 4-fold or greater rise in specific antibodies in paired sera, detected by commercially available EIA, also establishes the diagnosis. If laboratory tests are not available, epidemiological evidence may provide support for the diagnosis. HAV RNA can be detected in blood and stools of most persons during the acute phase of infection through nucleic acid amplification methods, but these are not generally used for diagnostic purposes.

2. Infectious agent—Hepatitis A virus (HAV), a 27-nanometer picornavirus (positive-strand RNA virus). It has been classified as a member of the family Picornaviridae.

3. Occurrence—Worldwide, geographic areas can be characterized by high, intermediate, or low levels of endemicity. Levels of endemicity are related to hygienic and sanitary conditions of geographic areas. In areas of high endemicity, adults are usually immune and epidemics of HA are uncommon. Improved sanitation in many parts of the world is leaving many young adults susceptible and the frequency of outbreaks is increasing. In industrialized countries, disease transmission is most frequent among household and sexual contacts of acute cases, and occurs sporadically in day care centers with diapered children, among travellers to countries where the disease is endemic, among injecting drug users and among men who have sex with men. Because most children have asymptomatic or unrecognized infections, they play an important role in HAV transmission and serve as a source of infection for others. Where environmental sanitation is poor, infection is common and occurs at an early age. In some southeastern Asian areas over 90% of the general population has serological evidence of prior HAV infection, vs. a rate of 33% in the USA.

Epidemics often evolve slowly in industrialized countries, cover wide geographic areas and last many months; common source epidemics may evolve rapidly. During some outbreaks, day care center employees or attenders, men with multiple male sex partners and injecting drug users may be at higher risk than the general population. In about half the cases no source of infection is identified. The disease is most common among school-age children and young adults. In recent years, community-wide outbreaks have accounted for most disease transmission, although common source outbreaks due to food contaminated by food handlers and contaminated produce continue to occur and require intensive public health efforts to control. These outbreaks are usually associated with contamination of food by an HAV-infected food handler during preparation, or with food (e.g. shellfish, raw produce) contaminated before entering the food chain. Outbreaks have been reported among susceptible persons working with nonhuman primates raised in the wild.

4. **Reservoir**—Humans, rarely chimpanzees and other primates.

5. **Mode of transmission**—Person-to-person by the fecal-oral route. The infectious agent is found in feces, reaches peak levels the week or two before onset of symptoms and diminishes rapidly after liver dysfunction or symptoms appear, which is concurrent with the appearance of circulating antibodies to HAV.

Common source outbreaks have been related to contaminated water; food contaminated by infected food handlers, including foods not cooked or handled after cooking; raw or undercooked molluscs harvested from contaminated waters; and contaminated produce such as lettuce and strawberries. Several outbreaks in the USA and Europe have been associated with injecting and noninjecting drug use. Transmission through transfusion of blood and clotting factor concentrates obtained from viraemic donors during incubation has been reported, albeit rarely.

6. **Incubation period**—Average 28-30 days (range 15-50 days).

7. **Period of communicability**—Studies of transmission in humans and epidemiological evidence indicate that maximum infectivity occurs during the latter half of incubation and continues for a few days after onset of jaundice (or during peak aminotransferase activity in anicteric cases). Most cases are probably noninfectious after the first week of jaundice, although prolonged viral excretion (up to 6 months) has been documented in infants and children. Chronic shedding of HAV in feces does not occur.

8. **Susceptibility**—General. Low incidence of manifest disease in infants and preschool children suggests that mild and anicteric infections are common. Homologous immunity after infection probably lasts for life.

9. **Methods of control**—

   A. *Preventive measures:*

   1) Educate the public about good sanitation and personal hygiene, with special emphasis on careful handwashing and sanitary disposal of feces.
   2) Provide proper water treatment and distribution systems and sewage disposal.
   3) There are at least 4 inactivated vaccines on the market, all of known good quality and in line with the WHO recommendations. The dose of vaccine, vaccination schedule, ages for which the vaccine is licensed, and whether there is a pediatric and adult formulation all vary from manufacturer to manufacturer, and they are not licensed for use in children

under 1. Clinical trials have shown these vaccines to be safe, immunogenic and efficacious. Protection against clinical hepatitis A may begin in some persons as soon as 14–21 days after a single dose of vaccine, and nearly all have protective levels of antibody by 30 days after receiving the first dose of vaccine. A second dose is felt to be necessary for long-term protection. Depending on the level of HAV endemicity, it may in some cases be cost-effective to screen for HAV antibody prior to immunization.

4) WHO has industrialized recommendations for the use of hepatitis A vaccine. In industrialized countries with low endemicity and with high rates of disease in specific high-risk populations, vaccination of these populations against hepatitis A may be recommended. High-risk groups include the following: a) persons at increased risk for HAV infection or its consequences (chronic liver disease or clotting factor disorders, men who have sex with men, injecting drug users, all susceptible persons travelling to or working in countries where HAV is endemic, persons who work with HAV infected primates or with HAV in research laboratory settings); b) children in communities that have consistently elevated rates of hepatitis A.

Close personal contacts (e.g. household, sexual) of hepatitis A patients should be given postexposure prophylaxis with IG within 2 weeks of last exposure, preferably simultaneously with hepatitis A vaccine given at a separate injection site. Recommendations for hepatitis A vaccination in outbreak situations depend on the epidemiology of hepatitis A in the community and the feasibility of rapidly implementing a widespread vaccination program. The use of hepatitis A vaccine to control community-wide outbreaks has been most successful in small self-contained communities when vaccination is started early in the course of the outbreak and with high coverage of multiple-age cohorts.

5) Although day care centers can be the source of outbreaks of hepatitis A in some communities, disease within those centers commonly reflects extended transmission in the community. Management of day care centers should stress measures to minimize the possibility of fecal-oral transmission, including thorough handwashing after every diaper change and before eating. If one or more hepatitis A cases are associated with a center, or if cases are recognized in two or more households of attenders, hepatitis A vaccine, possibly in combination with IG, should be administered to the staff and attenders. The same should be considered for family contacts of children in diapers attending centers where

outbreaks occur and cases are recognized in 3 or more families.

6) All susceptible travellers to intermediate or highly endemic areas, including Africa, the Middle East, Asia, eastern Europe and Central and South America should be given hepatitis A vaccine prior to departure, possibly together with IG if departure takes place in less than 2 weeks. If used, IG in a single dose of 0.02 ml/kg, or 2 ml for adults, is recommended for expected exposures of up to 3 months; for more prolonged exposures, 0.06 ml/kg or 5 ml should be given and repeated every 4–6 months if exposure continues (only if vaccine administration is contraindicated).

7) Hepatitis A vaccine should be considered for other populations with increased risk of hepatitis A infection, such as men who have sex with men, injecting drug users and persons who work with HAV-infected primates or HAV in a research laboratory setting.

8) Oysters, clams and other shellfish from contaminated areas should be heated to a temperature of 85°–90°C (185°–194°F) for 4 minutes or steamed for 90 seconds before eating. In endemic areas, travellers should take only hot or bottled beverages and hot, well-cooked food.

B. Control of patient, contacts and the immediate environment:

1) Report to local health authority: Obligatory in some, although not required in many countries; Class 2 (see Reporting).

2) Isolation: For proven hepatitis A, enteric precautions during the first 2 weeks of illness, but no more than 1 week after onset of jaundice; the exception is an outbreak in a neonatal intensive care setting, where prolonged enteric precautions must be considered.

3) Concurrent disinfection: Sanitary disposal of feces, urine and blood.

4) Quarantine: Not applicable.

5) Immunization of contacts: Active immunization should be given as soon as possible, but no later than 2 weeks after exposure. Passive immunization with IG (IM), 0.02 ml/kg of body weight, should be given as soon as possible after exposure, but also within 2 weeks. Because hepatitis A cannot be reliably diagnosed on clinical presentation alone, serological confirmation of HAV infection in index patients by IgM anti-HAV testing should be obtained before postexposure prophylaxis of contacts. Persons who have received 1 dose of hepatitis A vaccine at least 1 month prior to exposure do not need IG.

Hepatitis A vaccine and IG are not indicated for contacts in the usual office, school or factory settings. IG should be administered to previously unimmunized persons in the situations listed below, preferably together with hepatitis A vaccine given concurrently at a separate injection site: a) close personal contacts, including household, sexual, drug using and other close personal contacts; b) attenders at day care centers if one or more cases of hepatitis A are recognized in children or employees or if cases are recognized in 2 or more households of attenders—prophylaxis may be given to classroom contacts of an index case; c) in a common source outbreak, if a food handler is diagnosed with hepatitis A, hepatitis A vaccine and IG should be administered to other food handlers in the same establishment. Hepatitis A vaccine and IG is usually not offered to patrons; this may be considered if i) the food handlers were involved in the preparations of foods that were not heated; ii) deficiencies in personal hygiene are noted or the food handler has had diarrhea; and iii) the hepatitis A vaccine and IG can be given within 2 weeks after last exposure.

6) Investigation of contacts and source of infection: Search for missed cases and maintain surveillance of contacts in the patient's household or, in a common source outbreak, people exposed to the same risk.

7) Specific treatment: None.

C. Epidemic measures:

1) Determine mode of transmission (person-to-person or common vehicle) through epidemiological investigation; identify the population exposed. Eliminate common sources of infection.

2) Effective use of hepatitis A vaccine in community-wide outbreak situations requires the identification of an appropriate target group for immunization, the initiation of immunization early in the course of the outbreak and the rapid achievement of high (approximately 70% at least) first-dose vaccine coverage levels. Specific outbreak control measures must be tailored to the characteristics of hepatitis A epidemiology and of the existing hepatitis A immunization program, if any, in the community. Immunization of older children who have not previously received vaccine should be accelerated in communities with ongoing programs of routine hepatitis A immunization for young children; target immunization should be undertaken for groups or areas (age groups, risk groups, census tracts) where local surveillance and epidemiological data show the highest rates. In outbreak

settings such as day care, hospitals, institutions and schools, routine use of hepatitis A vaccine is not warranted. These immunization programs may reduce disease incidence only in the group(s) targeted.

3) Make special efforts to improve sanitary and hygienic practices to eliminate fecal contamination of foods and water.

4) Outbreaks in institutions may warrant mass prophylaxis with hepatitis A vaccine and IG.

D. Disaster implications: Hepatitis A is a potential problem in large collections of people with overcrowding, inadequate sanitation and water supplies; if cases occur, increased efforts should be exerted to improve sanitation and safety of water supplies. Mass administration of hepatitis A vaccine, which should be carefully planned, is not a substitute for environmental measures.

E. International measures: None.

II. VIRAL HEPATITIS B ICD-9 070.3; ICD-10 B16
(Type B hepatitis, Serum hepatitis, Homologous serum jaundice, Australia antigen hepatitis, HB)

1. Identification—A small proportion of acute hepatitis B virus (HBV) infections may be clinically recognized; less than 10% of children and 30%–50% of adults with acute hepatitis B virus (HBV) infection show icteric disease. In those with clinical illness, the onset is usually insidious, with anorexia, vague abdominal discomfort, nausea and vomiting, sometimes arthralgias and rash, often progressing to jaundice. Fever may be absent or mild. Severity ranges from inapparent cases detectable only by liver function tests to fulminating, fatal cases of acute hepatic necrosis. The case-fatality rate is about 1%; higher in those over 40. Fulminant HBV infection also occurs in pregnancy and among newborns of infected mothers.

Chronic HBV infection is found in 0.5% of adults in North America and in 0.1%–20% in other parts of the world. After acute HBV infection, the risk of developing chronic infection varies inversely with age; chronic HBV infection occurs among about 90% of infants infected at birth, 20%–50% of children infected from 1 to 5 years, and 1%–10% of persons infected as older children and adults. Chronic HBV infection is common in persons with immunodeficiency. Persons with chronic infection may or may not have a history of clinical hepatitis. About one-third have elevated aminotransferases; biopsy findings range from normal to chronic active hepatitis, with or without cirrhosis. An estimated 15%–25% of persons with chronic HBV infection will die prematurely of either cirrhosis or hepatocellular carcinoma. HBV may be the cause of up to 80% of all cases of hepatocellular carcinoma worldwide.

Demonstration in sera of specific antigens and/or antibodies confirms diagnosis. Three clinically useful antigen-antibody systems are identified for hepatitis B: 1) hepatitis B surface antigen (HBsAg) and antibody to HBsAg (anti-HBs); 2) hepatitis B core antigen (HBcAg) and antibody to HBcAg (anti-HBc); and 3) hepatitis B e antigen (HBeAg) and antibody to HBeAg (anti-HBe). Commercial kits are available for all markers except HBcAg. HBsAg can be detected in serum from several weeks before onset of symptoms to days, weeks or months after onset; it persists in chronic infections. Anti-HBc appears at the onset of illness and persists indefinitely. Demonstration of anti-HBc in serum indicates HBV infection, current or past; high titres of IgM anti-HBc occur during acute infection—IgM anti-HBc usually disappears within 6 months but can persist in some cases of chronic hepatitis; this test may reliably diagnose acute HBV infection. HbsAg is present in serum during acute infections and persists in chronic infections. The presence of HBsAg indicates that the person is potentially infectious. The presence of HBeAg is associated with relatively high infectivity.

2. Infectious agent—Hepatitis B virus (HBV), a hepadnavirus, is a 42-nanometer partially double-stranded DNA virus composed of a 27-nanometer nucleocapsid core (HBcAg), surrounded by an outer lipoprotein coat containing the surface antigen (HBsAg). HBsAg is antigenically heterogeneous, with a common antigen (designated a) and 2 pairs of mutually exclusive antigens (d, y, w (including several subdeterminants) and r), resulting in 4 major subtypes: adw, ayw, adr and ayr. The distribution of subtypes varies geographically; because of the common "a" determinant, protection against one subtype appears to confer protection against the other subtypes, and no differences in clinical features have been related to subtype. A genotype classification based on sequencing of genetic material has been introduced: HBV is currently classified into 8 main genotypes (A-H). There is growing evidence of differences in severity of liver disease between some HBV genotypes, which as of today are research tools.

3. Occurrence—Worldwide; endemic with little seasonal variation. WHO estimates that more than 2 billion persons have been infected with HBV (including 350 million chronically infected). Each year about a million persons die as a result of HBV infections and over 4 million new acute clinical cases occur. In countries where HBV is highly endemic (HBsAg prevalence 8% or higher), most infections occur during infancy and early childhood. Where HBV endemicity is intermediate (HBsAg prevalence from 2%-7%), infections occur commonly in all age groups, although the high rate of chronic infection is primarily maintained by transmission during infancy and early childhood. Where endemicity is low (HBsAg prevalence under 2%), most infections occur in young adults, especially those belonging to known risk groups. Even in countries with low HBV endemicity, a high proportion of chronic infections may be acquired during childhood because the development of chronic infection is age-dependent. Most of these infections would be prevented by perinatal vaccination against hepatitis B of all newborns or infants.

Serological evidence of previous infection may vary depending on age and socioeconomic class. Among the adult US population 5% have anti-HBc and 0.5% are HBsAg positive. Exposure to HBV may be common in certain high-risk groups, including injecting drug users, heterosexuals with multiple partners, men who have sex with men, household contacts and sex partners of HBV-infected persons, health care and public safety workers who have exposure to blood in the workplace, clients and staff in institutions for the developmentally disabled, hemodialysis patients and prisoners.

In the past, recipients of blood products were at high risk. In countries where pretransfusion screening of blood for HBsAg is required, and where pooled blood clotting factors (especially antihemophilic factor) are processed to destroy the virus, this risk has been virtually eliminated; however, it is still present in many developing countries. Contaminated and inadequately sterilized syringes and needles have resulted in outbreaks of hepatitis B among patients; this has been a major mode of transmission worldwide. Occasionally, outbreaks have been traced to tattoo parlours and acupuncturists. Rarely, transmission to patients from HBsAg-positive health care workers has been documented. Outbreaks have been reported among patients in dialysis centers in many countries through failure to adhere to recommended infection control practices against transmission of HBV and other bloodborne pathogens in these settings.

4. Reservoir—Humans. Chimpanzees are susceptible, but an animal reservoir in nature has not been recognized. Closely related hepadnaviruses are found in woodchucks, ducks, ground squirrels and other animals such as snow leopards and German herons; none cause disease in humans.

5. Mode of transmission—Body substances capable of transmitting HBV include: blood and blood products; saliva (although no outbreaks of HBV infection due to saliva alone have been documented); cerebrospinal fluid; peritoneal, pleural, pericardial and synovial fluid; amniotic fluid; semen and vaginal secretions and any other body fluid containing blood; and unfixed tissues and organs. The presence of antigen or viral DNA (HBV-DNA above 10^5 copies/mL) indicates high virus titre and higher infectivity of these fluids.

Transmission occurs by percutaneous (IV, IM, SC, intradermal) and permucosal exposure to infective body fluids. Because HBV is stable on environmental surfaces for at least 7 days, indirect inoculation of HBV can occur via inanimate objects. Fecal-oral or vector-borne transmission has not been demonstrated.

Major modes of HBV transmission include sexual or close household contact with an infected person, perinatal mother-to-infant transmission, injecting drug use and nosocomial exposure. Sexual transmission from infected men to women is about 3 times more efficient than that from infected women to men. Anal intercourse, insertive or receptive, is associated with an increased risk of infection. Transmission of HBV in households primarily occurs from child to child. Communally used razors and toothbrushes have been implicated as occasional vehicles of HBV transmission in this setting. Perinatal transmission is common, especially when HBV-infected mothers are also HBeAg-positive. The rate of transmission from HBsAg-positive, HBeAg-positive mothers is more than 70%; from HBsAg-positive, HBeAg-negative mothers it is less than 10%. Anti-HBe antibody-positive chronic hepatitis B was first described in patients of the Mediterranean Basin, where about 20% of HBsAg carriers were positive for anti-HBe antibodies and showed detectable serum levels of HBV DNA with liver necro-inflammation. The infecting HBV variants show mutations in the precore region that hamper HBeAg production. The HBeAg-negative form of chronic hepatitis B is present worldwide, and has been associated with transmission. Transmission through injecting drug use occurs though transfer of HBV-infected blood by sharing syringes and needles either directly or through contamination of drug preparation equipment. Nosocomial exposures such as transfusion of blood or blood products, hemodialysis, acupuncture and needlestick or other "sharps" injuries sustained by hospital personnel have resulted in HBV transmission. IG, heat treated plasma protein fraction, albumin and fibrinolysin are considered safe.

6. **Incubation period**—Usually 45–180 days, average 60–90 days. As short as 2 weeks to the appearance of HBsAg, and rarely as long as 6–9 months; variation is related in part to amount of virus in the inoculum, mode of transmission and host factors.

7. **Period of communicability**—All persons who are HBsAg-positive are potentially infectious. Blood from experimentally inoculated volunteers has been shown to be infective weeks before the onset of first symptoms and to remain infective through the acute clinical course of the disease. The infectivity of chronically infected individuals varies from high (HBeAg-positive) to modest (anti-HBe-positive).

8. **Susceptibility**—Susceptibility is general. Disease is often milder and anicteric in children; in infants it is usually asymptomatic. Protective immunity follows infection if antibodies to HBsAg (anti-HBs) develop and HBsAg is negative. Persons with Down syndrome, lymphoproliferative disease, HIV infection and those on hemodialysis appear more likely to develop chronic infection.

9. **Methods of control**—

   A. Preventive measures:

      1) Effective hepatitis B vaccines have been available since 1982. Two types of hepatitis B vaccines have been licensed and have been shown to be safe and highly protective against all

subtypes of HBV. The first, prepared from plasma from HBsAg-positive persons, is still widely used. The second, from recombinant DNA (rDNA), is produced by using HBsAg synthesized by yeast or cell-lines into which a plasmid containing the gene for HBsAg has been inserted. Combined passive-active immunoprophylaxis with hepatitis B immunoglobulin (HBIG) and vaccine has been shown comparable to vaccine alone in stimulating anti-HBs titres, but is expensive and not available in all countries.

a) In all countries, routine infant immunization should be the primary strategy to prevent HBV infection. Immunization of successive infant cohorts produces a highly immune population and suffices to interrupt transmission. In countries with high endemicity for HBV, routine infant immunization rapidly eliminates transmission because virtually all chronic infections are acquired among young children. Where HBV endemicity is low or intermediate, immunizing infants alone will not substantially lower disease incidence for about 15 years because most infections occur among adolescents and young adults; vaccine strategies for older children, adolescents and adults may be desirable. Strategies to ensure high vaccine coverage of successive age group cohorts are likely to be most effective in eliminating HBV transmission. In addition, immunization strategies can be targeted to high-risk groups, which account for most cases among adolescents and adults.

b) Testing to exclude people with pre-existing anti-HBs or anti-HBc is not required prior to immunization, but may be desirable as a cost-saving method among older children and adults in countries where the level of pre-existing infection is high.

c) Immunity against HBV is believed to persist for at least 15 years after successful immunization.

d) Vaccines licensed in different parts of the world may have varying dosages and schedules; in the USA they are most commonly administered in 3 IM doses: for infants, the first dose is given at birth or at 1–2 months of age with subsequent doses 1 to 2 and 6 to 18 months later. For infants born to HBsAg positive women, the schedule should be birth, 1–2 and 6 months of age. These infants should also receive 0.5 ml of HBIG (see 9B5a). The dose of vaccine varies by manufacturer. In mid-1999, it was announced that very small infants who receive multiple doses of vaccines containing thiomersal/thimerosal were at risk of receiving more than the recommended limits for mercury exposure as set out by industrialized guidelines. On the basis of a hypothetical risk of mercury exposure, reduction or elimination of thiomersal/thimerosal in vaccines as rapidly as possible was encouraged, although pharmacological and epidemiological data render it highly unlikely that such vaccines give rise to neurological adverse effects. Single antigen preservative-free hepatitis B vaccine is now available.

e) Pregnancy is not a contraindication for receiving hepatitis B vaccine.

2) The current WHO hepatitis B prevention strategy is based on routine universal newborn or infant immunization. The greatest fall in incidence and prevalence of hepatitis B is in countries with high vaccine coverage at birth or in infancy. Vaccination of adolescents is also valuable as it protects against transmission through sexual contact or injection drug use. The current hepatitis B prevention strategy in the USA includes: a) screening of all pregnant women for the presence of HBsAg, providing HBIG and hepatitis B vaccine to infants of HBsAg positive mothers, and providing hepatitis B vaccine to susceptible household contacts; b) providing routine hepatitis B immunization for all infants; c) providing catch-up immunization to children in groups with high rates of chronic HBV infection (Alaskan natives, Pacific Islanders and children of first generation immigrants from countries with high prevalence of chronic HBV infection); d) catch-up immunization of previously unimmunized children and adolescents, with highest priority for children aged 11–12 years; and e) intensified efforts to immunize adolescents and adults in defined risk groups.

3) Persons at high risk who should routinely receive pre-exposure hepatitis B immunization include: a) those who are diagnosed as having recently acquired other STDs and people who have a history of sexual activity with more than one partner in the previous 6 months; b) men who have sex with men; c) sexual partners and household contacts of HBsAg positive persons; d) inmates of juvenile detention facilities, prisons and jails; e) health care and public safety workers who perform tasks involving contact with blood or blood-contaminated body fluids; f) clients and staff of institutions for the developmentally disabled; g) hemodialysis patients; h) patients with bleeding disorders who receive blood products; and i) international travellers who plan to spend more than 6 months in areas with intermediate to high rates of chronic HBV infection (2% or greater) and who will have close contact with the local population.

4) Adequately sterilize all syringes and needles (including acupuncture needles) and lancets for finger puncture; use disposable equipment whenever possible. A sterile syringe and needle are essential for each individual receiving skin tests, parenteral inoculations or venepuncture. Discourage tattooing; enforce aseptic sanitary practices in tattoo parlours, including proper disposal of sharp or cutting tools.

5) In blood banks, all donated blood should be tested for HBsAg by sensitive tests; reject as donors all persons with a history of viral hepatitis, those who have a history of injecting drug use or show evidence of drug addiction or those who have received a blood transfusion or tattoo within the preceding 6 months. Use paid donors only in emergencies.

6) Limit administration of unscreened whole blood or potentially hazardous blood products to those in clear and immediate need of such therapeutic measures.

7) Maintain surveillance for all cases of posttransfusion hepatitis; keep a register of all people who donated blood for each case. Notify blood banks of potential carriers so that future donations may be identified promptly.

8) Although few public health authorities have established recommendations for HBV-positive health care workers, there is general consensus that HBeAg-positive HBV carriers should not perform exposure-prone surgery or similar treatment of patients. In the USA, medical and dental personnel infected with HBV and who are HBeAg-positive should not perform invasive procedures unless they have sought counsel from an expert review panel and have been advised under what circumstances, if any, they may continue to perform these procedures.

B. Control of patient, contacts and the immediate environment:

1) Report to local health authority: Official report obligatory in some countries; Class 2 (see Reporting).

2) Isolation: Universal precautions to prevent exposures to blood and body fluids.

3) Concurrent disinfection: Of equipment contaminated with blood or infectious body fluids.

4) Quarantine: Not applicable.

5) Immunization of contacts: Products available for postexposure prophylaxis include HBIG and hepatitis B vaccine. HBIG has high titres of anti-HBs (over 1:100 000). When indicated, administer HBIG as soon as possible after exposure.

   a) Infants born to HBsAg positive mothers should receive a single dose of vaccine within 12 hours of birth and, where available, HBIG (0.5 ml IM), the first dose of vaccine to be given concurrently with HBIG but at a separate site; second and third doses of vaccine (without HBIG) 1–2 and 6 months later. It is recommended to test the infant for HBsAg and anti-HBs at 9–15 months of age to monitor the success or failure of prophylaxis. Infants who are anti-HBs positive and HBsAg negative are protected and do not need further vaccine doses. Infants found to be anti-HBs negative and HBsAg negative should be reimmunized.

b) After percutaneous (e.g. needlestick) or mucous membrane exposures to blood that might contain HBsAg, a decision to provide postexposure prophylaxis must include consideration of: i) whether the source of the blood is available; ii) the HBsAg status of the source; iii) the hepatitis B immunization status of the exposed person. For previously unimmunized persons exposed to blood from an HBsAg positive source, a single dose of HBIG (0.06 ml/kg, or 5 ml for adults) should be given as soon as possible, but at least within 24 hours of high-risk needlestick exposure, and the hepatitis B vaccine series should be started. If active immunization cannot be given, another dose of HBIG should be given 1 month after the first. HBIG is not usually given for needlestick exposure to blood that is not known or highly suspected to be positive for HBsAg, since the risk of infection in these instances is small; however, initiation of hepatitis B immunization is recommended if the person has not previously been immunized. For previously immunized persons exposed to an HBsAg positive source, postexposure prophylaxis is not needed in cases with a protective antibody response to immunization (anti-HBs titre of 10 milli-IUs/mL or greater). For persons whose response to immunization is unknown, hepatitis B vaccine and/or HBIG should be administered.

c) After sexual exposure to a person with acute HBV infection, a single dose of HBIG (0.06 ml/kg) is recommended if it can be given within 14 days of the last sexual contact. For all exposed sexual contacts of persons with acute and chronic HBV infection, vaccine should be administered.

6) Investigation of contacts and source of infection: See 9C.

7) Specific treatment: No specific treatment available for acute hepatitis B. Alpha interferon, lamivudine and adefovir have been licensed for treatment of chronic hepatitis B in the USA and many other countries. Candidates for therapy should have liver biopsy evidence of chronic hepatitis B; treatment is most effective in individuals in the high-replicative phase

(HBeAg positive) of infection because they are the most likely to be symptomatic, infectious and at risk of long-term sequelae. Studies show that alpha interferon is successful in arresting viral replication in about 25%–40% of treated patients. Approximately 10% of patients who respond lose HBsAg 6 months after therapy. Clinical trials of long-term treatment with lamivudine have demonstrated sustained clearance of HBV DNA from serum, followed by improvements in serum aminotransferase levels and histological improvement. Lamivudine has fewer side-effects and is easier to administer, but has a modest efficacy rate, requires long-term treatment to maintain response, and is associated with a high rate of viral resistance, particularly when prolonged. Adefovir is an antiviral drug active against both wild-type and lamivudine-resistant HBV, and has an antiviral activity similar to that of lamivudine. There is no evidence that sustained responses and HBsAg clearance can be achieved with lamivudine or adefovir monotherapy.

C. *Epidemic measures:* When 2 or more cases occur in association with some common exposure, search for additional cases. Institute strict aseptic techniques. If a plasma derivative such as antihemophilic factor, fibrinogen, pooled plasma or thrombin is implicated, withdraw the lot from use and trace all recipients of the same lot in a search for additional cases.

D. *Disaster implications:* Relaxation of sterilization precautions and emergency use of unscreened blood for transfusions may result in an increased number of cases.

E. *International measures:* None.

III. VIRAL HEPATITIS C   ICD-9 070.5; ICD-10 B17.1
(Parenterally transmitted non-A non-B hepatitis [PT-NANB], Non-B transfusion associated hepatitis, Posttransfusion non-A non-B hepatitis, HCV infection)

1. **Identification**—Onset is usually insidious, with anorexia, vague abdominal discomfort, nausea and vomiting; progression to jaundice less frequent than with hepatitis B. Although initial infection may be asymptomatic (more than 90% of cases) or mild, a high percentage (50%–80%) develop a chronic infection. Of chronically infected persons, about half will eventually develop cirrhosis or cancer of the liver.

Diagnosis depends on detecting antibody to the hepatitis C virus (anti-HCV). Various tests are available for the diagnosis and monitoring of HCV infection. Tests that detect antibodies against the virus include the enzyme immunoassay (EIA) and the recombinant immunoblot assay. The same HCV antigens are used in both EIAs and the immunoblot assays. These tests do not distinguish between acute, chronic, or resolved infection. Reproducible and inexpensive EIA tests for the diagnosis of HCV are suitable for screening at-risk populations and recommended as the initial test for patients with clinical liver disease. A negative EIA test suffices to exclude a diagnosis of chronic HCV infection in immunocompetent patients. The high sensitivity and specificity of third-generation EIAs obviate the need for a confirmatory immunoblot assay in the diagnosis of individuals with clinical liver disease, particularly those with risk factors for HCV. Immunoblot assays are useful as a supplemental assay for persons screened in nonclinical settings and in persons with a positive EIA who test negative for HCV RNA.

Acute or chronic HCV infection in a patient with a positive EIA test should be confirmed by a sensitive HCV RNA assay. Confirmation may be unnecessary in a patient with evidence of liver disease and obvious risk factors for HCV. Target amplification techniques using polymerase chain reaction (PCR) or transcription-mediated amplification (TMA) have been developed as qualitative or quantitative tests for HCV RNA. Both target amplification (PCR) and signal amplification techniques (branched DNA) may be used to measure HCV RNA levels. A single positive qualitative assay for HCV RNA confirms active HCV replication, but a single negative assay does not exclude viraemia and may reflect a transient decline in viral level below the level of detection of the assay. A follow-up qualitative HCV RNA should be performed to confirm the absence of active HCV replication. Quantitative determination of HCV levels provides information on the likelihood of response to treatment in patients undergoing antiviral therapy. Liver biopsy can provide direct histological assessment of liver injury due to HCV but cannot be used to diagnose HCV infection.

2. Infectious agent—The hepatitis C virus is an enveloped RNA virus classified as a separate genus (*Hepacavirus*) in the Flaviviridae family. At least 6 different genotypes and approximately 100 subtypes of HCV exist. Evidence is limited regarding differences in clinical features, disease outcome or progression to cirrhosis or hepatocellular carcinoma (HCC) among persons with different genotypes. However, differences do exist in responses to antiviral therapy according to HCV genotypes.

3. Occurrence—Worldwide distribution. HCV prevalence is directly related to the prevalence of persons who routinely share injection equipment and to the prevalence of poor parenteral practices in health care settings. WHO estimates that some 130–170 million people (approximately 2%–3% of world population) are chronically infected with HCV, like HBV one of the most common global causes of chronic hepatitis, cirrhosis, and liver cancer. Most populations in Africa, the Americas, Europe and South East Asia have anti-HCV prevalence rates under 2.5%. Prevalence rates for the Western Pacific regions average 2.5 – 4.9%. In the Middle East, the prevalence of anti-HCV ranges from 1% to more than 12%.

The number of people with serological manifestation of HCV infection in Europe is estimated at 8.9 million and at 12.6 million in the Americas; the majority of infected individuals live in Asia (60 million in eastern Asia, 32 million in southeastern Asia) and Africa (28 million).

4. Reservoir—Humans; virus has been transmitted experimentally to chimpanzees.

5. Mode of transmission—HCV is primarily transmitted parenterally. Sexual and mother-to-child have been documented but appears far less efficient or frequent than the parenteral route.

6. Incubation period—Ranges from 2 weeks to 6 months; commonly 6–9 weeks. Chronic infection may persist for up to 20 years before the onset of cirrhosis or hepatoma.

7. Period of communicability—From one or more weeks before onset of the first symptoms; may persist in most persons indefinitely. Peaks in virus concentration appear to correlate with peaks in ALT activity.

8. Susceptibility—Susceptibility is general. The degree of immunity following infection is not known; repeated infections with HCV have been demonstrated in an experimental chimpanzee model.

9. Methods of control —

   A. *Preventive measures:* General control measures against HBV infection apply (see section II, 9A). Prophylactic IG is not effective. In blood bank operations, all donors should be routinely screened for anti-HCV and all donor units with elevated liver enzyme levels should be discarded. Routine virus inactivation of plasma-derived products, risk reduction counselling for persons uninfected but at high risk (e.g. health care workers) and nosocomial control activities must be maintained.

   B. *Control of patient, contacts and the immediate environment:* General control measures against HBV apply. Available data indicate that postexposure prophylaxis with IG is not effective in preventing infection. For the treatment of chronic hepatitis C, highest response rates (40–80%) have been achieved with a combination therapy of ribavirin and slow-release interferons ("pegylated interferons"), making it the treatment of choice. Genotype determinations influence treatment decisions. However, these medications have significant side-effects that require careful monitoring. Ribavirin is a teratogen; thus pregnancy should be avoided during treatment. Corticosteroids and acyclovir have not been effective.

   C. *Epidemic measures:* Same as for hepatitis B.

   D. *Disaster implications:* Same as for hepatitis B.

E. International measures: Ensure adequate virus inactivation for all internationally traded biological products.

IV. DELTA HEPATITIS   ICD-9 070.5; ICD-10 B17.0
(Viral hepatitis D, Hepatitis delta virus, \GD hepatitis, Delta agent hepatitis, Delta associated hepatitis)

1. Identification—Onset is usually abrupt, with signs and symptoms resembling those of hepatitis B; may be severe and always associated with a coexistent hepatitis B virus (HBV) infection. Delta hepatitis infection may occur as acute co-infection with hepatitis B virus, or as super-infection in persons with chronic HBV infection. In the former case the infection is usually self-limiting, in the latter it will usually progress to chronic hepatitis and delta hepatitis can be misdiagnosed as an exacerbation of chronic hepatitis B. Children may have a severe clinical course with usual progression to severe chronic hepatitis. In studies throughout Europe and the USA, 25%–50% of fulminant hepatitis cases thought to be caused by HBV were associated with concurrent HDV infection. Fulminant cases occur in super-infections rather than co-infections.

Diagnosis is through detection of total antibody to HDV (anti-HDV) by EIA. A positive IgM titre indicates ongoing replication; reverse transcription PCR is the most sensitive assay for detecting HDV viraemia.

2. Infectious agent—HDV is a virus-like particle of 35–37 nanometers consisting of a coat of HBsAg and a unique internal antigen, the delta antigen. Encapsulated with the delta antigen is the genome, a single-stranded RNA that can have a linear or circular conformation. The RNA does not hybridize with HBV DNA. HDV is unable to infect a cell by itself and requires co-infection with the HBV to undergo a complete replication cycle. Synthesis of HDV, in turn, results in temporary suppression of synthesis of HBV components. HDV is best considered in the new "satellite" family of sub-virions, some of which are pathogens of higher plants. Hepatitis D is the only agent in this family that infects animal species. Three genotypes of HDV have been identified: Genotype I is the most prevalent and widespread; genotype II is represented by 2 isolates from Japan and Taiwan (China); genotype III is reported only in the Amazon basin, causing severe fulminant hepatitis with microvesicular steatosis (spongiocytosis).

3. Occurrence—Worldwide, but prevalence varies widely. An estimated 10 million people are infected with hepatitis D virus and its helper virus HBV. It occurs epidemically or endemically in populations at high risk of HBV infection, such as where hepatitis B is endemic (highest in Africa and South America, southern Italy, Romania, parts of the Russian Federation); among hemophiliacs, injecting drug users and others who come in frequent contact with blood; in institutions for the developmentally disabled; and to a lesser extent among men who have sex with men.

Severe epidemics have been observed in tropical South America (Brazil, Colombia, Venezuela), in the Central African Republic and among injecting drug users in the USA. Dramatic changes have occurred in the epidemiology of HDV in the past years. Since HDV requires a concomitant HBV infection, the recent decrease in the prevalence of chronic HBsAg carriers in the general population has led to a rapid decline in both acute and chronic hepatitis D in the Mediterranean area (Greece, Italy, Spain) and in many other parts of the world. Better sanitation and social standards may also have contributed. New foci of high HDV prevalence continue to appear as in the case of Albania, areas of China, northern India and Japan (Okinawa).

4. Reservoir—Humans. Virus can be transmitted experimentally to chimpanzees and to woodchucks infected with HBV and woodchuck hepatitis virus, respectively.

5. Mode of transmission—Thought to be similar to that of HBV: exposure to infected blood and serous body fluids, contaminated needles, syringes and plasma derivatives such as antihemophilic factor, and through sexual transmission. Intrafamily contacts with HBsAg carriers are a major risk factor for the spreading of HDV.

6. Incubation period—Approximately 2–8 weeks.

7. Period of communicability—Blood is potentially infectious during all phases of active delta hepatitis infection. Peak infectivity probably occurs just prior to onset of acute illness, when particles containing the delta antigen are readily detected in the blood. Following onset, viraemia probably falls rapidly to low or undetectable levels. HDV has been transmitted to chimpanzees from the blood of chronically infected patients in whom particles containing delta antigen could not be detected.

8. Susceptibility—All people susceptible to HBV infection or who have chronic HBV can be infected with HDV. Severe disease can occur even in children.

9. Methods of control—

    A. ***Preventive measures:*** For people susceptible to HBV infection, same as for hepatitis B. Prevention of HBV infection with hepatitis B vaccine prevents infection with HDV. Among persons with chronic HBV, the only effective measure is avoidance of exposure to any potential source of HDV. HBIG, IG and hepatitis B vaccine do not protect persons with chronic HBV from infection by HDV. Studies suggest that measures decreasing sexual exposure and needle-sharing are associated with a decline in the incidence of HDV infection.

> *B., C., D.* and *E.* *Control of patient, contacts and the immediate environment, Epidemic measures, Disaster implications* and *International measures:* See hepatitis B.

V. VIRAL HEPATITIS E   ICD-9 070.5; ICD-10 B17.2
(Enterically transmitted non-A non-B hepatitis [ET-NANB], Epidemic non-A non-B hepatitis, Fecal-oral non-A non-B hepatitis)

1. Identification—Clinical course similar to that of hepatitis A; no evidence of a chronic form. The case-fatality rate is similar to that of hepatitis A except in pregnant women, where it may reach 20% among those infected during the third trimester of pregnancy. Epidemic and sporadic cases have been described.

Diagnosis depends on clinical and epidemiological features and exclusion of other causes of hepatitis, especially hepatitis A, by serological means. Acute hepatitis E is diagnosed in the presence of IgM anti-HEV. HEV RNA can be detected by PCR in acute phase feces in approximately 50% of cases. Western blot assays to detect anti-HEV IgM and IgG in serum can be used to confirm the results of EIA tests, along with PCR tests for the detection of HEV RNA in serum and feces, immunofluorescent antibody blocking assays to detect antibody to HEV antigen in serum and liver, and immune electron microscopy to visualize viral particles in feces.

2. Infectious agent—The hepatitis E virus (HEV), a spherical, nonenveloped, single-stranded RNA virus approximately 32 to 34 nanometers in diameter, provisionally classified in the Caliciviridae family. The organization of the HEV genome differs substantially from that of other caliciviruses and HEV may eventually be classified in a separate family.

3. Occurrence—HEV is the major causal agent of enterically transmitted non-A, non-B hepatitis worldwide. In recent years, serological tests for both IgM and IgG anti-HEV have allowed a comprehensive epidemiological survey of the distribution of HEV—the prevalence of HEV antibodies in suspected or documented endemic regions was much lower than expected (3%–26%), and it was higher than anticipated (1–3%) in nonendemic regions such as the USA. HEV infections account for >50% of acute sporadic hepatitis in some highly endemic areas. Outbreaks of hepatitis E and sporadic cases occur over a wide geographic area, primarily in countries with inadequate environmental sanitation. Outbreaks often occur as waterborne epidemics, but sporadic cases and epidemics not clearly related to water have been reported. The highest rates of clinically evident disease occur in young to middle aged adults; lower disease rates in younger age groups may be the result of anicteric and/or subclinical HEV infection. In most industrialized countries, hepatitis E cases have been documented only among travellers returning from HEV endemic areas. Outbreaks have also been reported from Algeria,

Bangladesh, China, Côte d'Ivoire, Egypt, Ethiopia, Greece, India, Indonesia, the Islamic Republic of Iran, Jordan, the Libyan Arab Jamahiriya, Mexico, Myanmar, Nepal, Nigeria, Pakistan, southern areas of the Russian Federation, Somalia, eastern Sudan and The Gambia. A large waterborne outbreak (3682 cases) occurred in 1993 in Uttar Pradesh.

4. Reservoir—Man is the natural host for HEV; some non-human primates, e.g. chimpanzees, cynomolgus monkeys, rhesus monkeys, pigtail monkeys, owl monkeys, tamarins and African green monkeys are reported as susceptible to natural infection with human strains of HEV. Natural infections have been described in pigs, chicken and cattle, particularly in highly endemic areas.

5. Mode of transmission—Primarily by the fecal-oral route; fecally contaminated drinking-water is the most commonly documented vehicle of transmission. Person-to-person transmission probably also occurs through the fecal-oral route, although secondary household cases are uncommon during outbreaks. Recent studies suggest that hepatitis E may in fact be a zoonotic infection with coincident areas of high human infection.

6. Incubation period—The range is 15 to 64 days; the mean incubation period has varied from 26 to 42 days in various epidemics.

7. Period of communicability—Not known. HEV has been detected in stools 14 days after the onset of jaundice and approximately 4 weeks after oral ingestion of contaminated food or water; it persists for about 2 weeks.

8. Susceptibility—Unknown. Over 50% of HEV infections may be anicteric; the expression of icterus appears to increase with increasing age. Women in the third trimester of pregnancy are especially susceptible to fulminant disease. The occurrence of major epidemics among young adults in regions where other enteric viruses are highly endemic and most of the population acquires infection in infancy remains unexplained.

9. Methods of control—

    A. Preventive measures: Provide educational programs to stress sanitary disposal of feces and careful handwashing after defecation and before handling food; follow basic measures to prevent fecal-oral transmission, as listed under Typhoid fever, 9A. Administration of immune serum globulin from endemic areas has not decreased infection rates during epidemics in India; encouraging advances have occurred in HEV vaccine development.

    B. Control of patient, contacts and the immediate environment:

        1), 2) and 3) Report to local health authority, Isolation and Concurrent disinfection: See hepatitis A.

4) Quarantine: Not applicable.
5) Immunization of contacts: No products are available to prevent hepatitis E. IG prepared from plasma collected in non- and high-HEV endemic areas were not effective in preventing clinical disease during hepatitis E outbreaks. A candidate vaccine using recombinant capsid protein is currently undergoing phase II/III clinical trials.
6) Investigation of contacts and source of infection: Same as for hepatitis A.
7) Specific treatment: None.

C. *Epidemic measures:* Determine mode of transmission through epidemiological investigation; investigate water supply and identify populations at increased risk of infection; special efforts to improve sanitary and hygienic practices in order to eliminate fecal contamination of foods and water.

D. *Disaster implications:* A potential problem where there is mass crowding and inadequate sanitation and water supplies. If cases occur, increased effort should be exerted to improve sanitation and the safety of water supplies.

E. *International measures:* None.

[D. Lavanchy]

HERPES SIMPLEX ICD-9 054; ICD-10 B00

ANOGENITAL HERPESVIRAL INFECTIONS ICD-10 A60
(Alphaherpesviral disease, Herpesvirus hominis, Human herpesviruses 1 and 2)

1. Identification—Herpes simplex is a viral infection characterized by a localized primary lesion, latency and a tendency to localized recurrence. The two causal agents— herpes simplex virus (HSV) types 1 and 2— generally produce distinct clinical syndromes, depending on the portal of entry. Either may infect the genital tract or oral mucosa.

Primary infection with HSV-1 may be mild and inapparent and occur in early childhood. In approximately 10% of primary infections, overt disease may appear as an illness of varying severity, marked by fever and malaise lasting a week or more; it may be associated with gingivostomatitis accompanied by vesicular lesions in the oropharynx, severe keratoconjunctivitis, a generalized cutaneous eruption complicating chronic eczema, meningoencephalitis or some of the fatal generalized infections in newborn infants (congenital herpes simplex, ICD-9 771.2, ICD-10 P35.2).

HSV-1 causes about 2% of acute pharyngotonsillitis, usually as a primary infection.

Reactivation of latent infection commonly results in herpes labialis (fever blisters, cold sores) manifested, usually on the face or lips, by superficial clear vesicles on an erythematous base that crust and heal within days. Reactivation is precipitated by various forms of trauma, fever, physiological changes or intercurrent disease, and may also involve other body tissues; it occurs in the presence of circulating antibodies, which are seldom elevated by reactivation. Severe and extensive spread of infection may occur in those who are immunodeficient or immunosuppressed.

CNS involvement may appear in association with either primary infection or recrudescence. HSV-1 is a common cause of meningoencephalitis. Fever, headache, leukocytosis, meningeal irritation, drowsiness, confusion, stupor, coma and focal neurological signs may occur and are frequently referable to one or the other temporal region. The condition may be confused with other intracranial lesions including brain abscess and tuberculous meningitis. Because antiviral therapy may reduce case-fatality, diagnostic PCR for DNA of herpes virus in the CSF or biopsy of cerebral tissue should be considered early in clinically suspected cases.

Genital herpes, usually caused by HSV-2, occurs mainly in adults and is sexually transmitted. Primary and recurrent infections occur, with or without symptoms. In women, the principal sites of primary disease are the cervix and the vulva; recurrent disease generally involves the vulva, perineal skin, legs and buttocks. In men, lesions appear on the glans penis or prepuce, and in the anus and rectum of those engaging in anal sex. Other genital or perineal sites, as well as the mouth, may be involved in men and women, depending on sexual practices. HSV-2 has been associated with aseptic meningitis and radiculitis rather than meningoencephalitis.

Neonatal infections can be divided into 3 clinical presentations: disseminated infections involving the liver, encephalitides and infections limited to the skin, eyes or mouth. The first two forms are often lethal. Infections are most frequently due to HSV-2, but HSV-1 is also common. Risk to the infant depends on two important maternal factors: stage of pregnancy at which the mother excretes HSV, and whether the infection is primary or secondary. Only excretion at the time of delivery is dangerous to the newborn, with the rare exception of intrauterine infections. Primary infection in the mother raises the risk of infection from 3% to over 30%, presumably because maternal immunity confers a degree of protection.

Diagnosis is suggested by characteristic cytological changes (multinucleated giant cells with intranuclear inclusions in tissue scrapings or biopsy), but confirmed through direct FA tests, isolation of the virus from oral or genital lesions, or a brain biopsy in cases of encephalitis or again by demonstration of HSV DNA in lesion or spinal fluid by PCR. A 4-fold titre rise in paired sera in various serological tests confirms the diagnosis of primary infection; the presence of herpes-specific IgM is suggestive but not conclusive evidence of primary infection. Reliable techniques to differentiate type 1 from type 2 antibody are now available in diagnostic laboratories; virus isolates can be distinguished readily from one another by DNA analysis. Type-specific serologic tests are not yet widely available.

2. Infectious agent—Herpes simplex virus in the virus family Herpesviridae, subfamily Alphaherpesvirinae. HSV types 1 and 2 can be differentiated immunologically (especially when highly specific or monoclonal antibodies are used) and differ with respect to their growth patterns in cell culture, embryonated eggs and experimental animals.

3. Occurrence—Worldwide; 50%–90% of adults possess circulating antibodies against HSV-1; initial infection with HSV-1 usually occurs before the fifth year of life, but more primary infections in adults are now being reported. HSV-2 infection usually begins with sexual activity and is rare before adolescence, except in sexually abused children. HSV-2 antibody occurs in 20%–30% of American adults. The prevalence is greater (up to 60%) in lower socioeconomic groups and persons with multiple sexual partners.

4. Reservoir—Humans.

5. Mode of transmission—Contact with HSV-1 in the saliva of carriers is probably the most important mode of spread. Infection on the hands of health care personnel (e.g. dentists) from patients shedding HSV results in herpetic whitlow. Transmission of HSV-2 is usually by sexual contact. Both types 1 and 2 may be transmitted to various sites by oral-genital, oral-anal or anal-genital contact. Transmission to the neonate usually occurs via the infected birth canal, less commonly in utero or postpartum.

6. Incubation period—From 2–12 days.

7. Period of communicability—HSV can be isolated for 2 weeks and up to 7 weeks after primary stomatitis or primary genital lesions. Both primary and recurrent infections may be asymptomatic. After either, HSV may be shed intermittently from mucosal sites for years and possibly lifelong, in the presence or absence of clinical manifestations. In recurrent lesions, infectivity is shorter than after primary infection, and usually the virus cannot be recovered after 5 days.

8. Susceptibility—Humans are probably universally susceptible.

9. Methods of control—

    A. Preventive measures:

        1) Health education and personal hygiene directed toward minimizing the transfer of infectious material.

2) Avoid contaminating the skin of eczematous patients with infectious material.

3) Health care personnel should wear gloves when in direct contact with potentially infectious lesions.

4) When primary genital herpes infections occur in late pregnancy, caesarean section is advised before the membranes rupture because of the risk of fatal neonatal infection (30%–50%). Use of scalp electrodes is contraindicated. The risk of fatal neonatal infection after a recurrent infection is much lower (3%–5%), and caesarean section advisable only when active lesions are present at delivery.

5) Use of latex condoms in sexual practice may decrease the risk of infection; no antiviral agent has yet been proved to be practical in prophylaxis of primary infection, although acyclovir may be used prophylactically to reduce the incidence of recurrences and of herpes infections in immunodeficient patients.

B. Control of patient, contacts and the immediate environment:

1) Report to local health authority: Official case report in adults not ordinarily justifiable, Class 5; neonatal infections reportable in some areas, Class 3 (see Reporting).

2) Isolation: Contact isolation for neonatal and disseminated or primary severe lesions; for recurrent lesions, drainage and secretion precautions. Patients with herpetic lesions should have no contact with newborns, children with eczema or burns, or immunodeficient patients.

3) Concurrent disinfection: Not applicable.

4) Quarantine: Not applicable.

5) Immmunization of contacts: Not applicable.

6) Investigation of contacts and source of infection: Seldom of practical value.

7) Specific treatment: The acute manifestations of herpetic keratitis and early dendritic ulcers may be treated with trifluridine or adenine arabinoside as an ophthalmic ointment or solution. Corticosteroids should never be used for ocular involvement unless administered by an experienced ophthalmologist. Acyclovir IV is of value in herpes simplex encephalitis, but may not prevent residual neurological problems. Acyclovir used orally, intravenously or topically has been shown to reduce shedding of virus, diminish pain and accelerate healing time in primary genital and recurrent herpes, rectal herpes and herpetic whitlow. The oral preparation is most convenient to use and may benefit patients with extensive recurrent infections. However, mutant strains of herpes virus resistant to acyclovir have been reported. Valacyclovir and famciclovir are recently licensed congeners

of acyclovir that have equivalent efficacy. Prophylactic daily administration of these drugs can reduce the frequency of HSV recurrences in adults. Neonatal infections should be treated with high-dose intravenous acyclovir.

C. *Epidemic measures:* Not applicable.

D. *Disaster implications:* None.

E. *International measures:* None.

MENINGOENCEPHALITIS DUE TO CERCOPITHECINE HERPES VIRUS 1   ICD-9 054.3; ICD-10 B00.4
(B-virus, Simian B disease)

HSV-1 (occasionally type 2) can cause meningoencephalitis; the picture is different with B-virus infection, which is a CNS disease caused by cercopithecine herpesvirus 1, a zoonotic virus closely related to HSV. This causes an ascending encephalomyelitis seen in veterinarians, laboratory workers and others in close contact with eastern Hemisphere monkeys or monkey cell cultures. After an incubation of 3 days to 3 weeks, there is acute febrile onset with headache, often local vesicular lesions, lympho-cytic pleocytosis and variable neurological patterns, ending in death in over 70% of cases, 1 day to 3 weeks after onset of symptoms. Occasional recoveries have been associated with considerable residual disability; a few cases, treated with acyclovir, have recovered completely. The virus causes a natural infection of monkeys analogous to HSV infection in humans; 30%–80% of rhesus monkeys (*Macaca mulatta*) are seropositive. During periods of stress (shipping and handling), they have high rates of viral shedding. Human illness, rare but highly fatal, is acquired through the bite of apparently normal monkeys, or exposure of naked skin or mucous membrane to infected saliva or monkey cell cultures. Prevention depends on proper use of protective gauntlets and care to minimize exposure to monkeys. All bite or scratch wounds incurred from macaques or from cages possibly contaminated with macaque secretions and that result in bleeding must be immediately and thoroughly scrubbed and cleaned with soap and water. Prophylactic treatment with an antiviral agent such as valacyclovir, acyclovir or famciclovir should be considered when an animal handler sustains a deep, penetrating wound that cannot be adequately cleaned, though it is not clear if this is as effective in humans as it is in rabbits. The B-virus status of the monkey should be determined to evaluate the risk. The appearance of any skin lesions or neurological symptoms, such as itching, pain, or numbness near the site of the wound calls for expert medical consultation for diagnosis and possible treatment.

[D. Lavanchy]

HISTOPLASMOSIS — ICD-9 115; ICD-10 B39

Two clinically different mycoses are designated as histoplasmosis; the pathogens that cause them cannot be distinguished morphologically when grown on culture media as moulds. Detailed information is given for the infection caused by *Histoplasma capsulatum* var. *capsulatum*, and a brief summary for that caused by *H. capsulatum* var. *duboisii*.

I. INFECTION BY *HISTOPLASMA CAPSULATUM* — ICD-9 115.0; ICD-10 B39.4

(Histoplasmosis capsulati, Histoplasmosis due to *H. capsulatum* var. *capsulatum*, American histoplasmosis)

1. Identification—A systemic mycosis of varying severity, with the primary lesion usually in the lungs. While infection is common, overt clinical disease is not. Five clinical forms are recognized:

1) Asymptomatic; although individuals manifest skin test reactivity to histoplasmin, this reagent is no longer commercially available.

2) Acute respiratory, which varies from a mild respiratory illness to temporary incapacity with general malaise, fever, chills, headache, myalgia, chest pains and nonproductive cough; occasional erythema multiforme and erythema nodosum. Multiple, small scattered calcifications in the lung, hilar lymph nodes, spleen and liver may be late findings.

3) Acute disseminated histoplasmosis with debilitating fever, GI symptoms, evidence of bone marrow suppression, hepatosplenomegaly, lymphadenopathy and a rapid course, most frequent in infants and young children and immunocompromised patients including AIDS cases. Without treatment, usually fatal.

4) Chronic disseminated disease with low-grade intermittent fever, weight loss, weakness, hepatosplenomegaly, mild hematological abnormalities and focal manifestations of disease (e.g. endocarditis, meningitis, mucosal ulcers of mouth, larynx, stomach or bowel and Addison disease). Subacute course progressing over 10–11 months and usually fatal unless treated.

5) Chronic pulmonary form, clinically and radiologically resembling chronic pulmonary tuberculosis with cavitation; occurs most often in middle-aged and elderly men with underlying

emphysema, progresses over months or years, with periods of quiescence and sometimes spontaneous cure.

Clinical diagnosis is confirmed by culture, DNA probe, or by visualizing the fungus in Giemsa- or Wright-stained smears of ulcer exudates, bone marrow, sputum or blood; demonstrating the fungus in biopsies of ulcers, liver, lymph nodes or lung requires special stains. The immunodiffusion test is the most specific and reliable of available serological tests. A rise in complement fixation titres in paired sera may occur early in acute infection and is suggestive evidence of active disease; a titre of 1:32 or greater is suggestive of active disease. False-negative tests are common, particularly in HIV-infected patients, and negative serology does not exclude the diagnosis. Detection of antigen in serum or urine is useful in making the diagnosis and following the results of treatment for disseminated histoplasmosis.

2. Infectious agent—*Histoplasma capsulatum* var. *capsulatum* (*Ajellomyces capsulatus*), a dimorphic fungus growing as a mould in soil and as a yeast in animal and human hosts.

3. Occurrence—Infections commonly occur in geographic foci over wide areas of the Americas, Africa, eastern Asia and Australia; rare in Europe. Hypersensitivity to histoplasmin (no longer manufactured) indicates antecedent infection and has been noted inasmuch as 80% of population in parts of eastern and central USA. Clinical disease is less frequent, severe progressive disease is rare. Prevalence increases from childhood to 15; the chronic pulmonary form is more common in males. Outbreaks have occurred in endemic areas in families, students and workers with exposure to bird, chicken or bat droppings or recently disturbed contaminated soil. Histoplasmosis occurs in dogs, cats, cattle, horses, rats, skunks, opossums, foxes and other animals, often with a clinical picture comparable to that in humans.

4. Reservoir—Soil with high organic content and undisturbed bird droppings, in particular that around and in old chicken houses, in bat-caves and around starling, blackbird and pigeon roosts.

5. Mode of transmission—Growth of the fungus in soil produces microconidia and tuberculate macroconidia; infection results from inhalation of airborne conidia. Person-to-person transmission can occur only if infected tissue is inoculated into a healthy person.

6. Incubation period—Symptoms appear within 3–17 days after exposure but this may be shorter with heavy exposure; commonly 10 days.

7. Period of communicability—Not transmitted from person to person.

8. Susceptibility—Susceptibility is general. Inapparent infections are common in endemic areas and usually result in increased resistance to infection. May be an opportunistic infection in those with compromised immunity.

9. Methods of control—

A. *Preventive measures:* Minimize exposure to dust in a contaminated environment, such as chicken coops and surrounding soil. Spray with water or oil to reduce dust; use protective masks.

B. *Control of patient, contacts and the immediate environment:*

1) Report to local health authority: In selected endemic areas; in many countries not a reportable disease, Class 3 (see Reporting).
2) Isolation: Not applicable.
3) Concurrent disinfection: Of sputum and articles soiled therewith. Terminal cleaning.
4) Quarantine: Not applicable.
5) Immmunization of contacts: Not applicable.
6) Investigation of contacts and source of infection: Household and occupational contacts for evidence of infection from a common environmental source.
7) Specific treatment: Itraconazole approved for pulmonary and disseminated histoplasmosis in non-HIV infected individuals. Ketoconazole approved for histoplasmosis in immunocompetent individuals. Neither should be used in patients with CNS involvement. For patients with acute disseminated histoplasmosis, IV amphotericin B is the drug of choice. Itraconazole constitutes effective chronic suppressive therapy in AIDS patients previously treated with amphotericin B.

C. *Epidemic measures:* Occurrence of grouped cases of acute pulmonary disease in or outside of an endemic area, particularly with history of exposure to dust within a closed space (caves or construction sites), should arouse suspicion of histoplasmosis. Suspected sites such as attics, basements, caves or construction sites with large amounts of bird droppings or bat guano must be investigated.

D. *Disaster implications:* None. Possible hazard if large groups, especially from nonendemic areas, are forced to move through or live in areas where the mould is prevalent.

E. *International measures:* None.

II. HISTOPLASMOSIS DUE TO
H. DUBOISII   ICD-9 115.1; ICD-10 B39.5
(Histoplasmosis due to *H. capsulatum* var. *duboisii*, African histoplasmosis)

This usually presents as a subacute granuloma of skin or bone. Infection, though usually localized, may be disseminated in the skin, subcutaneous tissue, lymph nodes, bones, joints, lungs and abdominal viscera. Disease is more common in males and may occur at any age, but especially in the second decade of life. Thus far, the disease has been recognized only in Africa and Madagascar. Diagnosis is made through culture or demonstration of yeast cells of *H. capsulatum* var. *duboisii* in tissue by smear or biopsy. These cells are much larger than the yeast cells of *H. capsulatum* var. *capsulatum*. The true prevalence of *H. duboisii*, its reservoir, mode of transmission and incubation period are unknown. It is not communicable from person to person. Treatment is the same as for histoplasmosis due to *H. capsulatum*.

HOOKWORM DISEASE   ICD-9 126; ICD-10 B76
(Ancylostomiasis, Uncinariasis, Necatoriasis)

1. Identification—A common chronic parasitic infection with a variety of symptoms, usually in proportion to the degree of anemia. In heavy infections, the bloodletting activity of the nematode leads to iron deficiency and hypochromic, microcytic anemia, the major cause of disability. Children with heavy long-term infection may have hypoproteinemia and may be retarded in mental and physical development. Occasionally, severe acute pulmonary and GI reactions follow exposure to infective larvae. Death is infrequent and usually can be attributed to other infections. Light hookworm infections generally produce few or no clinical effects.

Infection is confirmed by finding hookworm eggs in feces; early stool examinations may be negative until worms mature. Species differentiation requires microscopic examination of larvae cultured from the feces, or examination of adult worms expelled by purgation following a vermifuge. PCR-RFLP techniques allow species differentiation.

2. Infectious agents—*Ancylostoma duodenale*, *A. ceylanicum*, *A. braziliense*, *A. caninum* and *Necator americanus*.

3. Occurrence—Endemic in tropical and subtropical countries where sanitary disposal of human feces is not practised and soil, moisture and temperature conditions favor development of infective larvae. Also occurs in temperate climates under similar environmental conditions (e.g. mines). Both *Necator* and *Ancylostoma* occur in many parts of Asia (particularly southeastern Asia), the South Pacific and eastern Africa. *N. americanus* is the prevailing species throughout southeastern Asia, most of tropical Africa and America; *A. duodenale* prevails in North Africa, including the Nile Valley, northern India, northern parts of eastern Asia and the Andean areas of South America. *A. ceylanicum* occurs in southeastern Asia but is less common than either *N. americanus* or *A. duodenale*. *A. caninum* has been described in Australia as a cause of eosinophilic enteritis syndrome.

4. Reservoir—Humans for *A. duodenale* and *N. americanus*; cats and dogs for *A. ceylanicum*, *A. braziliense* and *A. caninum*.

5. Mode of transmission—Eggs in feces are deposited on the ground and hatch; under favorable conditions of moisture, temperature and soil type, larvae develop to the third stage, becoming infective in 7–10 days. Human infection occurs when infective larvae penetrate the skin, usually of the foot; in so doing, they produce a characteristic dermatitis (ground itch). The larvae of *A. caninum* and *A. braziliense* die within the skin, having produced cutaneous larva migrans. Normally, the larvae of *Necator*, *A. duodenale*, *A. ceylanicum* and other *Ancylostoma* enter the skin and pass via lymphatics and bloodstream to the lungs, enter the alveoli, migrate up the trachea to the pharynx, are swallowed and reach the small intestine where they attach to the intestinal wall, developing to maturity in 6–7 weeks (3–4 weeks in the case of *A. ceylanicum*) and typically producing thousands of eggs per day. Infection with *Ancylostoma* may also be acquired by ingesting infective larvae; possible vertical transmission through breastmilk has been reported.

6. Incubation period—Symptoms may develop after a few weeks to many months, depending on intensity of infection and iron intake of the host. Pulmonary infiltration, cough and tracheitis may occur during the lung migration phase of infection, particularly in *Necator* infections. After entering the body, *A. duodenale* may become dormant for about 8 months, after which development resumes, with a patent infection (stools containing eggs) a month later.

7. Period of communicability—No person-to-person transmission, but infected people can contaminate soil for several years in the absence of treatment. Under favorable conditions, larvae remain infective in soil for several weeks.

8. Susceptibility—Universal; no evidence that immunity develops with infection.

9. **Methods of control—**

   A. *Preventive measures:*

   1) Educate the public to the dangers of soil contamination by human, cat or dog feces, and in preventive measures, including wearing shoes in endemic areas.
   2) Prevent soil contamination by installation of sanitary disposal systems for human feces, especially sanitary latrines in rural areas. Night soil and sewage effluents are hazardous, especially where used as fertilizer.
   3) Examine and treat people migrating from endemic to receptive nonendemic areas, especially those who work barefoot in mines, construct dams or work in the agricultural sector.
   4) WHO recommends a strategy focused on high-risk groups for the control of morbidity due to soil-transmitted helminths, including community treatment (see Aseariasis), differentiated according to prevalence and severity of infections: i) universal medication of women (once a year, including pregnant women) and preschool children over 1 year (twice or thrice a year) if schoolchildren show 10% or more of heavy infections (4000+ hookworm eggs per gram of feces) whatever the prevalence; ii) yearly community medication targeted to risk groups (including pregnant women) if prevalence >50% and schoolchildren show <10% of heavy infections; iii) individual case management if prevalence <50% and schoolchildren show <10% of heavy infections. Extensive monitoring has shown no significant ill effects of administration to pregnant women under these circumstances.

   B. *Control of patient, contacts and the immediate environment:*

   1) Report to local health authority: Official report not ordinarily justifiable, Class 5 (see Reporting).
   2) Isolation: Not applicable.
   3) Concurrent disinfection: Safe disposal of feces to prevent contamination of soil.
   4) Quarantine: Not applicable.
   5) Immmunization of contacts: Not applicable.
   6) Investigate contacts and source of infection: Each infected contact and carrier is a potential or actual indirect spreader of infection.
   7) Specific treatment: Single dose oral treatment with mebendazole, albendazole (half dose for children 12–24 months), levamisole or pyrantel pamoate is recommended; adverse reactions are infrequent. Follow-up stool examination is indicated after 2 weeks, and treatment must be repeated if a heavy worm burden persists. Iron supplementation will correct the anemia

and should be used in conjunction with deworming. Transfusion may be necessary for severe anemia. As a general rule, pregnant women should not be treated in the first trimester unless there are specific medical or public health reasons.

C. *Epidemic measures:* Prevalence survey in highly endemic areas: provide periodic mass treatment. Health education in environmental sanitation and personal hygiene, and provide facilities for excreta disposal.

D. *Disaster implications:* None.

E. *International measures:* None.

[L. Savioli]

HYMENOLEPIASIS   ICD-9 123.6; ICD-10 B71.0

I. HYMENOLEPIASIS DUE TO *HYMENOLEPIS NANA*
(Dwarf tapeworm infection)

1. Identification—An intestinal infection with very small tapeworms; light infections are usually asymptomatic. Massive numbers of worms may cause enteritis with or without diarrhea, abdominal pain and other vague symptoms such as pallor, loss of weight and weakness.

Microscope identification of eggs in feces confirms diagnosis.

2. Infectious agent—*Hymenolepis nana* (dwarf tapeworm), the only human tapeworm without an obligatory intermediate host.

3. Occurrence—Cosmopolitan; more common in warm than cold, and in dry than wet climates. Dwarf tapeworm is the most common human tapeworm in the USA and Latin America; it is common in Australia, Mediterranean countries, the Near East and India.

4. Reservoir—Humans; possibly mice.

5. Mode of transmission—Eggs of *H. nana* are infective when passed in feces. Infection is acquired through ingestion of eggs in contaminated food or water; directly from fecally contaminated fingers (autoinfection or person-to-person transmission); or ingestion of insects bearing larvae that have developed from eggs ingested by the insect. *H. nana* eggs, once ingested, hatch in the intestine, liberating oncospheres that enter mucosal villi and develop into cysticercoids; these rupture into the lumen and grow into adult tapeworms. Some *H. nana* eggs are immediately infectious when released from the proglottids in the human gut, so autoinfections or person-to-person transmission can occur. If eggs are ingested by meal-worms, larval fleas, beetles or other insects, they may develop into cysticercoids that are infective to humans and rodents when ingested.

6. Incubation period—Onset of symptoms is variable; the development of mature worms requires about 2 weeks.

7. Period of communicability—As long as eggs are passed in feces. *H. nana* infections may persist for years.

8. Susceptibility—Universal; infection produces resistance to reinfection. Children are more susceptible than adults; intensive infection occurs in immunodeficient and malnourished children.

9. Methods of control—

A. *Preventive measures:*

1) Educate the public in personal hygiene and safe disposal of feces.
2) Provide and maintain clean toilet facilities.
3) Protect food and water from contamination with human and rodent feces.
4) Treat to remove sources of infection.
5) Eliminate rodents from home environment.

B. *Control of patient, contacts and the immediate environment:*

1) Report to local health authority: Official report not ordinarily justifiable, Class 5 (see Reporting).
2) Isolation: Not applicable.
3) Concurrent disinfection: Safe disposal of feces.
4) Quarantine: Not applicable.
5) Immunization of contacts: Not applicable.
6) Investigation of contacts and source of infection: Fecal examination of family or institution members.
7) Specific treatment: Praziquantel or niclosamide is effective. Albendazole may be considered where intestinal helminthiases coexist.

C. *Epidemic measures:* Outbreaks in schools and institutions can best be controlled through treatment of infected individuals and special attention to personal and group hygiene.

D. *Disaster implications:* None.

E. *International measures:* None.

II. HYMENOLEPIASIS DUE TO
HYMENOLEPIS DIMINUTA
ICD-9 123.6;
ICD-10 B71.0

(Rat tapeworm infection, Hymenolepiasis diminuta)

The rat tapeworm, *H. diminuta*, occurs accidentally in humans, usually in young children. The eggs passed in rodent feces are ingested by insects such as flea larvae, grain beetles and cockroaches in which cysticercoids develop in the hemocele. The mature tapeworm develops in rats, mice or other rodents when the insect is ingested. People are rare accidental hosts, usually of a single or few tapeworms; human infections are rarely symptomatic. Definitive diagnosis is based on finding characteristic eggs in the feces; treatment as for *H. nana*.

III. DIPYLIDIASIS
ICD-9 123.8; ICD-10 B71.1
(Dog tapeworm infection)

Toddler-age children are occasionally infected with the dog tapeworm (*Dipylidium caninum*), the adult of which is found worldwide in dogs and cats. It rarely if ever produces symptoms in the child but is disturbing to the parent who sees motile, seed-like proglottids (tapeworm segments) at the anus or on the surface of the stool. Infection is acquired when the child ingests fleas that, in their larval stage, have eaten eggs from proglottids. In 3–4 weeks the tapeworm becomes mature. Infection is prevented by keeping dogs and cats free of fleas and worms; niclosamide or praziquantel is effective for treatment.

[L. Savioli]

INFLUENZA
ICD-9 487; ICD-10 J10, J11

1. Identification—An acute viral disease of the respiratory tract characterized by fever, headache, myalgia, prostration, coryza, sore throat and cough. Cough is often severe and protracted; other manifestations are self-limited in most patients, with recovery in 2–7 days. Recognition is commonly by epidemiological characteristics (current quick tests lack sensitivity); only laboratory procedures can reliably identify sporadic cases. Influenza may be clinically indistinguishable from disease caused by other respiratory viruses, such as common cold, croup, bronchiolitis, viral pneumonia and undifferentiated acute respiratory disease. GI tract manifestations (nausea, vomiting, diarrhea) are uncommon, but may accompany the respiratory phase in children, and have been reported in up to 25% of children in school outbreaks of influenza B and A (H1N1).

Influenza derives its importance from the rapidity with which epidemics evolve, the widespread morbidity and the seriousness of complications, notably viral and bacterial pneumonias. In addition, emergence among humans of influenza viruses with new surface proteins can cause pandemics ranking as global health emergencies (e.g. 1918, 1957, 1968) with millions of deaths (c40 million in 1918). Severe illness and death during annual influenza epidemics occur primarily among the elderly and those debilitated by chronic cardiac, pulmonary, renal or metabolic disease, anemia or immunosuppression. The proportion of total deaths associated with pneumonia and influenza in excess of that expected for the time of year (excess mortality) varies and depends on the prevalent virus type. The annual global death toll is estimated to reach up to 1 million. In most epidemics, 80%–90% of deaths occur in persons over 65; in the 1918 pandemic, young adults showed the highest mortality rates. Reye syndrome, involving the CNS and liver, is a rare complication following virus infections in children who have ingested salicylates.

While the epidemiology of influenza is well understood in industrialized countries, information on influenza in developing countries is minimal.

During the early febrile stage, laboratory confirmation is through isolation of influenza viruses from pharyngeal or nasal secretions or washings on cell culture or in embryonated eggs; direct identification of viral antigens in nasopharyngeal cells and fluids (FA test or ELISA); rapid diagnostic tests (these differ in the influenza viruses they detect); or viral RNA amplification. Demonstration of a specific serological response between acute and convalescent sera may also confirm infection.

2. Infectious agents—Three types of influenza virus are recognized: A, B and C. Type A includes 15 subtypes of which only 2 (H1and H3) are associated with widespread epidemics; type B is infrequently associated with regional or widespread epidemics; type C with sporadic cases and minor localized outbreaks. The antigenic properties of the 2 relatively stable internal structural proteins, the nucleoprotein and the matrix protein, determine virus type.

Influenza A subtypes are classified by the antigenic properties of surface glycoproteins, hemagglutinin (H) and neuraminidase (N). Frequent mutation of the genes encoding surface glycoproteins of influenza A and influenza B viruses results in emergence of variants that are described by geographic site of isolation, year of isolation and culture number. Examples are A/New Caledonia/20/99(H1N1), A/Moscow/10/99(H3N2)-like virus, B/Hong Kong/330/2001.

Emergence of completely new subtypes—at irregular intervals and only for type A viruses—results from antigenic shift in HA gene or unpredictable recombination of human and mammalian or avian antigens, and leads to pandemics. The relatively minor antigenic changes (antigenic drift) of A and B viruses responsible for frequent epidemics and regional outbreaks occur constantly and require annual reformulation of influenza vaccine.

3. Occurrence—As pandemics (rare), epidemics (almost annual), localized outbreaks and sporadic cases. Clinical attack rates during epidemics range from 10% to 20% in the general community to more than 50% in closed populations (e.g. nursing homes, schools). During the initial phase of epidemics in industrialized countries, infection and illness appear predominantly in school-age children, with a sharp rise in school absences, physician visits, and pediatric hospital admissions. Schoolchildren infect family members, other children and adults. During a subsequent phase, infection and illness occur in adults, with industrial absenteeism, adult hospital admissions, and an increase in mortality from influenza-related pneumonia. Epidemics generally last 3–6 weeks, although the virus is present in the community for a variable number of weeks before and after the epidemic. The highest attack rates during type A epidemics occur among children aged 5–9, although the rate is also high in preschool children and adults.

Epidemics of influenza occur almost every year, caused primarily by type A viruses, occasionally influenza B viruses or both. In temperate zones, epidemics tend to occur in winter; in the tropics, they often occur in the rainy season, but outbreaks or sporadic cases may occur in any month.

Influenza viral infections with different antigenic subtypes also occur naturally in swine, horses, mink and seals, and in many other domestic species in many parts of the world. Aquatic birds are a natural reservoir and carrier for all influenza virus subtypes. Interspecies transmission (mainly transitory) and reassortment of influenza A viruses have been reported among swine, humans and some wild and domestic fowl.

Since 1997 influenza avian infections of the $A(H_3N_1)$ type have been identified in isolated human groups, with high fatality. Transmission gradually increased among poultry; in the first half of 2004, poultry outbreaks of influenza $A(H_3N_1)$ were occurring in several Asian countries, with transmission to humans in Thailand and Viet Nam. The cases fatality was high in human infections; there are no records of person-to-person transmission.

4. Reservoir—Humans are the primary reservoir for human infections; birds and mammalian reservoirs such as swine are likely sources of new human subtypes thought to emerge through genetic reassortment.

5. Mode of transmission—Airborne spread predominates among crowded populations in enclosed spaces; the influenza virus may persist for hours, particularly in the cold and in low humidity, and transmission may also occur through direct contact. New subtypes may be transmitted globally within 3–6 months.

6. Incubation period—Short, usually 1–3 days.

7. Period of communicability—Probably 3–5 days from clinical onset in adults; up to 7 days in young children.

8. Susceptibility—Size and relative impact of epidemics and pandemics depend upon level of protective immunity in the population, strain virulence, extent of antigenic variation of new viruses and number of previous infections. Infection produces immunity to the specific antigenic variant of the infecting virus; duration and breadth of immunity depend on the degree of antigenic similarity between viruses causing immunity.

Pandemics (emergence of a new subtype): Total population immunologically naive; children and adults equally susceptible, except for those who have lived through earlier pandemics caused by the same or an antigenically similar subtype.

Epidemics: Population partially protected because of earlier infections. Vaccines produce serological responses specific for the subtype viruses included and elicit booster responses to related strains with which the individual had prior experience.

Age-specific attack rates during an epidemic reflect persisting immunity from past experience with strains related to the epidemic subtype, so that incidence of infection is often highest in school-age children.

9. Methods of control—Detailed recommendations for the prevention and control of influenza are issued annually by national health agencies and WHO.

A. Preventive measures:

1) Educate the public and health care personnel in basic personal hygiene, especially transmission via unprotected coughs and sneezes, and from hand to mucous membrane.

2) Immunization with available inactivated and live virus vaccines may provide 70%–80% protection against infection in healthy young adults when the vaccine antigen closely matches the circulating strains of virus. Live vaccines, used in the Russian Federation for many years, have recently been licensed in the USA: registered for intranasal application in healthy individuals aged 5–49. In the elderly, although immunization may be less effective in preventing illness, inactivated vaccines may reduce severity of disease and incidence of complications by 50%–60% and deaths by approximately 80%. Influenza immunization should preferably be coupled with immunization against pneumococcal pneumonia (see Pneumonia).

   A single dose suffices for those with recent exposure to influenza A and B viruses; 2 doses more than 1 month apart are essential for children under 9. Routine immunization programs should be directed primarily towards those at greatest risk of serious complications or death (see Identification) and those who might spread infection (health care personnel and household contacts of high-risk persons). Immunization of children on long-term aspirin treatment is also recommended to prevent development of Reye syndrome after influenza infection.

The vaccine should be given each year before influenza is expected in the community; timing of immunization should be based on the seasonal patterns of influenza in different parts of the world (April to September in the southern hemisphere and rainy season in the tropics). Biannual recommendations for vaccine components are based on the viral strains currently circulating, as determined by WHO through global surveillance.

Contraindications: Allergic hypersensitivity to egg protein or other vaccine components is a contraindication. During the swine influenza vaccine program in 1976, the USA reported an increased risk of developing Guillain-Barré syndrome within 6 weeks after vaccination. Subsequent vaccines produced from other virus strains have not been clearly associated with an increased risk of Guillain-Barré.

3) Amantadine hydrochloride or rimantadine hydrochloride is effective in the chemoprophylaxis of influenza A, but not influenza type B. The CNS side-effects associated with amantadine in 5%–10% of recipients may be more severe in the elderly or those with impaired kidney function—the latter should receive reduced dosages that reflect the degree of renal impairment. Rimantadine is reported to cause fewer CNS side-effects. The use of these drugs should be considered in nonimmunized persons or groups at high risk of complications, such as residents of institutions or nursing homes for the elderly, when an appropriate vaccine is not available or as a supplement to vaccine when immediate maximal protection is desired against influenza A infection. The drug will not interfere with the response to influenza vaccine and should be continued throughout the epidemic. Inhibitors of influenza neuraminidase (oseltamivir) have been shown to be safe and effective for both prophylaxis and treatment of influenza A and B, although not yet approved in many countries for this use.

B. Control of patient, contacts and the immediate environment:

1) Report to local health authority: Reporting outbreaks or laboratory-confirmed cases assists disease surveillance. Report identity of the infectious agent as determined by laboratory examination if possible, Class 1 (see Reporting).

2) Isolation: Impractical under most circumstances because of the delay in diagnosis, unless rapid tests are available. In epidemics, because of increased patient load, it would be desirable to isolate patients (especially infants and young

children) believed to have influenza by placing them in the same room (cohorting) during the initial 5-7 days of illness.

3) Concurrent disinfection: Not applicable.

4) Quarantine: Not applicable.

5) Protection of contacts: A specific role has been shown for antiviral chemoprophylaxis with amantadine or rimantadine against type A strains (see 9A3). Neuraminidase inhibitors may also be considered for influenza A and B.

6) Investigation of contacts and source of infection: Of no practical value.

7) Specific treatment: Amantadine or rimantadine started within 48 hours of onset of influenza A illness and given for approximately 3-5 days reduces symptoms and virus titres in respiratory secretions. Dosages are 5 mg/kg/day in 2 divided doses for ages 1-9, 100 mg twice a day above 9 years (if weight less than 45 kg, 5 mg/kg/day in 2 doses) for 2-5 days. Doses should be reduced for those over 65 or with decreased hepatic or renal function. Neuraminidase inhibitors may also be considered for the treatment of influenza A and B.

During treatment with either drug, drug-resistant viruses may emerge late in the course of treatment and be transmitted to others; cohorting people on antiviral therapy should be considered, especially in closed populations with many high-risk individuals. Patients should be watched for bacterial complications and only then should antibiotics be administered. Because of the association with Reye syndrome, avoid salicylates in children.

C. Epidemic measures:

1) The severe and often disruptive effects of epidemic influenza on community activities may be reduced in part by effective health planning and education, particularly locally organized immunization programs for high-risk patients and their care providers. Surveillance by health authorities of the extent and progress of outbreaks and reporting of findings to the community are important.

The response to influenza pandemic must be planned at national level.

2) Closure of individual schools has not proven to be an effective control measure; it is generally applied too late and only because of high staff and students absenteeism.

3) Hospital administrators must anticipate the increased demand for medical care during epidemic periods and possible absenteeism of health care personnel as a result of

influenza. To prevent this, health care personnel should be immunized annually.

4) Maintaining adequate supplies of antiviral drugs would be desirable to treat high-risk patients and essential personnel in the event of the emergence of a new pandemic strain for which no suitable vaccine is available in time for the initial wave.

D. Disaster implications: Aggregations of people in emergency shelters will favor outbreaks of disease if the virus is introduced.

E. International measures: A disease under surveillance by WHO. The following are recommended:

1) Regularly report on epidemiological situation within a country to WHO (http://www.who.int/flunet).
2) Identify the causative virus in reports, and submit prototype strains to one of the WHO Centres for Reference and Research on Influenza in Atlanta, London, Melbourne and Tokyo (http://www.who.int/influenza). Throat secretion specimens, nasopharyngeal aspirates and paired blood samples may be sent to any WHO-recognized national influenza center.
3) Conduct epidemiological studies and promptly identify viruses to the national health agencies.
4) Ensure sufficient commercial and/or governmental facilities to provide rapid production of adequate quantities of vaccine and antiviral drugs; maintain programs for vaccine and antiviral drug administration to high-risk persons and essential personnel.

   Further information also on http://www.oms.b3e.jussieu.fr/flunet/.

[K. Stöhr]

KAWASAKI SYNDROME ICD-9 446.1; ICD-10 M30.3
(Kawasaki disease, Mucocutaneous lymph node syndrome, Acute febrile mucocutaneous lymph node syndrome)

1. Identification—An acute febrile, self-limited, systemic vasculitis of early childhood, presumably of infectious or toxic origin. Clinically characterized by a high, spiking fever, unresponsive to antibiotics, associated with pronounced irritability and mood change; usually solitary and frequently unilateral nonsuppurative cervical adenopathy; bilateral non-exudative bulbar conjunctival injection; an enanthem consisting of a "strawberry tongue", injected oropharynx or dry fissured or erythematous lips; limb changes consisting of oedema, erythema or periungual/generalized desquamation; and a generalized polymorphous erythematous exanthem that can be truncal or perineal and ranges from morbilliform maculopapular rash to urticarial rash or vasculitic exanthem.

Typically there are 3 phases: 1) acute febrile phase of about 10 days characterized by high, spiking fever, rash, adenopathy, peripheral erythema or oedema, conjunctivitis and enanthem; 2) subacute phase lasting about 2 weeks with thrombocytosis, desquamation, and resolution of fever; 3) lengthy convalescent phase during which clinical signs fade.

The case-fatality rate is 0.1%; half the deaths occur within 2 months of illness.

There is no pathognomonic laboratory test for Kawasaki syndrome, but an elevated ESR, C-reactive protein and platelet counts above 450 000/mm^3 (SI units 450 × 109/L) are common laboratory features.

According to *Diagnostic Guidelines of Kawasaki Disease* (Japan Kawasaki Disease Research Committee, 2002), at least 5 of the following 6 principal symptoms should be satisfied, although patients with 4 principal symptoms can be diagnosed when coronary aneurysm or dilatation is recognized by two-dimensional echocardiography or coronary angiography: 1) Fever persisting 5 days or more (including cases in whom the fever has subsided before the 5th day in response to treatment); 2) bilateral conjunctival congestion; 3) changes of lips and oral cavity: reddening of lips, strawberry tongue, diffuse injection of oral and pharyngeal mucosa, 4) polymorphous exanthema, 5) changes of peripheral extremities: reddening of palms and soles, indurative oedema in the initial stage, and membranous desquamation from fingertips in the convalescent stage, 6) acute nonpurulent cervical lymphadenopathy

2. Infectious agent—Unknown. Postulated to be a superantigen bacterial toxin secreted by *Staphylococcus aureus* or group A streptococci, but this has neither been confirmed nor generally accepted.

3. Occurrence—Worldwide; most cases (around 170 000) reported from Japan, with nationwide epidemics documented in 1979, 1982 and 1986. In the USA, the estimated number of new cases each year is about 2000. Approximately 80% of cases are diagnosed in children under 5, with a peak incidence at 1–2 years, more in boys than in girls. Cases are more frequent in the winter and spring. In Japan, where the disease has been tracked since 1970, peak incidence occurred in 1984–85. Since then, the incidence rate has been steady, about 140 per 100 000 children under 5.

4. Reservoir—Unknown, perhaps humans.

5. Mode of transmission—Unknown; no firm evidence of person-to-person transmission, even within families. Seasonal variation, limitation to the pediatric age group and outbreak occurrence in communities are all consistent with an infectious etiology.

6. Incubation period—Unknown.

7. Period of communicability—Unknown.

8. Susceptibility and resistance—In the USA, children, especially those of Asian ancestry, are most likely to develop the syndrome, but the majority of cases are reported among Caucasian children and American children of African origin. Recurrences appear infrequent (3% of reported patients in Japan).

9. Methods of control—

  A. Preventive measures: Unknown.

  B. Control of patient, contacts and the immediate environment:

  1) Report to local health authority: Clusters and epidemics should be reported immediately, Class 5 (see Reporting).
  2) Isolation: Not applicable.
  3) Concurrent disinfection: Not applicable.
  4) Quarantine: Not applicable.
  5) Immunization of contacts: Not applicable.
  6) Investigation of contacts: Not beneficial except in outbreaks and clusters.
  7) Specific treatment: High-dose IVIG, preferably as a single dose, within 10 days of onset of fever can reduce fever, inflammatory signs and aneurysm formation and should be considered even if the duration of fever exceeds 10 days. About 10% of patients may not respond and may require re-treatment. Recourse to high doses of aspirin is recommended during the acute phase, followed by low doses for at least 2 months. Measles and/or varicella vaccination should usually be deferred following receipt of IVIG.

  C. Epidemic measures: Investigate outbreaks and clusters to elucidate etiology and risk factors.

  D. Disaster implications: None.

  E. International measures: None.

[H.Yanagawa]

LASSA FEVER   ICD-9 078.8; ICD-10 A96.2

1. Identification—Acute viral illness of 1–4 weeks duration. Onset is gradual, with malaise, fever, headache, sore throat, cough, nausea, vomiting, diarrhea, myalgia and chest and abdominal pain; fever is persistent or spikes intermittently. Inflammation and exudation of the pharynx and conjunctivae are common. About 80% of human infections are mild or asymptomatic; the remaining cases have severe multisystem disease. Disease is more severe in pregnancy; fetal loss occurs in more than 80% of cases. In severe cases, hypotension or shock, pleural effusion, hemorrhage, seizures, encephalopathy and oedema of the face and neck are frequent, often with albuminuria and hemoconcentration. Early lymphopenia may be followed by late neutrophilia. Platelet counts are moderately depressed, but platelet function is abnormal. Transient alopecia and ataxia may occur during convalescence, and eighth cranial nerve deafness occurs in 25% of patients, of whom only half recover some function after 1–3 months. The overall case-fatality rate is about 1%, up to 15% among hospitalized cases and even higher in some epidemics. The rate is particularly high among women in the third trimester of pregnancy and fetuses. AST levels above 150 and high viraemia are of poor prognosis. Inapparent infections, diagnosed serologically, are common in endemic areas.

Diagnosis is through IgM antibody capture and antigen detection (ELISA) or detection of the viral genome by PCR; isolation of virus from blood, urine or throat washings; and IgG seroconversion by ELISA or IFA. Laboratory specimens must be handled with extreme care including BSL-4 containment, if available. Heating serum at 60°C (140°F) for 1 hour will largely inactivate the virus, and the serum can then be used to measure heat-stable substances such as electrolytes, blood urea nitrogen or creatinine.

2. **Infectious agent**—Lassa virus, an arenavirus, serologically related to lymphocytic choriomeningitis, Machupo, Junín, Guanarito and Sabiá viruses.

3. **Occurrence**—Endemic in Guinea, Liberia, regions of Nigeria, and Sierra Leone. Serologically related viruses of lesser virulence for laboratory hosts in Mozambique and Zimbabwe have not yet been associated with human infection or disease.

4. **Reservoir**—Wild rodents; in western Africa, the multimammate mouse of the *Mastomys* species complex.

5. **Mode of transmission**—Primarily through aerosol or direct contact with excreta of infected rodents deposited on surfaces such as floors and beds or in food and water. Laboratory infections occur, especially in the hospital environment, through inoculation with contaminated needles and through the patient's pharyngeal secretions or urine. Infection can also spread from person to person by sexual contact.

6. **Incubation period**—Commonly 6–21 days.

7. **Period of communicability**—Person-to-person spread may theo-

retically occur during the acute febrile phase when virus is present in the throat. Virus may be excreted in urine of patients for 3–9 weeks from onset of illness.

8. Susceptibility—All ages are susceptible; the duration of immunity following infection is unknown.

9. Methods of control —

    A. Preventive measures: Specific rodent control.

    B. Control of patient, contacts and the immediate environment:

      1) Report to local health authority: Individual cases should be reported, Class 2 (see Reporting).
      2) Isolation: Institute immediate strict isolation in a private hospital room away from traffic patterns. Entry of nonessential staff and visitors should be restricted. Nosocomial transmission has occurred, and strict procedures for isolation of body fluids and excreta must be maintained. Recourse to a negative pressure room and respiratory protection is desirable, if possible. Male patients should refrain from unprotected sexual activity until the semen has been shown to be free of virus or for 3 months. To reduce infectious exposure, laboratory tests should be kept to the minimum necessary for proper diagnosis and patient care, and only performed where full infection control measures are correctly implemented. Technicians must be alerted to the nature of the specimens and supervised to ensure application of appropriate specimen inactivation/isolation procedures. Dead bodies should be sealed in leakproof material and cremated or buried promptly in a sealed casket.
      3) Concurrent disinfection: Patient's excreta, sputum, blood and all objects with which the patient has had contact, including laboratory equipment used to carry out tests on blood, must be disinfected with 0.5% sodium hypochlorite solution or 0.5% phenol with detergent, and, as far as possible, effective heating methods, such as autoclaving, incineration, boiling or irradiation, as appropriate. Laboratory testing must be carried out in special high containment facilities; if there is no such facility, tests should be kept to a minimum and specimens handled by experienced technicians using all available precautions such as gloves and biological safety cabinets. When appropriate, serum may be heat-inactivated at 60°C (140°F) for 1 hour. Thorough terminal disinfection with 0.5% sodium hypochlorite solu-

tion or a phenolic compound is adequate; formaldehyde fumigation can be considered.

4) Quarantine: Only surveillance is recommended for close contacts (see 9B6).

5) Immmunization of contacts: Not applicable.

6) Investigation of contacts and source of infection: Identify all close contacts (people living with, caring for, testing laboratory specimens from or having noncasual contact with the patient) in the 3 weeks after the onset of illness. Establish close surveillance of contacts as follows: body temperature checks at least 2 times daily for at least 3 weeks after last exposure. In case of temperature above 38.3°C (101°F), hospitalize immediately in strict isolation facilities. Determine patient's place of residence during 3 weeks prior to onset; search for unreported or undiagnosed cases.

7) Specific treatment: Ribavirin, most effective within the first 6 days of illness, should be given IV, 30 mg/kg initially, followed by 15 mg/kg every 6 hours for 4 days and 8 mg/kg every 8 hours for 6 additional days.

C. Epidemic measures: Rodent control; adequate infection control and barrier nursing measures in hospitals and health facilities; availability of ribavirin; contact tracing and follow-up.

D. Disaster implications: *Mastomys* may become more numerous in homes and food storage areas and increase the risk of human exposures.

E. International measures: Notification of source country and to receiving countries of possible exposures by infected travellers. WHO Collaborating Centres.

[C. Roth]

LEGIONELLOSIS   ICD-9 482.8; ICD-10 A48.1
(Legionnaire disease; Legionnaire pneumonia)

NONPNEUMONIC
   LEGIONELLOSIS   ICD-10 A48.2
(Pontiac fever)

1. Identification—Acute bacterial disease with two distinct clinical and epidemiological manifestations: Legionnaire disease (ICD-10 A48.1) and Pontiac fever (ICD-10 A48.2). Both are characterized initially by anorexia, malaise, myalgia and headache. Within a day, there is usually a rapidly rising fever associated with chills. Temperatures commonly reach 39°C–40.5°C (102°F–105°F). Nonproductive cough, abdominal pain and diarrhea are common. In Legionnaire disease, a chest X-ray may show patchy or focal areas of consolidation that may progress to bilateral involvement and ultimately to respiratory failure; the case-fatality rate has been as high as 39% in hospitalized cases; it is generally higher in those with compromised immunity.

Pontiac fever has the same initial symptoms as pulmonary legionellosis (including productive cough) but is not associated with pneumonia or death; patients recover spontaneously in 2–5 days without treatment; this clinical syndrome may represent reaction to inhaled antigen rather than bacterial invasion.

Diagnosis depends on isolation of the causative organism on special media, its demonstration by direct IF stain of involved tissue or respiratory secretions, or detection of antigens of *Legionella pneumophila* serogroup 1 in urine through radioimmunoassay or through a rise (4-fold or greater) in IFA titre between acute phase serum and serum drawn 3–6 weeks later. The use of antigens in one sample of urine as a confirmatory test is under discussion by the European working Group for *Legionella* Infections (respedsc@PHIS.co.uk).

2. Infectious agent—Legionellae are poorly staining, Gram-negative bacilli that require cysteine and other nutrients to grow in vitro. Of the 18 serogroups of *L. pneumophila* currently recognized, *L. pneumophila* serogroup 1 is most commonly associated with disease. Related organisms, including *L. micdadei*, *L. bozemanii*, *L. longbeachae* and *L. dumoffii* have been isolated, predominantly from immunosuppressed patients with pneumonia. In all, 35 species of *Legionella* with at least 45 serogroups are currently recognized.

3. Occurrence—The earliest documented case occurred in 1947; the earliest documented outbreak in 1957 in Minnesota, USA. Since then, the disease has been identified throughout North America, as well as in Africa, Australia, Europe and South America. Although cases occur throughout the year, both sporadic cases and outbreaks are recognized more commonly in summer and autumn. In the few locations studied, antibodies to *L. pneumophila* serogroup 1 occur at a titre of 1:128 or greater in 1%–20% of the general population. The proportion of cases of community-acquired pneumonias due to *Legionella* ranges between 0.5% and 5.0%. A recent outbreak (France 2003–2004) led to 13 deaths among 85 cases.

Outbreaks of legionellosis usually occur with low attack rates (0.1%–5%) in the population at risk. Epidemic Pontiac fever has shown a high attack rate (about 95%) in several outbreaks.

4. Reservoir—Probably primarily aqueous. Hot water systems (showers), air conditioning cooling towers, evaporative condensers, humidifiers, whirlpool spas, respiratory therapy devices and decorative fountains have been implicated epidemiologically; the organism has been isolated from water in these, as well as from hot and cold water taps and showers, hot tubs and from creeks and ponds and the soil from their banks. It survives for months in tap and distilled water. An association of Legionnaire disease with soil disturbances or excavation has not been clearly established.

5. Mode of transmission—Epidemiological evidence supports airborne transmission; other modes are possible, including aspiration of water.

6. Incubation period—Legionnaire disease 2–10 days, most often 5–6 days; Pontiac fever 5–66 hours, most often 24–48 hours.

7. Period of communicability—Person-to-person transmission has not been documented.

8. Susceptibility—Illness occurs most frequently with increasing age (most cases are at least 50), especially in patients who smoke and those with diabetes mellitus, chronic lung disease, renal disease or malignancy; and in the immunocompromised, particularly those receiving corticosteroids or who had an organ transplant. The male:female ratio is about 2.5:1. The disease is rare under 20. Several outbreaks have occurred among hospitalized patients.

9. Methods of control—

    A. Preventive measures: Cooling towers should be drained when not in use, and mechanically cleaned periodically to remove scale and sediment. Appropriate biocides should be used to limit the growth of slime-forming organisms. Tap water should not be used in respiratory therapy devices. Maintaining hot water system temperatures at 50°C (122°F) or higher may reduce the risk of transmission.

    B. Control of patient, contacts and the immediate environment:

      1) Report to local health authority: In many countries, not a reportable disease, Class 3 (see Reporting).

      2) Isolation: Not applicable.

      3) Concurrent disinfection: Not applicable.

      4) Quarantine: Not applicable.

      5) Immmunization of contacts: Not applicable.

      6) Investigation of contacts and source of infection: Search (households, business) for additional cases due to infection from a common environmental source. Initiate an investigation for a hospital source should a single confirmed nosocomial case be identified.

      7) Specific treatment: Erythromycin appears to be the agent of choice; the newer macrolides, clarithromycin and azithromy-

cin, may be effective. Rifampicin may be a valuable adjunct but should not be used alone. Experience with fluoroquinolones is encouraging but limited. Penicillin, the cephalosporins and the aminoglycosides are ineffective.

C. *Epidemic measures:* Search for common exposures among cases and possible environmental sources of infection. Decontamination of implicated sources by chlorination and/or superheating water supplies has been effective.

D. *Disaster implications:* None known.

E. *International measures:* None.

LEISHMANIASIS ICD-9 085; ICD-10 B55

I. CUTANEOUS AND MUCOSAL
   LEISHMANIASIS ICD-9 085.1-085.5;
   ICD-10 B55.1, B55.2

(Aleppo evil, Baghdad or Delhi boil, Oriental sore; in the Americas, Espundia, Uta, Chiclero ulcer)

1. Identification—A polymorphic protozoan disease of skin and mucous membranes caused by several species of the genus *Leishmania*. These protozoa exist as obligate intracellular parasites in humans and other mammalian hosts. The disease starts with a macule then a papule that enlarges and typically becomes an indolent ulcer in the absence of bacterial infection. Lesions may be single or multiple, occasionally nonulcerative and diffuse. Lesions may heal spontaneously within weeks to months, or last for a year or more. In some individuals, certain strains (mainly from the Western Hemisphere) can disseminate to cause mucosal lesions (espundia), even years after the primary cutaneous lesion has healed. These sequelae, which involve nasopharyngeal tissues, are characterized by progressive tissue destruction and often scanty presence of parasites and can be severely disfiguring. Recurrence of cutaneous lesions after apparent cure may occur as ulcers, papules or nodules at or near the healed original ulcer.

Diagnosis is through microscope identification of the nonmotile, intracellular form (amastigote) in stained specimens from lesions, and through culture of the motile, extracellular form (promastigote) on suitable media. An intradermal (Montenegro) test with leishmanin, an antigen derived from the promastigotes is usually positive in established disease; it is not helpful with very early lesions, anergic disease or immunosuppressed patients. Serological (IFA or ELISA) testing can be done, but antibody levels typically are low or undetectable; this may not be helpful in diagnosis (except for mucosal leishmaniasis). Species identification is based on biological (development in sandflies, culture media and animals), immunological (monoclonal antibodies), molecular (DNA techniques) and biochemical (isoenzyme analysis) criteria. The WHO operational case definition is "a person showing clinical signs [of leishmaniasis] with parasitological confirmation and/or, *for mucosal leishmanaisis only*, serological diagnosis".

2. Infectious agents—Eastern hemisphere: *Leishmania tropica*, *L. major*, *L. aethiopica*; western hemisphere: *L. braziliensis* and *L. mexicana* complexes. Members of the *L. braziliensis* complex are more likely to produce mucosal lesions; *L. tropica* is the usual cause of "leishmaniasis recidivans" cutaneous lesions. Members of *L. donovani* complex usually cause visceral disease in the eastern hemisphere; in the western hemisphere the responsible organism is *L. infantum/chagasi*. Both may cause cutaneous leishmaniasis without concomitant visceral involvement, as well as post-kala-azar dermal leishmaniasis cases, which are considered residual reservoirs for the maintenance and dissemination of the parasite.

3. Occurrence—2 million new cases per year: China (recently), India and Pakistan; south-western Asia, including Afghanistan and the Islamic Republic of Iran; southern regions of former Soviet Union, the Mediterranean littoral; the sub-Saharan African savanna and Sudan, the highlands of Ethiopia and Kenya, Namibia; the Dominican Republic, Mexico (especially Yucatan), south central Texas, all of central America and every country of South America except Chile and Uruguay; leishmania have recently been reported among kangaroos in Australia. A nonulcerative, keloid-like form due to *L. infantum/chagasi* (atypical cutaneous leishmaniasis) has been observed with increasing frequency in central America, especially Honduras and Nicaragua. Numerous cases of diffuse cutaneous leishmaniasis have been reported in the past from the Dominican Republic and Mexico. In some areas in the eastern hemisphere, urban population groups, including children, are at risk for anthroponotic cutaneous leishmaniasis due to *L. tropica*. In rural areas, people are at risk for zoonotic cutaneous leishmaniasis due to *L. major*. In the western hemisphere, disease is usually restricted to special groups, such as those working in forested areas, those whose homes are in or next to a forest, and visitors to such areas from nonendemic countries. Generally more common in rural than urban areas.

4. Reservoir—Locally variable; humans (in anthroponotic cutaneous leishmaniasis), wild rodents (gerbils), hyraxes, edentates (sloths), marsupials and domestic dogs (considered victims more than real reservoirs); unknown hosts in many areas.

5. Mode of transmission—In zoonotic foci, from the animal reservoir through the bite of infective female phlebotomines (sandflies). Motile promastigotes develop and multiply in the gut of the sandfly after it has fed on an infected mammalian host; in 8–20 days, infective parasites develop and are injected during biting. In humans and other mammals, the organisms are taken up by macrophages and transform into amastigote forms, which multiply within the macrophages until the cells rupture, enabling spread to other macrophages. In anthroponotic foci person-to-person transmission occurs through sandfly bites and, very rarely, through transfusion.

6. Incubation period—At least a week, up to many months.

7. Period of communicability—Not directly transmitted from person to person, but infectious to sandflies as long as parasites remain in lesions in untreated cases, usually a few months to 2 years. Eventual spontaneous healing occurs in most cases. A small proportion of patients infected with *L. amazonensis* or *L. aethiopica* may develop diffuse parasite-rich cutaneous lesions that do not heal spontaneously. Infections with parasites of the *L. braziliensis* complex can heal spontaneously, but a small proportion (3%–5%) are followed, months or years later, by metastatic mucosal lesions.

8. Susceptibility—Susceptibility is probably general. Lifelong immunity may be present after lesions due to *L. tropica* or *L. major* heal but may not protect against other leishmanial species. Factors responsible for late mutilating disease, such as espundia, are still partly unknown; occult infections may be activated years after the primary infection. The most important factor in immunity is the development of an adequate cell-mediated response.

9. Methods of control—

    A. *Preventive measures:* Currently no vaccine available. Control measures vary according to the habits of mammalian hosts and phlebotomine vectors; they include the following:

        1) Case management: Detect cases systematically and treat rapidly. This applies to all forms of leishmaniasis and is one of the important measures to prevent development of destructive mucosal lesions in the western hemisphere and "recidivans form" in the eastern hemisphere, particularly where the reservoir is largely or solely human.

        2) Vector control: Apply residual insecticides periodically. Phlebotomine sandflies have a relatively short flight range and are highly susceptible to control by systematic spraying with residual insecticides. Spraying must cover exteriors and interiors of doorways and other openings if transmission occurs in dwellings. Possible breeding places of eastern

hemisphere sandflies, such as stone walls, animal houses and rubbish heaps, must be sprayed.

Exclude vectors by screening with a fine mesh screen (10–12 holes per linear cm or 25–30 holes per linear inch, an aperture not more than 0.89 mm or 0.035 inches). Insecticide-treated bednets are a good vector control alternative, especially in anthroponotic foci. In the focus of Aleppo (Syrian Arab Republic), they appeared particularly efficient in reducing the yearly incidence drastically (by 50% to 75%).

3) Eliminate rubbish heaps and other breeding places for eastern hemisphere phlebotomines.

4) Destroy gerbils (and their burrows) implicated as reservoirs in local areas by deep ploughing and removal of plants they feed on (chenopods).

5) In the western hemisphere, avoid sandfly infested and thickly forested areas, particularly after sundown; use insect repellents and protective clothing if exposure to sandflies is unavoidable.

6) Apply appropriate environmental management and forest clearance.

B. Control of patient, contacts and the immediate environment:

1) Report to local health authority: Official report not ordinarily justifiable, Class 5 (see Reporting).

2) Isolation: Not applicable, only of theoretical value.

3) Concurrent disinfection: Not applicable.

4) Quarantine: Not applicable.

5) Immmunization of contacts: Not applicable.

6) Investigation of contacts, source of infection, local transmission cycle (interrupt this in most practical fashion).

7) Specific treatment: Mainly pentavalent antimonials, either sodium stibogluconate, (available in USA from CDC) or meglumine antimonate, used in South America and some other areas. Pentamidine is used as a second line drug for cutaneous leishmaniasis. The imidazoles, ketoconazole and itraconazole may have moderate antileishmanial activity against some leishmanial species. Amphotericin B may be required in South American mucosal disease if this does not respond to antimonial therapy. An alkylphospholipid, the first oral drug active on visceral leishmaniasis, is currently tested for cutaneous leishmaniasis in Colombia and Guatemala. Topical formulations of 15% aminosidine (paramomycin) plus 10% urea have reduced the time of cure in cutaneous leishmaniasis cases due to *L. major*. Although spontaneous healing of simple cutaneous lesions occurs,

infections acquired in geographic regions where mucosal disease has been reported should be treated promptly.

C. *Epidemic measures:* In areas of high incidence, use intensive efforts to control the disease by provision of diagnostic facilities and appropriate measures directed against phlebotomine sand-flies and the mammalian reservoir hosts.

D. *Disaster implications:* None.

E. *International measures:* WHO Collaborating Centres. Further information: http://www.who.int/tdr/diseases/leish/default.htm

II. VISCERAL LEISHMANIASIS   ICD-9 085.0; ICD-10 B55.0
(Kala-azar)

1. Identification—A chronic systemic disease caused by intracellular protozoa of the genus *Leishmania*. The disease is characterized by fever, hepatosplenomegaly, lymphadenopathy, anemia, leukopenia, thrombocy-topenia and progressive emaciation and weakness. Untreated clinically evident disease is usually fatal. Fever is of gradual or sudden onset, persistent and irregular, often with two daily peaks, alternating periods of apyrexia and low-grade fever. Post-kala-azar dermal lesions may occur after apparent cure of systemic disease. They are particularly frequent in Sudan (up to 50% of visceral leishmaniasis cases). Leishmania/HIV co-infection is a well-known entity in southern Europe, and is currently emerging in eastern Africa and in Asia.

Parasitological diagnosis, based on invasive methods, is based preferably on culture of the organism from a biopsy specimen or aspirated material, or on demonstration of intracellular amastigotes in stained smears from bone marrow, spleen, liver, lymph nodes or blood (the latter is preferable in HIV-co-infected patients). The PCR technique is the most sensitive but remains expensive.

2. Infectious agents—Typically *Leishmania donovani*, *L. infantum* and *L. infantum/chagasi.*

Serological diagnosis is traditionally based on IFA and ELISA, tests that are expensive and difficult to decentralize. Recently, inexpensive, easy to use and reliable fieldtests such as freeze-dried antigen (DAT) and dipsticks (k39/k26) have become available. They are currently under comparative evaluation with an antigen detection test in urine that should be particularly relevant for Leishmania/HIV co-infected patients.

3. Occurrence—Visceral leishmaniasis occurs in 62 countries, with a yearly incidence of 500 000 cases and a population at risk of 120 million. A rural disease, occurring in foci in Bangladesh, China, India, Nepal, Pakistan, southern regions of the former Soviet Union, Middle East including Turkey, the Mediterranean basin, Mexico, central and South America (mostly Brazil), and in Ethiopia, Kenya, Sudan, Uganda and sub-Saharan savanna parts of Africa. In many affected areas, the disease occurs as scattered cases among infants, children and adolescents but occasionally in epidemic waves. Incidence is modified by the use of antimalarial insecticides. Where dog populations have been drastically reduced (e.g. China), human disease has also been reduced.

4. Reservoir—Known or presumed reservoirs include humans, wild Canidae (foxes and jackals) and domestic dogs. Humans are the only known reservoir in Bangladesh, India and Nepal.

5. Mode of transmission—Through bite of infected phlebotomine sandflies. In foci of anthroponotic visceral leishmaniasis, humans are the sole reservoir and transmission occurs from person to person through the sandfly bite. In foci of zoonotic visceral leishmaniasis, dogs, the domestic animal reservoir, constitute the main source of infection for sandflies. Person-to-person transmission has been reported in Leishmania/HIV co-infected intravenous drug users through exchange of syringes. Co-infected patients infect sandflies, acting as human reservoirs even in zoonotic foci.

6. Incubation period—Generally 2-6 months; range is 10 days to years.

7. Period of communicability—Not usually transmitted from person to person, but infectious to sandflies as long as parasites persist in the circulating blood or skin of the mammalian reservoir host. Infectivity for phlebotomines may persist after clinical recovery of human patients.

8. Susceptibility—Susceptibility is general. Kala-azar apparently induces lasting homologous immunity. Evidence indicates that asymptomatic and subclinical infections are common and that malnutrition predisposes to clinical disease and activation of inapparent infections. Manifest disease occurs among AIDS patients, presumably as reactivation of latent infections.

9. Methods of control—

    A. Preventive measures: See corresponding section I, 9A for cutaneous leishmaniasis. Dog control in zoonotic foci remains an unanswered question. In industrialized countries, dogs are usually treated but they often relapse. In many developing countries, massive culling of leishmanin-positive dogs has failed, except in China. A recent approach based on insecticide impregnated collars has proved effective in the Islamic Republic of Iran, reducing canine and human incidence of visceral leishmaniasis.

B. Control of patient, contacts and the immediate environment:

1) Report to local health authority: In selected leishmaniasis-endemic areas, Class 3 (see Reporting).
2) Isolation: Blood and body fluid precautions.
3) Concurrent disinfection: Not applicable.
4) Quarantine: Not applicable.
5) Immmunization of contacts: Not applicable.
6) Investigation of contacts and source of infection: Ordinarily none.
7) Specific treatment: Pentavalent antimonials (Sb5+) remain the first-line drugs in most countries. Sodium stibogluconate, available from CDC, and meglumine antimonate are effective. Cases that do not respond to antimony may be treated with amphotericin B or pentamidine; however these are not used routinely because of toxicity. In India, the disease is less and less responsive to first-line drugs (62% of visceral leishmaniasis patients do not respond to pentavalent antimonials) and requires alternative treatment. Some new drugs are available and/or are under development:
    - Amphotericin B included in liposomes is most efficient but its price restricts use to industrialized countries.
    - Aminosidine (paramomycin), a good candidate for combination therapy with Sb5+, still requires a completed dossier for registration and a producer.
    - An alkylphospholipid, the first oral drug active on visceral leishmaniasis, has been licensed in India (phase IV development).
    - Sitamaquine, a lepidine, is still under phase III development.

C. Epidemic measures: Effective control must include an understanding of the local ecology and transmission cycle, followed by adoption of practical measures to reduce mortality, stop transmission and avoid geographic extension of the epidemic, specially in anthroponotic foci.

D. Disaster implications: None.

E. International measures: Institute coordinated programs of control among neighboring countries where the disease is endemic. WHO Collaborating Centres. Further information: http://www.who.int/tdr/diseases/leish/default.htm.

[P. Desjeux]

LEPROSY
(Hansen disease)

ICD-9 030; ICD-10 A30

1. Identification—A chronic bacterial disease of the skin, peripheral nerves and (in lepromatous patients) the upper airway. The clinical manifestations of the disease vary in a continuous spectrum between 2 polar forms: i) lepromatous (multibacillary) leprosy: symmetrical and bilateral nodules, papules, macules and diffuse infiltrations, usually numerous and extensive; involvement of the nasal mucosa may lead to crusting, obstructed breathing and epistaxis; ocular involvement leads to iritis and keratitis; ii) tuberculoid (paucibacillary) leprosy: skin lesions single or few, sharply demarcated, anaesthesic or hypoaesthesic; bilateral asymmetrical involvement of peripheral nerves tends to be severe. Borderline leprosy has features of both polar forms and is more labile. Indeterminate leprosy is characterized by hypopigmented maculae with ill-defined borders; if untreated, it may progress to tuberculoid, borderline or lepromatous disease.

Case definition (WHO operational definition)

A case of leprosy is a person having one or more of the following, who has yet to complete a full course of treatment:

- Hypopigmented or reddish skin lesion(s) with definite loss of sensation
- Involvement of the peripheral nerves (definite thickening with loss of sensation)
- Skin smear positive for acid-fast bacilli.

The operational case definition includes retrieved defaulters with signs of active disease and relapsed cases who have previously completed a full course of treatment. It does not include cured persons with late reactions or residual disabilities.

Clinical diagnosis is based on complete skin examination. Search for signs of peripheral nerve involvement (hyperesthaesia, anesthaesia, paralysis, muscle wasting or trophic ulcers) with bilateral palpation of peripheral nerves (ulnar nerve at the elbow, peroneal nerve at the head of the fibula and the great auricular nerve) for enlargement and tenderness. Test skin lesions for sensation (light touch, pinprick, temperature discrimination).

The clinical manifestations can include "reactions" of leprosy, i.e. acute adverse episodes, which are termed erythema nodosum leprosum in lepromatous patients and reversal reactions in borderline leprosy.

Differential diagnosis includes many infiltrative skin diseases, including lymphomas, lupus erythematosus, psoriasis, scleroderma and neurofibromatosis. Diffuse cutaneous leishmaniasis, some mycoses, myxoedema and pachydermoperiostosis may resemble lepromatous leprosy, but acid-fast bacilli are not present. Several skin conditions, such as vitiligo, tinea versicolor, pityriasis alba, nutritional dyschromia, nevus and scars may resemble tuberculoid leprosy.

Laboratory criteria include the presence of alcohol-acid-fast bacilli in skin smears (scrape-incision method).

In the paucibacillary form the bacilli may be so few that they are not demonstrable. In view of the increasing prevalence of HIV and hepatitis B infection in many countries where leprosy remains endemic, the number of skin smear sites and the frequency of smear collection should be limited to the minimum necessary. In practice, laboratories are not essential for the diagnosis of leprosy.

Leprosy cases can be classified as follows:

- Multibacillary leprosy: more than 5 patches or lesions on the skin
- Paucibacillary leprosy: 1 to 5 patches or lesions on the skin.

2. Infectious agent—*Mycobacterium leprae*. This cannot be grown in bacteriological media or cell cultures.

3. Occurrence—During 2002, 620 000 persons were diagnosed with leprosy, 90% of them in Brazil, India, Madagascar, Mozambique, Nepal, and in the United Republic of Tanzania. Control has improved with the introduction of multidrug therapy (MDT). WHO has targeted the disease for elimination (less than 1 case/10 000 population) and this has been achieved in 110 out of the 122 countries endemic in 1985.

Newly recognized cases in the USA are few and diagnosed principally in California, Florida, Hawaii, Louisiana, Texas and in New York City, and in Puerto Rico. Most of these cases are in immigrants and refugees whose disease was acquired in their native countries; however, the disease remains endemic in California, Hawaii, Louisiana, Texas and Puerto Rico.

4. Reservoir—Humans are thought to be the only reservoir of proven significance. Feral armadillos in Louisiana and Texas (USA) have been found naturally affected with a disease identical to experimental leprosy in armadillos, and there have been reports suggesting that disease in armadillos has been naturally transmitted to humans. Naturally acquired leprosy has been observed in a mangabey monkey and in a chimpanzee captured in Nigeria and Sierra Leone, respectively.

5. Mode of transmission—Humans are the only significant reservoirs. The disease is in all likelihood transmitted from the nasal mucosa of a patient to the skin and respiratory tract of another person. Transmission requires close contact. Although the bacillus can survive up to 7 days in dried nasal secretions, indirect transmission is unlikely.

6. Incubation period—This ranges from 9 months to 20 years, the average is probably 4 years for tuberculoid leprosy and twice that for lepromatous leprosy. The disease is rarely seen in children under age 3;

however, more than 50 cases have been identified in children under 1, the youngest at 2.5 months.

7. Period of communicability—Clinical and laboratory evidence suggest that infectiousness is lost in most instances within a day of treatment with multidrug therapy.

8. Susceptibility—The persistence and form of leprosy depend on the ability to develop effective cell-mediated immunity. The high prevalence of *M. leprae*-specific lymphocyte transformation and antibodies specific for *M. leprae* among close contacts of leprosy patients suggests that infection is frequent, yet clinical disease occurs in only a small proportion of such close contacts. The immunological lepromin test used earlier should be reserved for research activities.

9. Methods of control—The availability of effective and time-limited ambulatory treatment, with rapid elimination of infectiousness, has changed management. Hospitalization should now be limited only to cases such as the surgical correction of deformities, treatment of ulcers resulting from anaesthesia, and severe leprosy reactions.

- *A.* **Preventive measures:** Early detection and treatment of cases. Dapsone chemoprophylaxis is not recommended (limited effectiveness and danger of resistance).

    The availability of drugs effective in treatment and in rapid elimination of infectiousness, such as rifampicin, has changed the management of the patient with leprosy, from societal isolation with attendant despair, to ambulatory treatment without the need for hospitalization.

    1) Health education together with counselling of patients and relatives must stress the availability of effective multidrug therapy, the absence of infectivity of patients under continuous treatment and the prevention of physical and social disabilities.
    2) BCG vaccination can induce protection against the tuberculoid form of the disease; this is part of the control of tuberculosis in some countries and must not be undertaken specifically to prevent leprosy.

- *B.* **Control of patient, contacts and the immediate environment:**

    1) Report to local health authority: Case report obligatory in many and countries and desirable in all, Class 2 (see Reporting).
    2) Isolation: Reducing contact with known leprosy patients is of dubious value and can lead to stigmatization. No restrictions in employment or attendance at school are indicated.
    3) Quarantine: Not applicable.
    4) Immunization of contacts: Not recommended

5) Investigation of contacts and source of infection: The initial examination of close contacts can be useful.

6) Specific treatment: Combined chemotherapy regimens are essential. The duration of therapy for multibacillary leprosy can be shortened to 12 months from the previously recommended 24 months. Patients under treatment should be monitored for drug side-effects, for leprosy reactions and for development of trophic ulcers. Some complications may need to be treated in a referral center. Ambulatory treatment by multidrug therapy (MDT) is given according to case classification.

Adults with multibacillary leprosy: the standard regimen is a combination of the following for 12 months:

- Rifampicin: 600 mg once a month

- Dapsone: 100 mg once a day

- Clofazimine: 50 mg once a day and 300 mg once a month.

Adults with paucibacillary leprosy: the standard regimen is a combination of the following for 6 months:

- Rifampicin: 600 mg once a month

- Dapsone: 100 mg once a day.

Children must receive appropriately scaled-down doses (in child blister-packs).

Patients must be advised to complete the full course of treatment and to seek care in the event of drug side-effects (allergic reaction) and immunological reactions (neuritis leading to damage of the peripheral nerve trunks).

Multiple drug therapy is available free of charge through WHO. MDT drugs must be given in blister packs, free of charge, to all patients.

Treatment of reactions: Corticosteroids are drugs of choice in the management of reactions associated with neuritis. During the 1960s thalidomide was reintroduced as treatment for Erythema nodosum leprosum (ENL). In view of the risk of deformed births among users, and despite its possible usefulness for other conditions, thalidomide has no place in the treatment of leprosy. Clofazimine is the drug of choice for the management of recurrent ENL reactions. Its presence in multidrug therapy (MDT) has significantly reduced the frequency and severity of ENL reactions worldwide.

C. Epidemic measures: Not applicable.

D. Disaster implications: Any interruption of treatment schedules is serious. During wars, diagnosis and treatment of leprosy patients has often been neglected.

E. International measures: Further information on http://www.who.int/lep/ and http://www.who.int/tdr/diseases/leprosy/default.htm

[D. Daumerie]

LEPTOSPIROSIS   ICD-9 100; ICD-10 A27
(Weil disease, Canicola fever, Hemorrhagic jaundice, Mud fever, Swineherd disease)

1. Identification—A group of zoonotic bacterial diseases with protean manifestations. Common features are fever with sudden onset, headache, chills, severe myalgia (calves and thighs) and conjunctival suffusion. Other manifestations that may be present are diphasic fever, meningitis, rash (palatal exanthem), hemolytic anemia, hemorrhage into skin and mucous membranes, hepatorenal failure, jaundice, mental confusion and depression, myocarditis and pulmonary involvement with or without hemorrhage and hemoptysis. In areas of endemic leptospirosis, a majority of infections are clinically inapparent or too mild to be diagnosed definitively.

The severity of illness tends to vary with the infecting serovar; the same serovar may cause mild or severe disease in different hosts. Cases are often misdiagnosed as meningitis, encephalitis or influenza; serological evidence of leptospiral infection occurs in 10% of cases with otherwise undiagnosed meningitis and encephalitis.

Clinical illness lasts from a few days to 3 weeks or longer. Generally, there are two phases in the illness: the leptospiraemic or febrile stage, lasting 4 to 9 days, followed by the convalescent or immune phase on the sixth to twelvth day. Recovery of untreated cases can take several months. Deaths are due predominantly to renal failure, cardiopulmonary failure and widespread hemorrhage, rarely to liver failure; the case-fatality rate is low but increases with advancing age and may reach 20% or more in patients with jaundice and kidney damage (Weil disease) who have not been treated with renal dialysis. Late sequelae may occur e.g. chronic fatigue, neuropsychiatric symptoms (paresis, depression) and occasionally uveitis.

Different serovars of leptospires may occur in different regions. Therefore, the standard serological test (microscopic agglutination test) preferably uses a panel of locally occurring leptospire serovars. Difficulties in diagnosis have compromised disease control in a number of settings and resulted in increased severity and elevated mortality. Diagnosis is confirmed by seroconversion or 4-fold or greater increase in leptospiraemic agglutination titres, and by isolation of leptospires from blood (first 7 days) or CSF (days 4–10) during acute illness, and from urine after the tenth day, with the use of special media. Inoculation of young guinea pigs, hamsters or gerbils is often positive. Techniques such as ELISA facilitate detection of leptospires in clinical and autopsy specimens.

2. Infectious agent—Leptospires, members of the order Spirochaetales. Pathogenic leptospires belong to the species *Leptospira interrogans*, subdivided into serovars. More than 200 pathogenic serovars have been identified, and these fall into 25 serogroups based on serologic relatedness. Important changes in leptospiral nomenclature are being made, based on DNA relatedness. Commonly identified serovars in the USA are *icterohaemorrhagiae*, *canicola*, *autumnalis*, *hebdomadis*, *ustralis* and *pomona*. In the United Kingdom, New Zealand and Australia, *L. interrogans* serovar *hardjo* infection in humans is the most common among those in close contact with infected livestock.

3. Occurrence—Worldwide; in all except polar regions. The disease is an occupational hazard for rice and sugarcane fieldworkers, farmers, fish workers miners, veterinarians, workers in animal husbandry, dairies and abattoirs, sewer workers, and military troops; outbreaks occur among those exposed to fresh river, stream, canal and lake water contaminated by the urine of domestic and wild animals, and to the urine and tissues of infected animals. The disease is a recreational hazard for bathers, campers and sportsmen in infected areas, and predominantly a disease of males, linked to occupation. It appears to be increasing as an urban hazard, especially during heavy rains when floods occur. A major outbreak in Nicaragua in 1995 caused extensive mortality. In recent years outbreaks have been reported from Asia, Europe, Australia and the Americas.

4. Reservoir—Pathogenic leptospires are maintained in the renal tubules of wild and domestic animals; serovars generally vary with the animal affected, e.g. rats (*icterohaemorrhagiae*), swine (*pomona*), cattle (*hardjo*), dogs (*canicola*) and racoons (*autumnalis*). In North America, swine appear to be the reservoir hosts for *bratislava*. Other animal hosts, some with a shorter carrier state, include feral rodents, insectivores, badgers, deer, squirrels, foxes, skunks, racoons and opossums. Reptiles and amphibians (frogs) have been found to carry pathogenic leptospires but are unlikely to play an important epidemiological role. In carrier animals, an asymptomatic infection occurs in the renal tubules, and leptospiruria persists for long periods or even for life, especially in reservoir species.

5. Mode of transmission—Contact of the skin, especially if abraded, or of mucous membranes with moist soil, vegetation—especially sugarcane—contaminated with the urine of infected animals, or contaminated water, as in swimming wading in floodwaters, accidental immersion or occupational abrasion; direct contact with urine or tissues of infected animals; occasionally through drinking of water and ingestion of food contaminated with urine of infected animals, often rats; also through inhalation of droplet aerosols of contaminated fluids.

6. Incubation period—Usually 10 days, with a range of 2–30 days.

7. Period of communicability—Direct person-to-person transmission is rare. Leptospires may be excreted in the urine, usually for 1 month, although leptospiruria has been observed in humans and in animals for months, even years, after acute illness.

8. Susceptibility—Susceptibility of humans is general; serovar-specific immunity follows infection or (occasionally) immunization, but this may not protect against infection with a different serovar.

9. Methods of control—

   A. Preventive measures:

   1) Educate the public on modes of transmission, to avoid swimming or wading in potentially contaminated waters and to use proper protection when work requires such exposure.
   2) Protect workers in hazardous occupations by providing boots, gloves and aprons.
   3) Recognize potentially contaminated waters and soil; drain such waters when possible.
   4) Control rodents in human habitations, urban or rural, and recreational areas. Management of sugarcane fields such as controlled preharvest burning reduces risks in harvesting.
   5) Segregate infected domestic animals; prevent contamination by the urine of infected animals for humans living, working or playing in potentially contaminated areas.
   6) Immunization of farm and pet animals prevents illness, but not necessarily infection and renal shedding. The vaccine must contain the dominant local strains.
   7) Immunization of people has been carried out against occupational exposures to specific serovars with varying degrees of success but is not a generalizable option at present.
   8) A systematic review concludes that doxycycline (e.g. 200 mg in one weekly dose for as long as necessary) may be effective in preventing leptospirosis in exposed persons in areas of high exposure.

   B. Control of patient, contacts and the immediate environment:

   1) Report to local health authority: Obligatory case report in many countries, Class 2 (see Reporting).
   2) Isolation: Blood and body fluid precautions.

3) Concurrent disinfection: Articles soiled with urine.

4) Quarantine: Not applicable.

5) Immmunization of contacts: Not applicable.

6) Investigation of contacts and source of infection: Search for exposure to infected animals and potentially contaminated waters.

7) Specific treatment: A systematic review of randomized controlled trials on antibiotics did not show sufficient evidence for the effectiveness of antibiotics in reducing mortality from leptospirosis. However, prompt specific treatment, as early in the illness as possible and preferably before the 5th day of illness, may reduce duration of fever and hospital stay. Penicillin (1.2 gram benzylpenicillin IV or IM every 4-6 hours) is probably the drug of choice for severe cases and is effective as late as 7 days into an illness. Jarisch-Herxheimer reactions may occur. Doxycycline (2 times a day 100 mg orally for 7 days), ampicillin or erythromycin can be used in patients allergic to penicillin and for less severe cases. Cephalosporins (e.g. cefotaxime and ceftriaxone) and quinolone antibiotics may also be effective.

C. *Epidemic measures:* Search for source of infection, such as a contaminated swimming pool or other water source; eliminate the contamination or prohibit use. Investigate industrial and occupational sources, including direct animal contact.

D. *Disaster implications:* A potential problem following flooding of certain areas with a high water table.

E. *International measures:* WHO Collaborating Centres.

[F. Meslin]

LISTERIOSIS   ICD-9 027.0; ICD-10 A32

1. **Identification**—A bacterial disease usually manifested as meningo-encephalitis and/or septicemia in new-borns and adults; in pregnant women, as fever and abortion. Those at highest risk are neonates, the elderly, immunocompromised individuals, pregnant women and alcoholic, cirrhotic or diabetic adults. The onset of meningoencephalitis (rare in pregnant women) can be sudden, with fever, intense headache, nausea, vomiting and signs of meningeal irritation, or subacute, particularly in immunocompromised or elderly hosts. Rhomboencephalitis may rarely occur. Delirium and coma may appear early; occasionally there is collapse and shock. Endocarditis, granulomatous lesions in the liver and other

organs, localized internal or external abscesses, and pustular or papular cutaneous lesions may occur on rare occasions.

The normal host acquiring infection may exhibit only an acute mild febrile illness; in pregnant women infection can be transmitted to the fetus. Infants may be stillborn, born with septicemia, or develop meningitis in the neonatal period even though the mother may be asymptomatic at delivery. The postpartum course of the mother is usually uneventful, but the case-fatality rate is 30% in newborns and approaches 50% when onset occurs in the first 4 days. In a recent epidemic, the overall case-fatality rate among nonpregnant adults was 35%: 11% in those below 40 and 63% in those over 60.

Diagnosis is confirmed only after isolation of the infectious agent from CSF, blood, amniotic fluid, placenta, meconium, lochia, gastric washings and other sites of infection. *Listeria monocytogenes* can be isolated readily from normally sterile sites on routine media, but care must be taken to distinguish this organism from other Gram-positive rods, particularly diphtheroids. Selective enrichment media improve rates of isolation from contaminated specimens. Microscopic examination of CSF or meconium permits presumptive diagnosis; serological tests are unreliable.

2. **Infectious agent**—*Listeria monocytogenes*, a Gram-positive rod-shaped bacterium; human infections are usually (>98%) caused by serovars 1/2a, 1/2b, 1/2c and 4b.

3. **Occurrence**—An uncommonly diagnosed infection that occurs worldwide; in the USA, the incidence of illness requiring hospitalization is about 1/200 000 population. In Europe, it is often associated with consumption of non-pasteurized milk or milk products including cheese. It often occurs sporadically; several outbreaks have been recognized in recent years. About 30% of clinical cases occur within the first 3 weeks of life; in nonpregnant adults, infection occurs mainly after 40. Nosocomial acquisition has been reported. Asymptomatic infections probably occur at all ages, although they are of importance only during pregnancy. Abortion can occur at any point in pregnancy, more usually in the second half; perinatal infection is acquired during the last trimester.

4. **Reservoir**—The organism mainly occurs in soil, forage, water, mud and silage. The seasonal use of silage as fodder is frequently followed by an increased incidence of listeriosis in animals. Animal reservoirs include infected domestic and wild mammals, fowl and people. Asymptomatic fecal carriage is common in humans (up to 10%) and can be higher in abattoir workers and laboratory workers who work with *Listeria monocytogenes* cultures. Soft cheeses may support the growth of *Listeria* during ripening and have caused outbreaks. Unlike most other foodborne pathogens, *Listeria* tends to multiply in refrigerated foods that are contaminated.

5. **Mode of transmission**—Outbreaks have been reported in associ-

ation with ingestion of raw or contaminated milk, soft cheeses, vegetables, and ready-to-eat meats, such as pâté. A substantial proportion of sporadic cases result from foodborne transmission. Papular lesions on hands and arms may occur from direct contact with infectious material.

In neonatal infections, the organism can be transmitted from mother to fetus in utero or during passage through the infected birth canal. There are rare reports of nursery outbreaks attributed to contaminated equipment or materials.

6. Incubation period—Variable; cases have occurred 3-70 days following a single exposure to an implicated product. Estimated median incubation is 3 weeks.

7. Period of communicability—Mothers of infected newborn infants can shed the infectious agent in vaginal discharges and urine for 7-10 days after delivery, rarely longer. Infected individuals can shed the organisms in their stools for several months.

8. Susceptibility—Fetuses and new-borns are highly susceptible. Children and young adults generally are resistant, adults less so after age 40, especially the immunocompromised and the elderly. Disease is usually superimposed on other debilitating illnesses such as cancer, organ transplantation, diabetes, cirrhosis and HIV infection. There is little evidence of acquired immunity, even after prolonged severe infection.

9. Methods of control—

A. Preventive measures:

1) Pregnant women and immunocompromised individuals should avoid ready-to-eat foods, smoked fish and soft cheeses made with unpasteurized milk. They should cook leftovers or foods such as hot dogs until steaming hot. They should also avoid contact with potentially infective materials, such as aborted animal fetuses on farms.
2) Ensure safety of foods of animal origin. Pasteurize all dairy products where possible. Irradiate soft cheeses after ripening or monitor nonpasteurized dairy products, such as soft cheeses, by culturing for *Listeria*.
3) Processed foods found to be contaminated by *Listeria monocytogenes* (e.g. during routine bacteriological surveillance) should be recalled.
4) Thoroughly wash raw vegetables before eating.
5) Thoroughly cook raw food from animal sources such as beef, pork, or poultry.
6) Wash hands, knives, and cutting boards after handling uncooked foods.
7) Avoid the use of untreated manure on vegetable crops.

8) Veterinarians and farmers must take proper precautions in handling aborted fetuses and sick or dead animals, especially sheep that died of encephalitis.

B. Control of patient, contacts and the immediate environment:

1) Report to local health authority: Obligatory case report required in many countries, Class 2; in others, report of clusters required, Class 4 (see Reporting).
2) Isolation: Enteric precautions.
3) Concurrent disinfection: Not applicable.
4) Quarantine: Not applicable.
5) Immmunization of contacts: Not applicable.
6) Investigation of contacts and source of infection: Case surveillance data— especially strain characteristics—should be analysed frequently (weekly) for possible clustering; all suspected clusters must be investigated for common-source exposures.
7) Specific treatment: Penicillin or ampicillin alone or together with aminoglycosides. For penicillin-allergic patients, trimethoprim-sulfamethoxazole or erythromycin is preferred. Cephalosporins, including third-generation cephalosporins, are not effective in the treatment of clinical listeriosis. Tetracycline resistance has been observed. A Gram-stain smear of meconium from clinically suspected newborns should be examined for short Gram-positive rods resembling *L. monocytogenes*. If positive, prophylactic antibiotics should be administered as a precaution.

C. Epidemic measures: Investigate outbreaks to identify a common source of infection, and prevent further exposure to that source.

D. Disaster implications: None.

E. International measures: None.

[P. Martin]

LOIASIS   ICD-9 125.2; ICD-10 B74.3
(*Loa loa* infection, Eyeworm disease of Africa, Calabar swelling)

1. Identification—A chronic filarial disease characterized by migration of the adult worm through subcutaneous or deeper tissues of the body, causing transient swellings several centimeters in diameter, located on any part of the body. The swellings may be preceded by localized pain with pruritus. Pruritus localized on arms, thorax, face and shoulders is a major symptom. Migration of the adult worm under the bulbar conjunctivae may be accompanied by pain and oedema. Allergic reactions with giant urticaria and fever may occur occasionally.

Infections with other filariae, such as *Wuchereria bancrofti*, *Onchocerca volvulus*, *Mansonella (Dipetalonema) perstans* and *M. streptocerca* (common in areas where *Loa loa* is endemic) should be considered in the differential diagnosis.

Larvae (microfilariae) are present in peripheral blood during the daytime and can be demonstrated in stained thick blood smears, stained sediment of blood where erythrocytes and hemoglobin have been separated (laking) or through membrane filtration. Eosinophilia is frequent. *Loa loa* specific DNA can be detected in the blood from symptomless infected individuals. A travel history is essential for diagnosis.

2. **Infectious agent**—*Loa loa*, a filarial nematode.

3. **Occurrence**—Widely distributed in the African rain forest, especially central Africa. In the Congo River basin, up to 90% of indigenous inhabitants of some villages are infected.

4. **Reservoir**—Humans. Primate *Loa loa* occur but the two have different transmission complexes and the disease is therefore not a zoonosis.

5. **Mode of transmission**—Transmitted by a deer fly of the genus *Chrysops*. *Chrysops dimidiata*, *C. silacea* and other species ingest blood containing microfilariae; the larvae develop to their infectious stage within 10–12 days in the fly and migrate to the proboscis whence they are transferred to a human host by the bite of the infective fly.

6. **Incubation period**—Symptoms usually appear several years after infection but may occur as early as 4 months. Microfilariae may appear in the peripheral blood as early as 6 months after infection.

7. **Period of communicability**—The adult worm may persist in humans, shedding microfilariae into the blood for as long as 17 years; in the fly, "communicability" starts from 10–12 days after its infection until all infective larvae have been released, or until the fly dies.

8. **Susceptibility**—Susceptibility is universal, with repeated infections; immunity, if present, has not been demonstrated.

9. **Methods of control—**

A. *Preventive measures:*

1) Measures directed against the fly larvae are effective but have not proven practical because the moist, muddy breeding areas are usually too extensive.
2) Diethyltoluamide or dimethyl phthalate applied to exposed skin are effective fly repellents.
3) Wear protective clothing (long sleeves and trousers), screen houses.
4) For temporary residents of endemic areas whose risk of exposure is high or prolonged, a weekly dose of diethylcarbamazine (300 mg) is prophylactic.

B. *Control of patient, contacts and the immediate environment:*

1) Report to local health authority: Official report not ordinarily required, Class 5 (see Reporting).
2) Isolation: As far as possible, patients with microfilaraemia should be protected from *Chrysops* bites to reduce transmission.
3) Concurrent disinfection: Not applicable.
4) Quarantine: Not applicable.
5) Immmunization of contacts: Not applicable.
6) Investigation of contacts and source of infection: None; a community problem.
7) Specific treatment: Diethylcarbamazine (DEC—5–10 mg/kg in 3 daily doses for 2–4 weeks) causes disappearance of microfilariae and may kill the adult worm with ensuing cure. During treatment, hypersensitivity reactions (sometimes severe) are common but may be controlled with steroids and/or antihistamines. Ivermectin (200 to 400 micrograms per kg body weight) also reduces microfilaraemia, and adverse reactions may be milder than with DEC. When microfilaraemia is heavy (greater than 2000/mL blood), there is a risk of meningoencephalitis and the advantages of treatment must be weighed against the risk of life-threatening encephalopathy; treatment with either drug must be individualized and undertaken under close medical supervision. Albendazole and mebendazole both cause a slow decrease in microfilaraemia with few side-effects and probably kills adult worms. Surgical removal of the migrating adult worm under the bulbar conjunctivae is indicated when feasible. *Loa loa* encephalopathy has been reported following ivermectin treatment for onchocerciasis, which is why the drug is not

recommended for mass treatment of onchocerciasis in areas where loiasis is endemic.

C. Epidemic measures: Not applicable.

D. Disaster implications: None.

E. International measures: None.

[M. Karam]

LYME DISEASE
ICD-9 104.8, 088.81; ICD-10 A69.2, L90.4
(Lyme borreliosis, Tick-borne meningopolyneuritis)

1. Identification—A tick-borne, spirochaetal, zoonotic disease characterized by a distinctive skin lesion, systemic symptoms and neurological, rheumatological and cardiac involvement occurring in varying combinations over months to years. Recent reports state that the optic nerve may be affected because of inflammation or increased intracranial pressure. Early symptoms are intermittent and changing. The illness typically begins in the summer; the first manifestation in about 80% of patients is a red macule or papule that expands slowly in an annular manner, often with central clearing. This lesion is called "erythema migrans" (EM; formerly "erythema chronicum migrans"). EM may be single or multiple. To be considered significant for case surveillance purposes, the EM lesion must reach 5 cm in diameter. With or without EM, early systemic manifestations may include malaise, fatigue, fever, headache, stiff neck, myalgia, migratory arthralgias and/or lymphadenopathy, all of which may last several weeks in untreated patients. In middle Europe and Scandinavia skin lesions called lymphadenosis benigna cutis and acrodermatitis chronica atrophicans are almost exclusively caused by *Borrelia afzelii*.

Within weeks to months after onset of the EM lesion, neurological abnormalities such as aseptic meningitis and cranial neuritis may develop–including facial palsy, chorea, cerebellar ataxia, motor or sensory radiculoneuritis, myelitis and encephalitis; symptoms fluctuate and may become chronic. Cardiac abnormalities (including atrioventricular block and, rarely, acute myopericarditis or cardiomegaly) may occur within weeks after onset of EM. Weeks to years after onset (mean, 6 months), intermittent episodes of swelling and pain in large joints, especially the knees, may develop and recur for several years; chronic arthritis may occasionally result. Treatment-resistant Lyme arthritis is a rare complication that may be result of cross reactivity between OspA and the human leukocyte function-associated antigen-1 (hlFA-1) following natural infection with *B. burgdorferi*. Similarly, following latent infection, chronic neurological manifestations may develop and include encephalopathy, polyneuropathy or leukoencephalitis; the CSF often shows lymphocytic pleocytosis and elevated protein levels, while the electromyogram is usually abnormal.

Diagnosis is currently based on clinical findings supported by two-stage serological tests, IFA, ELISA, then Western immunoblot. Serological tests are poorly standardized and must be interpreted with caution. They are insensitive during the first weeks of infection and may remain negative in people treated early with antibiotics. An ELISA for IgM antibodies that uses a recombinant outer surface protein C (rOspC) is more sensitive for early diagnosis than whole cell ELISA. VlsE (Vls locus expression site) or C6 recombinant antigens increase the sensitivity of IgG immunoblot. Test sensitivity increases when patients progress to later stages, but some chronic Lyme disease patients may remain seronegative. Cross-reacting IFA and ELISA antibodies may cause false-positive reactions in patients with syphilis, relapsing fever, leptospirosis, HIV infection, Rocky Mountain spotted fever, infectious mononucleosis, lupus or rheumatoid arthritis. The specificity of serological testing is enhanced by immunoblot testing of specimens that are positive or equivocal on IFA or ELISA. Diagnosis of nervous system Lyme disease requires demonstration of intrathecal antibody production. The causal agent is *Borrelia burgdorferi* sensu lato. The genotype present in North America, *Borrelia burgdorferi* sensu stricto, grows at 33°C (91.4°F) in the Barbour, Stoenner, Kelly (BSK) medium; other species causing Lyme-like disease may not grow well in this medium. Isolation from blood and tissue biopsies is difficult, but biopsies of the EM lesions may yield the organism in 80% of cases or more. PCR has identified *B. burgdorferi* genetic material *sensu lato* in synovial fluid, CSF, blood and urine, skin and other tissues; the usefulness of PCR in routine management of Lyme disease cases has yet to be verified. Recent real-time assays combining DNA amplification with species-specific probes allow single step identification of spirochaetal DNA to the species level.

2. Infectious agents—The causative spirochaete of North American Lyme disease, *B. burgdorferi*, was identified in 1982. Three genomic groups of *B. burgdorferi* have now been identified in Europe and named *B. burgdorferi sensu stricto*, *B. garinii* and *B. afzelii*. A few *B. bissetti*-like strains as well as *B. valaisiana* strains and one atypical A14S strain have been cultured from European patients with EM lesions.

3. Occurrence—In the USA, endemic foci exist along the Atlantic coast, in Wisconsin and Minnesota and in some areas of California and Oregon; increasing recognition of the disease have led to reports from 47 states and, in Canada, from Ontario and British Columbia, as well as from Europe, the former Soviet Union, China and Japan.

Initial infection occurs primarily during summer, with a peak in June and July, but may occur throughout the year, depending on the seasonal abundance of the tick locally. The distribution of most cases coincides with the distribution of *Ixodes scapularis* (formerly *I. dammini*) ticks in the eastern and midwestern USA, *I. pacificus* in western USA, *I. ricinus* in Europe and *I. persulcatus* in Asia. Dogs, cattle and horses develop systemic disease that may include the articular and cardiac manifestations seen in human patients. The explosive repopulation of the eastern USA by white-tailed deer has been linked to the spread of Lyme disease in this region.

4. Reservoir—Certain ixodid ticks through transstadial transmission. Wild rodents, especially *Peromyscus* spp. in the northeastern and midwestern USA and *Neotoma* spp. in the western USA maintain the enzootic transmission cycle. Deer serve as important mammalian maintenance hosts for vector tick species. Larval and nymphal ticks feed on small mammals, and adult ticks primarily on deer. The majority of Lyme disease cases result from bites by infected nymphs. Research in Europe supports the possible role of birds in dispersing *B. garinii* and *B. valaisiana*. Other studies support a relationship between *B. afzelii* and European rodents, notably *Clethrionomys* voles.

5. Mode of transmission—Tick-borne; in experimental animals, transmission by *I. scapularis* and *I. pacificus* usually does not occur until the tick has been attached for 24 hours or more; this may also be true in humans.

6. Incubation period—For EM, 3 to 32 days after tick exposure (mean 7 to 10 days); early stages of the illness may be inapparent and the patient may present with later manifestations.

7. Period of communicability—No evidence of natural person-to-person transmission. Despite rare case reports of congenital transmission, epidemiological studies have not shown a link between maternal Lyme disease and adverse outcomes of pregnancy.

8. Susceptibility—All persons are probably susceptible. Reinfection has occurred in those treated with antibiotics for early disease.

9. Methods of control—

   A. Preventive measures:

   1) Educate the public about the mode of tick transmission and the means for personal protection.
   2) Avoid tick-infested areas when feasible. To minimize exposure, wear light-colored clothing that covers legs and arms so that ticks may be more easily seen; tuck trousers into socks and apply tick repellent such as diethyltoluamide to the skin

or permethrin (repellent and contact acaricide) to sleeves and trouser legs.

3) If working or playing in an infested area, search the total body area daily, do not neglect hairy areas and remove ticks promptly; these may be very small. Remove ticks by using gentle, steady traction with forceps (tweezers) applied close to the skin, so as to avoid leaving mouth parts in the skin; protect hands with gloves, cloth or tissue when removing ticks. Following removal, cleanse the attachment site with soap and water.

4) Measures designed to reduce tick populations on residential properties (host management, habitat modification, chemical control) are usually impractical on a large-scale basis.

5) During the late 1990s, two Lyme disease vaccines were developed using recombinant *B. burgdorferi* stricto sensu lipidated outer-surface protein A (rOspA) as immunogen. In late 1999 one of these vaccines was licensed by the FDA for administration on a 3-dose schedule of 0, 1, and 12 months and was found to be safe and 76% effective in preventing overt Lyme disease after 3 doses. Information regarding vaccine safety and efficacy beyond the transmission season immediately after the third dose is not available. The duration of protective immunity and need for booster doses beyond the third dose is still unknown. The results of a large-scale safety study have not yet been finalized. After licensure, anecdotal reports of joint reactions associated with vaccination, accompanied by lawsuits, led to discontinuation of distribution in February 2002 because of low demand and sales.

a) Vaccine-induced anti-rOspA antibodies routinely cause false-positive ELISA results for Lyme disease. Experienced laboratory workers can usually discriminate between *B. burgdorferi* infection and previous rOspA immunization, because anti-OspA antibodies do not develop after natural infection.

b) Lyme disease vaccine does not protect all recipients against infection with *B. burgdorferi* and offers no protection against other tick-borne borrelioses. Decisions regarding the use of vaccine must be based on individual assessment of exposure risk, vaccine availability and consideration of the relative risks and benefits of the vaccine compared with other protective measures, including early diagnosis and treatment of Lyme disease. Few studies have investigated the effectiveness of such measures in actual use, and none has compared those measures to vaccination.

c) Risk assessment should include consideration of the geographic distribution of Lyme disease. The areas of highest risk in North America are concentrated within some northeastern and north-central states and provinces. However, the risk for Lyme disease differs even within counties and townships. Detailed information about the distribution of Lyme disease risk within specific areas is best obtained from public health authorities.

d) In areas of moderate to high risk, immunization had until 2002 been considered for persons aged 15-70 years who engaged in activities (recreational, property maintenance, occupational or leisure) resulting in frequent or prolonged exposure to tick-infested habitats. Future availability of vaccines against Lyme disease is uncertain.

B. Control of patient, contacts and the immediate environment:

1) Report to local health authority: Case report obligatory in some countries, Class 3 (see Reporting).

2) Isolation: Not applicable.

3) Concurrent disinfection: Carefully remove all ticks from patients.

4) Quarantine: Not applicable.

5) Immmunization of contacts: Not applicable.

6) Investigation of contacts and source of infection: Studies to determine source of infection when cases occur outside a recognized endemic focus.

7) Specific treatment: For adults, the EM stage can usually be treated effectively with doxycycline (100 mg twice daily) or amoxicillin (500 mg 3-4 times daily). For localized EM, 2 weeks of treatment usually suffice; for early disseminated infection, 3-4 weeks. Children under 9 can be treated with amoxicillin, 50 mg/kg/day in divided doses, for the same period of time as adults. Cefuroxime axetil or erythromycin can be used in those allergic to penicillin or who cannot receive tetracyclines. Lyme arthritis can usually be treated successfully with a 4-week course of the oral agents. However, objective neurological abnormalities, with the possible exception of isolated facial palsy, are best treated with IV ceftriaxone, 2 grams once daily, or IV penicillin, 20 million units in 6 divided doses, for 3-4 weeks. Treatment failures may occasionally occur with any of these regimens and retreatment may be necessary.

C. *Epidemic measures:* In hyperendemic areas, identify tick species involved and areas infested, see recommendations 9A1 through 9A3.

D. *Disaster implications:* None.

E. *International measures:* WHO Collaborating Centres.

[D. Húlínska]

LYMPHOCYTIC
CHORIOMENINGITIS   ICD-9 049.0; ICD-10 A87.2
(LCM, Benign [or serous] lymphocytic meningitis)

1. **Identification**—A viral infection of animals, especially mice, transmissible to humans, where they produce diverse clinical manifestations. There may be influenza-like symptoms, with myalgia, retroorbital headache, leukopenia and thrombocytopenia, followed by complete recovery; in some cases, the illness may begin with meningeal or meningoencephalomyelitic symptoms, or they may appear after a brief remission. Orchitis, parotitis, arthritis, myocarditis and rash occur occasionally. The acute course is usually short, very rarely fatal, and even with severe manifestations (e.g. coma with meningoencephalitis), prognosis for recovery without sequelae is usually good, although convalescence with fatigue and vasomotor instability may be prolonged. The CSF in cases with neurological involvement typically shows a lymphocytic pleocytosis and, at times, a low glucose level. The primary pathological finding in the rare human fatality is diffuse meningoencephalitis. Fatal cases of hemorrhagic fever-like disease have been reported. Transplacental infection of the fetus leading to hydrocephalus and chorioretinitis occurs and should be tested for in such cases.

Laboratory diagnostic methods include isolation of virus from blood or CSF early in the course of illness by intracerebral inoculation of LCM-free mice (3 to 5 week old) or cell cultures. Specific IgM in serum or CSF as evidenced by IgM capture ELISA or rising antibody titres by IFA in paired sera are considered diagnostic. LCM requires differentiation from other aseptic meningitides and viral encephalitides.

2. **Infectious agent**—Lymphocytic choriomeningitis virus, an arenavirus, serologically related to Lassa, Machupo, Junín, Guaranito and Sabiá viruses.

3. Occurrence—Not uncommon in Europe and the Americas; under-diagnosed. Loci of infection among feral mice often persist over long periods and results in sporadic clinical disease. Outbreaks have occurred from exposure to pet hamsters and laboratory animals. Nude mice, now extensively used in many research laboratories, are susceptible to infection and may be prolific chronic excreters of virus.

4. Reservoir—The infected house mouse, *Mus musculus*, is the natural reservoir; infected females transmit infection to the offspring, which become asymptomatic persistent viral shedders. Infection also occurs in mouse and hamster colonies and in transplantable tumour lines.

5. Mode of transmission—Virus excreted in urine, saliva and feces of infected animals, usually mice. Transmission to humans is probably through oral or respiratory contact with virus contaminated excreta, food or dust, or through contamination of skin lesions or cuts. Handling articles contaminated by naturally infected mice may place individuals at a high risk of infection.

6. Incubation period—Probably 8–13 days; 15–21 days until meningeal symptoms appear.

7. Period of communicability—Person-to-person transmission not demonstrated and unlikely.

8. Susceptibility—Recovery from the disease probably indicates immunity of long duration. Cell-mediated mechanisms are important, antibodies may play a secondary role

9. Methods of control—

    A. Preventive measures: Provide a clean home and place of work; eliminate mice and dispose of diseased animals. Keep foods in closed containers. Virological surveillance of commercial rodent breeding establishments, especially those producing hamsters and mice, is helpful. Ensure that laboratory mice are not infected and that personnel handling mice follow established procedures to prevent transmission from infected animals.

    B. Control of patient, contacts and the immediate environment:

        1) Report to local health authority: Reportable in selected endemic areas, Class 3 (see Reporting).
        2) Isolation: Not applicable
        3) Concurrent disinfection: Of discharges from the nose and throat, urine, feces and articles soiled therewith during acute febrile period. Terminal cleaning.
        4) Quarantine: Not applicable
        5) Immunization of contacts: Not applicable

6) Investigation of contacts and source of infection: Search home and place of employment for presence of house mice or rodent pets.

7) Specific treatment: None.

C. Epidemic measures: Not applicable.

D. Disaster implications: None.

E. International measures: None.

LYMPHOGRANULOMA VENEREUM   ICD-9 099.1; ICD-10 A55
(Lymphogranuloma inguinale, Climatic or tropical bubo, LGV)

1. Identification—A sexually acquired chlamydial infection beginning with a small, painless, evanescent erosion, papule, nodule or herpetiform lesion on the penis or vulva, frequently unnoticed. Regional lymph nodes undergo suppuration followed by extension of the inflammatory process to the adjacent tissues. In the male, inguinal buboes are seen that may become adherent to the skin, fluctuate and result in sinus formation. In the female, inguinal nodes are less frequently affected and involvement is mainly of the pelvic nodes with extension to the rectum and rectovaginal septum; the result is proctitis, stricture of the rectum and fistulae. Proctitis may result from rectal intercourse; lymphogranuloma venereum is a fairly common cause of severe proctitis in homosexual men. Elephantiasis of the genitalia may occur in both men and women. Fever, chills, headache, joint pains and anorexia are usually present during the bubo formation phase, probably due to systemic spread of *Chlamydia*. The disease course is often long and the disability great, but generally not fatal. Generalized sepsis with arthritis and meningitis is a rare occurrence.

Diagnosis is made by demonstration of chlamydial organisms by IF, EIA, DNA probe, PCR, culture of bubo aspirate or by specific micro-IF serologic test. CF testing is of diagnostic value if there is a 4-fold rise or a single titre of 1:64 or greater. A negative CF test rules out the diagnosis.

2. Infectious agent—*Chlamydia trachomatis*, immunotypes L-1, L-2 and L-3, related to but distinct from the immunotypes causing trachoma and oculogenital chlamydial infections.

3. Occurrence—Worldwide, especially in tropical and subtropical areas; more common than ordinarily believed. Endemic in parts of Asia and Africa. Age incidence corresponds with sexual activity. The disease is less commonly diagnosed in women, probably due to the frequency of asymptomatic infections; however, gender differences are not pronounced in countries with high endemicity. All races are affected. In temperate climates, it is seen predominantly among male homosexuals.

4. Reservoir—Humans; often asymptomatic (particularly in females).

5. Mode of transmission—Direct contact with open lesions of infected people, usually during sexual intercourse.

6. Incubation period—Variable, with a range of 3–30 days for a primary lesion; if a bubo is the first manifestation, 10–30 days to several months.

7. Period of communicability—Variable, from weeks to years during presence of active lesions.

8. Susceptibility and resistance—Susceptibility is general; status of natural or acquired resistance is unclear.

9. Methods of control—

   A. *Preventive measures:* Except for measures that are specific for syphilis, preventive measures are those for sexually transmitted diseases. See Syphilis, 9A, and Granuloma inguinale, 9A.

   B. *Control of patient, contacts and the immediate environment:*

   1) Report to local health authority: A reportable disease in selected endemic areas; not a reportable disease in most countries, Class 3 (see Reporting).
   2) Isolation: Refrain from sexual contact until all lesions are healed.
   3) Concurrent disinfection: Exercise care in disposal of discharges from lesions and of articles soiled therewith.
   4) Quarantine: Not applicable.
   5) Immmunization of contacts: Not applicable; prompt treatment on recognition or clinical suspicion of infection.
   6) Investigation of contacts and source of infection: Search for infected sexual contacts of patient. Recent contacts of confirmed active cases should receive specific therapy.
   7) Specific treatment: Tetracycline and doxycycline are effective for all stages, including buboes and ulcerative lesions; administer orally for at least 2 weeks. Erythromycin or sulfonamides may be used when tetracycline is contraindicated. Do not incise buboes; drain by aspiration through healthy tissue. Although oral azithromycin in a 1-gram dose has been proven effective for chlamydia urethritis and cervicitis its effectiveness in treatment is not known.

   C. *Epidemic measures:* Not applicable.

D. Disaster implications: None.

E. International measures: See Syphilis, 9E.

[F. Ndowa]

MALARIA   ICD-9 084; ICD-10 B50-B54

1. Identification—A parasitic disease; infections with the 4 human types of malaria can present symptoms sufficiently similar to make species differentiation impossible without laboratory studies. The fever pattern of the first few days of infection resembles that in early stages of many other illnesses (bacterial, viral and parasitic). Even the demonstration of para- sites, particularly in highly malarious areas, does not necessarily mean that malaria is the patient's sole illness (e.g. early yellow fever, Lassa fever, typhoid fever). The most serious malarial infection, falciparum malaria (ICD-9 084.0, ICD-10 B50) usually presents a protean clinical picture, including one or more of the following: fever, chills, sweats, anorexia, nausea, lassitude, headache, muscle and joint pain, cough and diarrhea. Anaemia and/or splenomegaly often develop after some days. If not treated adequately the disease may progress to severe malaria, of which the most important manifestations are: acute encephalopathy (cerebral malaria), severe anemia, icterus, renal failure (black-water fever), hypoglycaemia, respiratory distress, lactic acidosis and more rarely coagulation defects and shock. Severe malaria is a possible cause of coma and other CNS symptoms in any non-immune person recently returned from a tropical area. Prompt treatment of falciparum malaria is essential, even in mild cases, since irreversible complications may rapidly appear; case-fatality rates among untreated children and non-immune adults can reach 10%–40% or higher.

The other human malarias, vivax (ICD-9 084.1, ICD-10 B51), malariae (ICD-9 084.2, ICD-10 B52) and ovale (ICD-9 084.3, ICD-10 B53.0), are not usually life-threatening. Illness may begin with indefinite malaise and a slowly rising fever of several days' duration, followed by a shaking chill and rapidly rising temperature, usually accompanied by headache and nausea and ending in profuse sweating. After a fever-free interval, the cycle of chills, fever and sweating recurs daily, every other day or every third day. An untreated primary attack may last from a week to a month or longer and be accompanied by prostration, anemia and splenomegaly. True relapses following periods with no parasitaemia (in vivax and ovale infections) may occur at irregular intervals for up to 5 years. Infections with *P. malariae* may persist for life with or without recurrent febrile episodes.

Persons who are partially immune or who have been taking prophylac- tic drugs may show an atypical clinical picture and a prolonged incubation period.

Laboratory confirmation is through demonstration of malaria parasites in blood films. Repeated microscopic examinations every 12–24 hours may be necessary because the blood density of parasites varies and parasites are often not demonstrable in films from patients recently or actively under treatment. Several tests have been developed: the most promising are rapid diagnostic tests that detect plasmodial antigens in the blood. Diagnosis by PCR is the most sensitive method, but is not generally available in diagnostic laboratories. Antibodies, demonstrable by IFA or other tests, may appear after the first week of infection but may persist for years, indicating past malarial experience; thus antibody determinations are not helpful for diagnosis of current illness.

2. Infectious agents—*Plasmodium falciparum*, *P. vivax*, *P. ovale* and *P.malariae*; protozoan parasites with asexual and sexual phases. Mixed infections are not infrequent in endemic areas.

3. Occurrence—Endemic malaria no longer occurs in most temperate-zone countries and in many areas of subtropical countries, but is still a major cause of ill health in many tropical and subtropical areas. The disease causes over 1 million deaths per year in the world, most of these in young children in Africa; high transmission areas occur throughout tropical Africa, in the Southwestern Pacific, in forested areas of South America (e.g. Brazil) and southeastern Asia and in parts of the Indian sub-continent. Ovale malaria occurs mainly in sub-Saharan Africa where vivax malaria is much less frequent.

P. falciparum refractory to the 4-aminoquinolines (such as chloroquine) and other antimalarial drugs (such as sulfa-pyrimethamine combinations and mefloquine) occurs in the tropical portions of both hemispheres, particularly in the Amazon region and southeastern Asia, eastern Africa and increasingly also in central and western Africa. *P. vivax* refractory to chloroquine is present in Indonesia and Papua New Guinea ; it has been reported from Guyana, Myanmar and the Solomon Islands. The hepatic stages of some *P. vivax* strains may also be relatively resistant to treatment with primaquine. In the USA, a few episodes of locally acquired malaria have occurred since the mid-1980s. Current information on drug-resistant malaria is published annually by WHO in *International Travel and Health*, ISBN 92 4 158028 3 (http://whqlibdoc.who.int/publications/2003/9241580283.pdf), and can also be obtained from the Malaria Section, CDC, or by consulting http://www.cdc.gov/travel.

4. Reservoir—Humans are the only important reservoir of human malaria, except as regards *P.malariae*, which is common to man, the African apes and probably some South American monkeys. Non-human primates are naturally infected by some malaria parasite species, which can infect humans experimentally, although natural transmission to humans is rare.

5. Mode of transmission—Bite of an infective female *Anopheles* mosquito. Most species feed at night; some important vectors also bite at dusk or in the early morning. When a female *Anopheles* mosquito ingests blood containing sexual stages of the parasite (gametocytes), male and female gametes unite in the mosquito stomach to form an ookinete; this penetrates the stomach wall to form a cyst on the outer surface in which about a thousand sporozoites develop; this requires 8–35 days, depending on parasite species and on temperature. Sporozoites penetrate the wall of the oocyst, reach the salivary glands and are infective when injected into a person, as the insect takes its next blood-meal.

In the susceptible host, sporozoites enter hepatocytes and develop into exo-erythrocytic schizonts. When these mature, the infected hepatocytes rupture; asexual parasites reach the bloodstream and invade the erythrocytes to grow and multiply cyclically. Most will develop into asexual forms, from trophozoites to mature blood schizonts that rupture the erythrocyte within 48–72 hours, to release 8–30 erythrocytic merozoites (depending on the species) that invade other erythrocytes. At the time of each cycle, rupture of large numbers of erythrocytic schizonts induces clinical symptoms. Within infected erythrocytes, some of the merozoites may develop into male or female forms, gametocytes.

The period between an infective bite and detection of the parasite in a thick blood smear is the "prepatent period," which is typically 6–12 days for *P. falciparum*, 8–12 days for *P. vivax* and *P. ovale* and 12–16 days for *P. malariae*. Delayed primary attacks by some *P. vivax* strains may occur 6–12 months after exposure. Gametocytes usually appear in the blood stream within 3 days of overt parasitaemia with *P. vivax* and *P. ovale*, and after about 10 days with *P. falciparum*. In the liver, some sporozoites of *P. vivax* and *P. ovale* become dormant forms (hypnozoites) that remain in hepatocytes to mature months or years later and produce relapses. This phenomenon does not occur in falciparum or malariae malaria, and reappearance of these forms of the disease (recrudescence) is the result of inadequate treatment or of infection with drug-resistant strains. With *P. malariae*, low levels of erythrocytic parasites may persist for many years, to multiply at some future time to a level that may result again in clinical illness.

Injection or transfusion of infected blood or use of contaminated needles and syringes (e.g. injecting drug users) may also transmit malaria. Congenital transmission occurs rarely. However, pregnant women are more vulnerable than others to falciparum malaria (and possibly other *Plasmodium* species). In areas of intense transmission, *P. falciparum* may infect the placenta and cause low birth-weight as well as anemia, sometimes severe, of the pregnant mother. In low transmission areas, pregnant women are at high risk of severe malaria, abortion and premature delivery.

6. **Incubation periods**—The time between the infective bite and the appearance of clinical symptoms is approximately 9–14 days for *P. falciparum*, 12–18 days for *P. vivax* and *P. ovale*, and 18–40 days for

P. malariae. Some strains of *P. vivax*, mostly from temperate areas, may have an incubation period of 8-10 months and longer. With infection through blood transfusion, incubation periods depend on the number of parasites infused and are usually short, but may range up to about 2 months. Suboptimal drug suppression, such as from prophylaxis, may result in prolonged incubation periods.

7. Period of communicability—Humans may infect mosquitoes as long as infective gametocytes are present in the blood; this varies with parasite species and with response to therapy. Untreated or insufficiently treated patients may be a source of mosquito infection for several years in malariae, up to 5 years in vivax, and generally not more than 1 year in falciparum malaria; the mosquito remains infective for life. Transfusional transmission may occur as long as asexual forms remain in the circulating blood (with *P. malariae* up to 40 years or longer). Stored blood can remain infective for at least a month.

8. Susceptibility—Susceptibility is universal except in humans with specific genetic traits. Tolerance or refractoriness to clinical disease is present in adults in highly endemic communities where exposure to infective anophelines is continuous over many years. Most indigenous populations of Africa show a natural resistance to infection with *P. vivax*, which is associated with the absence of Duffy factor on their erythrocytes. Persons with sickle cell trait (heterozygotes) show relatively low parasitaemia when infected with *P. falciparum*, and thus are relatively protected from severe disease; homozygotes suffering from sickle cell disease are at increased risk of severe falciparum malaria, especially anemia. Persons infected with HIV are at increased risk of symptomatic falciparum malaria and its severe manifestations.

9. Methods of control—The control of malaria in endemic areas is based on early, effective treatment of all cases and a selection of preventive measures appropriate to the local situation.

Prompt and effective treatment of all cases is essential to reduce the risk of severe disease and prevent death. In areas of low transmission, this may also help reduce transmission. In areas of intense transmission, where children are the main risk group, formal health services are often not sufficient, and treatment needs to be available in or near the home. The increasing problems of drug resistance highlight the importance of selecting a locally effective drug. For falciparum malaria, it is now generally recommended to use antimalarial drug combinations, preferably including an artemisinin compound, in order to prolong the useful life of the treatments used.

While confirmatory diagnosis is in principle desirable, it may be of little use for young children in areas of intense transmission: they need to receive treatment when febrile as a matter of urgency and most of them may be parasite carriers, whether they are clinically ill or not.

A. *Preventive measures:*
I. Local community measures

1) Insecticide-treated mosquito nets (ITNs) are the most universally useful measure for the prevention of malaria. Although people may go to bed after mosquitoes have started biting, the partial protection is still useful; children, who are usually the most susceptible, generally go to bed earlier. Until recently the use of mosquito nets has been uncommon or absent among most affected populations, but since the mid-1990s a culture of using nets has been established in many areas through intense public and private promotion, even though high temperatures, small dwellings and cost may still be important constraints. The most acceptable nets are made of polyester or other synthetic materials; they should have fibre strength of at least 100 denier and a mesh size of at least 156 holes/in^2 (about 25 holes/cm^2). The nets must be carefully tucked under the mattress or mat. Insecticide treatment with pyrethrinoids should be repeated once or twice a year, depending on seasonality of transmission, net-washing habits and type of insecticide. Factory pretreated nets are now available, but achieving high re-treatment coverage rates is a major challenge to public health programs. One brand of pretreated nets is impregnated by a technique allowing the insecticide to remain effective for about 5 years despite washing; others (such as nets treated with two insecticides to prevent resistance) are under development.

2) Indoor residual spraying with insecticides (IRS) is another preventive method targeting adult mosquitoes with a wide range of applicability. This method is most effective where mosquitoes rest indoors on sprayable surfaces, where people are exposed in or near the home, and when it is applied before the transmission season or period of peak transmission. Coverage rates in the target area must be high: in contrast to ITN, IRS is ineffective at the household level. The susceptibility of vectors to the insecticide applied must be ascertained. When correctly applied on the basis of epidemiological and entomological data, IRS can be very effective, especially in areas of unstable (highly seasonal or irregular transmission) and epidemic malaria. The most important constraints are operational: difficulty of managing the operations once or twice a year, year after year, in areas with low human density and difficult terrain, as spraying often becomes less and less popular over time. One of the cheapest and most useful insecticides for this purpose is DDT, but because of possible environmental side-effects if

not used properly, programs deploying it are now expected, in accordance with the Stockholm Convention on Persistent Organic Pollutants, to reduce their reliance on it by adopting other effective products or methods. Pyrethroid insecticides are often selected as alternatives to DDT. Their duration of action is generally shorter, and thus they carry a lesser risk of environmental side-effects.

3) Control of larval stages by elimination of mosquito breeding sites, for example by filling and draining or by increasing the speed of water in natural or artificial channels, is of limited use in most of those areas where malaria transmission persists today. The same goes for chemical and biological (larvivorous fish) control methods applied to impounded water bodies—it is rarely possible to obtain the necessary level of coverage to reduce transmission in tropical areas. Nonetheless, these methods may be useful adjuncts in some situations such as arid, coastal and urban areas and refugee camps.

4) Intermittent preventive treatment with a full curative dose of an effective antimalarial drug is a highly effective measure for reducing the malaria burden among pregnant women in areas of moderate to intense *P. falciparum* transmission. This is promoted in Africa, but of limited use in other parts of the world, partly because transmission there is often less intense, partly because of widespread parasite resistance to the only drug that has been fully validated for this purpose, sulfadoxine-pyrimethamine.

5) In epidemic-prone areas, malaria surveillance should be based on weekly reporting and combined with monitoring of locally important factors regarding the genesis of epidemics, such as meteorological and environmental conditions and human population movements. The case definition for surveillance recommended within the national malaria control program should be used; as a minimum, confirmed cases must be distinguished from non-confirmed (probable) cases.

In non-endemic areas, blood donors should be questioned for a history of malaria or a history of travel to, or residence in, a malarious area. In most non-endemic areas, travellers who have not taken antimalarial drugs and have been free of symptoms may donate blood 6 months after return from an endemic area (in the USA, 1 year). Long-term (over 6 months) visitors to malarious areas who have been on antimalarials and have not had malaria, or persons who have immigrated or are visiting from an endemic area may be accepted as donors 3 years after cessation of prophylactic antimalarial drugs and departure from the endemic area, if they have remained asymptomatic. Immigrants or visitors from areas where *P. malariae* malaria is or has been endemic may be a source of transfusion-induced infection for many years. Such areas include malaria endemic countries of the Americas, tropical Africa, southwestern Pacific, and south and southeastern Asia.

II. Personal protective measures for non-immune travellers

Because of the resurgence of malaria, the following guidelines are presented in detail. Travellers to malarious areas must realize that: protection from biting mosquitoes is of paramount importance; no antimalarial prophylactic regimen gives complete protection; prophylaxis with antimalarial drugs should not automatically be prescribed for all travellers to malarious areas; and "standby" or emergency self-treatment is recommended when a febrile illness occurs in a falciparum malaria area where professional medical care is not readily available.

1) Measures to reduce the risk of mosquito bites include:

   a) Avoid going out between dusk and dawn when anopheline mosquitoes commonly bite. Wear long-sleeved clothing and long trousers when going out at night.

   b) Apply insect repellent to exposed skin; choose one containing either N, N-diethyl-m-toluamide (17.5% to 35%, effective for 4 to 12 hours) or dimethyl phthalate. Manufacturers' recommendations for use must not be exceeded, particularly with small children (not to exceed 10% of active product in the latter case).

   c) Stay in a well-constructed building, if possible air-conditioned, in the most developed part of town.

   d) Use screens over doors and windows; if no screens are available, close windows and doors at night.

   e) If accommodation allows entry of mosquitoes, use a mosquito net over the bed, with edges tucked in under the mattress; ensure that the net is not torn and that there are no mosquitoes inside it; sleep in the middle of the bed, avoiding contact between body and net. Impregnating the net with synthetic pyrethroid insecticides will increase protection.

   f) Use anti-mosquito sprays or insecticide dispensers (mains or battery operated) that contain tablets impregnated with pyrethroids, or burn pyrethroids, or pyrethroid mosquito coils in bedrooms at night.

2) People who are or will be exposed to mosquitoes in malarious areas should be given the following information:

a) The risk of malaria infection varies among countries and within different areas of each country. See country list in WHO's annual publication *International Travel and Health*, ISBN-92 4 158028 3, http://www.who.int/ith.

b) Pregnant women and young children when infected are highly susceptible to development of severe and complicated malaria.

c) Malaria can kill if treatment is delayed. Medical help must be sought promptly if malaria is suspected; a blood sample must be examined on more than one occasion and a few hours apart.

d) Symptoms of malaria may be mild; malaria should be suspected if, one week or more after entry into a transmission area, an individual suffers any fever, malaise with or without headache, backache, muscular aching and/or weakness, vomiting, diarrhea and cough. Seek prompt medical advice.

3) Pregnant women and parents of young children must be advised of the following:

a) Malaria in a pregnant woman increases the risk of maternal death, miscarriage, stillbirth and neonatal death.

b) Pregnant women should not visit malarious areas unless this is absolutely necessary.

c) Extra diligence is needed in using measures to protect against mosquito bites.

d) Take chloroquine (5.0 mg base/kg/week–the equivalent of 8.0 mg of diphosphate salt/kg/week; 6.8 mg of sulfate salt/kg/week and 6.1 of hydrochloride salt/kg/week) and proguanil (3.0 mg/kg/day–the equivalent of 3.4 mg of hydrochloride salt/kg/day) for prophylaxis. In areas with chloroquine-resistant *P. falciparum*, take chloroquine and proguanil during the first 3 months of pregnancy; mefloquine prophylaxis (5.0 mg/kg/week— equivalent to 5.48 mg of hydrochloride salt/kg/week) should be considered from the fourth month of pregnancy.

e) Doxycycline prophylaxis should not be taken.

f) Medical help should be sought immediately if malaria is suspected; emergency "standby" treatment should be taken only if no medical help is immediately available. Medical help must be sought as soon as possible after standby treatment (see 9AII4 and 9AII5c).

g) Malaria prophylaxis is important for the protection of young children. Chloroquine (5 mg base/kg/week) plus proguanil (3 mg/kg/day—not available in the USA) may safely be given to infants.

h) Women of childbearing age may take mefloquine prophylaxis (5 mg/kg/week), but should avoid pregnancy until 3 months after they have stopped the drug, which has a long half-life. There are limited data, but so far no firm evidence, for embryotoxic/teratogenic effects: in situations of inadvertent pregnancy, prophylaxis with mefloquine is not considered an indication for pregnancy termination.

i) Women of childbearing age may take doxycycline prophylaxis (1.5 mg dihydrochloride salt/kg/day), but pregnancy should be avoided until about 1 week after stopping the drug.

j) If pregnancy occurs during antimalarial prophylaxis (except with chloroquine plus proguanil), seek information about congenital risks from the drug manufacturer.

4) Standby treatment: The most important factors that determine the survival of patients with falciparum malaria are early diagnosis and immediate treatment. Most non-immune individuals exposed to or infected with malaria should be able to obtain prompt medical attention when malaria is suspected. A minority will be exposed to a high risk of infection while at least 12–24 hours away from competent medical attention. WHO recommends that prescribers issue antimalarial drugs to be carried by the persons who may be in such exposed situations for self-administration. Persons prescribed standby treatment must receive precise instructions on recognition of symptoms, complete treatment regimen to be taken, possible side-effects and action to be taken in the event of drug failure. They must be made aware that self-treatment is a temporary measure and medical advice is to be sought as soon as possible.

5) Prophylaxis: Non-immune individuals who will be exposed to mosquitoes in malarious areas must make use of protective measures against mosquito bites and will benefit from the use of suppressive drugs for chemoprophylaxis. The possible side-effects of long-term (up to 3 to 5 months) use of the drug or drug combination recommended for use in any particular area should be weighed against the actual likelihood of being bitten by an infected mosquito. The risk of exposure for visitors or residents in most urban areas in many malarious countries, including southeastern Asia and South America may be negligible, and suppressive drugs

may not be indicated. In some urban centers, notably in Indian subcontinent countries, there may be a risk of exposure. If there is a risk, protective measures must be used. The geographic distribution and specific drug sensitivities of malaria parasites can change rapidly: recent information about drug patterns must be sought before prescribing chemoprophylaxis.

a) For suppression of malaria in non-immune individuals temporarily residing in or travelling through endemic areas where, as of 2003, plasmodia are chloroquine-sensitive (Central America West of the Panama Canal, Haiti and Dominican Republic, malarious areas of the Middle East (except some in the Islamic Republic of Iran, Saudi Arabia and Yemen), and China (excepting Hainan and Yunnan Provinces): chloroquine 5 mg base/kg body weight (300 mg base or 500 mg chloroquine phosphate for the average adult) once weekly, or hydroxychloroquine 5 mg base/kg body weight to the adult dose of 310 mg base or 400 mg salt is recommended. Pregnancy is not a contraindication. The drug must be continued on the same schedule for 4 weeks after leaving endemic areas. Minor side-effects may occur at prophylactic doses and may be alleviated by taking the drug with meals or changing to hydroxychloroquine. Psoriasis may be exacerbated particularly in Africans and Americans of African origin; chloroquine may interfere with the immune response to intradermal rabies vaccine.

b) For suppressive malaria drug therapy for travellers who will be exposed to chloroquine-resistant *P. falciparum* infection (southeastern Asia, sub-Saharan Africa, rain forest areas of South America, and south-western Pacific Islands), mefloquine alone (5 mg/kg/week) is recommended. Suppressive drug treatment must be continued weekly, starting 1–2 weeks before travel and continued during travel or residence in malarious area and for 4 weeks after returning to non-malarious areas. Mefloquine is contraindicated in those with a known hypersensitivity to it. It is not recommended for women in the first trimester of pregnancy nor for individuals with cardiac arrhythmias, a recent history of epilepsy or severe psychiatric disorders. Data show no increased risk of serious side-effects with long-term use of mefloquine, but in general, for those with prolonged residence in high-risk areas, the seasonality of transmission and improved protective measures against mosquito bites should be weighed against the long-term risk of drug reactions.

For those who are unable to take mefloquine and for those going to malaria endemic areas of Cambodia, Myanmar and Thailand, doxycycline alone (100 mg once daily) is an alternative regimen. Doxycycline may precipitate *Candida* vaginitis, oesophageal irritation and photosensitivity. It should not be given to pregnant women and children under 8. Doxycycline prophylaxis can begin 1-2 days before travel to malarious areas and be continued daily during travel and for 4 weeks after leaving the malarious area. Atovaquone/proguanil offers an alternative prophylaxis for travellers who are making short trips to areas where there is chloroquine-resistance and who cannot take mefloquine or doxycycline. The daily adult dose is one tablet containing 250 mg atovaquone plus 100 mg proguanil, to be started 1 day before departure and continued for 7 days after return. It is registered in several European countries for prophylactic use, with restrictions on body weight (>40 kg) and duration of use (no more than 28 days)—in the USA these restrictions do not apply.

In areas of chloroquine resistance to both *P. vivax* and *P. falciparum*, a prophylactic regimen for adults who do not have G6PD deficiency and women who are neither pregnant nor nursing was proposed after clinical studies during the late 1990s. This consists of primaquine 0.5 mg base/kg/day, beginning on the first day of exposure and continued for 1 week after leaving the risk area. The most common side-effect was epigastric or abdominal pain and vomiting in less than 10% of recipients. Longer term exposure, up to 50 weeks of daily administration of primaquine, showed a slight increase of methemoglobin level to 5.8%, which declined by half within a week after ending primaquine administration.

Long-term travellers at risk of infection by chloroquine-resistant *P. falciparum* strains for whom none of the above regimens can be recommended should take all precautions to avoid mosquito bites at night and carry a treatment dose of a locally effective antimalarial, or artemether-lumefantrine (see 9B7c). In the event of a febrile illness, if professional care is not available, they must take the complete antimalarial dosage and obtain medical consultation as soon as possible. Such presumptive self-treatment is only a temporary measure and early medical evaluation is imperative.

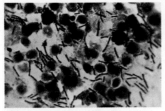

Photomicrograph of *Bacillus anthracis*; anthrax. **(Anthrax)**

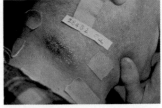

Cutaneous anthrax lesion on neck of man. **(Anthrax)**

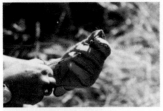

This clinician is shown extracting blood from a rodent for the purpose of testing the sample during a 1974 arbovirus study. Arthropod-borne viruses, such as arboviruses, are maintained in nature through biological transmission between susceptible vertebrate hosts by blood feeding arthropods, i.e mosquitoes, psychodids, ceratopogonids, and ticks. **(Arboviruses)**

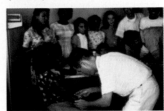

This is a clinician obtaining a human blood sample from a child during an arbovirus study. Arboviruses are a leading cause of viral encephalitis in the world. Recent outbreaks of St. Louis encephalitis and epizootics of eastern and western equine encephalitis in the U.S. demonstrate that arboviruses are still a public health problem. **(Arboviruses)**

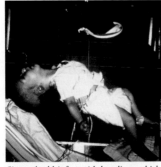

Six week old infant with botulism, which is evident as a marked loss of muscle tone, especially in the region of the head and neck. **(Botulism)**

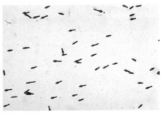

A photomicrograph of *Clostridium botulinum* type A viewed using a Gram stain technique.The bacterium produces a nerve toxin, which causes the rare, but serious paralytic illness Botulism. There are seven types of botulism toxin designated by the letters A through G; only types A, B, E and F cause illness in humans. **(Botulism)**

All Images courtesy of the CDC Public Health Image Library (unless otherwise indicated).

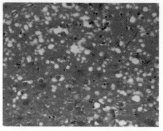

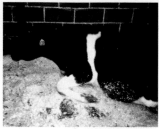

This micrograph of brain tissue reveals the cytoarchitectural histopathologic changes found in bovine spongiform encephalopathy. The presence of vacuoles, i.e. microscopic "holes" in the gray matter, gives the brain of BSE-affected cows a sponge-like appearance when tissue sections are examined in the lab. **(BSE)**

Cattle such as the one pictured here, which are affected by BSE experience progressive degeneration of the nervous system. Behavioral changes in temperament (e.g., nervousness or aggression), abnormal posture, incoordination and difficulty in rising, decreased milk production, and/or loss of weight despite continued appetite are followed by death in cattle affected by BSE. **(BSE)**

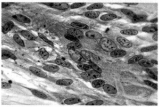

This photomicrograph reveals the intranuclear inclusions produced by varicella virus grown in a tissue culture; Magnified 500X. **(Chickenpox)**

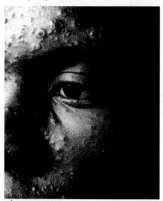

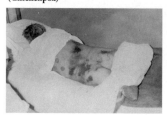

Isolated male patient diagnosed with Crimean-Congo hemorrhagic fever (C-CHF). Crimean-Congo Hemorrhagic Fever is a tickborne hemorrhagic fever with documented person-to-person transmission, and a case-fatality rate of approximately 30%. This widespread virus has been found in Africa, Asia, the Middle East, and eastern Europe. **(Crimean-Congo Hemorrhagic Fever)**

This slide of a patient with chickenpox, demonstrates the difference between smallpox and chickenpox on the 5th day of rash. **(Chickenpox)**

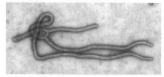

Transmission Electron Micrograph of the Ebola Virus; Photo Credit: C. Goldsmith **(Hemorrhagic Fever/Ebola)**

All images courtesy of the CDC Public Health Image Library (unless otherwise indicated).

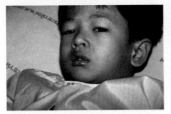

Sawanpracharuk hospital, Nakorn Sawan. A young boy with erythema, swollen face and full, very red lips, all signs of DHF; Thailand, 2000. Photographer: Andy Crump. WHO/TDR
(Dengue Hemorrhagic Fever)

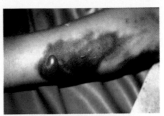

A large subcutaneous hemorrhage on the upper arm of a patient with dengue hemorrhagic fever. (Image courtesy of the Wellcome Trust). WHO/TDR/STI/Hatz
(Dengue Hemorrhagic Fever)

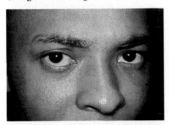

The viral disease Hepatitis A is manifested here as icterus, or jaundice of the conjunctivae and facial skin. HAV is usually spread from person to person by putting something in the mouth (even though it may look clean) that has been contaminated with the stool of a person with hepatitis A. Adults will have signs and symptoms more often than children. **(Hepatitis A Virus)**

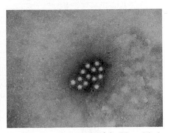

An electron micrograph of the Hepatitis A virus (HAV), an RNA virus that can survive up to a month at room temperature. This virus enters an organism by ingestion of water and food contaminated by human feces, and reaches the liver through the bloodstream. HAV infection is endemic in third world countries, and is prevalent in the Far East. **(Hepatitis A Virus)**

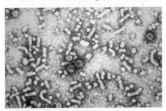

This electron micrograph reveals the presence of hepatitis-B virus HBV "Dane particles," or virions. These particles measure 42nm in their overall diameter, and contain a DNA-based core that is 27nm in diameter. **(Hepatitis B Virus)**

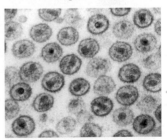

HIV-1. Transmission electron micrograph.HIV-1. Cone-shaped cores are sectioned in various orientations. Viral genomic RNA is located in the electron-dense wide end of core. **(HIV)**

All images courtesy of the CDC Public Health Image Library (unless otherwise indicated).

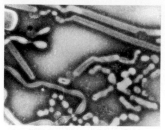

Transmission electron micrograph of influenza A virus, early passage. **(Influenza)**

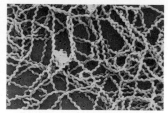

Scanning electron micrograph of Leptospira bacteria on 0.1 μm polycarbonate filter. Humans become infected by swallowing water contaminated by infected animals or through skin contact, especially with mucosal surfaces, such as the eyes or nose, or with broken skin. The disease is not known to be spread from person to person. Photo Credit: CDC/NCID/HIP/Janice Carr **(Leptospira)**

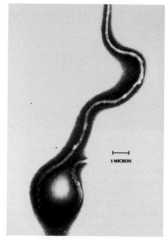

1 MICRON

Photomicrograph of *Borrelia burgdorferi*, the bacterium that cause Lyme disease. This is a spiral-shaped bacterium that is frequently carried by deer ticks of the genus *Ixodes*. **(Lyme Disease)**

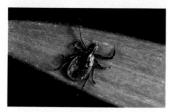

Black-legged ticks, *I. scapularis* are known to transmit Lyme disease, *Borrelia burgdorferi*, to humans and animals during feeding, when they insert their mouth parts into the skin of a host and slowly take in the nutrient-rich host blood. These ticks are found on a wide rage of hosts including mammals, birds and reptiles. Photo Credit: Jim Gathany **(Lyme Disease)**

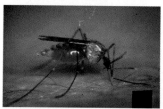

PA malaria vector mosquito (*Anopheles freeborni*) taking a blood meal. **(Malaria)**

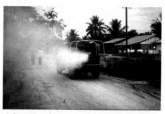

A Leco machine on a Landrover spraying with a pyrethroid insecticide to kill malaria vector mosquitos resting inside or outside houses. **(Malaria)**

All images courtesy of the CDC Public Health Image Library (unless otherwise indicated).

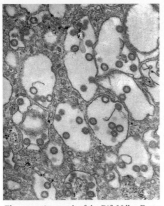

Electron micrograph of the Rift Valley Fever virus. Rift Valley Fever (RVF) virus is a member of the genus Phlebovirus in the family Bunyaviridae, first reported in livestock in Kenya around 1900. **(Rift Valley Fever)**

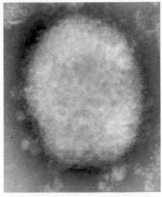

Negative stain electron micrograph reveals a "M" (mulberry type) monkeypox virus virion in human vesicular fluid. **(Monkeypox)**

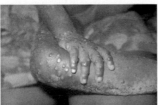

Human infection with monkeypox-like virus in 4 year-old female in Bondua, Grand Gedeh County, Liberia. This infection was caused by a pox virus of the vaccinia, variola, monkeypox type. **(Monkeypox)**

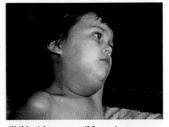

Child with mumps. **(Mumps)**

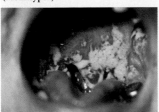

Oral thrush. Aphthae. Candida albican (often associated with low immune status such as cancer or AIDS). **(Oral Thrush)**

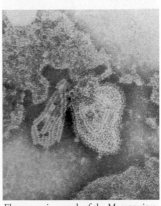

Electron micrograph of the Mumps virus. **(Mumps)**

All images courtesy of the CDC Public Health Image Library (unless otherwise indicated).

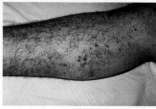

This photomicrograph depicts *Yersinia pestis* bacteria using a fluorescent antibody stain. Note the characteristic bipolar, close-pin shaped rods of the bacteria. **(Plague)**

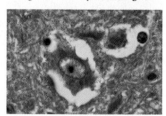

Capillary fragility is one of the manifestations of a plague infection, evident here on the leg of an infected patient. **(Plague)**

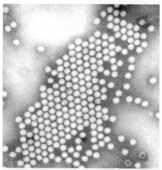

Transmission electron micrograph, negative stain image of the polio virus. **(Polio)**

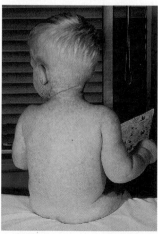

Photomicrograph of H&E stained brain tissue from a rabies encephalitis patient. Histopathologic brain tissue from a rabies patient displaying the pathognomonic finding of Negri Bodies within the neuronal cytoplasm, and stained using H&E stain. **(Rabies)**

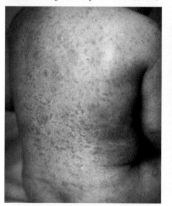

Rash of rubella on skin of child's back. Distribution is similar to that of measles but the lesions are less intensely red. **(Rubella)**

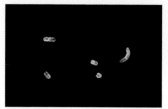

Back of boy with measles. Third day of rash. **(Measles)**

All images courtesy of the CDC Public Health Image Library (unless otherwise indicated).

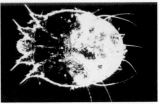

Coronaviruses are a group of viruses that have a halo, or crown-like (corona) appearance when viewed under a microscope. The coronavirus is now recognized as the etiologic agent of the 2003 SARS outbreak. Additional specimens are being tested to learn more about this coronavirus, and its etiologic link with Severe Acute Respiratory Syndrome. **(SARS)**

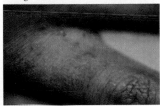

This is a Sarcoptes scabiei var. hominis or "itch mite," often associated with the transmission of human scabies. Scabies is usually transmitted by intimate interpersonal contact, often sexual in nature, but transmission through casual contact can occur. **(Scabies)**

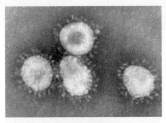

The pimple-like rash in the webbing between the fingers of this adult's hand was due to *Sarcoptes scabiei var. hominis.* **(Scabies)**

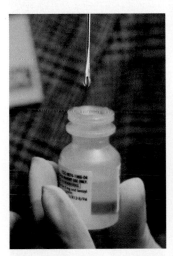

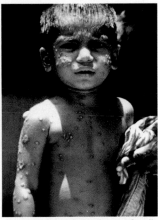

Bifurcated needle with saline solution used in smallpox vaccination during the 2002 Vaccinator Workshop. In December 2002, CDC Clinicians trained state licensed vaccine administers how to deliver smallpox vaccine safely and efficiently. Once training was completed, they provided additional smallpox vaccine administration training in their home states. **(Smallpox)**

Child with full-body distribution of smallpox eruptions, Pakistan, 1955. The scabs will eventually fall off leaving marks on the skin that will become pitted scars. The patient is contagious to others until all of the scabs have fallen off. **(Smallpox)**

All images courtesy of the CDC Public Health Image Library (unless otherwise indicated).

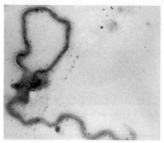

PA photomicrograph of a *Treponema pallidum* bacterium. **(Syphilis)**

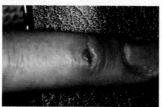

The ulcerative primary syphilitic lesion on this patient's finger was due to lab acquired disease. The primary stage of syphilis is usually marked by the appearance of a single sore known as a chancre, but there may be multiple sores. The chancre is usually firm, round, small, and painless. **(Syphilis)**

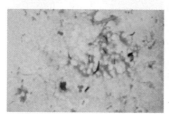

This photomicrograph reveals *Mycobacterium tuberculosis* bacteria using acid-fast Ziehl-Neelsen stain; Magnified 1000X. The acid-fast stains depend on the ability of mycobacteria to retain dye when treated with mineral acid or an acid-alcohol solution, such as the Ziehl-Neelsen or the Kinyoun stains that are carbolfuchsin methods specific for *M. tuberculosis*. **(Tuberculosis)**

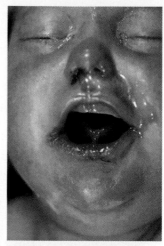

The face of a newborn infant displaying pathologic morphology indicative of "Congenital Syphilis." **(Syphilis)**

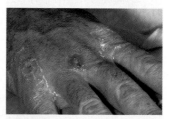

A Tularemia lesion on the dorsal skin of the right hand, caused by the bacterium *Francisella tularensis*. **(Tularensis)**

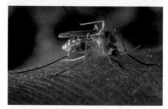

A *Culex quinquefasciatus* mosquito on a human finger. The mosquito is proven to be a vector associated with transmission of the West Nile Virus. Photo Credit: CDC/James Gathany. **(West Nile Virus)**

All images courtesy of the CDC Public Health Image Library (unless otherwise indicated).

c) With the exception of primaquine, chemosuppressive drugs do not eliminate intrahepatic parasites, so clinical relapses of vivax or ovale malaria may occur after the drug is discontinued. Primaquine, 0.3 mg base/kg/day for 14 days (15 mg base or 26.3 mg of primaquine phosphate for the average adult) is often effective and may be given after leaving endemic areas, concurrently with or following the suppressive drug. However, it can produce hemolysis, especially in those with G6PD deficiency. The decision to administer primaquine is made on an individual basis, after consideration of the potential risk of adverse reactions, and this drug is generally indicated only for persons with prolonged exposure, e.g. missionaries, aid workers and military personnel. Larger daily doses (30 mg base) are generally required for southwestern Pacific and some strains from southeastern Asia and South America.

Alternatively, primaquine, 0.75 mg base/kg, may be given once weekly for 8 doses (45 mg base or 79 mg primaquine phosphate for the average adult) after leaving endemic areas. Prior to primaquine administration, the patient should be tested for G6PD deficiency. Primaquine should not be administered during pregnancy; chloroquine chemosuppression should instead be continued weekly for the duration of the pregnancy.

B. Control of patient, contacts and the immediate environment:

1) In non-endemic areas, report to local health authority: Obligatory case report as a Disease under Surveillance by WHO, Class 1 (see Reporting), preferably limited to smear-confirmed cases; Class 3 (reporting of probable and confirmed cases) is the more practical procedure in endemic areas.

2) Isolation: For hospitalized patients, blood precautions. In non-endemic areas where malaria transmission is possible, patients should be in mosquito-proof areas from dusk to dawn, until microscopy shows that they have no gametocytes in the blood.

3) Concurrent disinfection: Not applicable.

4) Quarantine: Not applicable.

5) Immunization of contacts: Not applicable.

6) Investigation of contacts and source of infection: Determine history of previous infection or of possible exposure. If a history of sharing needles is obtained from the patient, investigate and treat all persons who shared the equipment. In transfusion-induced malaria, all donors must be located

and their blood examined for malaria parasites and for antimalarial antibodies; parasite-positive donors must receive treatment. Malaria cases in non-endemic areas are usually imported, but some cases with no travel history have been reported from areas near airports in recent years. These are believed to have been caused by infected mosquitoes air-transported from an endemic area. If the area is receptive to malaria (effective vectors present), household contacts should be screened, and persons living in the same community as well as health services should be advised about the risk of malaria; anybody developing malaria-like symptoms must be examined by blood microscopy or rapid diagnostic tests. The flight range of anopheline mosquitoes may reach 2 km, but in most cases it is only a few hundred meters. Vector control should only be considered if several cases occur in a small area.

7) Specific treatment for all forms of malaria:

a) *Plasmodium falciparum* is nowadays resistant to chloroquine in almost all endemic areas, and resistance to sulfadoxine-pyrimethamine, one of the few low-cost alternatives to chloroquine, is appearing where this was selected as replacement therapy. Identifying suitable antimalarial drug policies poses a major challenge to national programs. WHO recommends that falciparum-endemic countries where chloroquine or sulfadoxine-pyrimethamine treatments are failing or start to fail adopt combination treatments—where individual components can delay development of resistance to each other—as first-line treatment. WHO recommendations, products and drug policies can be found at http://www.rbm.who.int. The following is mainly designed for the management of malaria in travellers (during and after travel), taking into account the need for highly effective treatment for these patients, who generally have no immunity to the disease, and the products which may be available to them.

   The treatment of malaria due to infection with chloroquine-sensitive *P. falciparum*, *P. vivax*, *P. malariae* and *P. ovale* is the oral administration of a total of 25 mg of chloroquine base/kg administered over a 3-day period: 15 mg/kg the first day (10 mg/kg initially and 5 mg/kg 6 hours later; 600 and 300 mg doses for the average adult); 5 mg/kg the second day; and 5 mg/kg the third day.

b) For emergency treatment of adults with severe or complicated infections or for people unable to retain orally administered medication, quinine dihydrochloride, 20 mg salt/kg body weight to a maximum of 1200 mg, diluted in 10 ml/kg of isotonic fluid, may be administered by slow IV (over 4 hours); repeated if needed after 8 hours at a maintenance dose of 10 mg salt/kg given every 8 hours, until it can be supplanted by oral quinine. The total duration of quinine monotherapy should be 10 days. The pediatric dose is the same, but the interval between the doses is 12 hours. If no improvement within 48 hours, each dose should be reduced to 5–7 mg/kg; hypoglycaemia is a common side-effect, so plasma glucose should be monitored.

For infections acquired in areas where quinine resistance occurs (as of late 2003 in Thailand), use artemether IM (3.2 mg/kg the first day, followed by 1.6 mg/kg/day); or artesunate IV or IM (2.4 mg/kg on the first day, followed by 1.2 mg/kg/day). In hyperparasitacmic cases, artesunate 1.2 mg/kg may be given 4–6 hours after the first dose. Artemether and artesunate should be given for no more than 7 days, or until the patient can take another effective antimalarial drug, such as mefloquine, 25 mg/kg, by mouth. Oral artemether and artesunate and other artemisinin compounds should be used only in combination with other antimalarials. They are not recommended in the first trimester of pregnancy; and should be used later in pregnancy only if suitable alternatives are not available.

Where parenteral quinine and artemisinin compounds are not available, quinine can be substituted by parenteral quinidine, equally effective in the treatment of severe malaria. A loading dose of quinidine gluconate (15 mg base/kg) is administered by slow IV infusion over 4 hours, followed by a constant IV infusion of 0.02 mg base/kg/minute, preferably controlled by a constant-infusion pump, with monitoring of cardiac function and fluid balance through a central venous catheter; the quinidine infusion should be temporarily slowed or stopped for a QT interval greater than 0.6 seconds, an increase in the QRS complex by more than 50%, or hypotension unresponsive to fluid challenges. The infusion may continue for a maximum of 72 hours. All parenteral drugs should be discontinued as soon as oral drug administration can be initiated.

In extremely severe falciparum infections, particularly with a parasitaemia approaching or exceeding 10%, exchange transfusion should be considered. Details on the management of severe malaria can be found in: *Management of severe malaria. A practical Handbook*. Geneva, WHO, 2000. http://www.rbm.who.int/docs/hbsm_toc.htm

c) For *P. falciparum* infections acquired in areas where chloroquine-resistant strains are present, administer quinine, 30 mg salt/kg/day divided in 3 doses, for 7 days. (For severe infections, IV quinine as described above.) Along with oral quinine, administer doxycycline (2 mg/kg once a day, maximal 100 mg/dose), or tetracycline (5 mg/kg/dose, maximal 250 mg/dose) 4 times a day, for 7 days. If the patient is pregnant or under 8, doxycycline and tetracycline are contraindicated, and quinine should be given for 10 days. Mefloquine (25 mg/kg daily in 2 doses 12 hours apart) is effective for treatment of chloroquine-resistant *P. falciparum* from most parts of the world, but poorly effective on its own for *P. falciparum* in Thailand and neighboring countries. Failures have also been reported from Brazil. Currently, the best treatment for cases from these areas is mefloquine (25 mg/kg) combined with artesunate or artemether (4mg/kg/day) for 3 days, or artemether-lumefantrine (as artemether 1.3 mg/kg with lumefantrine 8 mg/kg twice daily) for 3 days, corresponding to a standard adult dose of 4 tablets of 20 mg artemether + 120 mg lumefantrine (also called co-artemether) twice daily for 3 days. This is not yet (2003) registered for children weighing less than 10 kg.

d) For *P. vivax* infections acquired in the southwestern Pacific or Indonesia, mefloquine is effective for treatment of the blood stages (15 mg/kg in a single dose). An alternative is chloroquine combined with primaquine (see 9B7e). Quinine, halofantrine and artemether-lumefantrine are possible alternatives; consult package inserts.

e) For prevention of relapses in mosquito-acquired *P. vivax* and *P. ovale* infections, administer primaquine, as described in 9A5c above, on completion of the treatment of an acute attack. It is desirable to test all patients (especially Africans, Americans of African origin, Asians and Mediterraneans) for G6PD deficiency to prevent drug-induced hemolysis. Many, particularly Africans and Americans of African origin, can tolerate hemolysis, but if it occurs during treatment, primaquine should be discontinued. Primaquine is not required in non-mosquito-transmitted disease (e.g. transfusion), since no liver phase occurs.

C. **Epidemic measures:** Determine the nature and extent of the epidemic situation. Malaria epidemics must be controlled through rapid and vigorous action and effective treatment of all cases; in advanced epidemics where a large part of the population is infected, mass treatment may be considered. In falciparum malaria epidemics the inclusion of an anti-gametocyte drug like primaquine in a single adult dose of 30–45 mg may be considered, but possible benefits must be weighed against possible side-effects in G6PD-deficient persons. As soon as possible, full coverage vector control measures should be instituted. Usually, indoor residual spraying is preferred because of its rapid effect; this may be followed by the use of insecticide-treated bednets and anti-larval measures.

D. **Disaster implications:** Disasters may lead to malaria epidemics as a result of population movements, ecological changes, breakdown of health services and other factors. In recent years in complex emergencies in Africa, malaria has presented with an epidemic pattern, taking an extraordinarily high toll among children and often adults. The drug resistance situation often turns out to be worse than had been assumed from national data. Control measures include early effective treatment and vector control (insecticide-treated nets, indoor residual spraying or other). In densely populated refugee camps, space spraying may be effective in the emergency phase; environmental measures may be relevant later. In areas of intense transmission in Africa, intermittent preventive treatment in pregnancy should be initiated. Health education, as in any context, is required to support these interventions and promote better malaria control.

E. **International measures:**

   1) Important international measures include the following:

      a) Disinsectization of aircraft before boarding passengers or in transit, using a residual spray application of an effective insecticide;
      b) Disinsectization of aircraft, ships and other vehicles on arrival if the health authority at the place of arrival has reason to suspect importation of malaria vectors;
      c) Enforcing and maintaining rigid anti-mosquito sanitation within the mosquito flight range of all ports and airports.

   2) In special circumstances, administer antimalarial drugs to potentially infected migrants, refugees, seasonal workers and persons taking part in periodic mass movement into an

area or country where malaria has been eliminated. Primaquine, 30 – 45 mg base (0.5 – 0.75 mg/kg), given as a single
dose, renders the gametocytes of falciparum malaria noninfectious, but should be avoided in persons with G6PD
deficiency.

3) As one of the world's major global public health problems,
malaria is a Disease under Surveillance by WHO. It is
addressed by the global Roll Back Malaria Initiative, by the
United Nations' Millennium Goals and by the Global Fund to
Combat AIDS, Tuberculosis and Malaria. National health
administrations in endemic countries are expected to notify
WHO annually of the following:

a) Recorded malaria cases/deaths, epidemics, coverage of
major interventions (see *Framework for Monitoring
Progress & Evaluating Outcomes and Impact* WHO/
CDS/RBM/2000.25 http://whqlibdoc.who.int/hq/2000/
WHO_CDS_RBM_2000.25.pdf);
b) The situation of antimalarial drug resistance;
c) Those international ports and airports free of malaria.
Further information on http://www.rbm.who.int and
http://who.int/diseases/malaria/default.htm

[A. Schapira]

MALIGNANT NEOPLASMS
ASSOCIATED WITH
INFECTIOUS AGENTS

Infectious agents are risk factors for several malignancies. Among the
agents implicated in the pathogenesis of various human malignancies,
either directly or indirectly, are parasites, viruses and the bacterium
Helicobacter pylori. The infectious agent is neither necessary nor sufficient cause for all cases of agent-related malignancy; other causes are
involved; cofactors, both external (environmental) and internal (genetic
and physiological at immunological and molecular levels), play important
roles in each of these malignancies, which usually represent the late
outcome of the infection.

Most of the infectious agents implicated in the etiology of tumours are
viruses. A common feature of most virus-related cancers is the persistence
of the virus following infection early in life or the presence of immunosuppression: this leads to integration and development of cancer, usually
in a single cell clone (monoclonal tumour). Both DNA and RNA viruses are
involved.

The 4 strongest DNA virus candidates as agents directly or indirectly involved in the pathogenesis of human malignancies are: (1) hepatitis B virus (HBV) and hepatitis C virus (HCV); (2) Epstein Barr virus (EBV); (3) human papillomaviruses (HPV, mainly types 16 and 18); (4) human herpesvirus-8 (HHV-8), also called Kaposi sarcoma-associated herpesvirus (KSHV). The first 3 occur worldwide and produce many more inapparent than apparent infections; most result in a latent virus state that is subject to reactivation. Monoclonality of the tumour cells and integration of the virus into the tumour cell indicate a causal association. The associated malignancies occur in special host and geographic settings.

Among RNA viruses, retroviruses—including human T-cell lymphotropic virus (HTLV-1) and human immunodeficiency virus (HIV)—are associated with human T-cell leukaemia/lymphoma. Evidence from serology, virology and epidemiology strongly implicates them in the causation of specific malignancies.

I. HEPATOCELLULAR
CARCINOMA   ICD-9 155.0; ICD-10 C22.0
(HCC, Primary liver cancer, Primary hepatocellular carcinoma)

Chronic infection with hepatitis B or C is an important risk factor for primary hepatocellular cancer (PHC or HCC). Prospective studies have shown a 100-fold higher risk of hepatocellular cancer in persons chronically infected with HBV than in noncarriers. Many patients go through stages of chronic hepatitis and cirrhosis before development of the tumour.

Periodic screening of carriers of hepatitis B virus (HBV) for alpha-fetoprotein—a serologic marker associated with hepatocellular cancer—and ultrasound screening can, in some cases, detect the tumour at an early, resectable stage.

Hepatocellular cancer is among the most common malignant neoplasms in many parts of Asia and Africa; it occurs with highest frequency in areas with high prevalence of HBV carriers, including most of Asia, Africa, the South Pacific and part of the Middle East. Rates are intermediate on the Indian subcontinent and relatively low in North America and western Europe. Case-control studies have shown hepatitis C virus (HCV) to be strongly associated with hepatocellular cancer among patients with and without HBV infections; in addition there is laboratory evidence for transforming properties of HCV. HCV infection may be the dominant cause of hepatocellular cancer in Japan.

See Viral hepatitis B and C for methods of control. The administration of hepatitis B (HB) vaccine alone or HB vaccine plus hepatitis B immune globulin (HBIG) to all newborns may help prevent development of the tumour; immunization interrupts mother-to-infant transmission. WHO recommends that all countries integrate HB vaccine into routine childhood immunization schedules. Many countries, including the USA, are implementing this recommendation, which should eventually lead to elimination of HBV and control of hepatocellular cancer caused by HBV. Hepatocellular cancer cases should be reported to a tumour registry. No vaccine is available for HCV infection but testing the blood supply for HCV antibody will prevent its transmission by transfusion.

[E. K. Yeoh]

II. BURKITT LYMPHOMA   ICD-9 200.2; ICD-10 C83.7
(BL, African Burkitt lymphoma, Endemic Burkitt lymphoma, Burkitt tumour)

Burkitt lymphoma (BL) is a monoclonal tumour of B cells occurring worldwide and hyperendemic in highly malarious areas below 1000 meters/3000 feet with heavy rainfall (above 1000 millimeters/40 inches a year), such as tropical Africa and lowland Papua New Guinea. African children commonly show jaw involvement. The tumour may also develop as a rare event in immunosuppressed patients (patients with organ transplant or familial X-linked immunodeficiency and more commonly in AIDS). The tumours may be monoclonal, polyclonal or mixed; not all are Burkitt-type, but all are acute lymphoblastic sarcomas.

Epstein-Barr virus (EBV), a herpesvirus responsible for infectious mononucleosis, plays an important pathogenic role in about 97% of cases in Africa and Papua New Guinea, where EBV infection occurs in infancy and where malaria, an apparent cofactor, is holoendemic. EBV is also associated with Burkitt lymphoma in about 30% of cases in nonmalarious areas and areas of low-endemicity for Burkitt lymphoma (American form). Regardless of the presence of EBV, there is a specific chromosomal translocation t(8;14) involving the proto-oncogene *c-myc* locus on the long arm of chromosome 8 and the immunoglobulin heavy chain locus on chromosome 14. Variant translocations t(2;8) and (8;22) involve the *c-myc* gene and the immunoglobulin kappa and lambda chain loci, located respectively on chromosomes 2 and 22. The subsequent activation of the *c-myc* gene plays an important role in malignant transformation. Recent studies suggest that the chromosomal breakpoint locations in African cases differ from those in American cases, suggesting a molecular heterogeneity in Burkitt lymphoma in general. Other genetic alterations include the inactivation of tumour suppressor gene p53. The estimated time range of tumour development is 2–12 years from primary EBV infection but is much shorter in AIDS patients in whom an EBV-related lymphoma (often CNS) develops. Evidence from serology, virology and epidemiology points to a strong role of EBV infection in the causation of the African form of the disease.

Burkitt lymphoma is a highly aggressive tumour but can nevertheless be cured in 90% of cases with intensive multiple chemotherapy. Prevention of EBV infection early in life and control of malaria (see Malaria, section 9) might reduce tumour incidence in Africa and Papua New Guinea. Subunit vaccines against EBV are in the trial stage. Chemotherapy is usually effective after the tumour develops. Cases should be reported to a tumour registry.

[E. K. Yeoh]

III. NASOPHARYNGEAL CARCINOMA   ICD-9 147.9; ICD-10 C11

Nasopharyngeal carcinoma (NPC) is a malignant tumour of the epithelial cells of the nasopharynx that usually occurs in adults aged 20–40. Incidence is particularly high (about 10-fold when compared with the general population) among groups from China (Taiwan and southern China), even in those who have moved elsewhere. This risk decreases in subsequent generations after emigration from Asia.

IgA antibody to the EBV viral capsid antigen in both serum and nasopharyngeal secretions is characteristic of the disease and has been used in China as a screening test for the tumour. Its appearance may precede the clinical appearance of nasopharyngeal carcinoma by several years and its reappearance after treatment heralds recurrence.

The serological and virological evidence relating EBV to NPC is similar to that for African Burkitt lymphoma (high EBV antibody titres, genome in tumour cells); this relationship has been found without respect to the geographical origin of the patient. The tumour occurs worldwide but is highest in southern China, southeastern Asia, northern and eastern Africa and the Arctic. Males outnumber females by about 2:1. Chinese with HLA-2 and SIN-2 antigen profiles have a particularly high risk.

EBV infection occurs early in life in settings where nasopharyngeal carcinoma is most common, yet the tumour does not appear until age 20–40, which suggests the occurrence of some secondary reactivating factor, with epithelial invasion later in life. Repeated respiratory infections or chemical irritants, such as nitrosamines in dried foods, may play a role. The higher frequency of the tumour in persons of southern Chinese origin, without respect to later residence, and the association with certain HLA haplotypes suggest a genetic susceptibility. A lower incidence among those who have migrated to the USA and elsewhere suggests that one or more environmental factor(s), such as the nitrosamines present in smoked fish and other foods, may be associated cofactors.

Early detection in highly endemic areas (screening for EBV IgA antibodies to viral capsid antigen) permits early treatment. A subunit vaccine against EBV infection is under study. Chemotherapy after early recognition is the only specific therapy. Cases should be reported to a tumour registry.

[B. Sylla]

IV. MALIGNANCIES POSSIBLY RELATED TO EBV

A. HODGKIN DISEASE   ICD-9 201; ICD-10 C81

Hodgkin disease (HD) is a tumour of the lymphatic system occurring in 4 histological subtypes–nodular sclerosis, lymphocyte predominance, mixed cellularity and lymphocyte depletion. The histology shows the presence of a highly specific but nonpathognomonic cell, the Reed-Sternberg cell, also seen in cases of infectious mononucleosis.

The cause of Hodgkin disease is not certain, but laboratory and epidemiological evidence implicates EBV in at least half the cases. The disease is more common in industrialized countries, but age-adjusted incidence is relatively low. It is more common in higher socioeconomic settings, in smaller families, and in Caucasians compared with Americans of African origin.

Cases that develop after infectious mononucleosis occur some 10 years later; cases in older adults, if EBV-related, are probably the result of virus reactivation in the presence of a deteriorating immune system. The high frequency of EBV found in cases of Hodgkin disease diagnosed among HIV-infected patients and the relatively short incubation period appear related to the severe immunodeficiency of HIV infection; whether the presence of EBV in the tumour cell is cause or effect is not known.

Among HIV-infected patients, particularly those infected through IV drug use, a higher proportion of Hodgkin disease cases are EBV-associated. Cases should be reported to a tumour registry.

B. NON-HODGKIN LYMPHOMAS   ICD-10 B21.2, C83.0, C83.8, C83.9, C85

The incidence of lymphomas in AIDS patients is about 50-100 times that in the general population. While these cases may be related to EBV, the virus most associated with non-Hodgkin lymphoma (NHL) tumours such as high grade and CNS lymphomas is HIV. Since 1980, NHL has shown a dramatic increase among young, single white men with AIDS in the USA. About 4% of AIDS patients present with lymphoma, and perhaps 30% will eventually develop one if survival is sufficiently long. Whether EBV is a causal factor in EBV-associated lymphomas in HIV-infected patients or simply enters the tumour cell after it has been formed is not clear, but accumulating evidence points to the former possibility.

A marked increase in NHL not explained by the increase in AIDS patients has been noted in recent years. The disease commonly occurs in the presence of other forms of immunodeficiency, such as that in posttransplant patients, those given immunosuppressive drugs and persons with inherited forms of immunodeficiency. There are few epidemiological clues to the risk factors responsible. Altered antibody patterns to EBV characteristic of those seen in immunodeficiency states occur in many cases of NHL; these changes have been shown to precede the development of NHL. Molecular techniques have evidenced the EBV genome in 10%-15% of tumour cells of the spontaneous form of NHL. Cases should be reported to a tumour registry.

[B. Sylla]

V. KAPOSI SARCOMA
ICD-9 173.0-173.9; ICD-10 C46.0-46.9

(Idiopathic multiple pigmented hemorrhagic sarcoma)

Kaposi sarcoma (KS) is a vascular neoplastic disorder that involves spindle cell proliferation, characterized by red-purple or blue-brown macules, plaques, and nodules of the skin and other organs. Skin lesions may be firm or compressible, solitary or multiple. First described in 1872, it was considered a rare tumour of unknown etiology before its frequent diagnosis in HIV-infected patients.

There are 4 epidemiological forms of KS. The classical form occurs in older males of mainly Mediterranean or eastern European Jewish backgrounds. An endemic form occurs in all age groups in parts of equatorial Africa; neither has a known precipitating environmental factor nor is associated with immune deficiency. The remaining types—in recipients of organ transplants who undergo immunosuppressive treatment or in HIV-infected persons—are accompanied by immune impairment. Overall, males are predominantly afflicted. The epidemic form presents the most aggressive clinical course and is seen almost exclusively in HIV-infected individuals. Despite differences in clinical manifestations and serostatus, it is appropriate to consider all forms of Kaposi sarcoma as one entity given the identical immunohistochemical features of the characteristic spindle cell of the tumour.

Kaposi sarcoma-associated herpesvirus (KSHV), or human herpesvirus 8 (HHV-8), is believed to be the causal agent of Kaposi sarcoma. Discovered in 1994, it is a new human *Gammaherpesvirus* related to an oncogenic herpesvirus of monkeys, *Herpesvirus saimiri*. Evidence of viral infection is found in virtually all cases and several lines of evidence point to a key etiologic role in this disease. KSHV infection precedes clinical sarcoma, is highly associated with increased risk in all populations studied thus far, and affects the endothelial (spindle) cell thought to be the prime determinant of tumourigenesis. KSHV has also been shown to induce transformation of primary endothelial cells.

Seroepidemiological analysis suggests that KSHV has a more limited distribution than any of the other 7 human herpesviruses. In North America, seroprevalence ranges from 0%-1% in blood donors to about 35%

in HIV-infected individuals and up to 100% in Kaposi patients with AIDS. In Milan, Italy, blood donors have a 4% seropositivity rate. Data suggest even higher KSHV rates in central Africa, where 58% of persons aged 14–84 were KSHV positive in one study and seroprevalence (similar in men and women) increased linearly with age.

Serological analyses also suggest that infection occurs primarily in sexually active people, particularly men who have sex with men. Differences in risk of Kaposi sarcoma for AIDS patients who acquired HIV via sexual transmission and those whose HIV infections derived from blood product exposure support the role of sexual transmission: only 1% to 3% of hemophilia- and transfusion-related AIDS patients develop Kaposi. Transplacental transmission of anti-KSHV antibody is almost certain and the virus may also be transmitted transplacentally since children of KSHV-positive mothers are at increased risk of infection after the neonatal period. In Africa, the high seroprevalence among adolescents and the relatively linear increase in prevalence with age suggest that nonsexual modes of transmission for KSHV may also be important.

There is no known cure for Kaposi sarcoma, but partial and complete remissions have been noted. Cases should be reported to a tumour registry.

[D. Parkin]

VI. LYMPHATIC TISSUE MALIGNANCY

ICD-9 202;
ICD-10 C84.1, C84.5, C91.4, C91.5

(Adult T-cell leukaemia [ATL], T-cell lymphosarcoma [TLCL], peripheral T-cell lymphoma [Sézary disease], Hairy cell leukaemia)

Adult T-cell leukaemia (ATL), a leukaemia/lymphoma of T-cell origin commonly seen in Japan, is identical to T-cell lymphoma sarcoma-cell leukaemia (TLCL) seen less commonly in the Caribbean, the Pacific coast of South America, equatorial Africa and southern USA. These malignancies primarily involve adults and are associated with human T-cell lymphotrophic virus (HTLV-1), a member of the family of retroviruses. The latent period between infection and the emergence of ATL is 20–30 years. Infection early in life, primarily through breastmilk, leads to tumour development in the adult, peaking at about age 50. This suggests the risk of ATL is lower should infection occur later in life through transfer of blood or blood products, IV drug use or sexual activity. The same virus causes tropical spastic paraparesis (also called HTLV-1-associated myelopathy in Japan). Adult Japanese and Afro-Caribbeans are at highest risk.

Serological, virological and epidemiological evidence strongly implicate HTLV-1 in the causation of leukaemia/lymphoma. Control measures are similar to those for prevention of AIDS (see AIDS, section 9). The effectiveness of screening donor blood for antibodies against HTLV-1 and

2 has yet to be demonstrated. In the USA, although the low overall virus prevalence renders transmission from blood donors a rare event, screening donor units for the virus is now a standard procedure. Cases should be reported to a tumour registry.

[E. K. Yeoh]

VII. CERVICAL CANCER   ICD-9 180; ICD-10 C53
(Carcinoma of the uterine cervix)

Cervical cancer is the second most common cancer in women worldwide, and the most common among women in Latin America, India and Sub-Saharan Africa. Cervical cancer risk is associated with lower socioeconomic status, early start of sexual activity, multiple sexual partners and smoking. Of all deaths from cervical cancer, 80% occur in developing countries.

Human papillomavirus (HPV) is now considered the necessary cause of cervical cancer. While so called "low risk" types of HPV cause benign warts and verrucae (see Warts, viral), "high risk" types, most notably HPV types 16, 18, 31, 33, and 45, have been found in tumour tissues of about 90% of cervical cancer cases worldwide. The strong association of cervical cancer with certain types of HPV opens good perspectives for a future prevention of the disease through immunization strategies. Phase-3 trials of prophylactic vaccines against HPV 16 and 18 infection are under way. For the moment, the best prevention tool against cervical cancer is organized screening programs based on cytological smears (Papanicolaou smears). Cases should be reported to a tumour registry.

[S. Franceschi]

MEASLES   ICD-9 055; ICD-10 B05
(Rubeola, Hard measles, Red measles, Morbilli)

1. Identification—An acute, highly communicable viral disease with prodromal fever, conjunctivitis, coryza, cough and small spots with white or bluish white centers on an erythematous base on the buccal mucosa (Koplik spots). A characteristic red blotchy rash appears on the third to seventh day; the rash begins on the face, then becomes generalized, lasts 4–7 days, and sometimes ends in brawny desquamation. Leukopenia is common. The disease is more severe in infants and adults than in children. Complications may result from viral replication or bacterial superinfection, and include otitis media, pneumonia, laryngotracheobronchitis (croup), diarrhea and encephalitis.

The case-fatality rates in developing countries are estimated to be

3%–5%, but are commonly 10%–30% in some localities. Acute and delayed mortality in infants and children have been documented. Measles is a more severe disease in the very young and in malnourished children, in whom it may be associated with hemorrhagic rash, protein-losing enteropathy, otitis media, oral sores, dehydration, diarrhea, blindness and severe skin infections. Children with clinical or subclinical vitamin A deficiency are at particularly high risk. In children whose nutrition status is borderline, measles often precipitates acute kwashiorkor and exacerbates vitamin A deficiency that may lead to blindness. Subacute sclerosing panencephalitis (SSPE) develops very rarely (about 1/100 000) several years after infection; over 50% of SSPE cases had measles diagnosed in the first 2 years of life. The WHO clinical case-definition reads "any person with fever and maculopapular rash and cough/coryza/conjunctivitis."

Diagnosis is usually on clinical and epidemiological grounds although laboratory confirmation is preferred. The detection of measles-specific IgM antibodies, present 3–4 days after rash onset, or a significant rise in antibody concentrations between acute and convalescent sera confirms the diagnosis. Techniques used less commonly include identification of viral antigen in nasopharyngeal mucosal swabs by FA techniques or virus isolation in cell culture from blood or nasopharyngeal swabs collected before day 4 of rash, or from urine specimens before day 8 of rash.

2. Infectious agent—Measles virus, a member of the genus *Morbillivirus* of the family Paramyxoviridae.

3. Occurrence—Prior to widespread immunization, measles was common in childhood, so that more than 90% of people had been infected by age 20; few went through life without becoming infected. In the prevaccine era, there was an estimated 100 million cases and 6 million measles deaths a year. Measles, endemic in large metropolitan communities, attained epidemic proportions about every second or third year. In smaller communities and areas, outbreaks tended to be more widely spaced and somewhat more severe. With longer intervals between outbreaks, as in some Sahelian populations, in the Arctic and some islands, measles outbreaks often involved a large proportion of the population with a high case-fatality rate. In temperate climates, measles occurs primarily in the late winter and early spring. In tropical climates, measles occurs primarily in the dry season.

With effective childhood immunization programs, measles cases in many industrialized countries have dropped by 99% and generally occur in young unimmunized children or older children, adolescents or young adults who received only one dose of vaccine.

In 1994, the countries of the western hemisphere established a regional target of elimination of indigenous measles transmission by the end of the year 2000 through a comprehensive measles immunization strategy, including the provision of measles vaccine to at least 95% of children aged 12–15 months through routine immunization services, with another opportunity for measles immunization to all children and careful measles surveillance. This second opportunity for measles immunization provides immunity to children who escaped routine immunization and those who failed to respond immunologically to the first vaccine. It is usually provided through Supplementary Immunization Activities (SIAs): a one-time to "catch-up" campaign targets all children 9 months to 14 years regardless of disease history or previous vaccination status. "Follow-up" campaigns are conducted every 3-4 years targeting all children 9 months-4 years. In Canada and USA, the second opportunity for measles immunization is provided through routine immunization services, gener-ally at school entry. By June 2003, over 6 months had passed without the strong regional measles surveillance systems having identified a single indigenous measles case in the Americas—strong evidence that measles virus circulation had been interrupted.

Despite the existence of a safe, effective and inexpensive measles vaccine for 40 years, measles remains the leading vaccine-preventable killer of children worldwide. WHO estimates that there were approxi-mately 35 million cases and 614 000 measles deaths worldwide in 2002. Over 98% of measles deaths occur in countries with per capita gross national products lower than $1000, over 75% in children under 5 years and over 50% in Africa. In 2003, the World Health Assembly adopted the target of reducing global measles deaths by 50% from the 1999 level of 875 000 before the end of 2005; it recommended that all countries fully implement the WHO/UNICEF comprehensive immunization strategy for sustainable measles mortality reduction.

4. Reservoir—Humans.

5. Mode of transmission—Airborne by droplet spread, direct contact with nasal or throat secretions of infected persons; less commonly by articles freshly soiled with nose and throat secretions. Measles is one of the most highly communicable infectious diseases.

6. Incubation period—About 10 days, but may be 7 to 18 days from exposure to onset of fever, usually 14 days until rash appears; rarely as long as 19-21 days. IG given for passive protection early in the incubation period may extend this period.

7. Period of communicability—From 1 day before the beginning of the prodromal period (usually about 4 days before rash onset) to 4 days after rash appearance; minimal after the 2nd day of rash. The vaccine virus has not been shown to be communicable.

8. Susceptibility—All persons who have not had the disease or who have not been successfully immunized are susceptible. Acquired immunity after illness is permanent. Infants born to mothers who have had the disease are protected against disease for the first 6-9 months or more, depending on the amount of residual maternal antibody at the time of pregnancy and the rate of antibody degradation. Maternal antibody interferes with response to vaccine. Immunization at 12–15 months induces immunity in 94%–98% of recipients; reimmunization increases immunity levels to about 99%. Children born to mothers with vaccine-induced immunity receive less passive antibody; they may become susceptible to measles and require measles immunization at an earlier age than is usually recommended.

9. **Methods of control—**

   A. *Preventive measures:*

   1) Public education by health departments and private physicians should encourage measles immunization for all susceptible infants, children, adolescents and young adults. Those for whom vaccine is contraindicated, and unimmunized persons identified more than 72 hours after exposure to measles in families or institutions may be partially or completely protected by IG given soon after exposure.

   2) Immunization: Live attenuated measles vaccine is the agent of choice, indicated for all persons not immune to measles, unless specifically contraindicated (see 9A2c). A single injection of live measles vaccine, usually combined with other live vaccines (mumps, rubella), can be administered concurrently with other inactivated vaccines or toxoids; it should induce active immunity in 94%–98% of susceptible individuals, probably for life, by producing a mild or inapparent noncommunicable infection. Another dose of measles vaccine may increase immunity levels up to 99%.

   About 5%–15% of nonimmune vaccinees may develop malaise and fever to 39.5°C (103°F) within 5–12 days post immunization; this lasts 1–2 days, with little disability. Rash, coryza, mild cough and Koplik spots may occasionally occur. Febrile seizures occur infrequently and without sequelae; the highest incidence is in children with a previous history or a close family (parents or siblings) history of seizures. Encephalitis and encephalopathy have been reported (at the rate of less than one case per million doses distributed) following measles immunization—this is lower than the background rate and consequently may not be caused by the vaccine.

   Current recommendations in the USA and other industrialized countries advise a routine 2-dose measles vaccination schedule, the initial dose at 12–15 months or as soon as possible thereafter; the following dose, usually at school entry (4–6 years), can be administered as early as 4 weeks after the initial dose where the risk of exposure to measles is high. Both doses are generally given as combined measles, mumps and rubella vaccine (MMR).

Routine immunization with MMR at 12 months is particularly important in areas where measles cases occur. During community outbreaks, the recommended age for immunization using monovalent vaccine can be lowered to 6–11 months. A second dose of measles vaccine is then given at 12–15 months and a third dose at school entry.

The optimal age for immunization in developing countries depends on the persistence of maternal antibodies in the infant and the increased risk of exposure to measles at a younger age. In most developing country settings, WHO recommends measles immunization of all children at 9 months with another opportunity for measles immunization, generally through SIAs. In Latin America, due to the markedly decreased risk of an infant being exposed to measles virus, PAHO recommends routine immunization at 12–15 months for all children, with another opportunity for measles immunization through periodic SIAs.

a) Vaccine shipment and storage: Immunization may not produce protection if the vaccine has been improperly handled or stored. Prior to reconstitution, freeze-dried measles vaccine is relatively stable and can be stored with safety for a year or more in a freezer or at refrigerator temperatures (2°–8°C/35.6°–46.4°F). Reconstituted vaccine must be kept at refrigerator temperatures and discarded after 8 hours; both freeze-dried and reconstituted vaccine must be protected from prolonged exposure to ultraviolet light, which may inactivate the virus.

b) Reimmunizations: In the USA and other industrialized countries, in addition to routine reimmunization of children entering school, measles reimmunization is offered at entry to high school and colleges, international travellers and health care workers, unless they have a documented history of measles disease or immunization with 2 doses of vaccine, or serological evidence of measles immunity. In those who received only inactivated vaccine, reimmunization may produce reactions such as local oedema and induration, lymphadenopathy and fever, but will protect against the atypical measles syndrome. Use of inactivated measles vaccine was discontinued more than 30 years ago.

c) Contraindications to the use of live virus vaccines:
   i) Patients with primary immune deficiency diseases affecting T-cell function or acquired immune deficiency due to leukaemia, lymphoma or generalized malignancy, or therapy with corticosteroids, irradiation,

alkylating drugs or antimetabolites should not receive live virus vaccines. Infection with HIV is not an absolute contraindication. WHO recommends measles immunization of all infants and children regardless of HIV status because of the greater risk of severe measles in such persons. The USA and other develop countries recommend measles vaccination only in asymptomatic HIV-positive individuals; low CD4+ counts are a contraindication to measles vaccine because of the risk of viral pneumonia.

ii) In patients with severe acute illness with or without fever, immunization should be deferred until recovery from the acute phase; minor febrile illnesses such as diarrhea or upper respiratory infections are not a contraindication.

iii) Persons with anaphylactic hypersensitivity to a previous dose of measles vaccine, gelatin or neomycin should not receive measles vaccine. Egg allergy, even if anaphylactic, is no longer considered a contraindication.

iv) Purely on theoretical grounds, vaccine should not be given to pregnant women; mothers should be advised of the theoretical risk of fetal damage if they become pregnant within 1 month after receipt of measles-containing vaccine.

v) Vaccine should be given at least 14 days before IG or blood transfusion. IG or blood products can interfere with the response to measles vaccine for varying periods depending on the dose of IG. The usual dose administered for hepatitis A prevention can interfere for 3 months; very large doses of intravenous IG can interfere for up to 11 months.

B. Control of patient, contacts and the immediate environment:

1) Report to local health authority: Obligatory case report in most countries, Class 2 (see Reporting). Early reporting (within 24 hours) provides opportunity for better outbreak control.

2) Isolation: Impractical in the community at large; children with measles should if practicable be kept out of school for 4 days after appearance of the rash. In hospitals, respiratory isolation from onset of catarrhal stage of the prodromal period through the 4th day of rash reduces the exposure of other patients at high risk.

3) Concurrent disinfection: Not applicable.

4) Quarantine: Usually impractical. Quarantine of institutions, wards or dormitories can sometimes be of value; strict segregation of infants if measles occurs in an institution.

5) Immunization of contacts: Live virus vaccine should be administered within 72 hours of exposure. Alternatively, IG may be given (0.25 ml/kg or 0.11 ml/lb)—for immunocompromised persons, 0.5 ml/kg or 0.22ml/lb up to a maximum of 15 ml within 72 hours of exposure for maximal protection. IG should be used within 6 days of exposure for susceptible household or other contacts with high risks of complications (contacts under 1 year of age, pregnant women or immunocompromised persons), or where measles vaccine is contraindicated. Live measles vaccine should be given 5–6 months later to those for whom vaccine is not contraindicated.

6) Investigation of contacts and source of infection: Search and immunize exposed susceptible contacts to limit the spread of disease. Carriers are unknown.

7) Specific treatment: None. During measles infection, vitamin A reserves fall rapidly (especially in malnourished children) which further weakens immunity. Vitamin A supplementation at the time of measles diagnosis replaces body reserves, prevents blindness due to corneal ulceration and keratomalacia and significantly reduces measles fatality. The following Vitamin A schedule is recommended:

Age	Immediately	Next day
<6 months	50 000 IU	50 000 IU
6–11 months	100 000 IU	100 000 IU
12 months+	200 000 IU	200 000 IU

A third dose of vitamin A should be given 2–4 weeks later if there are signs of vitamin A deficiency (night blindness, Bitot spots, conjunctival or corneal dryness, corneal clouding or ulceration) on diagnosis.

C. Epidemic measures:

1) Prompt reporting (within 24 hours) of suspected cases and comprehensive immunization programs for all susceptibles are needed to limit spread. In day care, school and college outbreaks in the USA, all persons without documentation of 2 doses of live virus vaccine at least 1 month apart on or after the first birthday should be immunized unless they have documentation of prior physician-diagnosed measles or laboratory evidence of immunity.

2) In institutional outbreaks, new admissions should receive vaccine or IG.

3) In many developing countries, measles has a relatively high case-fatality rate. If vaccine is available, prompt use at the beginning of an epidemic is essential to limit spread; if vaccine supply is limited, priority should be given to young children for whom the risk is greatest.

D. Disaster implications: Introduction of measles into refugee populations with a high proportion of susceptibles can result in devastating epidemics with high fatality rates. Providing measles vaccine to displaced persons living in camp settings within a week of entry is a public health priority.

E. International measures: Persons travelling to measles endemic areas should ensure that they are immune to measles.

[B. Hersh]

MELIOIDOSIS   ICD-9 025; ICD-10 A24.1–A24.4
(Whitmore disease)

1. Identification—An uncommon bacterial infection; clinical manifestations range from none or asymptomatic pulmonary consolidation to localised cutaneous or visceral abscesses, necrotizing pneumonia and/or a rapidly fatal septicemia. It may simulate typhoid fever or tuberculosis, with pulmonary cavitation, empyema, chronic abscesses and osteomyelitis.

Diagnosis depends on isolation of the causative agent; a rising antibody titre in serological tests is confirmatory. Direct immunofluorescent microscopy is 98% specific but only about 70% sensitive compared with culture. The possibility of melioidosis must be kept in mind in any unexplained suppurative disease, especially cavitating pulmonary disease, in patients living in or returned from endemic areas; disease may become manifest as long as 25 years after exposure.

2. Infectious agent—*Burkholderia pseudomallei*, the Whitmore bacillus.

3. Occurrence—Clinical disease is uncommon, generally occurring in individuals with impaired immunocompetence whose non-intact skin had intimate contact with contaminated soil or surface water. It may appear as a complication of overt wounds or follow aspiration of water. Cases have been recorded in many tropical and subtropical areas of Africa, America, Asia, Australia/Pacific Islands, India and the Middle East. In certain areas, 5%–20% of agricultural workers have demonstrable antibodies but no history of overt disease; in Thailand it is considered to be a disease of rice farmers.

4. Reservoir—The organism is saprophytic in certain soils and waters. Various animals, including sheep, goats, horses, swine, monkeys and rodents (plus various animals in zoological gardens) can become infected, without evidence that they are important reservoirs, except in the transfer of the agent to new foci.

5. Mode of transmission—Usually contact with contaminated soil or water through overt or inapparent skin wounds, aspiration or ingestion of contaminated water or inhalation of soil dust.

6. Incubation period—Can be as short as 2 days. However, years may elapse between presumed exposure and appearance of clinical disease.

7. Period of communicability—Person-to-person transmission has not been proven conclusively. Laboratory-acquired infections may rarely occur, especially if procedures produce aerosols.

8. Susceptibility—Disease in humans is uncommon even among people in endemic areas who have close contact with soil or water containing the infectious agent. Approximately two-thirds of cases have a predisposing medical condition such as diabetes, cirrhosis, alcoholism or renal failure, which may precipitate disease or recrudescence in asymptomatic infected individuals.

9. Methods of control—

A. *Preventive measures:*

1) Persons with debilitating disease, including diabetes, and those with traumatic wounds should avoid exposure to soil or water, such as rice paddies, in endemic areas.
2) In endemic areas, skin lacerations, abrasions or burns that have been contaminated with soil or surface water should be immediately and thoroughly cleaned.

B. *Control of patient, contacts and the immediate environment:*

1) Report to local health authority: No official report, Class 5 (see Reporting).
2) Isolation: Respiratory and sinus drainage precautions.
3) Concurrent disinfection: Safe disposal of sputum and wound discharges.
4) Quarantine: Not applicable.
5) Immmunization of contacts: Not applicable.
6) Investigation of contacts and source of infection: Human carriers are not known.
7) Specific treatment: The most effective treatment is IV ceftazidime or imipenem for at least 10 days followed by a 4-drug

combination of doxycycline, trimethoprim-sulfamethoxazole (for 20 weeks) and chloramphenicol (for the first 8 weeks). The infection may be slow to respond to treatment and even with 20 weeks of treatment, 10% relapse. Treatment for an inadequate length of time leads to a high probability of relapse. Abscesses should be drained if possible.

C. *Epidemic measures:* Usually a sporadic disease. Outbreaks should be investigated to determine if there is a point source.

D. *Disaster implications:* None, except as in C above.

E. *International measures:* None except as in C above. Risk of introduction should be considered when animals are moved to areas where the disease is unknown.

F. *Measures in the case of deliberate use:* B. pseudomallei is a potential agent for deliberate use that is moderately easy to disseminate and has low morbidity rates, although the case fatality rate among overt cases is high. Control measures include rapid identification (and control) of the point source. In the unlikely event of the spread of B. pseudomallei, the value of prophylactic medication is unproven but may be efficacious.

GLANDERS ICD-9 024; ICD-10 A24.0

Glanders is a highly communicable disease of horses, mules and donkeys; it has disappeared from most areas of the world, although enzootic foci are believed to exist in Asia and some eastern Mediterranean countries. Clinical glanders no longer occurs in the western hemisphere. Rare and sporadic human infections are reported almost exclusively in those whose occupations involve contact with animals or work in laboratories (e.g. veterinarians, equine butchers and pathologists). Infection with *Burkholderia mallei*, the glanders bacillus, cannot be differentiated serologically from infection with *B. pseudomallei*; characterization of the isolated organism alone can lead to specific diagnosis. Prevention depends on control of glanders in equine species and care in handling causative organisms. Treatment: see Melioidosis. *B. mallei*, like *B. pseudomallei*, is a potential agent for deliberate use.

[A. Plant]

I. VIRAL MENINGITIS   ICD-9 047.9; ICD-10 A87
(Aseptic meningitis, Serous meningitis, Nonbacterial or abacterial meningitis)
(Nonpyogenic meningitis: ICD-9 322.0; ICD-10 G03.0)

1. Identification—A relatively common but rarely serious clinical syndrome with multiple viral etiologies, characterized by sudden onset of febrile illness with signs and symptoms of meningeal involvement. CSF findings are pleocytosis (usually mononuclear, occasionally polymorphonuclear in early stages), increased protein, normal sugar and absence of bacteria. A rubella-like rash characterizes certain types caused by echoviruses and coxsackieviruses; vesicular and petechial rashes may also occur. Active illness seldom exceeds 10 days. Transient paresis and encephalitic manifestations may occur; paralysis is unusual. Residual signs lasting a year or more may include weakness, muscle spasm, insomnia and personality changes. Recovery is usually complete. GI and respiratory symptoms may be associated with enterovirus infection.

Various diseases caused by non-viral infectious agents may mimic aseptic meningitis: these include inadequately treated pyogenic meningitis, tuberculous and cryptococcal meningitis, meningitis caused by other fungi, cerebrovascular syphilis and lymphogranuloma venereum. Postinfectious and postvaccinal reactions require differentiation from sequelae to measles, mumps, varicella and immunization against rabies and smallpox; these syndromes are usually encephalitic in type. Leptospirosis, listeriosis, syphilis, lymphocytic choriomeningitis, viral hepatitis, infectious mononucleosis, influenza and other diseases may produce the same clinical syndrome, as discussed in individual chapters.

Infection by enteroviruses transmitted from the mother is a frequent cause of neonatal fever with neurological signs. In countries that are polio-free, the most prevalent infectious agent causing paralysis is enterovirus 71, responsible for outbreaks of meningitis and paralysis in many countries. Children and adults with B cell deficiencies are subject to chronic relapsing meningitis, usually caused by enteroviruses.

Under optimal conditions, specific identification is possible in about half the cases through serological and isolation techniques. Viral agents may be isolated in early stages from throat washings and stool, occasionally from CSF and blood, and through cell culture techniques and animal inoculation. PCR identification in CSF (and stool for enteroviruses) yields a more rapid diagnosis and probes are available for the identification of most viruses.

2. Infectious agents—A wide variety of infectious agents, many associated with other specific diseases. Several viruses can produce meningeal features. At least half the cases have no obvious cause. In epidemic periods, mumps may be responsible for more than 25% of cases of established etiology in nonimmunized populations. In the USA, enteroviruses (picornaviruses) cause most cases of known etiology, followed by coxsackievirus. These include coxsackievirus group B types 1-6 and echovirus types 2, 5, 6, 7, 9 (most), 10, 11, 14, 18 and 30, and enterovirus 71. Coxsackievirus group A (types 2, 3, 4, 7, 9 and 10), arboviruses, measles, herpes simplex and varicella viruses, lymphocytic choriomeningitis virus, adenovirus and others provide sporadic cases. Incidence of specific types varies with geographic location and time. *Leptospira* may cause up to 20% of cases of aseptic meningitis in various areas (see Leptospirosis).

3. Occurrence—Worldwide, as epidemics and sporadic cases; true incidence unknown. Seasonal increases in late summer and early autumn are due mainly to arboviruses and enteroviruses, while late winter outbreaks may be due primarily to mumps.

4., 5., 6., 7. and **8. Reservoir, Mode of transmission, Incubation period, Period of communicability** and **Susceptibility**—Vary with the specific infectious agent (refer to specific disease chapters).

9. Methods of control—

A. Preventive measures: Depend on causes (see specific disease).

B. Control of patient, contacts and the immediate environment:

1) Report to local health authority: In selected endemic areas; in many countries not a reportable disease, Class 3 (see Reporting). If laboratory-confirmed, specify infectious agent; otherwise, report as "cause undetermined".
2) Isolation: Specific diagnosis depends on laboratory data not usually available until after recovery. Therefore, enteric precautions are indicated for 7 days after onset of illness unless a nonenteroviral diagnosis is established.
3) Concurrent disinfection: No special precautions needed beyond routine sanitary practices.
4) Quarantine: Not applicable.
5) Immunization of contacts: See specific infectious agent.
6) Investigation of contacts and source of infection: Not usually indicated.
7) Specific treatment: Acyclovir may be given for herpes simplex meningitis. Pleconaril is available experimentally for enteroviral infections in Canada/USA and other industrialized countries. In the rare event of agammaglobulinaemia with chronic enteroviral meningitis patients should receive IG.

C. Epidemic measures: See specific infectious agent.

D. Disaster implications: None.

E. International measures: WHO Collaborating Centres.

[D. Lavanchy]

II. BACTERIAL MENINGITIS   ICD-9 320; ICD-10 G00

Neisseria meningitidis, *Streptococcus pneumoniae* and *Haemophilus influenzae* type b (Hib) constitute more than 75% of all cases of bacterial meningitis in most studies, and 90% of bacterial meningitis in children. Meningitis due to Hib, previously the most common cause of bacterial meningitis, has largely been eliminated in many industrialized countries through immunization programs. The agent causing disease varies by age group. In the United States and other countries, the medial age of persons with bacterial meningitis increased dramatically from 15 months in 1986 to 25 years or more in 1995, due to reduction in Hib disease. Meningococcal disease is unique among the major causes of bacterial meningitis in that it causes both endemic disease and also large epidemics. The less common bacterial causes of meningitis, such as staphylococci, enteric bacteria, group B streptococci and *Listeria*, occur in persons with specific susceptibilities (such as neonates and patients with impaired immunity) or as the consequence of head trauma.

II. A. MENINGOCOCCAL INFECTION   ICD-9 036; ICD-10 A39
(Meningococcaemia, not meningitis: ICD-10 A39.2-A39.4)
MENINGOCOCCAL MENINGITIS   ICD-9 036.0; ICD-10 A39.0
(Cerebrospinal fever)

1. **Identification**—An acute bacterial disease, characterized by sudden onset of fever, intense headache, nausea and often vomiting, stiff neck and photophobia. A petechial rash with pink macules or occasionally vesicles may be observed in Europe and North America but rarely in Africa. Case fatality rates formerly exceeded 50%. Antibiotics, intensive care units and improved supportive measures have decreased this but it remains high at 8%–15%. In addition, 10%–20% of survivors will suffer long-term sequelae including mental retardation, hearing loss and loss of limb use. Invasive disease is characterized by one or more clinical syndromes including bacteraemia, sepsis, or meningitis, the latter being the most common presentation. Meningococcaemia, or meningococcal sepsis, is the most severe form of infection with petechial rash, hypotension, disseminated intravascular coagulation and multiorgan failure. Other forms

of meningococcal disease such as pneumonia, purulent arthritis, and pericarditis are less common.

The gold standard for diagnosis is recovery of meningococci from a sterile site, primarily cerebrospinal fluid (CSF) or blood; however, the sensitivity of culture, especially in patients who have received antibiotics, is low. In culture-negative cases, identification of group-specific meningococcal polysaccharides in CSF by latex agglutination is of help but false-negative results are common, especially for serogroup B. Polymerase chain reaction offers the advantage of detecting meningococcal DNA in CSF or plasma and not requiring live organisms; it is not yet widely available in many countries. Microscopic examination of Gram-stained smears from petechiae may show *Neisseria*.

2. **Infectious agent**—*Neisseria meningitidis*, the meningococcus, is a Gram-negative, aerobic diplococcus. *Neisseria* are divided into serogroups according to the immunological reactivity of their capsular polysaccharide. Group A, B, and C organisms account for at least 90% of cases, although the proportion of groups Y and W135 is increasing in several regions. In most European and many Latin American countries, serogroups B and C cause the majority of disease while serogroup A causes the majority of disease in Africa and Asia. Serogroups A, B, C, Y, W-135 and X are all capable of causing outbreaks, most characteristically serogroup A, which is responsible for major epidemics, particularly in the so called African meningitis belt (see Occurrence). Outbreaks of *N. meningitidis* are usually caused by closely related strains. Molecular subtyping of isolates (multilocus enzyme electrophoresis or pulsed-field gel electrophoresis of enzyme-restricted DNA fragments) may allow identification of an "outbreak strain" and assist in better differentiation of outbreaks from endemic disease.

3. **Occurrence**—In Europe and North America the incidence of meningococcal disease is higher during winter and spring; in Sub-Saharan Africa the disease classically peaks during the dry season. Infants have the highest risk of meningococcal disease. Rates of disease decrease after infancy and then increase in adolescence and young adulthood. In addition to age, other individual risk factors for meningococcal disease include underlying immune deficiencies, such as asplenia, properdin deficiency, and a deficiency of terminal complement components. Crowding, low socioeconomic status, active or passive exposure to tobacco smoke and concurrent upper respiratory track tract infections increase the risk of meningococcal disease. In some countries males are at higher risk than females. New military recruits have also been consistently found to have higher risk of disease; it may be similar reasons that cause increased risk among university students living in dormitories.

The highest burden of the disease undoubtedly lies in the African meningitis belt, a large area that stretches from Senegal to Ethiopia and affects all or part of 21 countries. In this region, high rates of sporadic infections (1-20 cases per 100 000 population) occur in annual cycles with periodical superimposition of large-scale epidemics (usually caused by serogroup A, occasionally serogroup C, and more recently by serogroup W-135). In the countries of the African meningitis belt, epidemics with incidence rates as high as 1000 cases per 100 000 population have occurred every 8-12 years over at least the past 50 years. In addition, major epidemics have occurred in adjacent countries not usually considered part of the African meningitis belt (e.g. Kenya, the United Republic of Tanzania).

In 2000, an epidemic of serogroup W-135 meningococcal disease associated with the Hajj occurred in Saudi Arabia ; in 2000 and 2001, in several countries, cases of serogroup W-135 occurred among returning pilgrims and their close contacts. In 2002, the first major serogroup W 135 epidemic occurred in Burkina Faso with over 13 000 cases and 1400 deaths reported.

During the 1980s and 1990s, serogroup B has emerged as the most common cause of disease in Europe and most of the Americas. Epidemics characterized by a 5- to 10-fold increase in incidence for 10 - 20 years have been reported from many countries in Europe, Central and South America and most recently in New Zealand and the US Pacific northwest. Community outbreaks of group C disease have occurred with increasing frequency in Canada and the USA since 1990. During the late 1990s, group Y disease has become as common as groups B and C in parts of the USA.

4. **Reservoir**—Humans.

5. **Mode of transmission**—Direct contact, including respiratory droplets from nose and throat of infected people; infection usually causes only a subclinical mucosal infection. Up to 5%-10% of people may be asymptomatic carriers with nasopharyngeal colonization by *N. meningitidis*. Less than 1% of those colonized will progress to invasive disease. Carrier rates of 25% have been documented in some populations in the absence of any cases of meningococcal disease. In contrast, during some meningococcal outbreaks in industrialized countries, no carriers of the "outbreak stain" have been identified. Fomites transmission is insignificant.

6. **Incubation period**—2 to 10 days, commonly 3-4 days.

7. **Period of communicability**—Until live meningococci are no longer present in discharges from nose and mouth. Meningococci usually disappear from the nasopharynx within 24 hours after institution of antimicrobial treatment to which the organisms are sensitive and with substantial concentrations in oronasopharyngeal secretions. Penicillin will temporarily suppress the organisms, but does not usually eradicate them from the oronasopharynx.

8. **Susceptibility**—Susceptibility to the clinical disease is low and

decreases with age; this induces a high ratio of carriers to cases. Persons deficient in certain complement components are especially prone to recurrent disease; splenectomized persons are susceptible to bacteraemic illness. Group-specific immunity of unknown duration follows even subclinical infections.

9. **Methods of control—**

A. *Preventive measures:*

1) Educate the public on the need to reduce direct contact and exposure to droplet infection.

2) Reduce overcrowding in living quarters and workplaces, such as barracks, schools, camps and ships.

3) Vaccines containing groups A, C, Y and W-135 meningococcal polysaccharides are been available; two polysaccharide vaccines are currently available on the market although in most countries only one is available (quadrivalent ACYW-135 vaccine, and bivalent AC). Polysaccharide meningococcal vaccines against serogroups A and C are safe and effective in adults and children over 2, but do not elicit long-term protection, particularly in children under 5. The serogroup A polysaccharide can induce antibodies in children as young as 3 months, but the C polysaccharide is poorly immunogenic and ineffective in children under 2. Serogroup Y and W135 polysaccharides are also immunogenic in adults and children over 2 but immunogenicity and clinical protection have not been fully documented yet. Meningococcal polysaccharide vaccines are effective for outbreak control and for prevention among high-risk groups, such as travellers to countries where disease is epidemic, Hajj pilgrims, military groups, and individuals with underlying immune dysfunctions. Because these vaccines are often poorly immunogenic in young children and have limited duration of efficacy, they are not generally used in routine childhood immunization programs. Reimmunization may be considered within 3–5 years if indications still exist. No vaccine effective against group B meningococci is currently licensed, although several have been developed and show some efficacy in older children and adults.

Meningococcal serogroup C vaccines were first introduced in 1999 in the United Kingdom (mass vaccination for ages 2 months to 18 years). Early data suggest that these vaccines have high efficacy (>90%) in infants, children and teenagers, decrease nasopharyngeal carriage of the bacteria and induce herd immunity.

B. Control of patient, contacts and the immediate environment:

1) Report to local health authority: Obligatory case report in most countries, Class 2 (see Reporting).

2) Isolation: Respiratory isolation for 24 hours after start of chemotreatment.

3) Concurrent disinfection: Of discharges from the nose and throat and articles soiled therewith. Terminal cleaning.

4) Quarantine: Not applicable.

5) Protection of contacts: Close surveillance of household, day care, and other intimate contacts for early signs of illness, especially fever, to initiate appropriate therapy without delay; prophylactic administration of an effective chemotherapeutic agent to intimate contacts (household contacts, military personnel sharing the same sleeping space and people socially close enough to have shared eating utensils, e.g. close friends at school but not the whole class). Younger children in day care centers, even if not close friends, should all be given prophylaxis after an index case is identified. Rifampicin, ceftriaxone and ciprofloxacin are equally effective prophylactic agents. Rifampicin is administered twice daily for 2 days: adults 600 mg per dose; children over 1 month old, 10 mg/kg; under 1 month, 5 mg/kg. Rifampicin should not be given to pregnant women and may reduce the effectiveness of oral contraceptives.

   For adults, ceftriaxone, 250 mg IM, given in a single dose, is effective; 125 mg IM for children under 15. Ciprofloxacin, 500 mg PO, may be given as a single dose to adults. Because in most countries >50% of *N. meningitidis* isolates are resistant to sulfadiazine (no longer manufactured in the USA), the latter is rarely used for prophylaxis. If the organisms have been shown to be sensitive to sulfadiazine, it may be given to adults and older children at a dosage of 1 gram every 12 hours for 4 doses; for infants and children, the dosage is 125–150 mg/kg/day divided into 4 equal doses, on each of 2 consecutive days. Health care personnel are rarely at risk even when caring for infected patients; only intimate exposure to nasopharyngeal secretions (e.g. as in mouth-to-mouth resuscitation) warrants prophylaxis. Because of the efficacy of prophylaxis, immunization is generally not recommended.

6) Investigation of contacts and source of infection: Throat or nasopharyngeal cultures are of no value in deciding who should receive prophylaxis since carriage is variable and there is no consistent relationship between that found in the normal population and in an epidemic.

7) Specific treatment: Penicillin given parenterally in adequate doses is the drug of choice for proven meningococcal

disease; ampicillin and chloramphenicol are also effective. Penicillin-resistant strains have been reported in many countries, including Spain, the United Kingdom and the USA; strains resistant to chloramphenicol have been reported in France and in Viet Nam. Treatment should start as soon as the presumptive clinical diagnosis is made, even before meningococci have been identified. In children, until the specific agent has been identified, the drug chosen must be effective against *Haemophilus influenzae* type b (Hib) as well as *Streptococcus pneumoniae*. While ampicillin is the drug of choice for both as long as the organisms are ampicillin-sensitive, it should be combined with a third-generation cephalosporin, or chloramphenicol or vancomycin should be substituted in the many places where ampicillin-resistant *H. influenzae* b or penicillin-resistant *S. pneumoniae* strains are known to occur. Patients with meningococcal or Hib disease should receive rifampicin prior to discharge if neither a third-generation cephalosporin nor ciprofloxacin was given as treatment, to ensure elimination of the organism.

C. Epidemic measures:

1) When an outbreak occurs, major emphasis must be placed on careful surveillance, early diagnosis and immediate treatment of suspected cases. A high index of suspicion is invaluable. A threshold approach tailored to the epidemiology of the country is used in many countries to differentiate endemic disease from outbreaks. Thresholds (alert and epidemic) from a country with high rates of endemic disease (African meningitis belt) are given here as an example. When thresholds are passed, immunization campaigns must be implemented.

Alert threshold	Cases/week	
Population	>30 000	<30 000
	5/100 000	2 cases OR Increase in relation to previous non-epidemic years

Investigate, confirm agent, strengthen surveillance, enhance preparedness, treat cases.

Epidemic threshold	Cases/week	
Population	>30 000	<30 000
No epidemic for 3 years+ & vaccination <80% OR Alert threshold crossed early	10/100 000	5 cases OR Weekly doubling of cases over 3 weeks

Epidemic threshold		Cases/week
Other situations	15/100 000	Variable (e.g. mass gatherings, refugees, displaced persons): 2 confirmed cases in 1 week suffice.

Mass vaccination, provide drugs to health units, treat cases according to protocol, public education.

Specific actions are recommended at each stage of the epidemic: setting up an epidemic management committee, enhancing surveillance, undertaking field epidemiology and bacteriological investigations, ensuring supplies of drugs and laboratory material, social mobilization and mass vaccination if appropriate.

In the USA, the following steps are used to decide whether to declare an outbreak and initiate vaccination: a) determine whether it is an organization-based outbreak (e.g. school, university, prisons) or a community-based outbreak (town, city, county); b) investigate links between cases because secondary or co-primary cases are excluded from calculations; c) calculate attack rates with the outbreak strain among the population at risk; d) subtype *N. meningitidis* isolates, if available, from cases of disease, using molecular typing methods. If at least 3 cases have occurred during a 3 month period, the attack rate exceeds 10 cases per 100 000 in the population at risk, and the strain is vaccine preventable (serogroup A, C, Y or W-135), immunization of those in the group at risk should be considered.

2) Reduce overcrowding and ventilate living and sleeping quarters for all people exposed to infection because of living conditions (e.g. soldiers, miners and prisoners).

3) Mass chemoprophylaxis is usually not effective in controlling outbreaks; in outbreaks involving small populations (e.g. a single school), chemoprophylaxis to all members of the community may be considered, especially if the outbreak is caused by a serogroup not included in the available vaccine. If undertaken, chemoprophylaxis should be administered to all members at the same time. Intimate contacts should all be considered for prophylaxis, regardless of whether the entire small population is treated (see 9B5).

4) The use of vaccine in all age groups affected is strongly recommended if an outbreak occurs in a large institutional or community setting in which the cases are due to groups A, C, W-135 or Y (see 9A3). Meningococcal vaccine has

been very effective in halting epidemics due to A and C serogroups.

In countries where large-scale epidemics occur, mass vaccination of the entire population in affected areas should be considered when vaccine supply and administrative facilities allow. Geographical distribution of cases, age-specific attack rates and available resources all must be considered in estimating the target population. Decisions about vaccination should consider where the intervention is likely to have the largest impact in preventing disease and death.

D. Disaster implications: Epidemics may develop in situations of forced crowding.

E. International measures: WHO Collaborating Centres. Although the disease is not covered by *International Health Regulations*, some countries may require a valid certificate of immunization against meningococcal meningitis, e.g. Saudi Arabia for Hajj pilgrims. Further information at htt://www.who.int/emc/diseases/meningitis

II. B. HEMOPHILUS MENINGITIS   ICD-9 320.0; ICD-10 G00.0
(Meningitis due to *Haemophilus influenzae*)

1. Identification—Before widespread use of *Haemophilus* b conjugate vaccines, this was the most common bacterial meningitis in children aged 2 months to 5 years in the USA and many other industrialized countries. It is usually associated with bacteraemia. The onset can be subacute but is usually sudden, including fever, vomiting, lethargy and meningeal irritation, with bulging fontanelle in infants or stiff neck and back in older children. Progressive stupor or coma is common. Occasionally, there is a low-grade fever for several days, with more subtle CNS symptoms.

Diagnosis may be made through isolation of organisms from blood or CSF. Specific capsular polysaccharide may be identified by CIE or LA techniques.

2. Infectious agent—*H. influenzae* are Gram-negative coccobacilli that are divided into unencapsulated (nontypeable) and encapsulated strains. The encapsulated strains are further classified into serotypes a through f, based on the antigenic characteristics of their polysaccharide capsules. *H. influenzae* serotype b (Hib) is the most pathogenic.

3. Occurrence—Worldwide; most prevalent among children aged 2 months to 3 years; unusual over the age of 5. In developing countries, peak incidence is in children below 6 months; in Europe and the USA, generally in children 6-12 months. As of the late 1990s, with widespread vaccine use in early childhood, Hib meningitis has virtually disappeared in the USA. Most other industrialized countries have also now successfully implemented routine childhood immunization with Hib conjugate vaccines, with near elimination of Hib disease. Secondary cases in families and day care centers are rare. In industrialized countries, Hib most commonly presented as meningitis. Epiglottitis and bacteraemia without focus were the next most common presentations. In developing countries, the primary manifestation of Hib disease is lower respiratory tract infection. Hib may account for 5-8% of all pneumonia in children in these areas. In the developing world, *Haemophilus influenzae* (including all serotypes and nontypeable strains) causes an estimated 480 000 pneumonia deaths each year among children under 5.

4. **Reservoir**—Humans.

5. **Mode of transmission**—Droplet infection and discharges from nose and throat during the infectious period. The portal of entry is most commonly the nasopharynx.

6. **Incubation period**—Unknown; probably short, 2-4 days.

7. **Period of communicability**—As long as organisms are present, which may be for a prolonged period even without nasal discharge. Noncommunicable within 24-48 hours of starting effective antibiotherapy.

8. **Susceptibility**—Susceptibility assumed to be universal. Immunity associated with the presence of circulating bactericidal and/or anticapsular antibody, acquired transplacentally, from prior infection or through immunization.

9. **Methods of control**

   A. *Preventive measures:*

   1) Routine childhood immunization. Several protein polysaccharide conjugate vaccines have been shown to prevent meningitis in children more than 2 months of age and are licensed in many countries, both individually and combined with other vaccines. Immunization is recommended, starting at 2 months of age, followed by additional doses after an interval of 2 months; dosages vary with the vaccine in use. All vaccines require boosters at 12-15 months of age. Immunization is not routinely recommended for children over 5.

      Despite the availability of Hib conjugate vaccines since the 1980s and despite virtual elimination in most industrialized countries, Hib disease remains common in many developing countries, where cost and the non-recognition of Hib disease

burden constitute major obstacles to the introduction of Hib conjugate vaccine.
2) Monitor for cases occurring in susceptible population settings, such as day care centers and large foster homes.
3) Educate parents about the risk of secondary cases in siblings under 4 and the need for prompt evaluation and treatment if fever or stiff neck develops.

B. Control of patient, contacts and the immediate environment:

1) Report to local health authority: In selected endemic areas, Class 3 (see Reporting).
2) Isolation: Respiratory isolation for 24 hours after start of chemotherapy.
3) Concurrent disinfection: Not applicable.
4) Quarantine: Not applicable.
5) Protection of contacts: Recommended for Hib but not other serotypes of *H. influenzae*. Rifampicin prophylaxis (orally once daily for 4 days in a 20 mg/kg dose, maximal dose 600 mg/day) for all household contacts (including adults) in households with one or more children under 1 (other than the index case) or with a child of 1–3 who is inadequately immunized. When 2 or more cases of invasive disease have occurred within 60 days and unimmunized or incompletely immunized children attend the childcare facility, administration of rifampicin to all attenders and supervisory personnel is indicated. When a single case has occurred, the use of rifampicin prophylaxis is controversial.
6) Investigation of contacts and source of infection: Observe contacts under 6 years old, especially infants, for signs of illness, such as fever.
7) Specific treatment: Ampicillin has been the drug of choice (parenteral 200–400 mg/kg/day). However, about 30% of strains are now resistant due to beta-lactamase production: ceftriaxone, cefotaxime or chloramphenicol is thus recommended concurrently or singly until antimicrobial susceptibility has been ascertained. The patient should be given rifampicin prior to discharge from hospital to ensure elimination of the organism.

C. Epidemic measures: Not applicable.

D. Disaster implications: None.

E. International measures: None.

II. C. PNEUMOCOCCAL MENINGITIS   ICD-9 320.1; ICD-10 G00.1

1. Identification—Pneumococcal meningitis has a high case-fatality rate. It can be fulminant and occurs with bacteraemia but not necessarily with any other focus, although there may be otitis media or mastoiditis. Onset is usually sudden with high fever, lethargy or coma and signs of meningeal irritation. It is a sporadic disease in young infants, the elderly and other high-risk groups, including asplenic and hypogammaglobulinae-mic patients. Receipt of a cochlear implant and basilar fracture causing persistent communication with the nasopharynx are predisposing factors (See Pneumonia, pneumococcal.) Diagnosis may be made by isolation of organisms from blood or CSF. Pneumococcal capsular polysaccharide may be identified by CIE or LA techniques.

2. Infectious agent—*Streptococcus pneumoniae* is a Gram-positive diplococcus. Nearly all strains causing meningitis and other severe forms of pneumococcal disease are encapsulated; there are 90 known capsular serotypes. The distribution of serotypes varies regionally and with age. In the USA the 7 serotypes in pneumococcal conjugate vaccine are those that cause 80% of pneumococcal meningitis in children and the majority of pneumococcal meningitis in adults.

3. Occurrence—Worldwide; most prevalent among children 2 months to 3 years; in developing countries infants are at highest risk; in the USA peaks at 6-18 months. The elderly, and adults who are immunocom-promised or have certain chronic illness, are also at higher risk.

4. Reservoir—Humans. Pneumococci are often found in the upper respiratory tract of healthy persons. Carriage is more common in children than in adults.

5. Mode of transmission—Droplet spread and contact with respira-tory secretions; direct contract with a person with pneumococcal disease generally results in nasopharyngeal carriage of the organism rather than in disease.

6. Incubation period—Unknown; probably short, 1-4 days.

7. Period of communicability—As long as organisms are present, which may be for a prolonged period especially in immunocompromised hosts.

8. Susceptibility—Assumed to be universal. Immunity is associated with the presence of circulating bactericidal and/or anticapsular antibody, acquired transplacentally, from prior infection or from immunization.

9. **Methods of control**

A. *Preventive measures:* Vaccination is the mainstay of prevention. In the USA and other industrialized countries, a new pneumococcal conjugate vaccine is now recommended for all children under 2 and those 2–4 years with certain high-risk conditions, such as imunocompromising conditions, sickle cell disease, asplenia, heart or lung disease, or cochlear implantation. The vaccine covers the 7 serotypes most often causing pneumococcal meningitis in the United States and other industrialized countries. Other countries are currently using conjugate vaccine in selected high-risk populations. A polysaccharide vaccine containing 23 of the most common serotypes has been available since 1983 and is recommended in several countries for use in persons 65 and older and those 2–64 with immunocompromising conditions or certain chronic illnesses.

B. *Control of patient, contacts and the immediate environment:*

1) Report to local health authority: In selected areas, Class 3 (see Reporting).
2) Isolation: Standard precautions for hospitalized patients.
3) Concurrent disinfection: Of nasal and throat secretions.
4) Quarantine: Not applicable.
5) Protection of contacts: Not applicable, except in an outbreak setting (see Epidemic measures).
6) Investigation of contacts and source of infection: Generally not useful.
7) Specific treatment: Penicillin, ceftriaxone, or cefotaxime are the drugs of choice. Because resistance is common in many areas, blood and CSF culture should be performed for all patients with suspected bacterial meningitis and susceptibility testing performed on pneumococci. Where resistance is widespread, ceftriaxone or cefotaxime given along with vancomycin are recommended for empirical therapy until susceptibility results are known. Intravenous dexamethasone early in the course of the illness along with antibiotics has been shown to reduce the long-term complications of pneumococcal meningitis.

C. *Epidemic measures:* Pneumococcal meningitis can occur as part of a cluster of pneumococcal disease in institutional settings. Immunization using either the 23-valent polysaccharide vaccine or the 7-valent conjugate vaccine, depending on the setting, should be used to control outbreaks. Targeted antimicrobial prophylaxis (e.g. penicillin) may be useful in some outbreaks, especially those caused by non-vaccine type strains and when the outbreak strain is not resistant to antimicrobial agents. Widespread antimicrobial prophylaxis is not always effective and can induce resistance.

D. Disaster implications: None.

E. International measures: None.

II. D. NEONATAL MENINGITIS ICD-9 320.8, 771.8; ICD-10 P37.8, P35-P37, G00, G03

Infants with neonatal meningitis develop lethargy, seizures, apnoeic episodes, poor feeding, hypo- or hyperthermia and sometimes respiratory distress, usually in their first week of life. The WBC count may be elevated or depressed. CSF culture yields group B streptococci, *Listeria monocytogenes* (see Listeriosis), *E. coli* K-1 or other organisms acquired from the birth canal. Infants 2 weeks to 2 months of age may develop similar symptoms, with recovery from the CSF of group B streptococci or organisms of the Klebsiella-Enterobacter-Serratia group, acquired from the nursery environment. Meningitis in both groups is associated with septicemia. Treatment is with ampicillin, plus a third-generation cephalosporin or aminoglycoside, until the causal organism has been identified and its antimicrobial susceptibilities determined.

[W. Perea]

MOLLUSCUM CONTAGIOSUM ICD-9 078.0; ICD-10 B08.1

1. Identification—A viral disease of the skin resulting in smooth-surfaced, firm and spherical papules with umbilication of the vertex. The lesions may be flesh-colored, white, translucent or yellow. Most papules are 2-5 mm in diameter; giant-cell papules (above 15 mm diameter) are occasionally seen. Lesions in adults are most often on the lower abdominal wall, pubis, genitalia or inner thighs; on children most often on the face, trunk and proximal extremities. Immunocompetent hosts usually have 15-35 lesions; immunocompromised hosts (e.g. patients with HIV infection), may develop hundreds of disseminated lesions of the body and face. Occasionally the lesions itch and show a linear orientation, which suggests autoinoculation by scratching. In some patients, 50-100 lesions may become confluent and form a single plaque.

Without treatment, molluscum contagiosum persists for 6 months to 2 years. Any one lesion has a life span of 2-3 months. Lesions may resolve spontaneously or as a result of inflammatory response following trauma or secondary bacterial infection. Treatment (mechanical removal of the lesions) may shorten the course of illness.

Diagnosis can be clinical when multiple lesions are present. For confirmation, the core can be expressed onto a glass slide and examined by ordinary light microscopy for classic basophilic, Feulgen-positive, intracytoplasmic inclusions, the "molluscum" or "Henderson-Paterson bodies." Histology can confirm the diagnosis.

2. Infectious agent—Member of Poxviridae family, genus *Mollusci-poxvirus*; the genus comprises at least two species differentiated by DNA endonuclease cleavage maps. The virus has not been grown in cell culture.

3. Occurrence—Worldwide. Serological tests are not well standardized and skin inspection is the only screening technique available; epidemiological studies of the disease have therefore been limited. Population surveys have been conducted only in Fiji and Papua New Guinea, where the peak disease incidence occurs in childhood.

4. Reservoir—Humans.

5. Mode of transmission—Usually through direct contact. Transmission can be sexual or nonsexual, the latter includes spread via fomites. Autoinoculation is also suspected.

6. Incubation period—For experimental inoculation, 19–50 days; clinical reports give 7 days to 6 months.

7. Period of communicability—Unknown, probably as long as lesions persist.

8. Susceptibility—All ages may be affected; more often seen in children. Disease is more common in HIV-infected patients, in whom lesions may disseminate.

9. Methods of control—

A. *Preventive measures:* Avoid contact with affected patients.

B. *Control of patient, contacts and the immediate environment:*

1) Report to local health authority: Official report not ordinarily justifiable, Class 5 (see Reporting).
2) Isolation: Generally not indicated. Infected children with visible lesions should be excluded from close contact sports.
3) Concurrent disinfection: None.
4) Quarantine: None.
5) Immunization of contacts: None.
6) Investigation of contacts and source of infection: Examine sexual partners where applicable.

7) Specific treatment: Indicated to minimize risk of transmission. Curettage with local anesthaesia or topical application of cantharidin or peeling agents (salicylic or lactic acid). Freezing with liquid nitrogen has some advocates. Self-applied 0.5% podophyllotoxin cream has been effective. No therapy is effective in immunocompromised patients because of the rapid occurrence of new lesions as shown by the futility of both systemic and intralesional interferon.

C. Epidemic measures: Suspend direct contact activities.

D. Disaster implications: None.

E. International measures: None.

[F. Ndowa]

MONONUCLEOSIS, INFECTIOUS   ICD-9 075; ICD-10 B27
(Gammaherpesviral mononucleosis, Mononucleosis due to Epstein-Barr virus, Glandular fever, Monocytic angina)

1. Identification—An acute viral syndrome characterized clinically by fever, sore throat (often with exudative pharyngotonsillitis), lymphadenopathy (especially posterior cervical) and splenomegaly; characterized hematologically by mononucleosis and lymphocytosis of 50% or greater, including 10% or more atypical cells; and characterized serologically by the presence of heterophile and Epstein-Barr virus (EBV) antibodies. Recovery usually occurs in a few weeks, but a very small proportion of individuals can take months to regain their former level of energy. There is no evidence that this is due to abnormal persistence of the infection in a chronic form.

In young children the disease is generally mild and more difficult to recognize. Jaundice occurs in about 4% of infected young adults, although 95% will have abnormal liver function tests; splenomegaly occurs in 50%. Duration is from 1 to several weeks; the disease is rarely fatal. The disease is more severe in older adults.

The causal agent, EBV, is also closely associated with the pathogenesis of several lymphomas and nasopharyngeal cancer (see Malignant neoplasms associated with infectious agents). Fatal immunoproliferative disorders involving a polyclonal expansion of EBV infected B-lymphocytes may occur in persons with an X-linked recessive immunoproliferative disorder; they can also occur in persons with acquired immune defects, including patients infected with HIV, transplant recipients and persons with other conditions requiring long-term immunosuppressive therapy.

About 10%–15% of infectious mononucleosis cases are heterophile-negative. A heterophile-negative form of a syndrome resembling infectious mononucleosis is due to cytomegalovirus and accounts for 5% to 7% of the "mono syndrome" (see Cytomegalovirus infections); other rare causes are toxoplasmosis and herpesvirus type 6 (see Exanthema subitum following rubella). A mononucleosis-like illness may occur early in HIV-infected patients. Differentiation depends on laboratory results that include the EBV IgM test; only EBV elicits the "true" heterophile antibody. EBV accounts for over 80% of both heterophile positive and heterophile negative cases of the mononucleosis syndrome.

Laboratory diagnosis is based on the finding of a lymphocytosis exceeding 50% (including 10% or more abnormal forms), abnormalities in liver function tests (AST) or an elevated heterophile antibody titre after adsorption of the serum on guinea pig kidney. The most sensitive and commercially available test is the absorbed horse-RBC test; the most specific of the common tests the beef-cell hemolysin test; and the most frequently used procedure a commercial, qualitative slide agglutination assay. Very young children may not show an elevation of the heterophile titre, and heterophile-negative and clinically atypical forms rarely occur in the elderly. If available, the IFA test for IgM and IgA antibody specific for viral capsid antigen (VCA) or antibody against "early antigen" of the causal virus is helpful in diagnosis of heterophile-negative cases; antibody specific for the EBV nuclear antigen (EBNA) is usually absent during the acute phase of illness. Therefore, a positive anti-VCA titre and a negative anti-EBNA titre are diagnostic responses of an early primary EBV infection.

2. Infectious agent—Epstein-Barr virus, human (gamma) herpesvirus 4, closely related to other herpesviruses morphologically, but distinct serologically; it infects and transforms B-lymphocytes.

3. Occurrence—Worldwide. Infection is common and widespread in early childhood in developing countries and in socioeconomically depressed population groups, where it is usually mild or asymptomatic. Typical infectious mononucleosis occurs primarily in industrialized countries, where age of infection is delayed until older childhood and young adulthood, so that it is most commonly recognized in high school and college students. About 50% of those infected develop clinical infectious mononucleosis; the others are mostly asymptomatic.

4. Reservoir—Humans.

5. Mode of transmission—Person-to-person spread by the oropharyngeal route, via saliva. Young children may be infected by saliva on the hands of nurses and other attendants and on toys, or by prechewing of baby food by the mother, a practice in some countries. Kissing facilitates spread among young adults. Spread may also occur via blood transfusion to susceptible recipients, but ensuing clinical disease is uncommon. Reactivated EBV may play a role in the interstitial pneumonia of HIV infected infants and in hairy leukoplakia and B-cell tumours in HIV-infected adults.

6. Incubation period—From 4 to 6 weeks.

7. Period of communicability—Prolonged; pharyngeal excretion may persist in cell-free form for a year or more after infection; 15%–20% or more of EBV antibody-positive healthy adults are long-term oropharyngeal carriers.

8. Susceptibility—Susceptibility is general. Infection confers a high degree of resistance; immunity from unrecognized childhood infection may account for low rates of clinical disease in lower socioeconomic groups. Reactivation of EBV may occur in immunodeficient individuals and result in elevated antibody titres to EBV but not heterophile antibody, and possibly to the development of lymphomas.

9. Methods of control—

    A. Preventive measures: Undetermined. Use hygienic measures including handwashing to avoid salivary contamination from infected individuals; avoid drinking beverages from a common container to minimize contact with saliva.

    B. Control of patient, contacts and the immediate environment:

        1) Report to local health authority: Official report not ordinarily justifiable, Class 5 (see Reporting).

        2) Isolation: Not applicable.

        3) Concurrent disinfection: Of articles soiled with nose and throat discharges.

        4) Quarantine: Not applicable.

        5) Immunization of contacts: Not applicable.

        6) Investigation of contacts and source of infection: For the individual case, of little value.

        7) Specific treatment: None. Nonsteroidal anti-inflammatory drugs, or steroids given in small doses in decreasing amounts over about a week are of value in severe toxic cases and in patients with severe oropharyngeal involvement and airway encroachment.

    C. Epidemic measures: None.

    D. Disaster implications: None.

    E. International measures: None.

MUMPS
(Infectious parotitis)

ICD-9 072; ICD-10 B26

1. **Identification**—An acute viral disease characterized by fever, swelling and tenderness of one or more salivary glands, usually the parotid and sometimes the sublingual or submaxillary glands. Not all cases of parotitis are caused by mumps infection, but other parotitis-causing agents do not produce parotitis on an epidemic scale. Orchitis, most commonly unilateral, occurs in 20%–30% of affected postpubertal males. Testicular atrophy occurs in about one-third of patients, but sterility is extremely rare. Mumps orchitis has been reported to be a risk factor for testicular cancer. As many as 40%–50% of mumps infections have been associated with respiratory symptoms, particularly in children under 5. Mumps can cause sensorineural hearing loss in both children and adults. Pancreatitis, usually mild, occurs in 4% of cases; a suggested association with diabetes remains unproven.

Symptomatic aseptic meningitis occurs in up to 10% of mumps cases; patients usually recover without complications, though many require hospitalization. Mumps encephalitis is rare (1–2/10 000 cases), but can result in permanent sequelae, such as paralysis, seizures and hydrocephalus; the case-fatality rate for mumps encephalitis is about 1%. Mumps infection during the first trimester of pregnancy is associated with a high (25%) incidence of spontaneous abortion, but there is no firm evidence that mumps during pregnancy causes congenital malformations.

Acute mumps infection can be confirmed through: a positive serological test for mumps-specific IgM antibodies, by seroconversion or by a significant (at least 4-fold) rise in serum mumps IgG titre as determined by standard serological assay; or through isolation of mumps virus from an appropriate clinical specimen (throat swab, urine, CSF). In research settings, typing methods can distinguish wild-type mumps virus from vaccine virus.

2. **Infectious agent**—Mumps virus, a member of the family Paramyxoviridae, genus *Rubulavirus*.

3. **Occurrence**—About one-third of exposed susceptible people have inapparent infections; most infections in children under 2 are subclinical. In temperate climates, winter and spring are peak seasons. In the absence of immunization mumps is endemic, with an annual incidence usually greater than 100 per 100 000 population and epidemic peaks every 2–5 years. In many countries, mumps was a major cause of viral encephalitis. Serosurveys conducted prior to mumps vaccine introduction found that in some countries 90% of persons were immune by age 15 years, while in other countries a large proportion of the adult population remained

susceptible. In countries were mumps vaccine has not been introduced, the incidence of mumps remains high, mostly affecting children 5-9.

By the end of 2002, 121 countries/territories included mumps vaccine in their national immunization schedule. In countries where mumps vaccine coverage has been sustained at high levels the incidence of the disease has dropped tremendously.

4. Reservoir—Humans.

5. Mode of transmission—Airborne transmission or droplet spread; also direct contact with the saliva of an infected person.

6. Incubation period—About 16-18 days (range 14-25).

7. Period of communicability—Virus has been isolated from saliva (7 days before to 9 days after the onset of parotitis) and from urine (6 days before to 15 days after the onset of parotitis). Maximum infectiousness occurs between 2 days before to 4 days after onset of illness. Inapparent infections can be communicable.

8. Susceptibility—Immunity is generally lifelong and develops after either inapparent or clinical infections.

9. Methods of control—

    A. Preventive measures:

        Public education should encourage mumps immunization for susceptible individuals. Routine mumps vaccination is recommended in countries with an efficient childhood vaccination program and sufficient resources to maintain high levels of vaccine coverage. Mumps vaccination is recommended at age 12-18 months, as part of MMR. More than 90% of recipients develop immunity that is long-lasting and may be lifelong.

        Live attenuated mumps virus vaccines are available as monovalent vaccines or trivalent measles-mumps-rubella (MMR) vaccines. Hydrolysed gelatin and/or sorbitol are used as stabilisers in mumps vaccine, and neomycin as a preservative. Mumps vaccines are cold-chain dependent and should be protected from light.

        Different strains of live attenuated mumps vaccine have been developed in Japan, the Russian Federation, Switzerland and the USA. All licensed strains are judged acceptable by WHO for public health programs, except the Rubini strain, which is not recommended because of demonstrated low efficacy; persons who received this strain should be revaccinated with another strain.

        In the USA and other industrialized countries only the Jeryl Lynn strain or strains derived from it are accepted, because they show no confirmed association with aseptic meningitis. Those countries recommend 2 doses of MMR at the ages recommended for measles vaccination.

The reported incidence of adverse events depends on the strain of mumps vaccine. The most common adverse reactions are fever and parotitis. Rare adverse reactions include orchitis, sensorineural deafness, and thrombocytopenia. Aseptic meningitis, resolving spontaneously in less than one week without sequelae, has been reported at frequencies ranging from 0.1 to 100 cases per 100 000 vaccine doses. This reflects differences in vaccine strains and their preparation, as well as variations in study design and case ascertainment. Better data are needed to establish more precise estimates of aseptic meningitis incidence in recipients of different strains of mumps vaccine. The rates of aseptic meningitis due to mumps vaccine are at least 100-fold lower than rates of aseptic meningitis due to infection with wild mumps virus.

In addition to routine vaccination with a single dose of mumps vaccine at 12–18 months, some countries schedule another dose of mumps vaccine and some countries have conducted mass campaigns to reach broader target groups. Countries intending to use mumps or MMR vaccine during mass campaigns should give special attention to planning. The mumps vaccine strain should be carefully selected, health workers should receive training on expected rates of adverse events following immunization, and on community advocacy and health education activities.

Vaccine is contraindicated in the immunosuppressed; however, treatment with a low dose of steroids (less than 2 mg/kg/day) on alternate days, topical steroid use or aerosolized steroid preparations are no contraindication to administration of mumps vaccine. For theoretical reasons pregnant women or women planning a pregnancy in the next month (28 days in the USA) should not receive mumps vaccine, although no evidence exists that mumps vaccine causes fetal damage.

B. *Control of patient, contacts and the immediate environment:*

1) Report to local health authority: WHO recommends making mumps a notifiable disease in all countries, Class 3 (see Reporting).
2) Isolation: Respiratory isolation for 9 days from onset of parotitis. Exclusion from school or workplace until 9 days after onset of parotitis if susceptible contacts (those not immunized) are present.
3) Concurrent disinfection: Of articles soiled with nose and throat secretions.

4) Quarantine: Exclusion of susceptibles from school or the workplace from the 12th through the 25th day after exposure if other susceptibles are present.

5) Immunization of contacts: Immunization after exposure may not always prevent infection. IG is not effective and not recommended.

6) Investigation of contacts and source of infection: Immunization of susceptible contacts.

7) Specific treatment: None.

C. Epidemic measures: Immunize susceptibles, especially those at risk of exposure. Serological screening to identify susceptibles is impractical and unnecessary, since there is no risk in immunizing those who are already immune.

D. Disaster implications: None.

E. International measures: None.

[S. Robertson]

MYALGIA, EPIDEMIC   ICD-9 074.1; ICD-10 B33.0
(Epidemic pleurodynia, Bornholm disease, Devil's grippe)

1. Identification—An acute viral disease characterized by paroxysmal spasmodic pain in the chest or abdomen, which may be intensified by movement, usually accompanied by fever and headache. The pain tends to be more abdominal than thoracic in infants and young children, while the reverse applies to older children and adults. Most patients recover within 1 week of onset, but relapses occur; no fatalities have been reported. Localized epidemics are characteristic. It is important to differentiate from more serious medical or surgical conditions.

Complications occur infrequently and include orchitis, pericarditis, pneumonia and aseptic meningitis. During outbreaks of epidemic myalgia, cases of group B coxsackievirus myocarditis of the newborn have been reported; while myocarditis in adults is a rare complication, the possibility should always be considered.

Diagnosis is suggested by the appearance of similar symptoms among multiple family members; it is confirmed by a significant rise in antibody titre against specific etiologic agents in acute and convalescent sera, or isolation of the virus in cell culture or neonatal mice from throat secretions or patient feces.

2. Infectious agents—Group B coxsackievirus types 1-3, 5 and 6, and echoviruses 1 and 6 are associated with the illness. Many group A and B coxsackieviruses and echoviruses have been reported in sporadic cases.

3. Occurrence—An uncommon disease, occurring in summer and early autumn; usually in children and young adults aged 5-15, but all ages may be affected. Multiple cases in a household can occur frequently. Outbreaks have been reported in Europe, Australia, New Zealand and North America.

4. Reservoir—Humans.

5. Mode of transmission—Directly by fecal-oral or respiratory droplet contact with an infected person, or indirectly by contact with articles freshly soiled with feces or throat discharges of an infected person who may or may not have symptoms. Group B coxsackieviruses have been found in sewage and flies, though the relationship to transmission of human infection is not clear.

6. Incubation period—Usually 3-5 days.

7. Period of communicability—Apparently during the acute stage of disease; stools may contain virus for several weeks.

8. Susceptibility—Probably general; type-specific immunity presumably results from infection.

9. Methods of control—

    A. Preventive measures: None.

    B. Control of patient, contacts and the immediate environment:

      1) Report to local health authority: Obligatory report of epidemics, Class 4 (see Reporting).
      2) Isolation: Ordinarily limited to enteric precautions. Because of possible serious illness in the newborn, if a patient in a maternity unit or nursery develops an illness suggestive of enterovirus infection, precautions should be instituted at once. Individuals with suspected enterovirus infections (including health personnel) should be excluded from visiting maternity and nursery units and from contact with infants and women near term.
      3) Concurrent disinfection: Prompt and safe disposal of respiratory discharges and feces; wash or dispose of articles soiled therewith. Careful attention must be given to prompt, thorough handwashing when handling discharges, feces and articles soiled therewith.
      4) Quarantine: Not applicable.
      5) Immmunization of contacts: Not applicable.

6) Investigation of contacts and source of infection: Of no practical value.
7) Specific treatment: None.

C. Epidemic measures: General notice to physicians of the presence of an epidemic and the necessity for differentiation of cases from more serious medical or surgical emergencies.

D. Disaster implications: None.

E. International measures: None.

[D. Lavanchy]

MYCETOMA   ICD-9 039; ICD-10 B47

| ACTINOMYCETOMA | ICD-9 039; ICD-10 B47.1 |
| EUMYCETOMA | ICD-9 117.4; ICD-10 B47.0 |

(Maduromycosis, Madura foot)

1. Identification—A clinical syndrome caused by a variety of aerobic actinomycetes (bacteria) and eumycetes (fungi), characterized by swelling and suppuration of subcutaneous tissues and formation of sinus tracts with visible granules in the pus draining from the sinus tracts. Lesions are usually on the foot or lower leg, sometimes on the hand, shoulders and back, and rarely at other sites.

Mycetoma may be difficult to distinguish from chronic osteomyelitis and botryomycosis (a clinically and pathologically similar entity caused by a variety of bacteria, including staphylococci and Gram-negative bacteria).

Specific diagnosis depends on visualizing the granules in fresh preparations or histopathological slides and isolation of the causative actinomycete or fungus in culture.

2. Infectious agents—Eumycetoma is caused by *Madurella mycetomatis*, *M. grisea*, *Scedosporium apiospermum* (with a teleomorph, *Pseudallescheria boydii*), *Exophiala (Phialophora) jeanselmei*, *Acremonium (Cephalosporium) recifei*, *A. falciforme*, *Leptosphaeria senegalensis*, *Neotestudina rosatii*, *Pyrenochaeta romeroi* plus several other species. Actinomycetoma is caused by *Nocardia brasiliensis*, *N. asteroides*, *N. otitidiscaviarum*, *Actinomadura madurae*, *A. pelletieri*, *Nocardiopsis dassonvillei* or *Streptomyces somaliensis*.

3. Occurrence—Common in Mexico, Africa, southern Asia and other tropical and subtropical areas, especially where people go barefoot.

4. **Reservoir**—Soil and decaying vegetation.

5. **Mode of transmission**—Subcutaneous implantation of conidia or hyphal elements from a saprophytic source by penetrating wounds (thorns, splinters).

6. **Incubation period**—Usually months.

7. **Period of communicability**—No person-to-person transmission.

8. **Susceptibility**—Causal agents are widespread in nature, but clinical infection is rare, which suggests intrinsic resistance.

9. **Methods of control**—

A. *Preventive measures:* Protect against puncture wounds by wearing shoes and protective clothing.

B. *Control of patient, contacts and the immediate environment:*

1) Report to local health authority: Official report not ordinarily justifiable, Class 5 (see Reporting).
2) Isolation: Not applicable.
3) Concurrent disinfection: Not applicable. Ordinary cleanliness.
4) Quarantine: Not applicable.
5) Immmunization of contacts: Not applicable.
6) Investigation of contacts and source of infection: Not indicated.
7) Specific treatment: Some patients with eumycetoma may benefit from itraconazole or ketoconazole; some cases of actinomycetoma from clindamycin, trimethoprim-sufamethoxazole or long acting sulfonamides. Penicillin is usually not useful (unlike for actinomycosis). Resection of small lesions may be helpful; amputation may be required for an extremity with advanced lesions.

C. *Epidemic measures:* Not applicable, a sporadic disease.

D. *Disaster implications:* None.

E. *International measures:* WHO Collaborating Centres.

[L. Severo]

NAEGLERIASIS AND
ACANTHAMOEBIASIS   ICD-9 136.2; ICD-10 B60.2,
B60.1
(Primary amoebic meningoencephalitis)

1. Identification—In naegleriasis, a free-living amoeboflagellate invades the brain and meninges via the nasal mucosa and olfactory nerve; it causes a typical syndrome of fulminating pyogenic meningoencephalitis (primary amoebic meningoencephalitis [PAM]) with sore throat, severe frontal headache, occasional olfactory hallucinations, nausea, vomiting, high fever, nuchal rigidity and somnolence, and death within 10 days, usually on the fifth or sixth day. The disease occurs mainly in active immunocompetent young men and women.

Several species of *Acanthamoeba* and *Balamuthia mandrillaris* (leptomyxid amoebae) can invade the brain and meninges of immunocompromised individuals, probably after entry through a skin lesion and without involvement of the nasal and olfactory tissues; this causes a granulomatous disease (granulomatous amoebic encephalitis) of insidious onset and lasting from 8 days to several months; CFR may be high *Acanthamoeba*.

In addition to causing granulomatous amoebic encephalitis, species of (*A. polyphaga*, *A. castellanii*) have been associated with chronic granulomatous lesions of the skin, with or without secondary invasion of the CNS. Infections of the eye (Conjunctivitis due to *Acanthamoeba*, ICD-10 H13.1) and of the cornea (Keratoconjunctivitis due to *Acanthamoeba*, ICD-10 H19.2) have resulted in blindness.

Diagnosis of suspected primary or granulomatous amoebic encephalitis is made through microscopic examination of wet mount preparations of fresh CSF showing motile amoebae and of stained smears. In suspected *Acanthamoeba* infections, diagnosis is made by microscopic examination of scrapings, swabs or aspirates of the eye and skin lesions; or by culture on nonnutrient agar seeded with *Escherichia coli*, *Klebsiella aerogenes* or other suitable *Enterobacter* species. *Balamuthia* require mammalian cell cultures for isolation. The trophozoites of *Naegleria* may become flagellated after a few hours in water. Pathogenic *N. fowleri*, *Acanthamoeba* species and *Balamuthia* can be differentiated morphologically and through immunological testing. Amoebae have been misidentified as macrophages and have been mistaken for *Entamoeba histolytica* when microscopic diagnoses are made under low magnification.

2. Infectious agents—*Naegleria fowleri*, several species of *Acanthamoeba* (*A. culbertsoni*, *A. polyphaga*, *A. castellanii*, *A. astronyxis*, *A. hatchetti*, *A. rhysodes*) and *Balamuthia mandrillaris*.

3. **Occurrence**—The organisms are distributed globally in the environment. More than 160 cases of primary amoebic encephalitis in healthy people, over 100 cases of granulomatous in immunodeficient patients (including several with AIDS) and over 1000 cases of keratitis, primarily in contact lens wearers, have been diagnosed in many countries on all continents.

4. **Reservoir**—*Acanthamoeba* and *Naegleria* are free-living in aquatic and soil habitats. Little is known about the reservoir of *Balamuthia*.

5. **Mode of transmission**—*Naegleria* infection occurs through exposure of the nasal passages to contaminated water, most commonly by diving or swimming in fresh water, especially stagnant ponds or lakes in warm climate areas or during late summer; in thermal springs or bodies of water warmed by the effluent of industrial plants; in hot tubs, spas or inadequately maintained public swimming pools. *Naegleria* trophozoites colonize the nasal tissues, then invade brain and meninges by extension along the olfactory nerves.

Acanthamoeba and *Balamuthia* trophozoites reach the CNS through hematogenous spread, probably from a skin lesion or other site of primary colonization, frequently in chronically ill or immunosuppressed patients with no history of swimming or known source of infection. Eye infections have occurred primarily in soft contact lens wearers; homemade saline used as a cleaning or wetting solution and exposure to spas or hot tubs have been implicated as sources of corneal infection.

6. **Incubation period**—From 3 to 7 days in documented cases of *Naegleria* infection; usually longer in infections with *Acanthamoeba* and *Balamuthia*.

7. **Period of communicability**—No person-to-person transmission observed.

8. **Susceptibility**—Unknown. Apparently healthy individuals develop *Naegleria* infection; immunodeficient individuals have increased susceptibility to infection with *Acanthamoeba* and probably *Balamuthia*. *Naegleria* and *Balamuthia* have not been found in asymptomatic individuals; *Acanthamoeba* has been found in the respiratory tract of healthy people.

9. **Methods of control**—

   A. *Preventive measures:*

      1) Educate the public to the dangers of swimming in lakes and ponds where infection is known or presumed to have been acquired, and of allowing such water to be forced into the nose through diving or underwater swimming.

2) Protect nasopharynx from exposure to water likely to contain *N. fowleri*. In practice, this is difficult since the amoebae may occur in a wide variety of aquatic bodies, including swimming pools.

3) Swimming pools containing residual free chlorine of 1–2 ppm are considered safe. No infection is known to have been acquired in a standard chlorinated swimming pool.

4) Soft contact lens wearers should not wear lenses while swimming or in hot tubs and should strictly follow the wear and care procedures recommended by lens manufacturers and health care professionals.

B. *Control of patient, contacts and the immediate environment:*

1) Report to local health authority: Not reportable in most countries, Class 3 (see Reporting).

2) Isolation: Not applicable.

3) Concurrent disinfection: Not applicable.

4) Quarantine: Not applicable.

5) Immunization of contacts: Not applicable.

6) Investigation of contacts and source of infection: A history of swimming or introducing water into the nose within the week prior to onset of symptoms may suggest the source of infection.

7) Specific treatment: *N. fowleri* is sensitive to amphotericin B; recovery has followed intravenous and intrathecal administration of amphotericin B and miconazole in conjunction with oral rifampicin. Despite the sensitivity of the organisms to antibiotics in laboratory studies, recoveries have been rare. For eye infections, no standard treatment has been reported; topical propamidine isethionate has been reported to be effective; clotrimazole, miconazole and pimaricin have been used in small numbers of patients with some response.

C. *Epidemic measures:* Multiple cases may occur following exposure to an apparent source of infection. Any grouping of cases warrants prompt epidemiological investigation and the prohibition of swimming in implicated waters.

D. *Disaster implications:* None.

E. *International measures:* None.

F. *Measures in case of deliberate use:* *N. fowleri* can in principle be used as a biological agent against humans. Primary hazards are droplet or aerosol exposure of mucous membranes (eye, nose, or mouth) to trophozoites and tissue homogenates. Containment requirements correspond to biosafety level 2.

[L. Savioli]

NOCARDIOSIS   ICD-9 039.9; ICD-10 A43

1. Identification—A chronic bacterial disease of animals and humans which may be localised or disseminated. Members of the *Nocardia asteroides* complex are most likely to cause respiratory and disseminated infections, with high associated mortality, and a particular propensity to cause brain abscess. Other nocardiae (e.g. *N. brasiliensis*) may also cause cutaneous and/or lymphocutaneous disease of the extremities and actinomycotic mycetomas, predominantly in tropical and subtropical regions such as central and South America. *Streptomyces spp.* and *Actinomadura* are at least as important as causative agents of actinomycetoma (see Mycetoma, Actinomycetoma, Eumycetoma).

Microscopic examination of stained smears of sputum, pus or CSF may reveal beaded Gram-positive, weakly acid-fast, branched filaments; culture confirmation is desirable but often difficult and suspicion of nocardial infection should be notified to the microbiology laboratory in order to enhance diagnosis. Biopsy or autopsy usually clearly establishes involvement, although histopathology may be non-specific.

2. Infectious agents—*Nocardia asteroides* complex (includes *N. asteroides sensu stricto*, *N. farcinica* and *N. nova*), *N. brasiliensis*, *N. transvalensis* and *N. otitidiscaviarum*; aerobic actinomycetes.

3. Occurrence—An occasional sporadic disease in people and animals in all parts of the world. No evidence of age, gender, or racial differences.

4. Reservoir—Found worldwide as a soil saprophyte.

5. Mode of transmission—Typically acquired through inhalation or skin inoculation of skin, with some species and geographical variation in clinical manifestations.

6. Incubation period—Uncertain; probably a few days to a few weeks.

7. Period of communicability—Not directly transmitted from humans or animals to humans.

8. Susceptibility—Organism-specific virulence variation and host exposure are important determinants. Immunocompromised status (e. g., alcoholism, diabetes, steroid use) is a risk factor in more than 60% of infections, but the incidence in AIDS is lower than expected, even accounting for sulfamethoxazole prophylaxis.

9. **Methods of control—**

A. *Preventive measures:* None.

B. *Control of patient, contacts and the immediate environment:*

1) Report to local health authority: Official report not ordinarily justifiable, Class 5 (see Reporting).
2) Isolation: Not applicable.
3) Concurrent disinfection: Of discharges and contaminated dressings.
4) Quarantine: Not applicable.
5) Immmunization of contacts: Not applicable.
6) Investigation of contacts and source of infection: Most disease is sporadic. Occasional outbreaks may occur from environmental sources, and transmission through healthcare workers is probably rare.
7) Specific treatment: Trimethoprim-sulfamethoxazole, sulfisoxazole or sulfadiazine effective in systemic infections if given early and for prolonged periods. Imipenem and amikacin is an effective combination for intracerebral disease, but *N. farcinica* and *N. otidiscavarium* may be resistant to first-line treatments, including imipenem. *N. brasiliensis* is generally sensitive, except to imipenem. Minocycline may be tried in patients allergic to sulfonamides who do not have a brain abscess. Surgical drainage of abscesses may be needed in addition to antibiotherapy; intracerebral lesions in immunocompromised patients should be considered early for biopsy because of the wide differential diagnosis and variable antibiotic susceptibility

C. *Epidemic measures:* Not applicable, a sporadic disease.

D. *Disaster implications:* None.

E. *International measures:* None.

[J. Iredell]

ONCHOCERCIASIS
(River blindness)
ICD-9 125.3; ICD-10 B73

1. **Identification**—A chronic nonfatal filarial disease with fibrous nodules in subcutaneous tissues, particularly of the head and shoulders

(America) or pelvic girdle and lower extremities (Africa). Adult worms are found in these nodules, which occur superficially, and also in deep-seated bundles lying against the periosteum of bones or near joints. The female worm discharges microfilariae that migrate through the skin, often causing an intense pruritic rash when they die, with chronic dermatitis-altered pigmentation, oedema and atrophy of the skin. Pigment changes, particularly of the lower limbs, give the condition known as "leopard skin" while loss of skin elasticity and lymphadenitis may result in "hanging groin". Microfilariae frequently reach the eye, where their invasion and subsequent death causes visual disturbance and blindness. Microfilariae may be found in organs and tissues other than skin and eye, but the clinical significance of this is not yet clear; in heavy infections they may also be found in blood, tears, sputum and urine.

Laboratory diagnosis is made through microscopic examination of fresh superficial skin biopsy incubated in water or saline with observation of microfilariae; through evidence of microfilariae in urine; or through the finding of adult worms in excised nodules. Differentiation of the microfilariae from those of other filarial diseases is required where the latter are also endemic. Other diagnostic clues include evidence of ocular manifestations and slit-lamp observations of microfilariae in the cornea, anterior chamber or vitreous body. In low density infections, where microfilariae are not found in the skin and are not present in the eyes, the Mazzotti reaction (characteristic pruritus after oral administration of 25 mg of diethylcarbamazine citrate or topical application of the drug) may be used. This test may be dangerous in heavily infected individuals and has been abandoned in many countries. PCR on material obtained from skin scratches can be used to detect parasite DNA.

2. Infectious agent—*Onchocerca volvulus*, a filarial worm belonging to the class Nematoda.

3. Occurrence—Geographic distribution in the Western Hemisphere is limited to Guatemala (principally on the western slope of the continental divide); southern Mexico (states of Chiapas and Oaxaca); foci in northern and southern Venezuela; and small areas in Brazil (states of Amazonas and Roraima), Colombia and Ecuador. In sub-Saharan Africa, the disease occurs in an area extending from Senegal to Ethiopia down to Angola in the west and Malawi in the east; also in Yemen. In some endemic areas in western Africa, until recent years, a high percentage of the population was infected, and visual impairment and blindness were serious problems. People abandoned the river valleys and migrated to safer higher ground, where the soil was far less fertile. The disease thus had grave socioeconomic consequences. This problem has now been largely overcome through the activities of the Onchocerciasis Control Programme in western Africa and the African Programme for Onchocerciasis Control (APOC).

4. Reservoir—Humans. The disease can be transmitted experimentally to chimpanzees and has been found rarely in nature in gorillas. *Onchocerca* species found in animals cannot infect humans but may occur together with *O. volvulus* in the insect vector.

5. Mode of transmission—Only through the bite of infected female blackflies of the genus *Simulium*: in Central America, mainly *S. ochraceum*; in South America, *S. metallicum* complex, *S. sanguineum/amazonicum* complex, *S. quadrivittatum* and other species; in Africa and in Yemen, *S. damnosum* complex and *S. neavei* complex, as well as *S. albivirgulatum* in Congo. Microfilariae, ingested by a blackfly feeding on an infected person, penetrate thoracic muscles of the fly, develop into infective larvae, migrate to the cephalic capsule, are liberated on the skin and enter the bite wound during a subsequent blood-meal.

6. Incubation period—Microfilariae are found in the skin usually only after 1 year or more from the time of the infective bite; in Guatemala they have been found in children as young as 6 months. In Africa, vectors could be infective 7 days after a blood-meal; in Guatemala the extrinsic incubation period is measurably longer (up to 14 days) because of lower temperatures.

7. Period of communicability—People can infect flies as long as living microfilariae occur in their skin, i.e. for 10–15 years after last exposure to *Simulium* bites if untreated. No direct person-to-person transmission.

8. Susceptibility—Susceptibility is probably universal. Reinfection of infected people may occur; severity of disease depends on cumulative effects of the repeated infections.

9. Methods of control—

   A. Preventive measures:

   1) Avoid bites of *Simulium* flies by wearing protective clothing and headgear as much as possible or by use of an insect repellent such as diethyltoluamide.
   2) Identify vector species and their breeding sites; control vector larvae (which usually develop in rapidly running streams and artificial waterways) through use of biodegradable insecticides such as temefos at low concentrations, spraying 0.05 mg/L for 10 minutes weekly in the wet season and 0.1 mg/L for 10 minutes weekly in the dry season. B.t. H-14, a biological insecticide formulated as an aqueous suspension, can be used at a dose 2.5 times higher than temefos. In contrast to temefos, resistance is unlikely to develop against B.t. H-14, which has a much shorter carry and therefore needs numerous application points along the river. Aerial spraying may be used to ensure coverage of

breeding places in large-scale control operations such as in Africa. Because of mountainous terrain, such procedures generally are not feasible in the Americas. The use of insecticides has allowed elimination of *S. neavei* (which develop on crabs).

3) Provide facilities for diagnosis and treatment.

B. Control of patient, contacts and the immediate environment:

1) Report to local health authority: Official report not ordinarily justifiable, Class 5 (see Reporting).
2) Isolation: Not applicable.
3) Concurrent disinfection: Not applicable.
4) Quarantine: Not applicable.
5) Immmunization of contacts: Not applicable.
6) Investigation of contacts and source of infection: A community problem.
7) Specific treatment: A donation program provides Ivermectin free of charge for treatment of onchocerciasis in humans. Given in a single oral dose of 150 micrograms/kg, with annual retreatment, this reduces microfilarial load and morbidity; it kills microfilariae and also blocks release of microfilariae from the uterus of the adult worm, effectively reducing the number of microfilariae in the skin and eyes over a period of 6–12 months. In endemic communities, ivermectin treatment for whole eligible population at least once yearly is recommended.

Research is under way to develop safe and effective drugs that would sterilize or kill the adult worm; some of these are undergoing clinical trials. While diethylcarbamazine citrate (DEC) is effective against microfilariae, it may cause severe adverse reactions that only partially respond to corticosteroids. It is no longer recommended for treatment of onchocerciasis. In selected individual cases, suramin may be used in conjunction with invermectin (available in the USA from CDC, Atlanta). Suramin kills the adult worms and leads to gradual disappearance of microfilariae, but possible nephrotoxicity and other undesirable reactions require close medical supervision of its use. Neither suramin nor DEC is suited for mass treatment of onchocerciasis because of possible serious side-effects.

In Central America, where nodules commonly occur on the head, their excision is often carried out, as this may reduce symptoms and prevent blindness.

C. Epidemic measures: In areas of high prevalence, concerted efforts to reduce incidence, taking measures listed under 9A.

D. Disaster implications: None.

E. International measures: The Onchocerciasis Control Programme (OCP), a coordinated program in western Africa sponsored by the World Bank, UNDP, FAO and WHO, covered the area in 11 countries where primarily the savanna ("blinding") form of the infection is endemic. Control has been based mainly on antiblackfly measures, with insecticides applied systematically to breeding sites in the rivers of the area. Ivermectin is now being distributed to communities on an ever-increasing scale as a replacement for larviciding. OCP was phased out in 2002. The African Programme for Onchocerciasis Control (APOC) has been established to implement effective and sustainable community directed annual treatment with ivermectin throughout the remaining endemic areas in Africa, and to eliminate the disease by vector control in selected foci. The Onchocerciasis Elimination Program for the Americas (OEPA) is a multinational multiagency effort to eliminate new morbidity from onchocerciasis from the Americas by 2007. OEPA also aims to interrupt onchocerciasis transmission wherever feasible using a strategy of semi-annual mass distribution of ivermectin to at least 85% of the eligible population. Further information on http://www.who.int/tdr/diseases/oncho/default.htm.

[M. Behrend]

ORF VIRUS DISEASE   ICD-9 051.2; ICD-10 B08.0
(Contagious pustular dermatitis, Human orf, Ecthyma contagiosum)

1. Identification—A proliferative cutaneous viral disease transmissible to humans through contact with infected sheep and goats, and, occasionally, wild ungulates (deer, reindeer). The lesion in humans, usually solitary and located on hands, arms or face, is a red to violet vesiculonodule, maculopapule or pustule, progressing to a weeping nodule with central umbilication. There may be several lesions, each up to 3 cm in diameter and lasting 3–6 weeks. With secondary bacterial infection, lesions may become pustular. Regional adenitis occurs in a few cases. A maculopapular rash may occur on the trunk. Erythema multiforme and erythema multiforme bullosum are rare complications. Disseminated disease and serious ocular damage have been reported. The disease has been confused with cutaneous anthrax and malignancy.

Diagnosis is through a history of contact with sheep, goats or wild ungulates, in particular their young; in the presence of negative results of conventional bacteriology, through electron microscopy demonstration of ovoid parapoxvirions in the lesion or by growth of the virus in ovine, bovine or primate cell cultures; or through positive serological tests.

2. Infectious agent—Orf virus, a DNA virus belonging to the genus Parapoxvirus of Poxviruses (family Poxviridae). The agent is closely related to other parapoxviruses that can be transmitted to humans as occupational diseases such as milkers' nodule virus of dairy cattle and bovine papular stomatitis virus of beef cattle. Contagious ecthyma parapoxvirus of domesticated camels may infect people on rare occasions.

3. Occurrence—Probably worldwide among farm workers; a common infection among shepherds, veterinarians and abattoir workers in areas producing sheep and goats and an important occupational disease in New Zealand.

4. Reservoir—Probably in various ungulates (sheep, goats, reindeer, musk oxen). The virus is very resistant to physical factors, except UV light, and may persist for months in soil and on animal skin and hair.

5. Mode of transmission—Direct contact with the mucous membranes of infected animals, with lesions on udders of nursing dams, or through intermediate passive transfer from apparently normal animals contaminated by contact, knives, shears, stall manger and sides, trucks and clothing. Person-to-person transmission is rare. Human infection may follow production and administration of vaccines to animals.

6. Incubation period—Generally 3-6 days.

7. Period of communicability—Unknown. Human lesions show a decrease in the number of virus particles as the disease progresses.

8. Susceptibility—Susceptibility is probably universal; recovery produces variable levels of immunity.

9. Methods of control—

  A. Preventive measures: Good personal hygiene and washing the exposed area with soap and water. Domestic and wild ungulates should be considered a potential source of infection. Ensure general cleanliness of animal housing areas. The efficacy and safety of Parapoxvirus vaccines in animals has not been fully determined.

  B. Control of patient, contacts and the immediate environment:

  1) Report to local health authority: Not required, but desirable when a human case occurs in areas not previously known to have the infection, Class 5 (see Reporting).
  2) Isolation: Not applicable.

3) Concurrent disinfection: Boil, autoclave or incinerate dressings.
4) Quarantine: Not applicable.
5) Immmunization of contacts: Not applicable.
6) Investigation of contacts and source of infection: Secure history of contact.
7) Specific treatment: None.

C. Epidemic measures: None.

D. Disaster implications: None.

E. International measures: None for humans.

PARACOCCIDIOIDOMYCOSIS ICD-9 116.1; ICD-10 B41
(South American blastomycosis, Paracoccidioidal granuloma)

1. Identification—A serious and at times fatal mycosis (chronic form also known as adult type) characterized by patchy pulmonary infiltrates and/or ulcerative lesions of skin and mucosa (oral, nasal, GI). Lymphadenopathy is frequent. In disseminated cases all viscera may be affected; adrenal glands are especially susceptible. The less common juvenile (acute) form is characterized by reticuloendothelial system involvement and bone marrow dysfunction.

Keloidal blastomycosis (Lobo disease), a disease involving skin only, formerly confused with paracoccidioidomycosis, is caused by *Lacazia loboi*, a fungus known only in tissue form and not yet grown in culture.

Histology confirms the diagnosis, as does culture of the infectious agent. Serological techniques are useful in diagnosis.

2. Infectious agent—*Paracoccidioides brasiliensis*, a dimorphic fungus.

3. Occurrence—Endemic in tropical and subtropical regions of South America and, to a lesser extent, Central America and Mexico. Workers in contact with soil, such as farmers, laborers, and construction workers are especially at risk. Highest incidence in adults aged 30–50; more common in males than in females.

4. Reservoir—Presumably soil or fungus-laden dust.

5. Mode of transmission—Presumably through inhalation of contaminated soil or dust.

6. Incubation period—Highly variable, from 1 month to many years.

7. Period of communicability—Direct person-to-person transmission of clinical disease from is not known.

8. Susceptibility—Unknown.

9. Methods of control—

   A. Preventive measures: None.

   B. Control of patient, contacts and the immediate environment:

   1) Report to local health authority: Official report not ordinarily justifiable, Class 5 (see Reporting).
   2) Isolation: Not applicable.
   3) Concurrent disinfection: Of discharges and contaminated articles. Terminal cleaning.
   4) Quarantine: Not applicable.
   5) Immmunization of contacts: Not applicable.
   6) Investigation of contacts and source of infection: Not indicated.
   7) Specific treatment: Itraconazole appears to be the drug of choice for all but patients requiring hospitalization, who should receive intravenous amphotericin B followed by prolonged treatment with itraconazole. Sulfonamides are cheaper but less effective than azoles.

   C. Epidemic measures: Not applicable, a sporadic disease.

   D. Disaster implications: None.

   E. International measures: None.

[L. Severo]

PARAGONIMIASIS ICD-9 121.2; ICD-10 B66.4
(Pulmonary distomiasis, Lung fluke disease)

1. Identification—A trematode disease most frequently involving the lungs. Symptoms include cough, hemoptysis and pleuritic chest pain. X-ray findings may include diffuse and/or segmental infiltrates, nodules, cavities, ring cysts and/or pleural effusions. Extrapulmonary disease is not uncommon, with flukes found in such sites as the CNS, subcutaneous tissues, intestinal wall, peritoneal cavity, liver, lymph nodes and genitourinary tract. Infection usually lasts for years, and the infected person may appear well. The disease may be mistaken for tuberculosis, clinically and on chest X-rays.

The sputum generally contains orange-brown flecks, sometimes diffusely distributed, in which masses of eggs are seen microscopically and establish the diagnosis. However, acid-fast staining for tuberculosis destroys the eggs and precludes diagnosis. Eggs are also swallowed, especially by children, and may be found in feces by some concentration techniques. A highly sensitive and specific immunoblot serologic test is available at CDC.

2. Infectious agents—*Paragonimus westermani*, *P. skrjabini* and other species in Asia; *P. africanus* and *P. uterobilateralis* in Africa; *P. mexicanus* (*P. peruvianus*) and other species in the Americas; *P. kellicotti* in the USA and Canada.

3. Occurrence—The disease has been reported in eastern and southwestern Asia, India, Africa and the Americas. China, where an estimated 20 million people are infected, is now the major endemic area, followed by India (Manipur province), Lao People's Democratic Republic and Myanmar. The disease has been quasi-eliminated from Japan, while fewer than 1000 people are infected in the Republic of Korea. Of the Latin American countries, Ecuador is the most affected, with about 500 000 estimated infections; cases have also occurred in Brazil, Colombia, Costa Rica, Mexico, Peru and Venezuela. The disease is rarer in Canada and the USA.

4. Reservoir—Humans, dogs, cats, pigs and wild carnivores are definitive hosts and act as reservoirs.

5. Mode of transmission—Infection occurs through consumption of the raw, salted, marinated or partially cooked flesh of freshwater crabs, such as *Eriocheir* and *Potamon*, or crayfish, such as *Cambaroides*, containing infective larvae (metacercariae). Larvae excyst in the duodenum, penetrate the intestinal wall, migrate through the tissues, become encapsulated (usually in the lungs) and develop into egg-producing adults. Eggs are expectorated in sputum and, when this is swallowed, are passed in the feces, gain access to freshwater and embryonate in 2–4 weeks. Larvae (miracidia) hatch, penetrate suitable freshwater snails (*Semisulcospira*, *Thiara*, *Aroapyrgus* or other genera) and undergo a cycle of development of approximately 2 months. Larvae (cercariae) emerge from the snails to encyst in freshwater crabs and crayfish. Pickling of these crustaceans in wine, brine or vinegar, a common practice in Asia, does not kill encysted larvae. Many infections occur in tourists sampling "native" or exotic foods.

6. Incubation period—Flukes mature and begin to lay eggs approximately 6–10 weeks after ingestion of the infective larvae. The long, variable, poorly defined interval until symptoms appear depends on the organ invaded and the number of worms involved.

7. Period of communicability—Eggs may be discharged by those infected for up to 20 years; duration of infection in molluscan and crustacean hosts is not well defined. Not directly transmitted from person to person.

8. Susceptibility—Susceptibility is general.

9. Methods of control—

A. *Preventive measures:*

1) Educate the public in endemic areas about the life cycle of the parasite.
2) Stress thorough cooking of crustaceans.
3) Dispose of sputum and feces in a sanitary manner.
4) Control snails through molluscicides where feasible.

B. *Control of patient, contacts and the immediate environment:*

1) Report to local health authority: Official report not ordinarily justifiable, Class 5 (see Reporting).
2) Isolation: Not applicable.
3) Concurrent disinfection: Of sputum and feces.
4) Quarantine: Not applicable.
5) Immmunization of contacts: Not applicable.
6) Investigation of contacts and source of infection: None.
7) Specific treatment: Praziquantel, triclabendazole and bithionol. The less effective latter drug, no longer in production, is available in the USA from CDC for domestic distribution only.

C. *Epidemic measures:* In an endemic area, the occurrence of small clusters of cases, or even sporadic infections, is an important signal for examination of local waters for infected snails, crabs and crayfish, and determination of reservoir mammalian hosts, to establish appropriate controls.

D. *Disaster implications:* None.

E. *International measures:* WHO Collaborating Centres.

[D. Engels]

PEDICULOSIS AND PHTHIRIASIS   ICD-9 132; ICD-10 B85

1. Identification—Infestation by head lice (*Pediculus capitis*) occurs on hair, eyebrows and eyelashes; infestation by body lice (*P. corporis*) is of the clothing, especially along the seams of inner surfaces. Crab lice

(*Phthirus pubis*) usually infest the pubic area; more rarely facial hair (including eyelashes in heavy infestations), axillae and body surfaces. Infestation may result in severe itching and excoriation of the scalp or body. Secondary infection may lead to regional lymphadenitis (especially cervical).

2. Infesting agents—The ectoparaistes *Pediculus capitis* (head louse), *P. corporis* (body louse), *Phthirus pubis* (crab louse); adult lice, nymphs and nits (egg cases) infest people. Lice are host-specific and those of lower animals do not infest humans, although they may be present transiently. Both sexes feed on blood.

The body louse is the species involved in outbreaks of epidemic typhus caused by *Rickettsia prowazeki*, trench fever caused by *R. quintana* and epidemic relapsing fever caused by *Borrelia recurrentis.*

3. Occurrence—Worldwide. Outbreaks of head lice are common among children in schools and institutions everywhere. Body lice are prevalent among populations with poor personal hygiene, especially in cold climates where heavy clothing is worn and bathing is infrequent or when people cannot change clothes (e.g. in the case of refugees).

4. Reservoir—Humans.

5. Mode of transmission—For head and body lice, direct contact with an infested person and objects used by them; for body lice, indirect contact with the personal belongings of infested persons, especially shared clothing and headgear. Head and body lice can survive for only a week without a food source. Crab lice are most frequently transmitted through sexual contact. Lice leave a febrile host; fever and overcrowding increase transfer from person to person.

6. Incubation period—Life cycle of 3 stages: eggs, nymphs and adults. The most suitable temperature for the life cycle is 32°C (89.6°F). Eggs of head lice do not hatch at temperatures under 22°C (71.6°F). Under optimal conditions, lice eggs hatch in 7-10 days. The nymphal stages last about 7-13 days depending on temperatures. The egg-to-egg cycle averages about 3 weeks. The average life cycle of the body or head louse extends over a period of 18 days; that of the crab louse, 15 days.

7. Period of communicability—As long as lice or eggs remain alive on the infested person or on fomites. The adult's life span is approximately 1 month. Nits remain viable on clothing for 1 month. Body and head lice survive for a week without feeding off the host, crab lice only 2 days. Nymphs survive 24 hours without food.

8. Susceptibility—Any person may become infested under suitable conditions of exposure. Repeated infestations may result in dermal hypersensitivity.

9. **Methods of control—**

   A. *Preventive measures:*

   1) Educate the public on the value of destroying eggs and lice through early detection, safe and thorough treatment of the hair, laundering clothing and bedding in hot water (55°C or 131°F for 20 min), dry cleaning or dryers set at "hot cycle".
   2) Avoid physical contact with infested individuals and their belongings, especially clothing and bedding.
   3) Perform regular, direct inspection of children in a group setting for nits and head lice and, when indicated, of body and clothing for body lice.
   4) In high-risk situations, use appropriate repellents on hair, skin and clothing.

   B. *Control of patient, contacts and the immediate environment:*

   1) Report to local health authority: Official report not ordinarily justifiable; school authorities should be informed, Class 5 (see Reporting).
   2) Isolation: For body lice, contact isolation if possible until 24 hours after application of an effective insecticide.
   3) Concurrent disinfection: Clothing, bedding and fomites should be treated by laundering in hot water, dry cleaning or applying an effective chemical insecticide (see 9B7).
   4) Quarantine: Not applicable.
   5) Immunization of contacts: Not applicable.
   6) Investigation of contacts and source of infestation: Examine household and close personal contacts; treat those infested.
   7) Specific treatment: For head and pubic lice: 1% permethrin (a synthetic pyrethroid) cream rinse with 10 minutes' exposure; pyrethrins synergized with piperonyl butoxide (10 minutes); and malathion 1% and 5 %, an organophosphate (7–8 hours). None of these is 100 % effective; retreatment may be necessary after an interval of 7–10 days. Carbaryl 0.5 % and 1 % can also be used but is more toxic than above-mentioned products. Lindane and benzyl benzoate are no longer recommended or registered because of toxicity, side-effects and low efficacy.

      Resistance to permethrin and pyrethrins is widespread. Malathion resistance has been detected so far in France and the United Kingdom. Carbaryl resistance is emerging in the United Kingdom.

      For body lice: Clothing and bedding should be washed using the hot water cycle of an automatic washing machine or dusted with pediculicides using power dusters, hand dusters or 2-ounce sifter cans. Dusts recommended by WHO include 1% malathion and 0.5% permethrin.

C. *Epidemic measures:* Mass treatment as recommended in 9B7 above, using insecticides clearly known to be effective against prevalent strains of lice. In typhus epidemics, individuals may protect themselves by wearing silk or plastic clothing tightly fastened around wrists, ankles and neck, and by impregnating their clothes with repellents or permethrin.

D. *Disaster implications:* Diseases for which body and head lice are vectors are particularly prone to occur at times of social upheaval (see Typhus fever, section I, Epidemic louse-borne).

E. *International measures:* None.

[P. Guillet]

PERTUSSIS   ICD-9 033.0, 033.9; ICD-10 A37.0, A37.9

PARAPERTUSSIS   ICD-9 033.1; ICD-10 A37.1
(Whooping Cough)

1. Identification—An acute bacterial infection of the respiratory tract caused by *Bordetella pertussis*. The initial catarrhal stage has an insidious onset with an irritating cough that gradually becomes paroxysmal, usually within 1–2 weeks, and lasts for 1–2 months or longer. Paroxysms are characterized by repeated violent cough; each series of paroxysms has many coughs without intervening inhalation and can be followed by a characteristic crowing or high-pitched inspiratory whoop. Paroxysms frequently end with the expulsion of clear, tenacious mucus, often followed by vomiting. Infants under 6 months, vaccinated children, adolescents and adults often do not have the typical whoop or cough paroxysm.

The number of fatalities in vaccinated populations is low. The vast majority of deaths occur in infants under 6 months, often in those too young to have completed primary immunization. In recent years, all deaths from pertussis in most industrialized countries occurred in infants under 6 months. In nonimmunized populations, especially those with underlying malnutrition and multiple enteric and respiratory infections, pertussis is among the most lethal diseases of infants and young children. Complications include pneumonia, atelectasia, seizures, encephalopathy, weight loss, hernias and death. Pneumonia is the most common cause of death; fatal encephalopathy, probably hypoxic, and inanition from repeated vomiting occasionally occur.

Case-fatality rates in unprotected children are less than 1 per thousand in industrialized countries; in developing countries they are estimated at 3.7% for children under 1 and 1% for children 1 to 4 years. In several industrialized countries with high rates of infant immunization for many years an increasing proportion of cases has been reported in adolescents and adults, whose symptoms varied from a mild, atypical respiratory illness to the full-blown syndrome. Many such cases occur in previously immunized persons and suggest waning immunity following immunization.

Parapertussis is a similar but occasional and milder disease due to *Bordetella parapertussis*. The *Bordetella* are Gram-negative aerobic bacteria; *B. pertussis* and *B. parapertussis* are similar species but the latter lacks the expression of the gene coding for pertussis toxin.

Diagnosis is based on the recovery of the causal organism from nasopharyngeal specimens obtained during the catarrhal and early paroxysmal stages on appropriate culture media. WHO considers culture as the "gold standard" of laboratory confirmation. It is the most specific diagnosis but is not very sensitive (<60%). Polymerase chain reaction (PCR) is more sensitive and can be performed on the same biological samples as cultures. It is delicate to perform and requires more expensive equipment. Direct fluorescent antibody staining of nasopharyngeal secretions is not recommended because of frequent false-positive and false-negative results. Indirect diagnosis (serology) consists of detecting specific antibodies in the serum of infected individual, collected at the beginning of cough (acute serum) and on serum collected one month later (convalescent serum). The presence of high level of antibodies in the serum of a non-vaccinated individual indicates infection. Serology cannot be used for diagnosis during the year following vaccination since it does not differentiate between antibodies due to the vaccine or to natural infection

Differentiation between *B. parapertussis* and *B. pertussis* is based on culture, biochemical and immunological differences.

2. Infectious agents—*B. pertussis*, the bacillus of pertussis *stricto sensu*; *B. parapertussis* causes parapertussis.

3. Occurrence—An endemic disease common to children (especially young children) everywhere, regardless of ethnicity, climate or geographic location. Outbreaks occur typically every 3 to 4 years. A marked decline has occurred in incidence and mortality rates during the past 40 years, chiefly in communities with active immunization programs and where good nutrition and medical care are available. In 1999, despite a global vaccination coverage of around 80%, there were still an estimated 48.5 million pertussis cases in children worldwide with an estimated 295 000 deaths, nearly all in Africa. Incidence rates have increased in countries where pertussis immunization rates fell in the past (e.g. Japan in the early 1980s, Sweden and the United Kingdom), and rose again when immunization programs were reestablished. In countries with high vaccination coverage, the incidence rate in children under 15 is less than 1 per 100 000.

4. Reservoir—Humans are believed to be the only host for pertussis. *B. parapertussis* can also be isolated from ovines.

5. Mode of transmission—Direct contact with discharges from respiratory mucous membranes of infected persons by the airborne route, probably via droplets. In vaccinated populations, bacteria are frequently brought home by an older sibling and sometimes by a parent. Indirect spread through the air or contaminated objects occurs rarely if at all.

6. Incubation period—Average 9–10 days (range 6–20 days).

7. Period of communicability—Highly communicable in the early catarrhal stage and at the beginning of the paroxysmal cough stage (first 2 weeks). Thereafter, communicability gradually decreases and becomes negligible in about 3 weeks, despite persisting spasmodic cough with whoop. When treated with erythromycin, clarithromycin or azithromycin, patients are no longer contagious after 5 days of treatment.

8. Susceptibility—Susceptibility of nonimmunized individuals is universal. Secondary attack rate of up to 90% in non-immune household contacts. Although antibodies cross the placenta, transplacental immunity in infants has not been demonstrated. Incidence is highest in children under 5 years except where infant vaccination programs have been very effective and a shift has occurred toward adolescents. Milder and missed atypical cases occur in all age groups. There is a higher incidence and mortality in females. One attack usually confers prolonged immunity, although subsequent attacks (some of which may be attributable to *B. parapertussis*) can occur. Cases in previously immunized adolescents and adults in countries with long-standing and successful immunization programs occur because of waning immunity and are a source of infection for non immunized young children.

9. Methods of control—

   A. Preventive measures:

      1) Immunization is the most rational approach to pertussis control; and whole-cell vaccine against pertussis (wP) has been effective in preventing pertussis for more than 40 years. Educate the public, particularly parents of infants, about the dangers of whooping cough and the advantages of initiating immunization on time (between 6 weeks and 3 months depending on the country) and adhering to the immunization schedule. This continues to be important because of the wide negative publicity given to adverse reactions.

      2) Active primary immunization against *B. pertussis* infection with 3 doses of a vaccine consisting of either a suspension of killed bacteria (wP) or acellular preparations (aP) that contain 1–5 different components of *B. pertussis*. These are

usually given in combination with diphtheria and tetanus toxoids adsorbed on aluminium salts (Diphtheria and Tetanus Toxoids and Pertussis Vaccine Adsorbed, DTwP or DTaP). In terms of severe adverse effects aP and wP vaccines appear to have the same high level of safety; reactions (local and transient systemic) are less commonly associated with aP vaccines. Similar high efficacy levels (more than 80%) occur with the best aP and wP vaccines although the level of efficacy may vary within each group. Protection is greater against severe disease and begins to wane after about 5 years. Acellular pertussis vaccines do not protect against infection by *B. parapertussis*.

Although the use of aP vaccines is less commonly associated with local and systemic reactions such as fever, price considerations affect their use and wP vaccines are the vaccines of choice for most developing countries. Japan, USA and many other industrialized countries have completely replaced wP vaccines by aP vaccines. Schedules vary: North America vaccinates at 2, 4, 6 months, France at 3, 4, 5 months, Sweden at 3, 5, 12 months and the United Kingdom at 2, 3, 4 months; most developing countries vaccinate at 6, 10 and 14 weeks of age according to the WHO/EPI proposed schedule. In all countries and particularly where pertussis is still endemic and poses a serious health problem, the priority should be to reach at least 90% coverage with a primary series of 3 doses of DTP in infants in all areas. In countries where immunization programs have considerably reduced pertussis incidence, a booster dose approximately one year after the primary series is warranted. National programs should assess the need and timing for additional booster doses of DTP and their efficacy. The USA and some other countries recommend booster doses at 15–18 months of age and at school entry. Vaccines containing wP are not recommended after the seventh birthday since local reactions may be increased in older children and adults. Formulations of acellular pertussis vaccine for use in adolescents and adults have been licensed and are available in several countries.

DTaP/DTwP can be given simultaneously with oral poliovirus vaccine (OPV), inactivated poliovirus vaccine (IPV), *Haemophilus influenzae* type b (Hib), hepatitis B (HepB) vaccine and measles, mumps and rubella vaccine (MMR) at different sites. Combination vaccines with Hib, IPV and HepB are available and are widely used in Europe.

Minor adverse reactions such as local redness and swelling, fever and agitation often occur after immunization with wP vaccine (1 in 2–10). Prolonged crying and febrile seizures are less common (<1 in 100); hypotonic-hyporesponsive episodes are rare (<1 in 2000). Although febrile seizures and hypotonic-hyporesponsive episodes may follow DTwP and are disturbing to parents and physicians alike, there is no scientific evidence that these reactions have any permanent consequences. Recent detailed reviews of all available studies conclude that there is no demonstrable causal relationship between DTwP and chronic nervous system dysfunction in children. The only true contraindication to immunization with aP or wP is an anaphylactic reaction to a previous dose or to any constituent of the vaccine. In young infants with suspected evolving and progressive neurological disease, immunization may be delayed for some months to permit diagnosis in order to avoid possible confusion about the cause of symptoms

3) When an outbreak occurs, consider protection of health workers who have been exposed to pertussis cases, using a 7-day course of erythromycin. Clarithromycin and azithromycin are expensive but better tolerated alternatives.

B. *Control of patient, contacts and the immediate environment:*

1) Report to local public health authorities Class 2 (See Reporting). Early reporting permits better outbreak control. The WHO-recommended clinical case definition is: A case diagnosed as pertussis by a physician or a person with a cough lasting at least 2 weeks and at least one of the following symptoms: paroxysms (fits) of coughing, inspiratory "whooping", post-tussive vomiting (vomiting immediately after coughing) without other apparent cause.

2) Isolation: Respiratory isolation for known cases. Suspected cases should be removed from the presence of young children and infants, especially nonimmunized infants, until the patients have received at least 5 days of a minimum 7-day course of antibiotics. Suspected cases who do not receive antibiotics should be isolated for 3 weeks after onset of paroxysmal cough or till the end of cough, whichever comes first.

3) Concurrent disinfection: Disinfection measures are of little impact.

4) Quarantine: Inadequately immunized household contacts under 7 may be excluded from schools, day care centers and public gatherings for 21 days after last exposure or until the cases and contacts have received 5 days of a minimum 7-day course of appropriate antibiotics.

5) Protection of contacts: All contacts must have their immunization status verified and brought up to date. Passive immunization has not been demonstrated to be effective and there

is no product currently commercially available. The initiation of active immunization following recent exposure is not effective against infection but should be undertaken to protect the child against further exposure in case it has not been infected. Close contacts under 7 who have not received 4 DTP doses or have not received a DTP dose within 3 years should be given a dose as soon after exposure as possible. A 7-day course of erythromycin, clarithromycin or azithromycin for household and other close contacts, regardless of immunization status and age, is recommended for households where there is a child under 1. Prophylactic antibiotherapy in the early incubation period may prevent disease, but difficulties of early diagnosis, costs involved and concerns related to the occurrence of drug resistance all limit prophylactic treatment to selected individual conditions:
- children under 1 year and pregnant women in the last 3 weeks of pregnancy (because of the risk of transmission to the newborn);
- stopping infection among household members, particularly if there are children aged under 1 and pregnant women in the last 3 weeks of pregnancy.

6) Investigation of contacts and source of infection: A search for early, missed and atypical cases is indicated where a nonimmune infant or young child is or might be at risk.

7) Specific treatment: Erythromycin, clarithromycin and azithromycin shorten the period of communicability, but do not reduce symptoms except when given during the incubation period, in the catarrhal stage or early in the paroxysmal stage.

C. *Epidemic measures:* A search for unrecognized and unreported cases may be indicated to protect preschool children from exposure and to ensure adequate preventive measures for exposed children under 7. Accelerated immunization, with the first dose at 4 – 6 weeks of age and the second and third doses at 4-week intervals, may be indicated; immunizations should be completed for those whose schedule is incomplete.

D. *Disaster implications:* Pertussis is a potential problem if introduced into crowded refugee camps with many non-immunized children.

E. *International measures:* Ensure completion of primary immunization of infants and young children before they travel to other countries; review need for a booster dose.

[P. Duclos]

PINTA
(Carate)

ICD-9 103; ICD-10 A67

1. **Identification**—An acute and chronic nonvenereal treponemal skin infection. A scaling painless papule with satellite lymphadenopathy appears 1–8 weeks after infection, usually on the hands, legs or dorsum of the feet. Within 3–12 months a maculopapular, erythematous secondary rash appears and may evolve into tertiary splotches of altered (dyschromic) skin pigmentation of variable size. These treponema-containing macules pass through stages of blue to violet to brown pigmentation, finally becoming treponema-free depigmented (achromic) scars. Lesions coexist at different stages of evolution and are most common on the face and extremities. Organ systems are not involved; physical disability and death do not occur.

Spirochaetes are demonstrable in dyschromic (but not achromic) lesions through darkfield or direct FA microscopic examination. Serological tests for syphilis usually become reactive before or during the secondary rash and thereafter behave as in venereal syphilis.

2. **Infectious agent**—*Treponema carateum*, a spirochaete.

3. **Occurrence**—Found only among isolated rural populations living under crowded unhygienic conditions in the American tropics. Predominantly a disease of older children and adults. Surveys carried out during the mid-1990s by PAHO/WHO in targeted Amazonian populations in Brazil, Peru and Venezuela found few cases, mostly inactive. WHO concludes that pinta is a residual problem and that the infection is on its way to elimination and eradication. Isolated foci may still exist in Central America and Cuba.

4. **Reservoir**—Humans.

5. **Mode of transmission**—Presumably person-to-person through direct and prolonged contact with initial and early dyschromic skin lesions. The location of primary lesions suggests that trauma provides a portal of entry; lesions in children occur in those body areas most scratched. Various biting and sucking arthropods, especially blackflies, are suspected but are not proven as biological vectors.

6. **Incubation period**—Usually 2–3 weeks.

7. **Period of communicability**—Unknown; potentially communicable while dyschromic skin lesions are active, sometimes for many years. Not highly contagious; several years of intimate contact may be necessary for transmission.

8. Susceptibility—Undefined; presumably as in other treponematoses.

9. Methods of control—

A. *Preventive measures:* Those applicable to other nonvenereal treponematoses apply to pinta; see Yaws, 9A.

B. *Control of patient, contacts and the immediate environment:*

1) Report to local health authority: In selected endemic areas; in most countries, not a reportable disease, Class 3 (see Reporting).

2), 3), 4), 5), 6) and 7) Isolation, Concurrent disinfection, Quarantine, Immunization of contacts, Investigation of contacts and source of infection and Specific treatment: See Yaws, 9B2 through 9B7.

C., D. and E. *Epidemic measures, Disaster implications* and *International measures:* See Yaws, C, D and E.

[G. Antal]

PLAGUE
(Pestis)

ICD-9 020; ICD-10 A20

1. Identification—A specific zoonosis involving rodents and their fleas, which transfer the bacterial infection to various animals and to people. Initial signs and symptoms may be nonspecific with fever, chills, malaise, myalgia, nausea, prostration, sore throat and headache. Lymphadenitis often develops in those lymph nodes that drain the site of the bite, where there may be an initial lesion. This is bubonic plague, and it occurs more often (90%) in lymph nodes in the inguinal area and less commonly in those in the axillary and cervical areas. The involved nodes become swollen, inflamed and tender and may suppurate. Fever is usually present. All forms, including instances in which lymphadenopathy is not apparent, may progress to septicemic plague with bloodstream dissemination to diverse parts of the body that include the meninges. Endotoxic shock and disseminated intravascular coagulation (DIC) may occur without localizing signs of infection. Secondary involvement of the lungs results in pneumonia; mediastinitis or pleural effusion may develop. Secondary pneumonic plague is of special significance, since respiratory droplets may serve as the source of person-to-person transfer with resultant primary pneumonic or pharyngeal plague; this can lead to localized outbreaks or devastating epidemics. Though naturally acquired plague usually presents as bubonic plague, purposeful aerosol dissemination as a result of deliberate use would be manifest primarily as pneumonic plague.

Untreated bubonic plague has a case-fatality rate of about 50%–60%. Plague organisms have been recovered from throat cultures of asymptomatic contacts of pneumonic plague patients. Untreated primary septicemic plague and pneumonic plague are invariably fatal. Modern therapy markedly reduces fatality from bubonic plague; pneumonic and septicemic plague also respond if recognized and treated early. However, one report stated that patients who had not received adequate therapy for primary pneumonic plague within 18 hours after onset of respiratory symptoms were less likely to survive.

Visualization of characteristic bipolar staining, "safety pin" ovoid, Gram-negative organisms in direct microscopic examination of material aspirated from a bubo, sputum or CSF are each suggestive, but not conclusive, evidence of plague infection. Examination by FA test or antigen capture ELISA is more specific and is particularly useful in sporadic cases. Diagnosis is confirmed by culture and identification of the causal organism from exudate aspirated from buboes, from blood, CSF or sputum, or by a 4-fold or greater rise or fall in antibody titre. Slow growth of the organism at normal incubation temperatures may lead to misidentification by automated systems. The passive hemagglutination test (PHA) using *Yersinia pestis* Fraction-1 antigen is most frequently used for serodiagnosis. Medical personnel should be aware of areas where the disease is endemic and entertain the diagnosis of plague early; unfortunately, plague is often misdiagnosed, especially in travellers who develop illness after returning from an endemic area.

2. Infectious agent—*Yersinia pestis*, the plague bacillus.

3. Occurrence—Plague continues to be a threat because of vast areas of persistent wild rodent infection; contact of wild rodents with domestic rats occurs frequently in some enzootic areas. Wild rodent plague exists in the western half of the USA; large areas of South America; central, eastern and southern Africa; central, southwestern and southeastern Asia, and extreme southeastern Europe near the Caspian Sea. While urban plague has been controlled in most of the world, human plague has occurred in the 1990s in several African countries that include Botswana, the Democratic Republic of the Congo, Kenya, Madagascar, Malawi, Mozambique, the United Republic of Tanzania, Uganda, Zambia and Zimbabwe. Plague is endemic in China, India, Lao People's Democratic Republic, Mongolia, Myanmar and Viet Nam. In the Americas, foci in northeastern Brazil and the Andean region (Brazil, Ecuador and Peru) continue to produce sporadic cases and occasional outbreaks including an outbreak of pneumonic plague in Ecuador in 1998.

Human plague in the western USA is sporadic (12–14 cases a year since 1900), with only single cases or small common source clusters in an area, usually following exposure to wild rodents or their fleas. No person-to-person transmission has occurred in the USA since 1925, although secondary plague pneumonia has occurred in about 20% of bubonic cases in recent years; 5 instances of primary plague pneumonia through cat-to-human transmission have been recorded.

4. Reservoir—Wild rodents (especially ground squirrels) are the natural vertebrate reservoir of plague. Lagomorphs (rabbits and hares), wild carnivores and domestic cats may also be a source of infection to people.

5. Mode of transmission—Naturally acquired plague in people occurs as a result of human intrusion into the zoonotic (also termed sylvatic or rural) cycle during or following an epizootic, or by the entry of sylvatic rodents or their infected fleas into human habitat; infection in commensal rodents and their fleas may result in a domestic rat epizootic and flea-borne epidemics of bubonic plague. Domestic pets, particularly house cats and dogs, may carry plague infected wild rodent fleas into homes, and cats may occasionally transmit infection through bites, scratches or respiratory droplets; cats develop plague abscesses that have been a source of infection to veterinary personnel.

The most frequent source of exposure that results in human disease worldwide has been the bite of infected fleas (especially *Xenopsylla cheopis*, the oriental rat flea).

Other important sources include the handling of tissues of infected animals, especially rodents and rabbits, but also carnivores; rarely airborne droplets from human patients or household cats with plague pharyngitis or pneumonia; or careless manipulation of laboratory cultures. Person-to-person transmission by *Pulex irritans* fleas ("human" flea), is presumed to be important in the Andean region of South America and in other places where plague occurs and this flea is abundant in homes or on domestic animals. Certain occupations and lifestyles (including hunting, trapping, cat ownership and rural residence) carry an increased risk of exposure. In the case of deliberate use plague bacilli would possibly be transmitted as an aerosol.

6. Incubation period—From 1 to 7 days; may be a few days longer in those immunized who develop illness. For primary plague pneumonia, 1–4 days, usually short.

7. Period of communicability—Fleas may remain infective for months under suitable conditions of temperature and humidity. Bubonic plague is not usually transmitted directly unless there is contact with pus from suppurating buboes. Pneumonic plague may be highly communicable under appropriate climatic conditions; overcrowding facilitates transmission.

8. Susceptibility—Susceptibility is general. Immunity after recovery is relative; it may not protect against a large inoculum.

9. **Methods of control—**

   A. *Preventive measures:* The basic objective is to reduce the likelihood of people being bitten by infected fleas, having direct contact with infective tissues and exudates, or of being exposed to patients with pneumonic plague.

     1) Educate the public in enzootic areas on the modes of human and domestic animal exposure; on rat-proofing buildings, preventing access to food and shelter by peridomestic rodents through appropriate storage and disposal of food, garbage and refuse; and the importance of avoiding flea bites by use of insecticides and repellents. In sylvatic or rural plague areas, the public should be advised to use insect repellents and warned not to camp near rodent burrows and to avoid handling of rodents, but to report dead or sick animals to health authorities or park rangers. Dogs and cats in such areas should be protected periodically with appropriate insecticides.

     2) Survey rodent populations periodically to determine the effectiveness of sanitary programs and to evaluate the potential for epizootic plague. Rat suppression by poisoning (see 9B6) may be necessary to augment basic environmental sanitation measures; rat control should always be preceded by measures to control fleas. Maintain surveillance of natural foci by bacteriologic testing of sick or dead wild rodents and by serological studies of wild carnivore and outdoor ranging dog and cat populations in order to define areas of plague activity. Collection and testing of fleas from wild rodents and their nests or burrows may also be appropriate.

     3) Control rats on ships and docks and in warehouses by rat-proofing or periodic fumigation, combined when necessary with destruction of rats and their fleas in vessels and in cargoes, especially containerized cargoes, before shipment and on arrival from locations endemic for plague.

     4) Wear gloves when hunting and handling wildlife.

     5) Active immunization with a vaccine of killed bacteria confers some protection against bubonic plague (but not primary pneumonic plague) in most recipients if administered in a primary series of 3 doses with doses 1 and 2 given 1-3 months apart followed by dose 3 after 5-6 months; booster injections are necessary every 6 months if high risk exposure continues. After the third booster dose, the intervals can be extended to every 1 to 2 years. Immunization of visitors to epidemic localities and of laboratory and fieldworkers handling plague bacilli or infected animals is justifiable but should not be relied upon as the sole preventive measure;

routine immunization is not indicated for most persons resident in enzootic areas. Live attenuated vaccines are used in some countries; they may produce more adverse reactions, without evidence that they are more protective. Commercial plague vaccine is no longer available in the USA.

B. Control of patient, contacts and the immediate environment:

1) Report to local health authority: Case report of suspected and confirmed cases universally required by *International Health Regulations*, Class 1 (see Reporting). Because of the rarity of naturally acquired primary plague pneumonia, even a single case should initiate prompt suspicion by both public health and law enforcement authorities of deliberate use.

2) Isolation: Rid patients, and especially their clothing and baggage, of fleas, using an insecticide effective against local fleas and known to be safe for people; hospitalize if practical. For patients with bubonic plague (if there is no cough and the chest X-ray is negative) drainage and secretion precautions are indicated for 48 hours after start of effective treatment. For patients with pneumonic plague, strict isolation with precautions against airborne spread is required until 48 hours of appropriate antibiotherapy have been completed and there has been a favorable clinical response (see 9B7).

3) Concurrent disinfection: Disinfect sputum and purulent discharges and articles soiled therewith. Terminal cleaning of bodies and carcases should be handled with strict aseptic precautions.

4) Quarantine: Those who have been in household or face-to-face contact with patients with pneumonic plague should be provided chemoprophylaxis (see 9B5) and placed under surveillance for 7 days; those who refuse chemoprophylaxis should be maintained in strict isolation with careful surveillance for 7 days.

5) Protection of contacts: In epidemic situations where human fleas are known to be involved, contacts of bubonic plague patients should be disinfested with an appropriate insecticide. All close contacts should be evaluated for chemoprophylaxis. Close contacts of confirmed or suspected plague pneumonia cases (including medical personnel) should be provided with chemoprophylaxis using tetracycline (15–30 mg/kg) or chloramphenicol (30 mg/kg) daily in 4 divided doses for 1 week after exposure ceases.

6) Investigation of contacts and source of infection: Search for people with household or face-to-face exposure to pneumonic plague, and for sick or dead rodents and their fleas. Flea

control must precede—or coincide with—antirodent measures. Dust rodent runs, harbourages and burrows in and around known or suspected plague areas with an insecticide labelled for flea control and known to be effective against local fleas. If nonburrowing wild rodents are involved, insecticide bait stations can be used. If urban rats are involved, disinfest by dusting the houses, outhouses and household furnishings; dust the bodies and clothing of all residents in the immediate vicinity. Suppress rat populations by well-planned and energetic campaigns of poisoning and with vigorous concurrent measures to reduce rat harbourages and food sources.

7) Specific treatment: Streptomycin is the drug of choice, gentamicin can be used when streptomycin is not readily available; tetracyclines and chloramphenicol are alternative choices. Chloramphenicol is required for treatment of plague meningitis. All are highly effective if used early (within 8–18 hours after onset of pneumonic plague). After a satisfactory response to drug treatment, reappearance of fever may result from a secondary infection or a suppurative bubo that may require incision and drainage.

C. Epidemic measures:

1) Investigate all suspected plague deaths with autopsy and laboratory examinations when indicated. Develop and carry out case-finding. Establish the best possible facilities for diagnosis and treatment. Alert existing medical facilities to report cases immediately and to use full diagnostic and therapeutic services.

2) Attempt to prevent or mitigate public hysteria by appropriate informational and educational releases through the press and news media.

3) Institute intensive flea control in expanding circles from known foci.

4) Implement rodent destruction within affected areas only after satisfactory flea control has been accomplished.

5) Protect all contacts as noted in 9B5.

6) Protect fieldworkers against fleas; dust clothing with insecticide powder and use insect repellents daily. Antibiotic prophylaxis should be undertaken for those with close documented exposure (see 9B5).

D. Disaster implications:
Plague could become a significant problem in endemic areas when there are social upheavals, crowding and unhygienic conditions. See preceding and following paragraphs for appropriate actions.

E. International measures:

1) Notification within 24 hours by governments to WHO and to adjacent countries of the first imported, first transferred or first nonimported case of plague in any area previously free of the disease. Report newly discovered or reactivated foci of plague among rodents.

2) Measures applicable to ships, aircraft and land transport arriving from plague areas are specified in *International Health Regulations* (currently under revision).

3) All ships should be free of rodents or periodically deratted.

4) Rat-proof buildings at seaports and airports; apply appropriate insecticides; eliminate rats with effective rodenticides.

5) For international travellers, international regulations require that prior to their departure on an international voyage from an area where there is an epidemic of pulmonary plague, those suspected of significant exposure shall be placed in isolation for 6 days after last exposure. On arrival of an infested or suspected infested ship, or an infested aircraft, travellers may be disinsected and kept under surveillance for a period of not more than 6 days from the date of arrival. Immunization against plague cannot be required as a condition of admission to a territory. These measures, outlined in the *International Health Regulations*, are currently under revision.

6) WHO Collaborating Centres.

F. Measures in the case of deliberate use:

Y. pestis is distributed worldwide; techniques for mass production and aerosol dissemination are thought to exist; the fatality rate of primary pneumonic plague is high and there is a real potential for secondary spread. For these reasons, a biological attack with plague is considered to be of serious public health concern. In some countries, a few sporadic cases may be missed or not attributed to a deliberate act. Any suspect case of pneumonic plague should be reported immediately to the local health department. The sudden appearance of many patients presenting with fever, cough, a fulminant course and high case-fatality rate should provide a suspect alert for anthrax or plague; if cough is primarily accompanied by hemoptysis, this presentation favors the tentative diagnosis of pneumonic plague. For a suspected or confirmed outbreak of pneumonic plague, follow the treatment and containment measures outlined in 9B. Depending on the extent of dissemination, mass prophylaxis of potentially exposed populations may be considered.

[E. Bertherat]

PNEUMONIA

I. PNEUMOCOCCAL
PNEUMONIA   ICD-9 481; ICD-10 J13

1. Identification—An acute lower respiratory tract bacterial infection, this is the most common community-acquired pneumonia at all ages. In Europe and North America, pneumococcal pneumonia is estimated to affect approximately 100 per 100 000 adults each year. Clinical manifestations typically include sudden onset, high fever (with shaking chill or rigor and/or other systemic symptoms like myalgia, arthralgia, headache, malaise), pleural pain, dyspnoea, tachypnoea and cough productive of "rusty" sputum. Laboratory findings include leukocytosis (neutrophilia), elevated C-reactive protein and accelerated ESR. The onset may be less abrupt, especially in the elderly, and fever, shortness of breath or altered mental status may provide first evidence of pneumonia. In infants and young children, fever, vomiting and convulsions may be the initial manifestations. Typical chest X-ray shows lobar or segmental consolidation; consolidation may be bronchopneumonic, especially in children and the aged. Pneumococcal pneumonia is an important cause of death in infants and the aged. Persons suffering from chronic conditions and immune deficiencies are at increased risk. The case-fatality rate, formerly 20%–40% among hospitalized patients, has fallen to 5%–10% with antimicrobial therapy, but remains 20%–40% among patients with substantial underlying disease or alcoholism (it may exceed 50% in the high-risk groups). In developing countries the case-fatality rates in children are often over 10% and as high as 60% in infants under 6 months. Secondary pneumococcal pneumonia is often observed in the vulnerable population and among previously healthy individuals, following other respiratory infections (e.g. influenza, RSV), with severe outcomes.

Early causal diagnosis is important for guiding specific treatment. The presence in sputum of many Gram-positive diplococci together with polymorphonuclear leukocytes suggests the diagnosis, which can be confirmed through isolation of pneumococci from blood or, exceptionally, from lower respiratory tract secretions obtained in adults by percutaneous transtracheal aspiration. For severe cases suspected to have bacterial pneumonia, treatment should not be delayed and empiricial antimicrobial therapy should start before microbiological confirmation. It is important to identify the etiological agent together with its antimicrobial susceptibility.

2. Infectious agent—*Streptococcus pneumoniae* (pneumococcus), a Gram-positive encapsulated coccus often colonizing the human nasopharynx, where it can be carried asymptomatically. Children carry *S. pneumoniae* more often than adults do. Current data suggest that the 11 most common serotypes cause at least 75% of invasive disease in all regions.

3. Occurrence—A disease of continuing endemicity, particularly in infancy and old age and in individuals with underlying medical conditions; more frequent in malnourished populations, the lower socioeconomic groups and in developing countries. It occurs in all climates and seasons, incidence being highest in winter and spring in temperate zones. It may occur in epidemics in closed populations and during rapid urbanization. Recurring epidemics have been described among South African miners; incidence is high in certain geographic areas (e.g. Papua New Guinea) and among children in many developing countries. An increased incidence often accompanies epidemics of influenza. High-level antibiotic resistance to essential anti-microbials such as penicillin, cephalosporins and macrolides is a serious and rapidly increasing problem worldwide.

4. Reservoir—Humans. Pneumococci are commonly found in the upper respiratory tract of healthy people worldwide.

5. Mode of transmission—Droplet spread, direct oral contact, or indirectly through articles freshly soiled with respiratory discharges. Person-to-person transmission of the organisms is common, but illness among casual contacts and attendants is infrequent.

6. Incubation period—Not well determined; may be as short as 1–3 days.

7. Period of communicability—Presumably until discharges of mouth and nose no longer contain virulent pneumococci in significant numbers. Penicillin will render patients with susceptible strains noninfectious within 24–48 hours.

8. Susceptibility—Susceptibility is general and disease may occur in persons susceptible to the serotype involved. Even a previously healthy adult can develop pneumococcal pneumonia. Susceptibility to symptomatic pneumococcal infection is increased by processes affecting the integrity of the lower respiratory tract, including influenza, pulmonary oedema, aspiration following alcoholic intoxication or other causes, chronic lung disease or exposure to irritants (e.g. cigarettes, cooking fire smoke). Elderly persons and persons with the following chronic medical conditions are at increased risk: anatomical or functional asplenia, sickle cell disease, chronic cardiovascular disease, diabetes mellitus, cirrhosis, Hodgkin disease, lymphoma, multiple myeloma, chronic renal failure, nephrotic syndrome, HIV infection and recent organ transplantation. Immunity, specific for the infecting capsular serotype, usually follows an attack and may last for years. Malnutrition and low birthweight are important risk cofactors for pneumonia among infants and young children in developing countries.

9. **Methods of control—**

   A. *Preventive measures:*

   1) Avoid crowding in living quarters whenever practical, particularly in institutions, barracks and ships. Avoid malnutrition and encourage physical activity. Bedridden patients should be fed or lie in upright position.

   2) Because risk of infection and case-fatality rates increase with age, the benefits of immunization also increase. Administer to high risk persons (individuals 65 and older and those with anatomic or functional asplenia, sickle cell disease, HIV infection and a variety of chronic systemic illnesses, including heart and lung disease, cirrhosis of the liver, renal insufficiency and diabetes mellitus) a polyvalent vaccine containing the capsular polysaccharides of the 11 most common serotypes that cause 75% of invasive disease in all regions; this vaccine is not effective in children under 2 and has no impact on pneumococcal carriage. In February 2000 a new 7-valent conjugate vaccine, which apparently reduces invasive disease by about 70%, was approved for use in children even under 2.

   For most eligible patients, vaccine need be given only once; however, reimmunization is generally safe, and vaccine should be offered to eligible patients whose immunization status cannot be determined. Reimmunization is recommended once for persons over 2 who are at highest risk for serious pneumococcal infection (e.g. asplenic patients) and those likely to have a rapid decline in pneumococcal antibody levels, provided that 5 years or more have elapsed since receipt of the 1st dose of vaccine. Reimmunization after 3 years should also be considered for children with functional or anatomic asplenia and those who present conditions associated with rapid antibody decline after initial immunization (e.g. nephrotic syndrome, renal failure, renal transplantation) who would be 10 or older at reimmunization. In addition, persons 65 and older should be given another dose of vaccine if they received the vaccine more than 5 years previously and were under 65 at the time of primary immunization. Most of the pneumococcal antigen types in the vaccine are poor immunogens in children under 2. Because of differences in serotype prevalence, the vaccine may have lower efficacy in developing countries. A 7-valent glycoprotein conjugate vaccine has been approved for routine infant use in the USA. This has been effective in preventing pneumococcal pneumonia and meningitis in young children and infants. The vaccine has some efficacy against otitis media and against carriage of vaccine-included pneumococcal serotypes.

Prophylactic use of xylitol, a sugar that inhibits pneumococcal growth, may also represent a feasible intervention against non-invasive disease and resistance in developing countries.

B. Control of patient, contacts and the immediate environment:

1) Report to local health authority: Obligatory report of epidemics in some countries; no individual case report, Class 4 (see Reporting).

2) Isolation: Respiratory isolation may be warranted for hospitalized patients with antibiotic resistant infection who may transmit it to patients at high risk of pneumococcal disease.

3) Concurrent disinfection: Of discharges from nose and throat. Terminal cleaning.

4) Quarantine: Not applicable.

5) Immunization of contacts: Not applicable (See 9C).

6) Investigation of contacts and source of infection: Of no practical value.

7) Specific treatment: Where diagnostic facilities are limited and a delay in treatment could prove fatal, antibiotherapy of infants and young children must start on a presumptive diagnosis based on clinical signs, in particular tachypnoea and chest indrawing. Infants under 2 months should be transferred to hospital care without delay. Penicillin G, parenterally, is the preferred treatment (erythromycin for those hypersensitive to penicillin). Because pneumococci resistant to penicillin and other antimicrobials are increasingly recognized, sensitivities of strains isolated from normally sterile sites, including blood or CSF, should be determined. For pneumonia and other pneumococcal infections, parenteral beta-lactam antibiotics are likely to be effective in most cases. Where beta-lactam resistance is common, vancomycin should be included in initial regimens for the treatment of meningitis possibly due to pneumococci until susceptibilities can be determined (in some counties use of vancomycin is limited because of concern for adverse effects). Vancomycin is rarely if ever indicated for pneumococcal infections not involving the CNS. In developing countries, WHO guidelines recommend trimethoprim-sulfamethazole, ampicillin or amoxicillin for home-treatment of nonsevere pneumonia for children under 5. WHO guidelines are not intended for industrialized countries, most of which have no unified guidelines for the treatment of pneumococcal disease, although professional

societies have published recommendations for the treatment of community-acquired pneumonia in adults (first line agent for outpatient treatment include macrolides and tetracyclines).

C. **Epidemic measures:** In outbreaks in institutions or in other closed groups, immunization may be carried out unless it is known that the type causing disease is not included in the vaccine.

D. **Disaster implications:** Crowding of populations in temporary shelters bears a risk of disease, especially for the very young and the elderly.

E. **International measures:** None.

II. MYCOPLASMAL PNEUMONIA

(Primary atypical pneumonia)

ICD-9 483; ICD-10 J15.7

1. Identification—Predominantly a febrile lower respiratory infection causing about 20% of pneumonias; less often, a pharyngitis that sometimes progresses to bronchitis or pneumonia. Onset is gradual with headache, malaise, cough (often paroxysmal), sore throat and sometimes chest discomfort that may be pleuritic. Sputum, scant at first, may increase later. Early patchy infiltration of the lungs is often more extensive on X-rays than clinical findings suggest. In severe cases, the pneumonia may progress from one lobe to another and become bilateral. Leukocytosis occurs after the first week in approximately one-third of cases. Duration varies from a few days to a month or more. Secondary bacterial infection and other complications such as CNS involvement and Stevens-Johnson syndrome are infrequent; fatalities are rare.

Differentiation is required from atypical pneumonitis due to many other agents: bacteria, adenoviruses, influenza, respiratory syncytial virus, parainfluenza, measles, Q fever, psittacosis, certain mycoses, severe acute respiratory syndrome (SARS) and tuberculosis.

Diagnosis is based on a rise in antibody titres between acute and convalescent sera; titres rise after several weeks. The ESR is almost always high. Nonspecific development of cold hemagglutinins may occur in up to two-thirds of hospitalized cases; the level of titre increase may reflect the severity of disease. Rapid diagnosis through PCR and direct immunofluorescence assay (IFA) using throat swabs/sputum is possible in some countries. The infectious agent may be cultured on special media.

2. Infectious agent—*Mycoplasma pneumoniae* belongs to the Mycoplasmas (Molicutes), placed between bacteria and viruses. Mycoplasmas lack cell walls, cell wall synthesis inhibitors such as the penicillins and cephalosporines are therefore not effective in treatment. With *Streptococ-*

cus pneumoniae and *Haemophilus influenzae, Mycoplasma pneumoniae* is one of the most common agents of community-acquired pneumonia.

3. Occurrence—Worldwide; sporadic, endemic and occasionally epidemic, especially in institutions and military populations. Outbreaks often occur in schools and households. Attack rates vary from 5 to more than 50/1000/year in military populations and 1 to 3/1000/year in civilians. Epidemics occur more often in late summer and autumn; endemic disease is not seasonal, but there can be variation from year to year and among different geographic areas. Men and women of all ages are equally affected. The disease is asymptomatic or mild in children under 5; recognized disease is most frequent among school-age children and young adults.

4. Reservoir—Humans.

5. Mode of transmission—Probably droplet inhalation, direct contact with an infected person (probably including those with subclinical infections) or with articles freshly soiled with nose and throat discharges from an acutely ill and coughing patient. Secondary cases of pneumonia among contacts, family members and attendants are frequent.

6. Incubation period—6 to 32 days.

7. Period of communicability—Probably less than 20 days. Treatment does not eradicate the organism from the respiratory tract, where it may persist for as long as 13 weeks.

8. Susceptibility—Clinical pneumonia occurs in about 3%–30% of infections with *M. pneumoniae*. Disease varies from mild afebrile pharyngitis to febrile illness of the upper or lower respiratory tract. Duration of immunity is uncertain. Second attacks of pneumonia may occur. Resistance has been correlated with humoral antibodies that persist up to 1 year.

9. Methods of control—

> **A. Preventive measures:** Avoid crowded living and sleeping quarters whenever possible, especially in institutions, barracks and ships.

> **B. Control of patient, contacts and the immediate environment:**

> 1) Report to local health authority: Obligatory report of epidemics in some countries; no individual case report, Class 4 (see Reporting).
> 2) Isolation: Not applicable. Respiratory secretions may be infectious.

3) Concurrent disinfection: Of discharges from nose and throat. Terminal cleaning.
4) Quarantine: Not applicable.
5) Immunization of contacts: Not applicable.
6) Investigation of contacts and source of infection allows for treatment of clinical disease among family members.
7) Specific treatment: Erythromycin or other macrolides, or a tetracycline. Erythromycin or other macrolides are preferred for children under 9 to avoid tetracycline staining of immature teeth. Neither antibiotic eliminates organisms from the pharynx; treatment may select erythromycin-resistant mycoplasmas. Ketolides, a new class of antibiotics, may be useful.

C. *Epidemic measures:* No reliably effective measures for control are available.

D. *Disaster implications:* None.

E. *International measures:* WHO Collaborating Centres.

III. *PNEUMOCYSTIS*
PNEUMONIA   ICD-9 136.3; ICD-10 B59
(Interstitial plasma-cell pneumonia, PCP)

1. Identification—An acute to subacute, often fatal, pulmonary disease, especially in malnourished, chronically ill and premature infants. In older children and adults, opportunistic illness associated with diseases of the immune system and the use of immunosuppressants. It can be a major problem for people with HIV infection, although incidence has fallen with the use of highly active antiretroviral therapy (HAART). Clinically, there is progressive dyspnoea, tachypnoea and cyanosis; sometimes without fever. About 60% of patients have non-productive cough; productive cough is less common. Auscultatory signs, other than rales, are usually minimal or absent. Chest X-ray images typically show bilateral hilar-dominant diffuse interstitial infiltrates.

Demonstration of the causative agent in material from bronchial brushings, open lung biopsy and lung aspirates or in smears of tracheobronchial mucus establishes the diagnosis. IFA, or staining with methenamine silver, toluidine blue O, Giemsa, Gram-Weigert, cresyl-echt-violet identify the organisms. There is no satisfactory routine culture method or serological test at present.

2. Infectious agent—*Pneumocystis carinii.* Generally considered a protozoan parasite; recent studies have shown that its DNA sequence closely resembles that of a fungus.

3. Occurrence—Worldwide; may be endemic and epidemic in debilitated, malnourished or immunosuppressed infants. It affected approximately 60% of patients with HIV infection in the USA, Europe and Australia before the routine use of prophylactic medication and HAART.

4. Reservoir—Humans. Organisms have been demonstrated in rodents, cattle, dogs and other animals, but the ubiquitous presence of the organism and its subclinical persistence in man renders these potential animal sources of human infection of little public health significance.

5. Mode of transmission—Airborne animal-to-animal transmission has occurred in rats. The mode of transmission in people is not known. In one USA study, approximately 75% of normal individuals were reported to have humoral antibody to *P. carinii* by the age of 4, suggesting that subclinical infection is common. Pneumonitis in the compromised host may result from either a reactivation of latent infection or a newly acquired infection.

6. Incubation period—Unknown. Analysis of data from institutional outbreaks and animal studies indicates that the onset of disease often occurs 1–2 months after establishment of the immunosuppressed state.

7. Period of communicability—Unknown

8. Susceptibility—Susceptibility is enhanced by prematurity, chronic debilitating illness and disease or treatments that impair immune mechanisms. Infection with HIV is a predominant risk factor.

9. Methods of control—

    A. Preventive measures: Among immunosuppressed patients, especially those with HIV infection, those treated for lymphatic leukaemia and those with organ transplants, prophylaxis with either oral trimethoprim-sulfamethoxazole or aerosolized pentamidine and atovaquone is effective—for as long as the patient receives the drug—in preventing endogenous reactivation.

    B. Control of patient, contacts and the immediate environment:

        1) Report to local health authority: Official report not ordinarily justifiable, Class 5; when cases occur in people with evidence of HIV infection, case report may be required in some countries, Class 2 (see Reporting).

        2) Isolation: Not applicable.

        3) Concurrent disinfection: Insufficient knowledge.

        4) Quarantine: Not applicable.

        5) Immunization of contacts: Not applicable.

        6) Investigation of contacts and source of infection: Not applicable.

        7) Specific treatment: Trimethoprim-sulfamethoxazole is the drug of choice. Alternate drugs are pentamidine (IM or IV), dapsone-trimethoprim, atovaquone, clindamycin-primaquine

and trimeterxate with leucovorin; several drugs are currently under intensive evaluation.

C. *Epidemic measures:* Knowledge of the source and mode of transmission is so incomplete that there are no generally accepted measures.

D. *Disaster implications:* None.

E. *International measures:* None.

IV. CHLAMYDIAL PNEUMONIAS
IV.A. PNEUMONIA DUE TO *CHLAMYDIA TRACHOMATIS*   ICD-9 482.8; ICD-10 P23.1
(Neonatal eosinophilic pneumonia, Congenital pneumonia due to *Chlamydia*)

1. Identification—A subacute chlamydial pulmonary disease occurring in early infancy among infants whose mothers have chlamydial infection of the uterine cervix. Clinically, the disease is characterized by insidious onset, cough (characteristically staccato), lack of fever, patchy infiltrates on chest X-ray with hyperinflation, eosinophilia and elevated IgM and IgG. About half of infant cases show prodromal rhinitis and conjunctivitis. Duration of illness is commonly 1–3 weeks but may extend as long as 2 months. The spectrum of illness is broad, ranging from rhinitis to severe pneumonia. Many infants with pneumonia ultimately develop asthma or obstructive lung disease.

Diagnosis is usually made by direct IF technique. Definition of the infecting immunotype is based on cell culture isolation of the causative agent from the posterior nasopharynx or demonstration of specific serum antibody at a titre of 1:32 or greater by micro-IF. A high titre of specific IgG antibody supports the diagnosis.

2. Infectious agent—*Chlamydia trachomatis* of immunotypes D to K (excluding immunotypes that cause lymphogranuloma venereum).

3. Occurrence—Probably coincides with the worldwide distribution of genital chlamydial infection. The disease has been recognized in many countries. Epidemics have not been recognized.

4. Reservoir—Humans. Experimental infection with *C. trachomatis* has been induced in nonhuman primates and mice; animal infections are not known to occur in nature.

5. Mode of transmission—From the infected cervix to an infant during birth, with resultant nasopharyngeal infection (and occasionally chlamydial conjunctivitis). Respiratory transmission has not been established.

6. Incubation period—Not known; pneumonia may occur in infants from 1 to 18 weeks of age (more commonly between 4 and 12 weeks). Nasopharyngeal infection is usually not recognized before 2 weeks of age.

7. Period of communicability—Unknown.

8. Susceptibility—Unknown. Maternal antibody does not protect the infant from infection.

9. Methods of control—

   A. Preventive measures: See Chlamydial Conjunctivitis (Conjunctivitis, section IV).

   B. Control of patient, contacts and the immediate environment:

   1) Report to local health authority: Official report not ordinarily justifiable, Class 5 (see Reporting).
   2) Isolation: Universal precautions in hospitals and nurseries.
   3) Concurrent disinfection: Of discharges from nose and throat.
   4) Quarantine: Not applicable.
   5) Immunization of contacts: Not applicable.
   6) Investigation of contacts and source of infection: Examine parents for infection and treat if positive.
   7) Specific treatment: Oral erythromycin (50 mg/kg/day) is the drug of choice for these infants. Sulfisoxazole is a possible alternative.

   C. Epidemic measures: No epidemic occurrence recognized.

   D. Disaster implications: None.

   E. International measures: None.

IV.B. PNEUMONIA DUE TO *CHLAMYDIA PNEUMONIAE*   ICD-9 482.8; ICD-10 J16.0

1. Identification—An acute chlamydial respiratory disease with cough, frequently a sore throat and hoarseness, and fever at the onset; sputum is scanty and chest pain is rare. Inflammatory signs are sometimes not obvious. Pulmonary rales are usually present. The clinical picture is similar to other atypical pneumonias. Radiographic abnormalities include bilateral infiltrates, sometimes with pleural effusions. Age distribution has 2 peaks: one in the pediatric population and one in those aged 60 or over. Outbreaks in community, household, daycare centers, and schools are often reported. Illness is usually mild, but recovery is slow, with cough persisting for 2–6 weeks; in older adults, bronchitis and sinusitis may become chronic. Death is very rare in uncomplicated cases.

Laboratory diagnosis is primarily serological: the CF test detects antibodies to chlamydia group antigens, and a specific micro-IF test for IgM and IgG (on sera obtained 3 weeks after initial infection) identifies antibodies to the agent. In cases of reinfection, IgG antibodies appear early and rise to a high level. Those treated early with tetracycline may have a poor antibody response. The organism can be isolated from throat swab specimens in the yolk sac of embryonated eggs, and cultured in special cell lines.

2. Infectious agent—*Chlamydia pneumoniae*, strain TWAR, is the species name for the organism with distinct morphological and serological differences from *C. psittaci* and *C. trachomatis*.

3. Occurrence—Presumably worldwide. Antibodies are rare in children under 5; prevalence increases among teenagers and young adults to a plateau of about 50% by age 20-30; prevalence remains high into old age. While clinical disease is encountered most frequently in young adults, disease has occurred in all age groups. No seasonality has been noted.

4. Reservoir—Presumably humans. No avian association has been found; no isolations or antibodies were found in pigeons and other birds captured at the site of an outbreak, nor in dogs or cats.

5. Mode of transmission—Not defined; possibilities include direct contact with secretions, spread via fomites and airborne spread.

6. Incubation period—Unknown; may be 3-4 weeks.

7. Period of communicability—Not defined but presumably long; some military outbreaks have lasted as long as 8 months.

8. Susceptibility—Presumably universal with increased likelihood of clinical disease in the presence of pre-existing chronic disease. Serological evidence of recall type immune response suggests immunity after infection; second episodes of pneumonia have been observed in military recruits, with a secondary type of serological response to the second attack.

9. Methods of control—

   A. Preventive measures:

   1) Avoid crowding in living and sleeping quarters.
   2) Apply personal hygiene measures: cover mouth when coughing and sneezing, dispose of discharges from mouth and nose in a sanitary manner and wash hands frequently.

   B. Control of patient, contacts and the immediate environment:

   1) Report to local health authority: Obligatory report of epidemics; no individual case report, Class 4 (see Reporting).

2) Isolation: Not applicable. Universal precautions should be practised.
3) Concurrent disinfection: Of discharges from nose and throat.
4) Quarantine: Not applicable.
5) Immunization of contacts: Not applicable.
6) Investigation of contacts and source of infection: Examine all members of the family for infection and treat if positive.
7) Specific treatment: A definite diagnosis is difficult at the early stages of illness, and empirical treatment should be based on the clinical picture. Oral tetracycline or erythromycin, 2 grams/day for 10–14 days. The new macrolides, azithromycin and clarithromycin may also be used, as can the new fluoroquinolones.

C. Epidemic measures: Case-finding and appropriate treatment.

D. Disaster implications: None.

E. International measures: None.

OTHER PNEUMONIAS
ICD-9 480, 482;
ICD-10 J12, J13, J15, J16.8, J18

Among the known viruses, adenoviruses, respiratory syncytial virus, parainfluenza viruses and probably others as yet unidentified may produce a pneumonitis. Because these agents cause upper respiratory disease more often than pneumonia, they are presented under Respiratory Disease, Acute Viral. Viral pneumonia occurs in measles, influenza and chickenpox. Infection by *Chlamydia psittaci* is presented as Psittacosis (q.v.). Pneumonia is also caused by infection with rickettsiae (see Q fever) and *Legionella* (see Legionellosis). It can be associated with the invasive phase of nematode infections, such as ascariasis, and with mycoses such as aspergillosis, histoplasmosis and coccidioidomycosis.

Various pathogenic bacteria commonly found in the mouth, nose and throat, such as *Haemophilus influenzae, Staphylococcus aureus, Klebsiella pneumoniae, Streptococcus pyogenes* (group A hemolytic streptococci), *Neisseria meningitidis, Bacteroides species, Moraxella catarrhalis* and anaerobic cocci may produce pneumonia, especially in association with influenza, as superinfection following broad-spectrum antibiotherapy, as a complication of chronic pulmonary disease and after aspiration of gastric contents or tracheostomy. With increased use of antimicrobial and immunosuppressive treatment, pneumonias caused by enteric Gram-negative bacilli have become more common, especially those caused by *Escherichia coli, Pseudomonas aeruginosa* and *Proteus* species. Management depends on the organism involved.

[N. Shindo]

POLIOMYELITIS, ACUTE   ICD-9 045; ICD-10 A80
(Polioviral fever, Infantile paralysis)

1. Identification—A viral infection most often recognized by the acute onset of flaccid paralysis. Poliovirus infection occurs in the GI tract with spread to the regional lymph nodes and, in a minority of cases, to the central nervous system. Flaccid paralysis occurs in less than 1% of poliovirus infections; over 90% of infections are either inapparent or result in a nonspecific fever. Aseptic meningitis occurs in about 1% of infections. A minor illness is recognized in 10% of infections with symptoms including fever, malaise, headache, nausea and vomiting. If the disease progresses to major illness, severe muscle pain and stiffness of the neck and back with flaccid paralysis may occur. The paralysis of poliomyelitis is usually asymmetric, with fever present at the onset. The maximum extent of paralysis is reached in a short period, usually within 3–4 days. The site of paralysis depends on the location of nerve cell destruction in the spinal cord or brain stem. The legs are affected more often than the arms. Paralysis of the respiration and/or swallowing muscles can be life threatening. Some improvement in paralysis may occur during convalescence, but paralysis still present after 60 days is likely to be permanent. Infrequently, recurrence of muscle weakness following recovery may occur many years after the original infection has resolved ("postpolio syndrome"); this is not believed to be related to persistence of the virus itself. Given the progress made towards global eradication, poliomyelitis must now be distinguished from other paralytic conditions by isolation of virus from stool. Other enteroviruses (notably types 70 and 71), echoviruses and coxsackieviruses can cause an illness simulating paralytic poliomyelitis.

The most frequent cause of acute flaccid paralysis (AFP) that must be distinguished from poliomyelitis is Guillain-Barré syndrome (GBS). Paralysis in GBS is typically symmetrical and may progress for periods as long as 10 days. The fever, headache, nausea, vomiting and pleocytosis characteristic of poliomyelitis are usually absent in GBS; high protein and low cell counts in the CSF and sensory changes are seen in the majority of GBS cases. Acute motor axonal neuropathy ("China paralytic syndrome") is an important cause of AFP in northern China and is probably present elsewhere; it is seasonally epidemic and closely resembles poliomyelitis. Fever and CSF pleocytosis are usually absent, but paralysis may persist for several months. Other causes of AFP include transverse myelitis, traumatic neuritis, infectious and toxic neuropathies, tick paralysis, myasthenia gravis, porphyria, botulism, insecticide poisoning, polymyositis, trichinosis and periodic paralysis.

Differential diagnosis of acute nonparalytic poliomyelitis includes other forms of acute nonbacterial meningitis, purulent meningitis, brain abscess, tuberculous meningitis, leptospirosis, lymphocytic choriomeningitis, infectious mononucleosis, the encephalitides, neurosyphilis and toxic encephalopathies.

Definitive laboratory diagnosis requires isolation of the wild poliovirus from stool samples, CSF or oropharyngeal secretions in cell culture systems of human or monkey origin (primate cells). Specialized laboratories can differentiate "wild" from vaccine virus strains. Rises in antibody levels (4-fold or greater) are now less helpful in the diagnosis of wild poliomyelitis infection, since type-specific neutralizing antibodies may already be present when paralysis develops and significant titre rises may not be demonstrable in paired sera. Furthermore, the antibody response following immunization mimics the response following infection with wild type viruses and the widespread use of live polio vaccines makes interpretation of antibody levels difficult, although it may help in ruling out polio in cases where no antibody has developed in immunocompetent children.

2. **Infectious agent**—Poliovirus (genus *Enterovirus*) types 1, 2 and 3; all types can cause paralysis. Type 1 is isolated from paralytic cases most often and type 3 less so. Circulating wild type 2 poliovirus has not been detected since October 1999. Type 1 most frequently causes epidemics. Most vaccine-associated cases are due to type 2 or 3.

3. **Occurrence**—Prior to the advent of immunization, poliomyelitis occurred worldwide. As a result of improved immunization worldwide and the global initiative to eradicate poliomyelitis, circulation of polioviruses is limited to a decreasing number of countries. The last culture-confirmed cases of poliomyelitis due to indigenous wild poliovirus were detected in the Western Hemisphere in Peru in August 1991, in the WHO Region of the Western Pacific (Cambodia) in 1997, and in Europe (Turkey) in November 1998. Poliomyelitis may be on the verge of worldwide eradication: only 7 countries remained endemic at end 2002 (Afghanistan, Egypt, India, Niger, Nigeria, Pakistan, Somalia). The greatest risks of polio are now on the Indian subcontinent (89% of cases in 2002) and in West Africa (10% of cases in 2002).

Although wild poliovirus transmission has ceased in the majority of countries, importation remains a threat. A large outbreak of poliomyelitis occurred in 1992–1993 in the Netherlands among members of a religious group that refuse immunization. The virus was also found among members of a related religious group in Canada, although no cases occurred. Imported wild poliovirus has recently caused paralytic cases in countries as diverse as Algeria, Bulgaria, Burkina Faso, Georgia, Ghana, the Islamic Republic of Iran, Lebanon, Togo and Zambia. With the exception of rare imported cases, the few cases of poliomyelitis recognized in industrialized countries, until recent changes in immunization policy, were caused by vaccine virus strains. About half the vaccine-associated paralytic poliomyelitis (VAPP) cases occurred among adult contacts of vaccinees.

Historically, in endemic areas, cases of poliomyelitis occurred both sporadically and as epidemics, with an increase during the late summer and autumn in temperate countries. In tropical countries, a less pronounced seasonal peak occurred in the hot and rainy season.

Poliomyelitis remains primarily a disease of infants and young children. In the few remaining endemic countries, 80%–90% of cases are under 3 and virtually all cases are under 5. Clusters of susceptible persons, including groups that refuse immunization, minority populations, migrants and other unregistered children, nomads, refugees and urban poor are at high risk.

4. Reservoir—Humans, most frequently people with inapparent infections, especially children. No long-term carriers of wild type poliovirus has been detected.

5. Mode of transmission—Primarily person-to-person spread, principally through the fecal-oral route; virus is detectable more easily and for a longer period in feces than in throat secretions. Where sanitation levels are high, pharyngeal spread may be relatively more important. In rare instances, milk, foodstuffs and other materials contaminated with feces have been incriminated as vehicles. No reliable evidence of spread by insects exists; water and sewage are rarely implicated.

6. Incubation period—Commonly 7–14 days for paralytic cases; reported range of 3 to possibly 35 days.

7. Period of communicability—Not precisely defined, but transmission is possible as long as the virus is excreted. Poliovirus is demonstrable in throat secretions as early as 36 hours and in feces 72 hours after exposure to infection in both clinical and inapparent cases. Virus typically persists in the throat for approximately 1 week and in feces for 3–6 weeks. Cases are most infectious during the days before and after onset of symptoms.

8. Susceptibility—Susceptibility to infection is universal; paralysis occurs in only about 1% of infections. Residual paralysis is observed in 0.1% to 1% of cases, depending on the virulence of the strain and perhaps on genetic factors. The rate of paralysis among infected nonimmune adults is higher than that among nonimmunized infants and young children. Type-specific immunity, apparently of lifelong duration, follows both clinically recognizable and inapparent infections. Second attacks are rare and result from infection with a poliovirus of a different type. Infants born of immune mothers have transient passive immunity.

Intramuscular injections, trauma or surgery during the incubation period or prodromal illness may provoke paralysis in the affected extremity. Tonsillectomy increases the risk of bulbar involvement. Excessive muscular activity in the prodromal period may predispose to paralysis.

9. **Methods of control—**

A. *Preventive measures:*

1) Educate the public on the advantages of immunization in early childhood.

2) Both a trivalent live, attenuated oral poliovirus vaccine (OPV) and an injectable, inactivated poliovirus vaccine (IPV) are commercially available. Their use varies in different circumstances.

OPV simulates natural infection by inducing both circulating antibody and resistance to infection of the pharynx and intestine, and also immunizes some susceptible contacts through secondary spread. In developing countries, lower rates of seroconversion and reduced vaccine efficacy for OPV have been reported; this can be overcome by administration of numerous extra doses in immunization programs and/or supplemental campaigns. Breastfeeding does not cause a significant reduction in the protection provided by OPV. WHO recommends the use of OPV alone for immunization programs in developing countries because of low cost, ease of administration and superior capacity to provide population immunity through community spread.

IPV, like OPV, provides excellent individual protection by inducing circulating antibody that blocks the spread of virus to the CNS. Although IPV also protects against pharyngeal infection, it does not induce intestinal immunity of the level induced by OPV. Many industrialized countries, including the USA, switched to IPV alone for routine immunization when it was clear that wild type polioviruses had been eliminated.

Since OPV was introduced 40 years ago, 19 individuals with underlying primary immune deficiency disorders have been identified who excreted an OPV-derived poliovirus for longer than 6 months. As of June 2003 only 2 were known to continue to excrete. The significance of these cases with regard to the possibility of eventually stopping poliomyelitis immunization is under review and studies are in place to look for instances in developing countries. No secondary cases were associated with long-term excretors of vaccine-derived polioviruses.

More troublesome have been epidemics of poliomyelitis caused by vaccine-derived polio viruses, which are often recombinants with other neurovirulent enteric viruses capable of spreading through populations. These viruses become manifest in non-vaccinated or incompletely vaccinated individuals. The extent of this problem is being evaluated.

3) Recommendations for routine immunization:

In developing countries, WHO recommends 4 doses of OPV at 6, 10 and 14 weeks of age, with an additional dose at birth or at the measles contact (usually 9 months of age), depending on the endemicity and/or risk of polio in the country. In endemic countries, WHO recommends the use of national supplemental immunization campaigns administering 2 doses of OPV, 1 month apart, to all children under 5 regardless of prior immunization status. These campaigns should be conducted during the cool, dry season to achieve maximum effect. On the attainment of a high level of control in a country, targeted house-to-house mop-up immunization campaigns in high-risk areas are recommended to interrupt the final chains of transmission.

Where polio is still endemic or at high risk of importation and spread, WHO recommends the use of OPV for all infants, including those who may be infected with HIV. Diarrhea is not a contraindication to OPV. In industrialized countries, contraindications to OPV frequently include congenital immunodeficiency (B-lymphocyte deficiency, thymic dysplasia), current immunosuppressive treatment, disease states associated with immunosuppression (e.g. lymphoma, leukaemia, and generalized malignancy) and the presence of immunodeficient individuals in the household of potential vaccine recipients. IPV should be used in such people.

OPV causes paralytic poliomyelitis in vaccine recipients or their healthy contacts at a rate of approximately one in every 2.5 million doses administered, or 1 in 800 000 first vaccinations. In Romania, multiple injections of antibiotics were associated with an increased risk of vaccine-associated poliomyelitis (VAPP).

With progress towards the international goal of eradication, the risk profile of paralytic poliomyelitis is changing, particularly in industrialized and high/middle income countries. Many of these have decided that the risks of paralytic poliomyelitis due to adverse events associated with continued use of OPV in routine immunization are greater than those due to the handling or circulation of wild poliovirus, and have adopted one of 2 approaches to prevent or minimize immunization-related adverse events: 1) replacement of OPV by inactivated poliovirus vaccine (IPV) for routine immunization 2) introduction of a mixed OPV/IPV schedule. For example, effective January 2000, all children in the USA were to receive 4 doses of IPV at ages 2, 4, 6-18 months and 4-6 years. In those countries, OPV is now reserved only for circumstances such as mass campaigns to control possible outbreaks

Immunization of adults: Routine immunization for adults is not considered necessary. Primary immunization is advised for previously nonimmunized adults travelling to endemic countries, members of communities or population groups in which poliovirus disease is present, laboratory workers handling specimens containing poliovirus, and health care workers who may be exposed to patients excreting wild type polioviruses. In most industrialized countries, IPV is recommended for adult primary immunization; e.g. 2 doses at 1–2 months interval and a third dose 6–12 months later. Those having previously completed a course of immunization and currently at increased risk of exposure are often given an additional dose of IPV.

B. Control of patient, contacts and the immediate environment:

1) Report to local health authority: Obligatory case report of paralytic cases as a Disease under surveillance by WHO, Class 1. In countries undertaking poliomyelitis eradication, each case of acute flaccid paralysis (AFP), including Guillain-Barré syndrome, in children under 15 years must be reported and fully investigated. Results of virus culture of stools, demographic information, immunization history, clinical examination and examination for residual paralysis after 60 days will be covered in supplemental reports. Immunization history should be recorded. Nonparalytic cases are also reported to the local health authority, Class 2 (see Reporting).

2) Isolation: Enteric precautions in the hospital for wild virus disease; of little value under home conditions because many household contacts are infected before poliomyelitis has been diagnosed.

3) Concurrent disinfection: Throat discharges, feces and articles soiled therewith. In communities with modern and adequate sewage disposal systems, feces and urine can be discharged directly into sewers without preliminary disinfection. Terminal cleaning.

4) Quarantine: Of no community value.

5) Protection of contacts: Immunization of familial and other close contacts is recommended but may not contribute to immediate control; the virus has often infected susceptible close contacts by the time the initial case is recognized.

6) Investigation of contacts and source of infection: Occurrence of a single case of poliomyelitis due to wild poliovirus must be recognized as a public health emergency prompting immediate investigation and planning for a large-scale response. A thorough search for additional cases of AFP in the

area around the case assures early detection, facilitates control and permits appropriate treatment of unrecognized and unreported cases.

7) Specific treatment: None; attention during acute illness to complications of paralysis requires expert knowledge and equipment, especially for patients in need of respiratory assistance. Physical therapy is used to attain maximum function after paralytic poliomyelitis and can prevent many deformities that are late manifestations of the illness.

C. *Epidemic measures:* In any country, a single case of poliomyelitis must now be considered a public health emergency, requiring an extensive supplementary immunization response over a large geographic area.

D. *Disaster implications:* Overcrowding of nonimmune groups and collapse of the sanitary infrastructure pose an epidemic threat.

E. *International measures:*

1) Poliomyelitis is a Disease under surveillance by WHO and is targeted for eradication by 2005. National health administrations are expected to inform WHO immediately of individual cases and to supplement these reports as soon as possible with details of the nature and extent of virus transmission. Planning a large scale immunization response must begin immediately and, if epidemiologically appropriate, in coordination with bordering countries. Primary isolation of the virus is often best accomplished in a laboratory designated to be part of the Global Polio Eradication Laboratory Network. Once a wild poliovirus is isolated, molecular epidemiology can often help trace the source. Countries should submit monthly reports on case of poliomyelitis AFP cases and AFP surveillance performance to their respective WHO offices.

   An independent international commission has certified that no locally acquired cases of polio have occurred in the Americas since August 1991. Subsequently, independent international commissions have also certified the WHO Regions of the Western Pacific and Europe as polio-free in the years 2000 and 2002, respectively.

2) International travellers visiting areas of high prevalence must be adequately immunized.

3) WHO Collaborating Centres. Further information on http://www.who.int/gpv/

[R. B. Aylward]

PSITTACOSIS   ICD-9 073; ICD-10 A70
(*Chlamydia psittaci* infection, Ornithosis, Parrot fever, Avian chlamydiosis)

   1. Identification—Acute generalized chlamydial disease with variable clinical presentations; fever, headache, rash, myalgia, chills and upper or lower respiratory tract disease are common. Respiratory symptoms are often mild when compared with the extensive pneumonia demonstrable by X-ray examination. Cough is initially absent or nonproductive; when present, sputum is mucopurulent and scant. Pleuritic chest pain and splenomegaly occur infrequently; pulse may be slow in relation to temperature. Encephalitis, myocarditis and thrombophlebitis are occasional complications; relapses may occur. Although usually mild or moderate, human disease can be severe, especially in untreated elderly persons.

   The diagnosis may be suspected in patients with appropriate symptoms, a history of exposure to birds and elevated or increasing antibody titres to chlamydial antigens in sera collected 2–3 weeks apart. Isolation of the infectious agent from sputum, blood or postmortem tissues in mice, eggs or cell culture, under safe laboratory conditions only, confirms the diagnosis. Recovery of the agent may be difficult, especially if the patient has received broad-spectrum antibiotics.

   2. Infectious agent—*Chlamydia psittaci*.

   3. Occurrence—Worldwide. May be associated with obviously sick or apparently healthy pet birds. Outbreaks occasionally occur in households, pet shops, aviaries, avian exhibits and pigeon lofts. Most human cases are sporadic; many infections are probably not diagnosed.

   4. Reservoir—Mainly in birds of the parrot family (a.k.a. psittacine birds—including parakeets, parrots and love birds); less often in poultry, pigeons, canaries and sea birds. Apparently healthy birds can be carriers and shed the infectious agent, particularly when subjected to stress through crowding and shipping.

   5. Mode of transmission—By inhaling the agent from desiccated droppings, secretions and dust from feathers of infected birds. Imported psittacine birds are the most frequent source of exposure, followed by turkey and duck farms; processing and rendering plants have also been sources of occupational disease. Geese and pigeons are occasionally responsible for human disease. Laboratory infections can occur. Rarely, person-to-person transmission may occur during acute illness with paroxysmal coughing; these cases may have been caused by the recently described *C. pneumoniae* rather than *C. psittaci*.

6. Incubation period—From 1 to 4 weeks.

7. Period of communicability—Birds (diseased or seemingly healthy) may shed the agent intermittently, and sometimes continuously, for weeks or months.

8. Susceptibility—Susceptibility is general, post-infection immunity incomplete and transitory. Older adults may be more severely affected. There is no evidence that persons with antibodies are protected.

9. Methods of control—

A. Preventive measures:

1) Educate the public to the danger of exposure to infected pet birds. Medical personnel responsible for occupational health in processing plants should be aware that febrile respiratory illness with headache or myalgia among the employees may be psittacosis.

2) Regulate the importation of, raising of and trafficking in birds of the parrot family. Prevent or eliminate avian infections through quarantine and appropriate antibiotics.

3) Psittacine birds offered for sale should be raised under psittacosis-free conditions and handled in such manner as to prevent infection. Tetracyclines can be effective in controlling disease in psittacines and other companion birds if properly administered to ensure adequate intake for at least 30 and preferably 45 days.

4) Conduct surveillance of pet shops and aviaries where psittacosis has occurred or where birds epidemiologically linked to cases were obtained, and of farms or processing plants to which human psittacosis was traced. Infected birds must be treated or destroyed and the area where they were housed thoroughly cleaned and disinfected with a phenolic compound.

B. Control of patient, contacts and the immediate environment:

1) Report to local health authority: Obligatory case report in many countries, Class 2 (see Reporting).

2) Isolation: Not applicable. Coughing patients should be instructed to cough into paper tissue.

3) Concurrent disinfection: Of all discharges.

4) Quarantine: Of infected farms (or premises with infected birds) until the buildings have been disinfected and diseased birds destroyed or adequately treated with tetracycline.

5) Immunization of contacts: Not applicable.

6) Investigation of contacts and source of infection: Trace origin of suspected birds. If they cannot be killed, ship swab-cultures of their cloacae or droppings to the laboratory in appropriate

transport media and shipping containers, in compliance with postal regulations; after the cultures are taken, the birds should be treated with a tetracycline drug. If they can, immerse bodies after slaughter in 2% phenolic or equivalent disinfectant. Place in plastic bags, close securely and ship frozen (on dry ice) to nearest laboratory capable of isolating *Chlamydia*.

7) Specific treatment: Antibiotics of the tetracycline group, given until 10–14 days after temperature returns to normal. Erythromycin is an alternative when tetracycline is contraindicated (pregnancy, children under 9).

C. Epidemic measures: Cases are usually sporadic or confined to family outbreaks, but epidemics related to infected aviaries or bird suppliers may be extensive. Report outbreaks of avian psittacosis to agriculture and health authorities. In poultry flocks, large doses of tetracycline can suppress, but not eliminate, infection and thus may complicate investigations.

D. Disaster implications: None.

E. International measures: Compliance with national regulations to control importation of psittacine birds.

Q FEVER
(Query fever)

ICD-9 083.0; ICD-10 A78

1. Identification—An acute febrile rickettsial disease; onset may be sudden with chills, retrobulbar headache, weakness, malaise and severe sweats. There is considerable variation in severity and duration; infections may be inapparent or present as a nonspecific fever of unknown origin. A pneumonitis may be found on X-ray examination, but cough, expectoration, chest pain and physical findings in the lungs are not prominent. Abnormal liver function tests are common. Acute and chronic granulomatous hepatitis, which can be confused with tuberculous hepatitis, has been reported. Chronic Q fever manifests primarily as endocarditis and this form of the disease can occur in up to half the people with antecedent valvular disease. Q fever endocarditis can occur on prosthetic or abnormal native cardiac valves; these infections may have an indolent course, extending over years, and can present up to 2 years after initial infection. Other rare clinical syndromes, including neurological syndromes, have been described. The case-fatality rate in untreated acute cases is usually less than 1% but has been reported as high as 2.4%; it is negligible in treated cases, except for individuals who develop endocarditis, in whom protracted antibiotic courses are the rule. A post- Q fever fatigue syndrome has been described.

Laboratory diagnosis is made by demonstration of a rise in specific antibodies between acute and convalescent stages by IF or CF, or by IgM detection through IF or ELISA; high antibody titres to phase I of the infective organism may indicate chronic infection, such as endocarditis. Recovery of the infectious agent from blood is diagnostic but poses a hazard to laboratory workers. Q fever Coxiellae may be identified in tissues (liver biopsy or heart valve) by immunostains and EM.

2. Infectious agent—*Coxiella burnetii*, an organism with 2 antigenic phases: the antibodies to phase I antigens are found at lower levels than Phase II antibodies in the acute period and the reverse is true in chronic disease. The organism has unusual stability, can reach high concentrations in animal tissues, particularly placenta, and is highly resistant to many disinfectants.

3. Occurrence—Reported from all continents; the real incidence is greater than that reported because of the mildness of many cases, limited clinical suspicion and nonavailability of testing laboratories. It is endemic in areas where reservoir animals are present, and affects veterinarians, meat workers, sheep (and occasionally dairy) workers and farmers. Epidemics have occurred among workers in stockyards, meatpacking and rendering plants, laboratories and in medical and veterinary centers that use sheep (especially pregnant ewes) in research. Individual cases may occur where no direct animal contact can be demonstrated. Evidence of previous infection is common among researchers working with *C. burnetii* and cases have occurred among casual visitors to such facilities.

4. Reservoir—Sheep, cattle, goats, cats, dogs, some wild mammals (bandicoots and many species of feral rodents), birds and ticks are natural reservoirs. Transovarial and transstadial transmission are common in ticks that participate in wildlife cycles in rodents, larger animals and birds. Infected animals, including sheep and cats, are usually asymptomatic, but shed massive numbers of organisms in placental tissues at parturition.

5. Mode of transmission—Commonly through airborne dissemination of Coxiellae in dust from premises contaminated by placental tissues, birth fluids and excreta of infected animals; in establishments processing infected animals or their byproducts and in necropsy rooms. Airborne particles containing organisms may be carried downwind for a distance of one kilometer or more; contamination also occurs through direct contact with infected animals and other contaminated materials, such as wool, straw, fertilizer and laundry. Raw milk from infected cows contains organisms and may be responsible for some cases. Direct transmission by blood or marrow transfusion has been reported.

6. Incubation period—Depends on the size of the infecting dose; usually 2–3 weeks.

7. Period of communicability—Direct person-to-person transmission occurs rarely, if ever. However, contaminated clothing may be a source of infection.

8. Susceptibility—Susceptibility is general. Immunity following recovery from clinical illness is probably lifelong, with cell-mediated immunity lasting longer than humoral. Antibodies detected by CF persist for 3–5 years: antibodies detected by IF may persist as long as 10–15 years.

9. Methods of control—

A. Preventive measures:

1) Educate persons in high risk occupations (sheep and dairy farmers, veterinary researchers, abbatoir workers) on sources of infection and the necessity for adequate disinfection and disposal of animal products of conception; restrict access to cow and sheep sheds, barns and laboratories with potentially infected animals, and stress the value of inactivation procedures such as pasteurization of milk.

2) Pasteurizing milk from cows, goats and sheep at 62.7°C (145°F) for 30 minutes or at 71.6°C (161°F) for 15 seconds, or boiling, inactivates Q fever Coxiellae.

3) No commercially available vaccine currently in general use (except for Australia and some other coutnries). Immunization with inactivated vaccines prepared from *C. burnetii* phase I-infected yolk sac is useful in protecting laboratory workers and is strongly recommended for those knowingly working with live *C. burnetii*. It should also be considered for abattoir workers and others in hazardous occupations, including those carrying out medical research with pregnant sheep. To avoid severe local reactions, vaccine administration should be preceded by a skin sensitivity test with a small dose of diluted vaccine; vaccine should not be given to individuals with a positive skin or antibody test or a documented history of Q fever. In the USA, vaccine may be obtained from Fort Detrick, Frederick, MD 21702-5009 (301-619-2051).

4) Research workers using pregnant sheep should be identified and enrolled in a health education and surveillance program. This should include a baseline serum evaluation, followed by periodic evaluations. Persons at risk (i.e. those with valvular heart disease, women of childbearing age, persons who are immunosuppressed) should be advised of the risk of serious illness that may result from Q fever. Animals used in research

should also be assessed for Q fever infection through serology. Laboratory clothes must be appropriately bagged and washed to prevent infection of laundry personnel. Sheep-holding facilities should be away from populated areas and measures should be implemented in order to prevent air flow to other occupied areas; no casual visitors should be permitted.

B. Control of patient, contacts and the immediate environment:

1) Report to local health authority: In the USA, in areas where disease is endemic; in many countries not a reportable disease, Class 3 (see Reporting).
2) Isolation: Not applicable.
3) Concurrent disinfection: Of sputum and blood and articles freshly soiled by these substances, using 0.05% hypochlorite, 5% peroxide or a 1:100 solution of a triphenyl-based disinfectant such as Lysol®. Use precautions at postmortem examination of suspected cases in humans or animals.
4) Quarantine: Not applicable.
5) Immunization of contacts: Unnecessary.
6) Investigation of contacts and source of infection: Search for history of contact with sheep, cattle or goats on farms or in research facilities, parturient cats, consumption of raw milk, or direct or indirect association with a laboratory that handles *C. burnetii*.
7) Specific treatment: Acute disease: Tetracyclines (particularly doxycycline) administered orally and continued for 15–21 days; doxycycline and hydroxychloroquine in patients with acute Q fever and valvulopathy. In cases of pregnancy: cotrimoxazole throughout the pregnancy. Chronic disease (endocarditis): Doxycycline in combination with hydroxychloroquine for 18 to 36 months. Surgical replacement of the infected valve may be necessary in some patients for hemodynamic reasons.

C. Epidemic measures: Outbreaks are generally of short duration; control measures are limited essentially to elimination of sources of infection, observation of exposed people and provision of antibiotics to those becoming ill. Detection is particularly important in pregnant women and patients with cardiac valve lesions.

D. Disaster implications: None.

E. International measures: Measures to ensure the safe importation of goats, sheep and cattle, and their products (e.g. wool). WHO Collaborating Centres.

F. Measures in case of deliberate use: *C. burnetii* is easy to produce in animals, can be dessicated and transmitted through aerosol. Armies and organizations have worked on its possible use. Immunocompromised patients, people with valvular diseases and pregnant women should be actively diagnosed and treated.

[D. Raoult]

RABIES   ICD-9 071; ICD-10 A82
(Hydrophobia, Lyssa)

1. Identification—An almost invariably fatal acute viral encephalomyelitis; onset generally heralded by a sense of apprehension, headache, fever, malaise and indefinite sensory changes often referred to the site of a preceding animal bite. Excitability and aerophobia are frequent symptoms. The disease progresses to paresis or paralysis; spasms of swallowing muscles leads to fear of water (hydrophobia); delirium and convulsions follow. Without medical intervention, the usual duration is 2–6 days, sometimes longer; death is often due to respiratory paralysis.

Diagnosis is made through specific FA staining of brain tissue or virus isolation in mouse or cell cultures. Presumptive diagnosis by specific FA staining of frozen skin sections taken from the back of the neck at the hairline. Serological diagnosis based on neutralization tests in mice or cell culture.

2. Infectious agent—Rabies virus, a rhabdovirus of the genus *Lyssavirus*. All members of the genus are antigenically related, but use of monoclonal antibodies and nucleotide sequencing shows differences according to animal species or geographical location of origin. Rabies-related viruses in Africa (Mokola and Duvenhage) have been associated, rarely, with fatal rabies-like human illness. A new lyssavirus, first identified in 1996 in several species of flying foxes and bats in Australia, has been associated with 2 human deaths from rabies-like illnesses. This virus, provisionally named Australian bat lyssavirus, is closely related to, but not identical to classical rabies virus. Some of the illnesses due to rabies related viruses may be diagnosed as rabies by the standard FA test.

3. Occurrence—Worldwide, with an estimated 65 000–87 000 deaths a year, almost all in developing countries, particularly Asia (an estimated 38 000 to 60 000 deaths) and Africa (estimated 27 000 deaths). Most human deaths follow dog bites for which adequate post-exposure prophylaxis was not or could not be provided. In Latin America a regional dog rabies control program coordinated by PAHO since 1981 has led to a reduction by 84% in the number of human deaths with only 56 cases reported in 2001. During the past 10 years drastic decrease of the numbers of human deaths have also been reported by several Asian countries particularly China, Thailand and Viet Nam. Western, central and eastern Europe including the Russian Federation report less than 50 rabies deaths annually. From 1958 through 2000, in the USA, 35 of 57 human deaths from rabies were acquired domestically. Of those infected within the USA, almost all were bat-associated rabies (strain analysis).

Rabies is a disease primarily of animals. The areas currently free of autochthonous rabies in the animal population (excluding bats) include most of Australasia and western Pacific, many countries in Western Europe (insular and continental), part of Latin America including the Caribbean. Dogs transmit urban (or canine) rabies, whereas sylvatic rabies is a disease of wild carnivores and bats, with sporadic spillover to dogs, cats and livestock. In western Europe, fox rabies, once widespread, has decreased considerably since oral rabies immunization of foxes began in the early 1990s. Since 1985 bat rabies cases have been reported in Denmark, Finland, France, Germany, Luxembourg, the Netherlands, Spain, Switzerland and the United Kingdom. In the USA and Canada, wildlife rabies most commonly involves racoons, skunks, foxes, coyotes and bats. There has been a progressive epizootic among racoons in the eastern USA and among coyotes and dogs in south Texas.

4. Reservoir—Wild and domestic Canidae, including dogs, foxes, coyotes, wolves and jackals; also skunks, racoons, mongooses and other biting mammals. In developing countries, dogs remain the principal reservoir. Infected populations of vampire, frugivorous and insectivorous bats occur in Mexico, Central and South America; infected insectivorous bats in Canada, the USA and Europe. Rabbits, opossums, squirrels, chipmunks, rats and mice are rarely infected: their bites rarely call for rabies prophylaxis.

5. Mode of transmission—Virus-laden saliva of rabid animal introduced though a bite or scratch (very rarely into a fresh break in the skin or through intact mucous membranes). Person-to-person transmission is theoretically possible, but rare and not well documented. Organ (corneal) transplants from persons dying of undiagnosed CNS disease have resulted in rabies in the recipients. Airborne spread has been demonstrated in a cave where bats were roosting and in laboratory settings, but this occurs very rarely. Transmission from infected vampire bats to domestic animals is common in Latin America. In the USA, rabid insectivorous bats rarely transmit rabies to terrestrial animals, wild or domestic.

6. Incubation period—Usually 3–8 weeks, rarely as short as 9 days or as long as 7 years; depends on wound severity, wound site in relation to nerve supply and distance from the brain, amount and strain of virus, protection provided by clothing and other factors.

7. Period of communicability—In dogs and cats, usually for 3-7 days before onset of clinical signs (rarely over 4 days) and throughout the course of the disease. Longer periods of excretion before onset of clinical signs (14 days) have been observed with Ethiopian dog rabies strains. In one study, bats shed virus for 12 days before evidence of illness; in another, skunks shed virus for at least 8 days before onset of clinical signs. Skunks may shed virus for up to 18 days before death.

8. Susceptibility—All mammals are susceptible to varying degrees, which may be influenced by the virus strain. Humans are more resistant to infection than several animal species; a study in the Islamic Republic of Iran showed that, of those bitten by proven rabid animals and not treated, about 40% developed the disease.

9. Methods of control—

   A. *Preventive measures:* Many preventive measures are possible at the level of the main animal main host(s) and transmitter(s) of rabies to humans. They are all part of a comprehensive rabies control program.

   1) Register, license and immunize all dogs in enzootic countries; collect and sacrifice ownerless animals and strays. Immunize all cats. Educate pet owners and the public on the importance of restrictions for dogs and cats (e.g. pets must be leashed in congested areas when not confined on owner's premises; strange-acting or sick animals of any species, domestic or wild, should not be picked up/handled; reporting of such animals and of animals that have bitten a person or another animal to police/local health department; confinement and observation of such animals as a preventive measure; wild animals should not be kept as pets). Where dog control is sociologically impractical, repetitive total dog population immunization has been effective.

   2) Maintain active surveillance for rabies in animals. Laboratory capacity should be developed to perform FA testing on all wild animals involved in human or domestic animal exposures and all domestic animals clinically suspected of having rabies. Get physicians, veterinarians and animal control officials to obtain/sacrifice/test animals involved in human and domestic animal exposures.

   3) Detain and clinically observe for 10 days any healthy-appearing dog or cat known to have bitten a person (unwanted dogs and cats may be sacrificed immediately and examined for rabies by fluorescent microscopy); dogs and cats showing suspicious signs of rabies should be sacrificed and tested for rabies. If the biting animal was infective at the time of bite, signs of rabies will usually follow within 4-7 days, with a

change in behaviour and excitability or paralysis, followed by death. All wild mammals that have bitten a person must be sacrificed immediately and the brain examined for evidence of rabies. In the case of bites by a normally behaving valuable pet or zoo animal, it may be appropriate to consider postexposure prophylaxis for the human victim, and, instead of sacrificing the animal, hold it in quarantine for 3–12 weeks.

4) Immediately submit to a laboratory the intact head of animals that die of suspected rabies, packed in ice (not frozen), for viral antigen testing by FA staining, or, if not available, by microscopic examination for Negri bodies, followed by mouse inoculation.

5) Immediately sacrifice unimmunized dogs or cats bitten by known rabid animals; if detention is elected, hold the animal in a secure pound or kennel for at least 6 months under veterinary supervision, and immunize against rabies 30 days before release. If previously immunized, reimmunize and detain (leashing and confinement) for at least 45 days.

6) Oral immunization of wildlife animal reservoirs, using air-drops of bait containing attenuated or recombinant vector vaccine, has eliminated fox rabies from parts of Europe and Canada. The technique is being evaluated within the USA.

7) Cooperative programs with wildlife conservation authorities to reduce fox, skunk, racoon and other terrestrial wildlife hosts of sylvatic rabies may be used in circumscribed enzo-otic areas near campsites and areas of human habitation. If such focal depopulation is undertaken, it must be maintained to prevent repopulation from the periphery.

8) Individuals at high risk (e.g. veterinarians, wildlife conservation personnel and park rangers in enzootic or epizootic areas, staff of quarantine kennels, laboratory and field personnel working with rabies, long-term travellers to rabies-endemic areas) should receive pre-exposure immunization, using potent and safe cell-culture vaccines. Vaccine can be given in 3 doses of 1.0 ml (IM) on days 0, 7 and 21 or 28: Post-immunization serological testing may be advisable for groups at high risk of exposure or immuno-deficient persons. Results with ID immunization for Human Diploid Cell rabies Vaccine (HDCV) have generally been good, but the mean antibody response is somewhat lower and may be of shorter duration than for the 1.0 ml dose given IM. Antibody response to ID immunization has been erratic in some groups on chloroquine for antimalar-ial chemoprophylaxis. Although immune response has not been evaluated for antimalarials structurally related to

chloroquine (e.g. mefloquine, hydroxychloroquine), similar precautions for individuals receiving these drugs should be followed. Other cell-culture vaccines fulfilling WHO requirements for the ID route, such as vero cell vaccine and chick embryo cell vaccine, are widely used in rabies-endemic countries.

If risk of exposure continues, single booster doses are given, or preferably serum is tested for neutralizing antibody every 2 years, with booster doses given when indicated.

9) Prevention of rabies after animal bites ("postexposure prophylaxis") consists of the following (*8th Report of WHO Expert Committee on Rabies*, 1992; Recommendations of the Advisory Committee for Immunization Practices, *MMWR* **48**(RR-1): 1–21, 1999):

a) *First aid:* Clean and flush the wound immediately with soap or detergent and water (or water alone) then apply either 70% ethanol, tincture of aqueous solution of iodine or povidone iodine. The wound should not be sutured unless unavoidable. Sutures, if required, should be placed after local infiltration of antiserum (see 9b); they should be loose and not interfere with free bleeding and drainage.

b) *Specific treatment (serum and vaccine):* Specific immunological protection in humans is provided by administration of human (HRIG) or equine (ERIG) rabies immune globulin at site of bite as soon as possible after exposure to neutralize the virus, and then by giving vaccine at a different site to elicit active immunity. Animal studies suggest that human disease caused by the Australian bat lyssavirus may be prevented by rabies vaccine and rabies immune globulin, and such post-exposure prophylaxis is recommended for persons bitten or scratched by any bat in Australia. Although rabies vaccine may not always be effective for the treatment of African bat lyssaviruses, it should be administered.

Passive immunization: HRIG should be used in a single dose of 20 IU/kg and ERIG in a single dose of 40 IU/kg. As much as possible of this must be infiltrated into and around the bite wound and the rest, if any, given IM. If serum of animal origin is used, an intradermal or subcutaneous test dose should precede its administration to detect allergic sensitivity. Modern cell-culture vaccines should be given in 5 IM doses of 0.5 or 1.0 ml (see manufacturer's instructions) in the deltoid region; to start as soon as possible after exposure and the last dose within 28 days for IM (0, 3, 7, 14, 28) and 90 days for ID (0, 3, 7, 28, 90) vaccination.

Although the ID dose/route at multiple sites has not been approved in the USA, it may be used for postexposure prophylaxis when vaccine is in short supply or out of reach for patients; WHO recommends 2 ID multisite regimens with cell-culture vaccines known to be safe and immunogenic when they are given ID: i) 2-site regimen (2-2-20-1-1); ii) 8-site regimen (8-0-4-0-1-1)—see *WHO Recommendations on Rabies Post-Exposure Treatment and the Correct Technique of Intradermal immunization against Rabies* (http://whqlibdoc.who.int/hq/1996/WHO_EMC_ZOO_96.6.pdf).

In individuals with possible immunodeficiency, a serum specimen should be collected at the time the last dose of vaccine is administered and tested for rabies antibodies. If sensitization reactions appear in the course of immunization, consult the health department or infectious disease consultants for guidance. If the person has had a previous full course of antirabics immunization with an approved vaccine, or had developed neutralizing antibodies after pre-exposure immunization (see 9A8) or after a postexposure regimen, only 2 doses of vaccine need to be given–one immediately and one 3 days later. With severe exposure (e.g. head bites), a third dose may be given on day 7. Neither HRIG nor ERIG is used with this regimen.

c) The combination of local wound treatment, passive immunization with HRIG or ERIG and vaccination is recommended for all severe exposures (category III, see end of this item), virtually guaranteeing complete protection. In the US, passive immunization is standard for all postexposure vaccination. Pregnancy and infancy are never contraindications to post-exposure rabies vaccination. Persons presenting even months after the bite must be dealt with in the same way as recent exposures. Factors to be considered in the initiation of post-exposure treatment are: nature of the contact; rabies endemicity at site of encounter or origin of animal; animal species involved; vaccination/clinical status and availability of animal for observation plus type of vaccine used; laboratory results of animal for rabies if available.

d) Immunization with current rabies vaccines has occasionally been followed by Guillain-Barré syndrome, but too rarely to be certain of causal association. Local reactions, such as pain, erythema, swelling or itching at the injection site have been reported in 25% of those receiving 5 doses of 1.0 ml. Mild systemic reactions of headache, nausea, muscle aches, abdominal pain and dizziness were reported in about 20%. "Serum sickness-like" reactions, including primarily urticaria with generalized itching and wheezing, have been reported infrequently.

Among those receiving booster doses for pre-exposure prophylaxis, hypersensitivity reactions occur in approximately 6% of recipients 2–21 days after HDCV, presenting as a generalized pruritic rash, urticaria, possible arthralgia, arthritis, angioedema, nausea, vomiting, fever and malaise. These symptoms have responded to antihistamines; a few have required corticosteroids or epinephrine. Persons exposed to rabies who develop these symptoms should complete the required number of injections using a rabies vaccine prepared with another cell type. This reaction has not been definitely associated with other rabies vaccines. Systemic allergic reactions in those receiving booster doses have been rare. No significant adverse reactions have been attributed to HRIG; however, antiserum from a nonhuman source produces serum sickness in 5%–40% of recipients. Newer commercially produced purified animal globulins, in particular equine globulin, have only a 1% risk of adverse reactions. The risk of contracting fatal rabies usually outweighs the risks of allergic reactions.

B. Control of patient, contacts and the immediate environment:

1) Report to local health authority: Obligatory case report required in most countries, Class 2 (see Reporting).
2) Isolation: Contact isolation for respiratory secretions for duration of the illness.
3) Concurrent disinfection: Of saliva and articles soiled therewith. Although transmission from a patient to attending personnel has not been documented, immediate attendants should be warned of the potential hazard of infection from saliva, and wear rubber gloves, protective gowns, and protection to avoid exposure from a coughing patient.
4) Quarantine: Not applicable.
5) Immunization of contacts: Contacts who have an open wound or mucous membrane exposure to the patient's saliva must receive specific antirabies treatment (see 9A9b).
6) Investigation of contacts and source of infection: Search for rabid animal and for people and other animals bitten.
7) Specific treatment: For clinical rabies, intensive supportive medical care.

C. Epidemic (epizootic) measures: Applicable only to animals; a sporadic disease in humans.

1) Establish area control under authority of laws, regulations and ordinances, in cooperation with appropriate wildlife conservation and animal health authorities.
2) Immunize dogs and cats through officially sponsored, intensified mass programs that provide immunizations at temporary and emergency stations. For protection of other domestic animals, use approved vaccines appropriate for each animal species.
3) In urban areas of industrialized countries, strict enforcement of regulations requiring collection, detention and killing of ownerless and stray dogs, and of nonimmunized dogs found off owners' premises; control of the dog population by castration, spaying or drugs have been effective in breaking transmission cycles.
4) Immunization of wildlife through baits containing vaccine has successfully contained fox rabies in western Europe and Canada and is investigated in the USA.

D. Disaster implications: A potential problem if the disease is freshly introduced or enzootic in an area where there are many stray dogs or wild reservoir animals.

E. International measures:

1) Strict compliance by common carriers and travellers with national laws and regulations in rabies-free countries. Immunization of animals, certificates of health and origin, or microchip identification of animals may be required.
2) WHO Collaborating Centres. Further information on http://www.oms2.b3e.jussieu.fr/rabnet

POSTEXPOSURE PROPHYLAXIS GUIDE

Consult local or state health officials if questions arise about the need for rabies prophylaxis. In addition to treatment as described under A9a, b.

WHO recommendations for post-exposure rabies management follow:

Category of exposure	Type of contact with a suspect or confirmed rabid domestic or wild[a] animal or animal unavailable for observation	Recommended treatment
I	Touching or feeding of animal Licks on intact skin	None, if reliable case history available
II	Nibbling of uncovered skin Minor scratches or abrasion without bleeding	Administer vaccine immediately[b] Stop treatment if animal remains healthy throughout observation[c] (10 days) or is killed and found to be negative for rabies by appropriate laboratory techniques
	Licks on broken skin	
III	Single or multiple transdermal bites or scratches	Administer vaccine immediately[b]
	Contamination of mucous membrane with saliva (licks)	Stop treatment if animal remains healthy throughout observation[c] (10 days) or is killed and found to be negative for rabies by appropriate laboratory techniques

[a]Exposure to rodents, rabbits and hares seldom if ever requires specific anti-rabies treatment

[b]The placing of an apparently healthy dog or cat in or from a low-risk area under careful supervision may warrant delaying treatment

[c]Applicable only to dogs and cats. Except for threatened or endangered species, other animals suspected of rabies must be killed and their tissues examined using appropriate laboratory techniques

USA recommendations for post-exposure management follow (ACIP):

Human Rabies Prevention - United States, 1999: Recommendations of Advisory Committee on Immunization Practices (ACIP). *MMWR*, **48**:(RR) 1–21, 1999.

Vaccination Status	Treatment	Regimen*
Not previously vaccinated	Wound cleansing	All postexposure treatment to begin with immediate thorough cleansing of all wounds with soap and water. If available, a virucidal agent such as a povidone-iodine solution should be used to irrigate the wounds.
	HRIG	Administer 20 IU/kg body weight. If anatomically feasible, *the full dose* should be infiltrated around the wound(s); any remaining volume should be administered intramuscularly (IM) at an anatomic site distant from that of vaccine administration. RIG should not be administered in the same syringe as the vaccine. Because HRIG may partially suppress active production of antibody, no more than the recommended dose should be given.
	Vaccine	HDCV, RVA, or PCECV, 1.0 ml, IM (deltoid area[†]), one each on days 0**, 3, 7, 14, and 28.
Previously vaccinated[§]	Wound cleansing	All postexposure treatment to begin with immediate thorough cleansing of all wounds with soap and water. If available, a virucidal agent such as a povidone-iodine solution should be used to irrigate the wounds.
	RIG	RIG should *not* be administered.
	Vaccine	HDCV, RVA (rabies vaccine, adsorbed), or PCEV, 1.0 mL, IM (deltoid area[†]), one each on days 0** and 3.

*Regimens are applicable for all age groups, including children.

[†]The deltoid area is the only acceptable site of vaccination for adults and older children. For younger children, the outer aspect of the thigh may be used. Never administer vaccine in the gluteal area.

**Day 0 is the day the 1st dose of vaccine is administered.

[§]History of pre-exposure vaccination with HDCV, RVA, or PCVEC; prior postexposure prophylaxis with HDCV, RVA, or PCECV; or previous vaccination with any other type of rabies vaccine and a documented history of antibody response to the prior vaccination.

[F. Meslin]

RAT-BITE FEVER   ICD-9 026; ICD-10 A25

The general term of rat-bite fever covers 2 bacterial diseases. Strepto-bacillosis is caused by *Actinobacillus muris* (formerly *Streptobacillus moniliformis* or *Haverbillia multiformis*) and spirillary fever or sodoku by *Spirillum minus* (*minor*). Because of their clinical and epidemiological similarities, only streptobacillosis is presented in detail; variations manifested by *Spirillum minus* infection are noted in a brief summary.

I. STREPTOBACILLOSIS   ICD-9 026.1; ICD-10 A25.1
(Streptobacillary fever, Haverhill fever, Epidemic arthritic erythema)

1. Identification—An abrupt onset of chills and fever, headache and muscle pain, is followed within 1–3 days by a maculopapular rash most marked on the extremities. The rash may also be petechial, purpuric or pustular. One or more large joints usually become swollen, red and painful. There is usually a history of a rat bite within the previous 10 days that healed normally. Relapses are common. Bacterial endocarditis, pericarditis, parotitis, tenosynovitis and focal abscesses of soft tissues or the brain may occur late in untreated cases, with a case-fatality rate of 7%–10%.

Laboratory confirmation is through isolation of the organism by inoculating material from the primary lesion, lymph node, blood, joint fluid or pus into the appropriate bacteriological medium or laboratory animals (guinea pigs or mice that are not naturally infected). Serum antibodies may be detected by agglutination tests.

2. Infectious agent—*Actinobacillus muris* (*Streptobacillus moniliformis*).

3. Occurrence—Worldwide, but uncommon in North and South America and most European countries. Cases have followed bites by laboratory rats and rarely by pet rats.

4. Reservoir—An infected rat, rarely other animals (squirrel, weasel, gerbil).

5. Mode of transmission—Urine or secretions of mouth, nose or conjunctival sac of an infected animal, most frequently introduced through biting. Sporadic cases may occur without history of a bite. Blood from an experimental laboratory animal has infected humans. Direct contact with rats is not necessary; infection has occurred in people working or living in rat-infested buildings. In outbreaks, contaminated milk or water has usually been suspected as the vehicle of infection.

6. **Incubation period**—From 3 to 10 days, rarely longer.

7. **Period of communicability**—No direct person-to-person transmission.

8. **Susceptibility**—No information.

9. **Methods of control**—

A. *Preventive measures:* Rat-proof dwellings and reduce rat populations. Penicillin or doxycycline could be used as prophylaxis following a rat bite.

B. *Control of patient, contacts and the immediate environment:*

1) Report to local health authority: Obligatory report of epidemics in most countries; no case report required, Class 4 (see Reporting).
2) Isolation: No special precautions are recommended.
3) Concurrent disinfection: Not applicable.
4) Quarantine: Not applicable
5) Immunization of contacts: Not applicable
6) Investigation of contacts and source of infection: To establish whether there are additional unrecognized cases.
7) Specific treatment: Penicillin or tetracyclines for 7–10 days.

C. *Epidemic measures:* A cluster of cases requires search for a common source, possibly contaminated food and water.

D. *Disaster implications:* None.

E. *International measures:* None.

II. SPIRILLOSIS   ICD-9 026.0; ICD-10 A25.0
(Spirillary fever, Sodoku, Rat bite fever due to *Spirillum minus*)

Rat bite fever caused by *Spirillum minus* is the common form of sporadic rat bite fever in Asia, predominantly in Japan. Untreated, the case-fatality rate is approximately 10%. Clinically, *Spirillum minus* disease differs from streptobacillary fever in the rarity of arthritic symptoms and the distinctive rash of reddish or purplish plaques. The incubation period is 1–3 weeks, and the previously healed bite wound reactivates when symptoms appear. Laboratory methods are essential for differentiation; animal inoculation is used for isolation of the *Spirillum*.

RELAPSING FEVER   ICD-9 087; ICD-10 A68

1. Identification—A systemic louse-borne epidemic or tick-borne sporadic spirochaetal disease in which periods of fever lasting 2–9 days alternate with afebrile periods of 2–4 days; the number of relapses varies from 1 to 10 or more. Each febrile period terminates by crisis. Total duration of the louse-borne disease averages 13–16 days; usually longer for the tick-borne disease. Transitory petechial rashes are common during the initial febrile period. Symptoms vary with host immunity, strain of *Borrelia* involved and phase of the epidemic. Hematuria is rare but epistaxis has been reported. Gastrointestinal involvement is common; respiratory symptoms are frequently observed in the USA, southern Europe and western Mediterranean countries, and meningeal symptoms in Spain. Neuropsychiatric symptoms are more common in tick-borne than in louse-borne epidemics. Predisposing factors (thiamine and vitamin B deficiency) may lead to neuritis or encephalitis. Severity varies according to individual susceptibility (in Africa infections are severe for Europeans but milder for the local population) and to geography (tick-borne infections may be severe in Egypt, Israel, Lebanon, the Syrian Arab Republic, Pakistan and mild in Poland, Romania and the Russian Federation). The overall case-fatality rate in untreated cases is between 2% and 10%.

Diagnosis is made during the attack through demonstration of the infectious agent in darkfield preparations of fresh blood or stained thick or thin blood films, through intraperitoneal inoculation of laboratory rats or mice with blood taken during the febrile period or through blood culture in special media. Borreliae are usually absent from the blood between relapses.

2. Infectious agents—In louse-borne disease, *Borrelia recurrentis*, a Gram-negative spirochaete. In tick-borne disease, different strains have been distinguished by area of first isolation and/or vector rather than by inherent biological differences. Strains isolated during a relapse often show antigenic differences from those obtained during the immediately preceding paroxysm. The classical agent of relapsing fever in Europe is *B. hispanica*. A "Spain strain" has recently been implicated in severe human disease. New relapsing fever-like spirochetes transmitted by hard ticks (*Ixodes*, *Amblyomma*) cause a tick-associated rash (Master disease) different from that transmitted by soft ticks (*Ornithodoros*).

3. Occurrence—Characteristically, epidemic where spread by lice; endemic where spread by ticks. Louse-borne relapsing fever occurs in limited areas in Asia, eastern Africa (Burundi, Ethiopia and Sudan), highlands of central Africa and South America. Tick-borne disease is endemic throughout tropical Africa, with other foci in India, the Islamic

Republic of Iran, Portugal, Saudi Arabia, Spain, northern Africa, central Asia, as well as North and South America. Sporadic human cases and occasional outbreaks of tick-borne disease occur in limited areas of western Canada and Europe. Relapsing fever has been observed in all parts of the world except Australia and New Zealand.

4. Reservoir—For *B. recurrentis*, humans; for tick-borne relapsing fever Borreliae, wild rodents and argasid (soft) ticks.

5. Mode of transmission—Vector-borne; no direct person-to-person transmission. Louse-borne relapsing fever is acquired by crushing an infective louse, *Pediculus humanus*, so that it contaminates the bite wound or an abrasion of the skin. In tick-borne disease, people are infected by the bite or coxal fluid of an argasid tick, principally *Ornithodoros moubata* and *O. hispanica* in Africa, *O. rudis* and *O. talaje* in Central and South America, *O. tholozani* in the Near and Middle East, *O. hermsi* and *O. turicata* in the USA. These ticks usually feed at night, rapidly engorge and leave the host; they live 2–5 years and remain infective throughout their lifespan.

6. Incubation period—Louse-borne relapsing fever: 5 to 15 days; usually 8 days. A short 2–4 days incubation has been observed in North Africa.

7. Period of communicability—The louse becomes infective 4–5 days after ingestion of blood from an infective person and remains so for life (20–40 days). Infected ticks can live and remain infective for several years without feeding; they pass the infection transovarially to their progeny.

8. Susceptibility—Susceptibility is general. Duration and degree of immunity after clinical attack unknown; repeated infections may occur.

9. Methods of control—

A. Preventive measures:

1) Control lice using measures prescribed for louse-borne typhus fever (see Typhus fever, Epidemic louse-borne, 9A).
2) Control ticks by measures prescribed for Rocky Mountain spotted fever, 9A. Tick-infested human habitations may present problems, and eradication may be difficult. Rodent-proofing structures to prevent future colonization by rodents and their soft ticks is the mainstay of prevention and control. Spraying with approved acaricides such as diazinon, chlorpyrifos, propoxur, pyrethrum or permethrin may be tried.
3) Use personal protective measures, including repellents and permethrin on clothing and bedding for people with expo-

sure in endemic foci. Dimethyl phthalate (5%) and 10% carbolic soap are effective.

4) Antibiotic chemoprophylaxis with tetracyclines may be taken after exposure (arthropod bites) when the risk of acquiring the infection is high. Vaccines against borreliae are not yet available for human use.

B. Control of patient, contacts and the immediate environment:

1) Report to local health authority: Report of louse-borne relapsing fever required as a Disease under Surveillance by WHO, Class 1; tick-borne disease, in selected areas, Class 3 (see Reporting).

2) Isolation: Blood/body fluid precautions. Patients, clothing, household contacts and immediate environment must be deloused or freed of ticks.

3) Concurrent disinfection: Not applicable, if disinfestation has been carried out correctly.

4) Quarantine: Not applicable.

5) Immmunization of contacts: Not applicable.

6) Investigation of contacts and source of infection: For individual tick-borne cases, search for additional associated cases and sources of infection; for louse-borne disease, application of appropriate lousicidal preparation to infested contacts (see Pediculosis, 9B6 and 9B7).

7) Specific treatment: Tetracyclines.

C. Epidemic measures: For louse-borne relapsing fever, when reporting has been good and cases are localized, dust or spray contacts and their clothing with 1% permethrin (residual effect insecticide), and apply permethrin spray at 0.03– 0.3 kg/hectare (2.47 acres) to the immediate environment of all reported cases. Provide facilities for washing clothes and for bathing to affected populations; establish active surveillance. Where infection is known to be widespread, apply permethrin systematically to all people in the community. For tick-borne relapsing fever, apply permethrin or other acaricides to target areas where vector ticks are thought to be present; for sustained control, a treatment cycle of 1 month is recommended during the transmission season. Since animals (horses, camels, cows, sheep, pigs, and dogs) also play a role in tick-borne relapsing fever, persons entering tick-infested areas (hunters, soldiers, vacationers and others) should be educated regarding tick-borne relapsing fever.

D. Disaster implications: A serious potential hazard among louse-infested populations. Epidemics are common in wars, famine and other situations with increased prevalence of pediculosis (e.g. overcrowded, malnourished populations with poor personal hygiene) especially with important population movements.

E. International measures:

1) Prompt notification by governments to WHO and adjacent countries of an outbreak of louse-borne relapsing fever in any areas of their territories, with further information on the source and type of the disease and the number of cases and deaths.

2) Louse-borne relapsing fever is not a disease subject to the International Health Regulations, but WHO considers it a Disease under Surveillance and the measures outlined under 9E1 should be followed.

[D. Hulínská]

RESPIRATORY DISEASE, ACUTE VIRAL
(Excluding influenza)
(Acute viral rhinitis, Pharyngitis, Laryngitis)

Numerous acute respiratory illnesses of known and presumed viral etiology are grouped here. Clinically, infections of the upper respiratory tract (above the epiglottis) can be designated as acute viral rhinitis or acute viral pharyngitis (common cold, upper respiratory infections) and infections involving the lower respiratory tract (below the epiglottis) can be designated as croup (laryngotracheitis), acute viral tracheobronchitis, bronchitis, bronchiolitis or acute viral pneumonia. These respiratory syndromes are associated with a large number of viruses, each of which can produce a wide spectrum of acute respiratory illness and differ in etiology between children and adults.

The illnesses caused by known agents have important common epidemiological attributes, such as reservoir and mode of transmission. Many of the viruses invade any part of the respiratory tract; others show a predilection for certain anatomical sites. Some predispose to bacterial complications. Morbidity and mortality from acute respiratory diseases are especially significant in children. In adults, relatively high incidence and resulting disability, with consequent economic loss, make acute respiratory diseases a major health problem worldwide. As a group, acute respiratory diseases are one of the leading causes of death from any infectious disease.

Several other infections of the respiratory tract are presented as separate chapters because they are sufficiently distinctive in their manifestations and occur in regular association with a single infectious agent: influenza, psittacosis, hantavirus pulmonary syndrome, chlamydial pneumonia, vesicular pharyngitis (herpangina) and epidemic myalgia (pleurodynia) are examples. Particularly in pediatric practice, influenza must be considered in cases of acute respiratory tract disease.

Symptoms of upper respiratory tract infection, mainly pharyngotonsillitis, can be produced by bacterial agents, among whom A streptococcus is the most common. Viral infections should be differentiated from bacterial or other infections for which specific antimicrobial measures are available. For instance, although viral pharyngotonsillitis is more common, group A streptococcal infection should be ruled out by rapid streptococcal antigen test and culture, particularly in children over 2. In nonstreptococcal outbreaks, it is important to identify the cause in a representative sample of cases through appropriate clinical and laboratory methods in order to rule out other diseases (e.g. mycoplasmal pneumonia, chlamydial pneumonia, legionellosis and Q fever) for which specific treatments may be effective.

I. ACUTE VIRAL
RHINITIS–COMMON COLD   ICD-9 460; ICD-10 J00
(Rhinitis, Coryza [acute])

1. Identification—An acute catarrhal infection of the upper respiratory tract characterized by coryza, sneezing, lacrimation, irritation of the nasopharynx, chilliness and malaise lasting 2-7 days. Fever is uncommon in children over 3 and rare in adults. No fatalities have been reported, but disability is important because it affects work performance and industrial and school absenteeism; illness may be accompanied by laryngitis, tracheitis or bronchitis and may predispose to more serious complications such as sinusitis and otitis media. WBC counts are usually normal, and bacterial flora of the respiratory tract within normal limits in the absence of complications.

Cell or organ culture studies of nasal secretions may show a known virus in 20%-35% of cases. Specific clinical, epidemiological and other manifestations aid differentiation from similar diseases due to toxic, allergic, physical or psychological stimuli.

2. Infectious agents—Rhinoviruses, of which there are more than 100 recognized serotypes, are the major known causal agents of the common cold in adults; they account for 20%-40% of cases, especially in the autumn. Coronaviruses, such as 229E, OC43 and B814, are responsible for about 10%-15% and influenza for 10%-15% of the common colds in adults; they appear especially important in the winter and early spring, when the prevalence of rhinoviruses is low. Other known respiratory viruses account for a small proportion of common colds in adults. In infants and children, parainfluenza viruses, respiratory syncytial viruses (RSV), influenza, adenoviruses, certain enteroviruses and coronaviruses cause illnesses similar to common cold. The cause of about half of common colds has not been identified.

3. Occurrence—Worldwide, both endemic and epidemic. In temperate zones, incidence rises in autumn, winter and spring; in tropical settings, incidence is highest in the rainy season. Many people, except in small isolated communities, have 1–6 colds yearly. Incidence is highest in children under 5 years and gradually declines with increasing age.

4. Reservoir—Humans.

5. Mode of transmission—Presumably direct contact or inhalation of airborne droplets; more importantly, indirect transmission through hands and articles freshly soiled by nose and throat discharges of an infected person. Contaminated hands carry rhinovirus, RSV and probably other similar viruses to the mucous membranes of the eye or nose.

6. Incubation period—Between 12 hours and 5 days, usually 48 hours, varying with the agent.

7. Period of communicability—Nasal washings taken 24 hours before onset and for 5 days after onset have produced symptoms in experimentally infected volunteers.

8. Susceptibility—Susceptibility is universal. Inapparent and abortive infections occur; frequency of healthy carriers is undetermined but known to be rare with some viral agents, notably rhinoviruses. Frequently repeated attacks are most likely due to the multiplicity of agents, but may be due to the short duration of homologous immunity against different serotypes of the same virus or to other causes.

9. Methods of control—

A. Preventive measures:

1) Educate the public in personal hygiene, such as frequent handwashing, covering the mouth when coughing and sneezing, and safe disposal of oral and nasal discharges.
2) When possible, avoid crowding in living and sleeping quarters, especially in institutions, in barracks and on board ships. Provide adequate ventilation.
3) Oral live adenovirus vaccines have proven effective against adenovirus 4, 7 and 21 infections in military recruits, but are not indicated in civilian populations because of the low incidence of specific disease.
4) Avoid smoking in households with children, whose risk of pneumonia increases when exposed to passive smoke.

B. Control of patient, contacts and the immediate environment:

1) Report to local health authority: Official report not ordinarily justifiable, Class 5 (see Reporting).

2), 3), 4), 5), 6) and 7): Isolation, Concurrent disinfection, Quarantine, Immunization of contacts, Investigation of contacts and source of infection and Specific treatment: See section II, 9B2 through 9B7.

C, D. and **E. Epidemic measures, Disaster implications** and **International measures:** See section II, 9C, 9D and 9E

II. ACUTE FEBRILE RESPIRATORY
DISEASE   ICD-9 461–466; 480; ICD-10 J01-J06; J12
(Excluding Streptococcal pharyngitis, q.v., JO2.0)

1. Identification—Viral diseases of the respiratory tract may be characterized by fever, cough, increased respiratory rate and one or more systemic reactions, such as chills or chilliness, headache, general aching, malaise and anorexia; occasionally in infants by GI disturbances. Localizing signs also occur at various sites in the respiratory tract, either alone or in combination, such as rhinitis, pharyngitis or tonsillitis, laryngitis, laryngotracheitis, bronchitis, bronchiolitis, pneumonitis or pneumonia. There may be associated conjunctivitis. Symptoms and signs usually subside in 2-5 days without complications; infection may, however, be complicated by bacterial sinusitis, otitis media or more rarely bacterial pneumonia. WBC counts and respiratory bacterial flora are within normal limits unless modified by complications.

In very young infants, it may be difficult to distinguish between pneumonia, sepsis and meningitis. Specific diagnosis depends on isolation of the causal agent from respiratory secretions in appropriate cell or organ cultures, identification of viral antigen in nasopharyngeal cells by FA, ELISA and RIA tests and/or antibody studies of paired sera.

2. Infectious agents—Parainfluenza virus, types 1, 2, 3 and rarely type 4; respiratory syncytial virus (RSV); adenovirus, especially types 1-5, 7, 14 and 21; rhinoviruses; certain coronaviruses; certain types of coxsackievirus groups A and B; and echoviruses are considered etiologic agents of acute febrile respiratory illnesses. Influenza virus (see Influenza) can produce the same clinical picture, especially in children. Some of these agents tend to cause more severe illnesses; others have a predilection for certain age groups and populations. RSV, the major viral respiratory tract pathogen of early infancy, produces illness with greatest frequency during the first 2 years of life; it is the major known causal agent of bronchiolitis and is a cause of pneumonia, croup, bronchitis, otitis media and febrile upper respiratory illness. The parainfluenza viruses are the major known causal agents of croup and also cause bronchitis, pneumonia, bronchiolitis and febrile upper respiratory illness in pediatric populations. RSV and the parainfluenza viruses may cause symptomatic disease in adults, particularly the debilitated elderly. Adenoviruses are associated with several forms of respiratory disease; types 4, 7 and 21 are common causes of acute respiratory disease in nonimmunized military recruits; in young infants, adenoviruses are the most aggressive viral agents to cause significant mortality.

3. Occurrence—Worldwide. Seasonal in temperate zones, with greatest incidence during autumn and winter and occasionally spring. In tropical zones, respiratory infections tend to be more frequent in wet and in colder weather. In large communities, some viral illnesses are constantly present, usually with little seasonal pattern (e.g. adenovirus type 1); others tend to occur in sharp outbreaks (e.g. RSV).

Annual incidence is high, particularly in infants and children, with 2–6 episodes per child per year, and depends on the number of susceptibles and the virulence of the agent. During the season where prevalence is high, attack rates for preschool children may average 2% per week, as compared to 1% per week for school-age children and 0.5% per week for adults. Under special host and environmental conditions, certain viral infections may disable more than half a closed community within a few weeks (e.g. outbreaks of adenovirus type 4 or 7 in military recruits).

4. Reservoir—Humans. Many known viruses produce inapparent infections; adenoviruses may remain latent in tonsils and adenoids. Viruses of the same group cause similar infections in many animal species but are of minor importance as sources of human infections.

5. Mode of transmission—Directly by oral contact or droplet spread; indirectly by hands, handkerchiefs, eating utensils or other articles freshly soiled by respiratory discharges of an infected person. Viruses discharged in the feces, including enteroviruses and adenoviruses, may be transmitted by the fecal-oral route. Outbreaks of illness due to adenovirus types 3, 4 and 7 have been related to swimming pools.

6. Incubation period—From 1 to 10 days.

7. Period of communicability—Shortly prior to and for the duration of active disease; little is known about subclinical or latent infections. Especially in infants, RSV shedding may very rarely persist several weeks after clinical symptoms subside.

8. Susceptibility—Susceptibility is universal. Illness is more frequent and more severe in infants, children and the elderly. Infection induces specific antibodies that are usually short lived. Reinfection with RSV and parainfluenza viruses is common, but illness is generally milder. Individuals with compromised cardiac, pulmonary or immune systems are at increased risk of severe illness.

9. **Methods of control—**

A. *Preventive measures:* See section I, 9A. Infants at high risk of RSV-related complications include infants and children under 2 with chronic lung disease who have required medical treatment for lung disease within 6 months of the RSV season, and premature infants 32 to 35 weeks gestation at birth. These high-risk infants may benefit from intravenous RSV immune globulin (RSV-IGIV). In addition, palivizumab, an RSV monoclonal antibody preparation that is given IM, has reduced RSV-related hospitalization by about half in these infants. RSV-IGIV is however contraindicated and palivizumab is not recommended for those with cyanotic congenital heart disease because of possible safety concerns.

B. *Control of patient, contacts and the immediate environment:*

1) Report to local health authority: Obligatory report of epidemics in some countries; no individual case report, Class 4 (see Reporting).

2) Isolation: Contact isolation is desirable in children's hospital wards. Outside hospitals, ill people should avoid direct and indirect exposure of young children, debilitated or aged people or patients with other illnesses.

3) Concurrent disinfection: Of eating and drinking utensils; sanitary disposal of oral and nasal discharges.

4) Quarantine: Not applicable.

5) Immmunization of contacts: Not applicable.

6) Investigation of contacts and source of infection: Not generally indicated.

7) Specific treatment: None. Indiscriminate use of antibiotics is to be discouraged; they should be reserved for patients with group A streptococcal pharyngitis and patients with identified bacterial complications such as otitis media, pneumonia or sinusitis. There is a lack of consensus regarding appropriate management of the infant with RSV infection, specifically with respect to the use of aerosolized ribavirin. Despite studies in the USA and Canada, no clear improvement in clinical outcomes attributed to the use of aerosolized ribavirin is consistent across all studies. Cough medicines, decongestants and antihistaminics are of questionable effectiveness and may be hazardous, especially in children.

C. *Epidemic measures:* No effective measures known. Some nosocomial transmission can be prevented by good infection control procedures, including handwashing; procedures such as ultraviolet irradiation, aerosols and dust control have not proven useful. Avoid crowding (see section I, 9A2).

D. *Disaster implications:* None.

E. *International measures:* WHO Collaborating Centres.

[O. Fontaine]

RICKETTSIOSES, TICK-BORNE   ICD-9 082; ICD-10 A77
(Spotted fever group)

Rickettsioses are a group of clinically similar diseases caused by closely related rickettsiae. They are transmitted by ixodid (hard) ticks, which are widely distributed throughout the world; tick species differ markedly by geographical area. For all of these rickettsial fevers, control measures are similar, and doxycycline is the reference treatment. IFA tests become positive generally in the second week of illness. The Weil-Felix tests using Proteus OX-19 and Proteus OX-2 antigens are much less specific and should be confirmed by more specific serologic tests.

I. ROCKY MOUNTAIN SPOTTED
   FEVER   ICD-9 082.0; ICD-10 A77.0
(North American tick typhus, New World spotted fever, Tick-borne typhus fever, Sao Paulo fever)

1. Identification—This prototype disease of the spotted fever group rickettsiae is characterized by sudden onset of moderate to high fever, which ordinarily persists for 2–3 weeks in untreated cases, significant malaise, deep muscle pain, severe headache, chills and conjunctival injection. A maculopapular rash generally appears on the extremities on the 3rd to 5th day; this soon includes the palms and soles and spreads rapidly to much of the body. A petechial exanthem occurs in 40% to 60% of patients, generally on or after the 6th day. The case-fatality rate ranges between 13% and 25% in the absence of specific treatment; with prompt recognition and treatment, death is uncommon, yet 3%–5% of cases reported in the USA during recent years have been fatal. Risk factors associated with more severe disease and death include delayed antibiotherapy and patient age over 40. Absence or delayed appearance of the typical rash or failure to recognize it, especially in dark-skinned individuals, contribute to delay in diagnosis and increased fatality.

The early stages of Rocky Mountain spotted fever (RMSF) may be confused with ehrlichiosis, meningococcaemia (see Meningitis) and enteroviral infection.

The serological response to specific antigens confirms the diagnosis. During the early stages, rickettsiae may be detected in blood by PCR and in skin biopsies using immunostains or PCR.

2. Infectious agent—*Rickettsia rickettsii*.

3. Occurrence—Throughout the USA, primarily from April through September, mainly from the south Atlantic and western south-central regions; the highest incidence rates are seen in North Carolina and Oklahoma. Few cases are reported from the Rocky Mountain region. In the western USA, adult males are infected most frequently, while in the east, the incidence is higher in children; the difference relates to conditions of exposure to infected ticks. Infection also has been documented in Argentina, Brazil, Canada, Colombia, Costa Rica, western and central Mexico, and Panama.

4. Reservoir—Maintained in nature among ticks by transovarial and transstadial passage. The rickettsiae can be transmitted to dogs, various rodents and other animals; animal infections are usually subclinical, but disease in rodents and dogs has been observed.

5. Mode of transmission—Ordinarily through the bite of an infected tick. At least 4–6 hours of attachment and feeding on blood by the tick are required before the rickettsiae become reactivated and infectious for people. Contamination of breaks in the skin or mucous membranes with crushed tissues or feces of the tick may also lead to infection. In eastern and southern USA, the common vector is the American dog tick, *Dermacentor variabilis*, and in northwestern USA, the Rocky Mountain wood tick, *D. andersoni*. The principal vector in Latin America is *Amblyomma cajennense*.

6. Incubation period—From 3 to about 14 days.

7. Period of communicability—Not directly transmitted from person to person. The tick remains infective for life, commonly as long as 18 months.

8. Susceptibility—Susceptibility is general. One attack probably confers lasting immunity.

9. Methods of control—

A. Preventive measures:

1) See also Lyme disease, 9A. Remove attached or crawling ticks after exposures to tick-infested habitats.
2) Deticking dogs and using tick-repellent collars on them minimizes the tick population near residences.
3) A trial of a conventional killed organism vaccine failed to prevent infection in 75% of challenged recipients.

B. *Control of patient, contacts and the immediate environment:*

1) Report to local health authority: Case report obligatory in most countries, Class 2 (see Reporting).
2) Isolation: Not applicable.
3) Concurrent disinfection: Carefully remove all ticks from patients.
4) Quarantine: Not applicable.
5) Immunization of contacts: Unnecessary.
6) Investigation of contacts and source of infection: Not beneficial except as a community measure. See Lyme disease, 9C.
7) Specific treatment: Tetracyclines (usually doxycyline) in daily oral or intravenous doses for 5–7 days and for at least 48 hours once the patient is afebrile. Chloramphenicol may also be used, but only when there is an absolute contraindication for using tetracyclines. Treatment should be initiated on clinical and epidemiological considerations without waiting for laboratory confirmation of the diagnosis.

C. *Epidemic measures:* See Lyme disease, 9C.

D. *Disaster implications:* None.

E. *International measures:* WHO Collaborating Centres.

II. BOUTONNEUSE FEVER   ICD-9 082.1; ICD-10 A77.1
(Mediterranean tick fever, Mediterranean spotted fever, Marseilles fever, Kenya tick typhus, India tick typhus, Israeli tick typhus)

1. **Identification**—A mild to severe febrile illness of a few days to 2 weeks; there may be a primary lesion or eschar at the site of a tick bite. This eschar (tache noire), often evident at the onset of fever, is a small ulcer 2–5 mm in diameter with a black center and red areola; regional lymph nodes are often enlarged. In some areas, such as the Negev in Israel, primary lesions are rarely seen. A generalized maculopapular erythematous rash usually involving palms and soles appears about the 4th to 5th day and persists for 6–7 days; with antibiotherapy, fever lasts no more than 2 days. The case-fatality rate is low (less than 3%) even without specific treatment.

Diagnosis is confirmed by serological tests or PCR or immunostains of biopsied tissues. Culturing blood on human fibroblast monolayers permits demonstration of the organisms by DFA testing.

2. **Infectious agent**—*Rickettsia conorii* and closely related organisms.

3. **Occurrence**—Widely distributed throughout the African continent, in India and in those parts of Europe and the Middle East adjacent to the

Mediterranean and the Black and Caspian seas. Expansion of the European endemic zone to the north occurs because tourists often carry their dogs with them; the dogs acquire infected ticks, which establish colonies when the dogs return home, with subsequent transmission. In more temperate areas, the highest incidence is during warmer months when ticks are numerous; in tropical areas, disease occurs throughout the year.

4. Reservoir—As in RMSF (see section I, 4).

5. Mode of transmission—In the Mediterranean area, bite of infected *Rhipicephalus sanguineus*, the brown dog tick.

6. Incubation period—Usually 5-7 days.

7., 8. and **9. Period of communicability, Susceptibility** and **Methods of control**—As in RMSF (see section I, 7, 8 and 9).

III. AFRICAN TICK BITE FEVER   ICD-9 082.8; ICD-10 A77.8

1. Identification—The disease is milder than other rickettsioses. Clinically similar to Boutonneuse fever (see above), but fever less common, rash noticed in only half the cases and may be vesicular. Aphthous stomatitis is common. Multiple eschars, lymphangitis, lymphadenopathy, and oedema localized to the eschar site are seen more commonly than with Boutonneuse fever. Outbreaks of disease may occur when groups of travellers (such as persons on safari in Africa) are bitten by ticks. Cases are often imported to United States and Europe.

2. Infectious agent—*Rickettsia africae*.

3. Occurrence—Sub-Saharan Africa, including Botswana, South Africa, Swaziland and Zimbabwe,

4. Reservoir—As in RMSF (see section 1, 4).

5. Mode of transmission—As in Rocky Mountain Spotted Fever (see section 1, 5 above). *Amblyomma hebraeum* and *A. africanum* appear to be the major vectors.

6. Incubation period—1 to 15 days (median 4 days after tick bite).

7., 8. and **9. Period of communicability, Susceptibility** and **Methods of control**—As in RMSF (see section 1, 7, 8 and 9).

IV. QUEENSLAND TICK TYPHUS   ICD-9 082.3; ICD-10 A77.3

1. Identification—Clinically similar to Boutonneuse fever (see section II); the rash could be vesicular.

2. Infectious agent—*Rickettsia australis*.

3. Occurrence—Queensland, New South Wales, Tasmania and coastal areas of eastern Victoria, Australia.

4. Reservoir—As in RMSF (see section I, 4).

5. Mode of transmission—As in RMSF (see section I, 5). *Ixodes holocyclus*, which infests small marsupials and wild rodents, is probably the major vector.

6. Incubation period—About 7-10 days.

7., 8. and **9. Period of communicability, Susceptibility** and **Methods of control**—As in RMSF (see section I, 7, 8 and 9).

V. NORTH ASIAN TICK FEVER   ICD-9 082.2; ICD-10 A77.2
(Siberian tick typhus)

1. Identification—Clinically similar to Boutonneuse fever (see section II); lymphadenitis is common.

2. Infectious agent—*Rickettsia sibirica*.

3. Occurrence—North China, Mongolia and Asiatic areas of the former Soviet Union.

4. Reservoir—As in RMSF (see section I, 4).

5. Mode of transmission—Through the bite of ticks in the genera *Dermacentor* and *Haemaphysalis*, which infest certain wild rodents.

6. Incubation period—2 to 7 days.

7., 8. and **9. Period of communicability, Susceptibility** and **Methods of control**—As in RMSF (see section I, 7, 8 and 9).

VI. RICKETTSIALPOX   ICD-9 083.2; ICD-10 A79.1
(Vesicular rickettsiosis)

An acute febrile illness transmitted by mites. An initial skin lesion at the site of a mite bite, often associated with lymphadenopathy, is followed by fever; a disseminated vesicular skin rash appears, which generally does not involve the palms and soles and lasts only a few days. It may be confused with chickenpox. Death is uncommon and the infection is responsive to tetracyclines. Diagnosis is made by serology or by PCR or immunostains of biopsied tissues. The disease, caused by *Rickettsia akari*, a member of the spotted fever group of rickettsiae, is transmitted to humans from mice (*Mus musculus*) by a mite (*Liponyssoides sanguineus*). It occurs primarily in urban areas of the eastern USA; most cases have been described from New York City and in the former Soviet Union. Incidence has been markedly reduced by changes in management of garbage in tenement housing, so that few cases have been diagnosed in recent years. *R. akari* has also been isolated in Africa and the Republic of Korea. In the former Soviet Union, commensal rats are reported to be the reservoir. Prevention includes rodent elimination and mite control.

[D. Raoult]

RUBELLA   ICD-9 056; ICD-10 B06
(German measles)

CONGENITAL RUBELLA   ICD-9 771.0; ICD-10 P35.0
(Congenital rubella syndrome)

    1. Identification—Rubella is a mild febrile viral disease with a diffuse punctate and maculopapular rash. Clinically, this is usually indistinguishable from febrile rash illness due to measles, dengue, parvovirus B19, human herpesvirus 6, Coxsackie virus, Echovirus, adenovirus or scarlet fever. Children usually present few or no constitutional symptoms, but adults may experience a 1–5 day prodrome of low grade fever, headache, malaise, mild coryza and conjunctivitis. Postauricular, occipital and posterior cervical lymphadenopathy is the most characteristic clinical feature and precedes the rash by 5–10 days. Leukopenia is common and thrombocytopenia can occur, but hemorrhagic manifestations are rare. Arthralgia and, less commonly, arthritis complicate a substantial proportion of infections, particularly among adult females. Encephalitis is a more common complication than generally appreciated, and occurs with a higher frequency in adults. Up to 50% of rubella infections are subclinical.

    For surveillance purposes, the WHO-recommended case definition of a suspected rubella case is any person with fever, non-vesicular (maculopapular) rash and adenopathy (cervical, suboccipital or post-auricular). Laboratory diagnosis of rubella is required, since clinical diagnosis is often inaccurate. Laboratory confirmation is usually based on a positive rubella-specific IgM ELISA test on a blood specimen obtained within 28 days after the rash onset. An epidemiologically confirmed rubella case is a patient with suspected rubella with an epidemiological link to a laboratory-confirmed case. Other methods for rubella diagnosis include paired serum specimens that show seroconversion or at least a 4-fold rise in rubella-specific IgG antibody titre, positive rubella PCR test, and virus isolation; most of these methods are only available in higher level reference laboratories.

Rubella is important because of its ability to produce anomalies in the developing fetus. Congenital rubella syndrome (CRS) occurs in up to 90% of infants born to women who are infected with rubella during the first trimester of pregnancy; the risk of a single congenital defect falls to approximately 10%-20% by the 16th week; defects are rare when maternal infection occurs after the 20th week of gestation. Congenital malformations and fetal death may occur following inapparent maternal rubella.

Fetuses infected early are at greatest risk of intrauterine death, spontaneous abortion and congenital malformations of major organ systems. These include single or combined defects such as deafness, cataracts, microphthalmia, congenital glaucoma, microcephaly, meningoencephalitis, mental retardation, patent ductus arteriosus, atrial or ventricular septal defects, purpura, hepatosplenomegaly, jaundice and radiolucent bone disease. Moderate and severe cases of CRS are usually recognizable at birth; mild cases with only slight cardiac involvement or deafness may not be detected for months or even years after birth. Insulin-dependent diabetes mellitus is recognized as a frequent late manifestation of CRS.

Laboratory confirmation of CRS in an infant is based on a positive rubella-specific IgM ELISA test on a blood specimen; or the persistence of a rubella-specific IgG antibody titre in a blood specimen beyond the time expected from passive transfer of maternal IgG antibody; or isolation of the virus from a throat swab or urine specimen. Almost all infants with CRS will have a positive rubella IgM test in the first 6 months of life, and 60% will be positive during the second 6 months of life. Rubella virus has been isolated from throat and urine specimens from infants with CRS, and from cataract surgery aspirates in children up to 3.

2. Infectious agent—Rubella virus (family Togaviridae; genus *Rubivirus*).

3. Occurrence—In the absence of generalized immunization rubella occurred worldwide at endemic levels with epidemics every 5-9 years. Large rubella epidemics resulted in very high levels of morbidity. For example, the USA epidemic in 1964-1965 led to an estimated 12.5 million cases of rubella, over 20 000 cases of CRS, and 11 000 fetal deaths; the incidence rate of CRS during endemic periods was 0.1-0.2 per 1000 live births and during epidemics 1-4 per 1000 live births. In countries where rubella vaccine has not been introduced, rubella remains endemic. An estimated 100 000 CRS cases at least occur each year in developing countries.

By the end of 2002, 124 countries/territories (58% of the world total) were using rubella vaccine in their national immunization program with the highest levels in the Americas (94% of countries), Europe (84%) and the Western Pacific (59%). Of these 124 countries, 89 include 2 doses in the routine schedule. In many countries, sustained high levels of rubella immunization have drastically reduced or practically eliminated rubella and CRS.

4. Reservoir—Humans.

5. Mode of transmission—Contact with nasopharyngeal secretions of infected people. Infection is by droplet spread or direct contact with patients. Infants with CRS shed large quantities of virus in their pharyngeal secretions and urine, and serve as a source of infection to their contacts.

6. Incubation period—From 14–17 days with a range of 14–21 days.

7. Period of communicability—For about 1 week before and at least 4 days after onset of rash; highly communicable. Infants with CRS may shed virus for months after birth.

8. Susceptibility—Immunity is usually permanent after natural infection and thought to be long-term, probably lifelong, after immunization, but this may depend on contact with endemic cases. Infants born to immune mothers are ordinarily protected for 6–9 months, depending on the amount of maternal antibodies acquired transplacentally.

9. Methods of control—Rubella control is needed primarily to prevent defects in the offspring of women who acquire the disease during pregnancy.

    *A. **Preventive measures:***

        1) Educate the general public on modes of transmission and stress the need for rubella immunization. Health care providers must be aware of the risk of rubella in pregnancy.

        2) WHO recommends that all countries assess their rubella situation and, if appropriate, make plans for the introduction of rubella vaccine. This can be done using combined vaccines (MR or MMR). Two approaches are recommended to prevent the occurrence of CRS: (a) prevention of CRS only, through immunization of adolescent girls or women of childbearing age; or (b) elimination of rubella as well as CRS, through universal immunization of infants and ensuring immunity in women of childbearing age. For increased impact men should also be vaccinated. Decisions on which approach is taken will be based on level of susceptibility in women of childbearing age, burden of disease due to CRS, strength of the basic immunization program as indicated by routine measles vaccine coverage, infrastructure and resources for child and adult immunization programs, assurance of injection safety, and priorities linked to other diseases. A policy of rubella vaccination of adults is unlikely to alter rubella transmission dynamics and is difficult to implement in practice with high coverage rates, whereas inadequately implemented childhood vaccination runs the risk of

increasing the number of susceptibles among women—and the possibility of increased numbers of cases of CRS—until immunized child cohorts become adults. Consequently, it is essential that childhood rubella vaccination programs achieve and maintain high levels of coverage (above 80%) on a long-term basis.

A single dose of live, attenuated rubella virus vaccine elicits a significant antibody response in about 95%–100% of susceptible individuals aged 9 months or older. Rubella vaccines are cold-chain dependent and should be protected from light. Several rubella vaccines are available as single antigen, measles-rubella (MR), or measles-mumps-rubella (MMR) vaccines. Most of the currently licensed vaccines are based on the live attenuated RA2/73 strain of rubella virus; other live attenuated rubella virus strains are used in China and Japan.

Following the introduction of large-scale rubella vaccination, coverage should be measured periodically by age and locality. In addition, surveillance is needed for rubella and CRS. If resources permit, longitudinal serological surveillance can be used to monitor the impact of the immunization program, especially through assessing rubella IgG antibody in serum samples from women attending antenatal clinics.

Rubella vaccine should be avoided in pregnancy because of the theoretical, but never demonstrated, teratogenic risk. No cases of CRS have been reported in more than 1000 susceptible pregnant women who inadvertently received rubella vaccine in early pregnancy. If pregnancy is being planned, then an interval of one month should be observed after rubella immunization. Receipt of rubella vaccine during pregnancy is not an indication for abortion.

Rubella vaccine should not be given to anyone with an immunodeficiency or who receives immunosuppressive therapy. Asymptomatic HIV-infected persons can be immunized.

3) In case of infection with wild rubella virus early in pregnancy, culturally appropriate counselling should be provided. Abortion may be considered in those countries where this is an option.

4) IG given after exposure early in pregnancy may not prevent infection or viraemia, but it may modify or suppress symptoms. It is sometimes given in huge doses (20 ml) to a susceptible pregnant woman exposed to the disease who would not be in a position to consider abortion, but the value of this has not been established.

B. Control of patient, contacts and the immediate environment:

1) Report to local health authority: All cases of rubella and of CRS should be reported. In many countries, reporting is obligatory, Class 3 (see Reporting). Early reporting of suspected cases will permit early establishment of control measures.

2) Isolation: In hospitals, patients suspected of having rubella should be managed under contact isolation precautions; attempts should be made to prevent exposure of nonimmune pregnant women. Exclude children from school and adults from work for 7 days after onset of rash. Infants with CRS may shed virus for prolonged periods of time. All persons having contact with infants with CRS should be immune to rubella (naturally or through immunization); contact between these infants and pregnant women should be avoided. In hospitals, contact isolation precautions should be applied to infants under 12 months with CRS, unless urine and pharyngeal virus cultures are negative for rubella virus after 3 months of age.

3) Concurrent disinfection: Not applicable.

4) Quarantine: Not applicable.

5) Immunization of contacts: Immunization of contacts will not necessarily prevent infection or illness. Passive immunization with IG is not indicated (except possibly as in 9A4).

6) Investigation of contacts and source of infection: Identify pregnant female contacts, especially those in the first trimester. Such contacts should be tested serologically for susceptibility or early infection (IgM antibody) and advised accordingly.

7) Specific treatment: None.

C. Epidemic measures:

1) Prompt reporting of all confirmed and suspected cases. A limited number (5-10) of suspected cases (see definition earlier) should be investigated with laboratory tests periodically during an outbreak to confirm that it is due to rubella.

2) The medical community and general public should be informed about rubella epidemics in order to identify and protect susceptible pregnant women. Active surveillance for infants with CRS should be carried out until 9 months after the last reported rubella case.

D. Disaster implications: None.

E. International measures: None.

[S. Robertson]

SALMONELLOSIS   ICD-9 003; ICD-10 A02

1. Identification—A bacterial disease commonly manifested by acute enterocolitis, with sudden onset of headache, abdominal pain, diarrhea, nausea and sometimes vomiting. Dehydration, especially among infants or in the elderly, may be severe. Fever is almost always present. Anorexia and diarrhea often persist for several days. Infection may begin as acute enterocolitis and develop into septicemia or focal infection. Occasionally, the infectious agent may localize in any tissue of the body, produce abscesses and cause septic arthritis, cholecystitis, endocarditis, meningitis, pericarditis, pneumonia, pyoderma or pyelonephritis. Deaths are uncommon, except in the very young, the very old, the debilitated and the immunosuppressed. However, morbidity and associated costs of salmonellosis may be high.

In cases of septicemia, *Salmonella* may be isolated on enteric media from feces and blood during acute stages of illness. In cases of enterocolitis, fecal excretion usually persists for several days or weeks beyond the acute phase; administration of antibiotics may not decrease this duration. For detection of asymptomatic infections, 3-10 grams of fecal material is preferred to rectal swabs and this should be inoculated into an appropriate enrichment medium; specimens should be collected over several days since excretion of the organisms may be intermittent. Serological tests are not useful in diagnosis.

2. Infectious agents—In the recently proposed nomenclature for *Salmonella* the agent formerly known as *S. typhi* is called *S. enterica* subsp. *enterica* serovar Typhi (commonly *S.* Typhi, the latter word not italicized).

Numerous serotypes of *Salmonella* are pathogenic for both animals and people (strains of human origin that cause typhoid and paratyphoid fevers are presented in a separate chapter). There is much variation in the relative prevalence of different serotypes from country to country; in most countries that maintain *Salmonella* surveillance, *Salmonella enterica* subsp. *enterica* serovar Typhimurium (commonly *S.* Typhimurium) and *Salmonella enterica* subsp. *enterica* serovar Enteritidis (*S.* Enteritidis) are the most commonly reported. In most areas, a small number of serotypes account for the majority of confirmed cases.

3. Occurrence—Worldwide; more extensively reported in North America and Europe because of better reporting systems. Salmonellosis is classified as a foodborne disease because contaminated food, mainly of animal origin, is the predominant mode of transmission. Only a proportion of cases are recognized clinically; in industrialized countries as few as 1% of clinical cases are reported. The incidence rate of infection is highest in infants and young children. Epidemiologically, *Salmonella* gastroenteritis may occur in small outbreaks in the general population. About 60%–80% of all cases occur sporadically; however, large outbreaks in hospitals, institutions for children, restaurants and nursing homes are not uncommon, usually arising from food contaminated at its source, or less often through handling by an ill person or a carrier; person-to-person spread can also occur. An epidemic in the USA that involved 25 000 cases resulted from a nonchlorinated municipal water supply; the largest single epidemic due to improperly pasteurized milk affected 285 000 persons.

4. Reservoir—Domestic and wild animals, including poultry, swine, cattle, rodents and pets such as iguanas, tortoises, turtles, terrapins, chicks, dogs and cats; also humans, i.e. patients, convalescent carriers and, especially, mild and unrecognized cases. Chronic carriers are rare in humans but prevalent in animals and birds.

5. Mode of transmission—Ingestion of the organisms in food derived from infected animals or contaminated by feces of an infected animal or person. This includes contaminated raw and undercooked eggs/egg products, raw milk/milk products, contaminated water, meat/meat products, poultry/poultry products. In addition, pet turtles, iguanas and chicks, and unsterilized pharmaceuticals of animal origin are potential sources of infection. Several outbreaks of salmonellosis have been traced to consumption of raw fruits and vegetables that were contaminated during slicing. Infection is transmitted to farm animals by feeds and fertilizers prepared from contaminated meat scraps, tankage, fish meal and bones; the infection spreads by bacterial multiplication during rearing and slaughter. Person-to-person fecal-oral transmission is important, especially when diarrhea is present; infants and stool-incontinent adults pose a greater risk of transmission than do asymptomatic carriers. With several serotypes, a few organisms ingested in vehicles that buffer gastric acid can suffice to cause infection, but over 100 to 1000 organisms are usually required.

   Epidemics are usually traced to foods such as processed meat products, inadequately cooked poultry/poultry products; uncooked or lightly cooked foods containing eggs/egg products, raw milk and dairy products, including dried milk, and foods contaminated by an infected food handler. Epidemics may also be traced to foods such as meat and poultry products processed or prepared with contaminated utensils or on work surfaces contaminated in previous use. *S.* Enteritidis infection of chickens and eggs has caused outbreaks and single cases and is responsible for the majority of cases of this serotype in the USA. The organisms can multiply in a variety of foods, especially milk, to attain a very high infective dose; temperature abuse of food during its preparation and cross-contamination during food handling are the most important risk factors. Hospital epidemics tend to be protracted, with organisms persisting in the environment; they often start with contaminated food and continue through person-to-person transmission via the hands of personnel or contaminated instruments. Maternity units with infected (at times asymptomatic) infants are sources of further spread. Fecal contamination of nonchlorinated public water supplies has caused some extensive outbreaks. In recent years, geographically widespread outbreaks due to ingestion of tomatoes or melons from single suppliers have been recognized.

6. Incubation period—From 6 to 72 hours, usually about 12-36 hours.

7. Period of communicability—Throughout the course of infection; extremely variable, usually several days to several weeks. A temporary carrier state occasionally continues for months, especially in infants. Depending on the serotypes, approximately 1% of infected adults and 5% of children undere 5 may excrete the organism for >1 year.

8. Susceptibility—Susceptibility is general and usually increased by achlorhydria, antacid treatment, gastrointestinal surgery, prior or current broad-spectrum antibiotherapy, neoplastic disease, immunosuppressive treatment and other debilitating conditions including malnutrition. Severity of the disease is related to serotype, number of organisms ingested and host factors. HIV infected persons are at possible risk for recurrent nontyphoidal *Salmonella* septicemia. Septicaemia in people with sickle-cell disease increases the risk of focal systemic infection, e.g. osteomyelitis.

9. Methods of control—

  A. Preventive measures:

   1) Educate all food handlers about the importance of a) handwashing before, during and after food preparation; b) refrigerating prepared foods in small containers; c) thoroughly cooking all foodstuffs derived from animal sources, particularly poultry, pork, egg products and meat dishes; d) avoiding recontamination within the kitchen after cooking is completed; and e) maintaining a sanitary kitchen and protecting prepared foods against rodent and insect contamination.

   2) Educate the public against consuming raw or incompletely cooked eggs ("over easy" or "sunny side up", eggnogs or homemade ice cream), and using dirty or cracked eggs.

   3) Use pasteurized or irradiated egg products to prepare dishes in which eggs would otherwise be pooled before cooking or when the dish containing eggs is not subsequently cooked.

   4) Exclude individuals with diarrhea from food handling and from care of hospitalized patients, the elderly and children.

   5) Indoctrinate known carriers on the need for careful handwashing after defecation (and before handling food) and

discourage them from handling food for others as long as they shed organisms.

6) Recognize the risk of *Salmonella* infections in pets. Chicks, ducklings and turtles are particularly dangerous pets for small children.

7) Establish the facilities for, and encourage the use of, food irradiation for meats and eggs.

8) Inspect for sanitation and adequately supervise abattoirs, food-processing plants, feed-blending mills, egg grading stations and butcher shops.

9) Establish *Salmonella* control programs (feed control, cleaning and disinfection, vector control and other sanitary and hygienic measures).

10) Adequately cook or heat-treat (including pasteurization or irradiation) animal-derived foods prepared for animal consumption (meat or bone or fish meal, pet foods) to eliminate pathogens; follow by measures to avoid recontamination.

B. *Control of patient, contacts and the immediate environment:*

1) Report to local health authority: Obligatory case report, Class 2 (see Reporting).

2) Isolation: Proper handwashing should be stressed. For hospitalized patients, enteric precautions in handling feces and contaminated clothing and bed linen. Exclude symptomatic individuals from food handling and from direct care of infants, elderly, immunocompromised and institutionalized patients. Exclusion of asymptomatic infected individuals is indicated for those with questionable hygienic habits and may be required by local or state regulations. When exclusion is mandated, release to return to work handling food or in patient care generally requires 2 consecutive negative stool cultures for *Salmonella* collected not less than 24 hours apart; if antibiotics have been given, the initial culture should be taken at least 48 hours after the last dose.

3) Concurrent disinfection: Of feces and articles soiled therewith. In communities with adequate sewage disposal systems, feces can be discharged directly into sewers without preliminary disinfection. Terminal cleaning.

4) Quarantine: Not applicable.

5) Immunization of contacts: Not applicable.

6) Investigation of contacts and source of infection: Culture stools of household contacts who are involved in food handling, direct patient care, or care of young children or elderly people in institutional settings.

7) Specific treatment: For uncomplicated enterocolitis, none generally indicated except rehydration and electrolyte re-

placement with oral rehydration solution (see Cholera, 9B7). Antibiotics may not eliminate the carrier state and may lead to resistant strains or more severe infections. However, infants up to 2 months, the elderly, the debilitated, those with sickle-cell disease, persons infected with HIV or patients with continued/high fever or manifestations of extraintestinal infection should receive antibiotherapy. Antimicrobial resistance of nontyphoidal salmonellae is variable; in adults, ciprofloxacin is highly effective but its use is not approved for children; ampicillin or amoxicillin may also be used. Trimethoprim-sulfamethoxazole and chloramphenicol are alternatives when antimicrobial resistant strains are involved. Patients infected with HIV may require lifelong treatment to prevent *Salmonella* septicemia.

C. *Epidemic measures:* See Foodborne diseases, Staphylococcal food intoxication, Typhoid fever 9C. Search for a history of food handling errors, such as use of unsafe raw ingredients, inadequate cooking, time-temperature abuses and cross-contamination. In *S.* Enteritidis outbreaks in which dishes containing eggs are implicated, initiate trace back to the egg source; report to the Department of Agriculture is advised.

D. *Disaster implications:* A danger in a situation with mass feeding and poor sanitation.

E. *International measures:* WHO Collaborating Centres. Also see *WHO Golden Rules for Safe Food Preparation,* and WHO Global Salm-Surv Network (http://www.who.int/salmsurv)

[P. Braam]

SCABIES   ICD-9 33.0; ICD-10 B86
(Sarcoptic itch, Acariasis)

1. **Identification**—A parasitic infestation of the skin caused by a mite whose penetration is visible as papules, vesicles or tiny linear burrows containing the mites and their eggs. Lesions are prominent around finger webs, anterior surfaces of wrists and elbows, anterior axillary folds, belt line, thighs and external genitalia in men; nipples, abdomen and the lower portion of the buttocks are frequently affected in women. In infants, the head, neck, palms and soles may be involved; these areas are usually spared in older individuals. Itching is intense, especially at night, but complications are limited to lesions secondarily infected by scratching. In immunodeficient individuals and in senile patients, infestation often

appears as a generalized dermatitis more widely distributed than the burrows, with extensive scaling and sometimes vesiculation and crusting ("Norwegian scabies"); the usual severe itching may be reduced or absent. When scabies is complicated by beta-hemolytic streptococcal infection, there is a risk of acute glomerulonephritis.

Diagnosis may be established by recovering the mite from its burrow and identifying it microscopically. Care should be taken to choose lesions for scraping or biopsy that have not been excoriated by repeated scratching. Prior application of mineral oil facilitates collecting the scrapings and examining them under a cover slip. Applying ink to the skin and then washing it off will disclose the burrows.

2. Etiologic agent—*Sarcoptes scabiei*, a mite.

3. Occurrence—Widespread. Past epidemics were attributed to poverty, poor sanitation and crowding due to war, movement of refugees and economic crises. The recent wave of infestation in the USA and Europe has evolved in the absence of major social disturbances and has affected people of all socioeconomic levels, groups and standards of personal hygiene. Endemic in many developing countries.

4. Reservoir—Humans; *Sarcoptes* species and other animal mites can live on humans but do not reproduce on them.

5. Mode of transmission—Transfer of parasites commonly occurs through prolonged direct contact with infested skin and also during sexual contact. Transfer from undergarments and bedclothes occurs only if these have been contaminated by infested people immediately beforehand. Mites can burrow beneath the skin surface in 2.5 minutes. Persons with the Norwegian scabies syndrome are highly contagious because of the large number of mites present in the exfoliating scales.

6. Incubation period—In people without previous exposure, 2–6 weeks before onset of itching. People who have been previously infested develop symptoms 1–4 days after reexposure.

7. Period of communicability—Until mites and eggs are destroyed by treatment, ordinarily after 1 or occasionally 2 courses of treatment, a week apart.

8. Susceptibility—Some resistance is suggested; fewer mites succeed in establishing themselves on people previously infested than on those with no prior exposure but immunologically compromised people are susceptible to hyperinfestation.

9. Methods of control—

    A. *Preventive measures:* Educate the public and medical community on mode of transmission, early diagnosis and treatment of infested patients and contacts.

B. *Control of patient, contacts and the immediate environment:*

1) Report to local health authority: Official report not ordinarily justifiable, Class 5 (see Reporting).
2) Isolation: Exclude infested individuals from school or work until the day after treatment. For hospitalized patients, contact isolation for 24 hours after start of effective treatment.
3) Concurrent disinfestation: Laundering underwear, clothing and bedsheets worn or used by the patient in the 48 hours prior to treatment, using hot cycles of both washer and dryer, will kill mites and eggs but may not be needed for most infestations. Laundering bedding and clothing is important for patients with Norwegian scabies because potential for fomites transmission is high.
4) Quarantine: Not applicable.
5) Immmunization of contacts: Not applicable.
6) Investigation of contacts and source of infestation: Search for unreported and unrecognized cases among companions and household members; single infestations in a family are uncommon. Treat prophylactically those who have had skin-to-skin contact with infested people (including family members and sexual contacts).
7) Specific treatment: The treatment of choice for children is topical 5% permethrin. Alternatively, topical applications of 1% gamma benzene hexachloride (lindane is contraindicated in premature neonates and must be used with caution in children under 1 and pregnant women); chromatin; tetra-ethylthiuram monosulfide in 5% solution twice daily; or an emulsion of benzyl benzoate to the whole body except head and neck. Treatment details vary with the drug. On the following day, a cleansing bath is taken and a change made to fresh clothing and bedclothes. All affected members of a household or close community must be treated at the same time to avoid reinfestation. Itching may persist for 1–2 weeks; this should not be regarded as a sign of drug failure or reinfestation. Overtreatment is common and should be avoided because of toxicity of some of these agents, especially gamma benzene hexachloride. In about 5% of cases, a repeat course of treatment may be necessary after 7–10 days if eggs survived the initial treatment. Close supervision of treatment, including bathing, is necessary.

C. *Epidemic measures:*

1) Provide treatment and educate infested individuals and others at risk. Cooperation of non-health authorities is often needed.

2) Treatment is undertaken on a coordinated mass basis.
3) Case-finding efforts are extended to screen whole families, military units or institutions, with segregation of infested individuals if possible.
4) Soap and facilities for mass bathing and laundering are essential. Tetmosol soap, where available, helps prevent infestation.

D. Disaster implications: A potential nuisance in situations of overcrowding.

E. International measures: None.

[F. Ndowa]

SCHISTOSOMIASIS
(Bilharziasis, Snail fever)

ICD-9 120; ICD-10 B65

1. Identification—A blood fluke (trematode) infection with adult male and female worms living within mesenteric or vesical veins of the host over a life span of many years. Eggs produce minute granulomata and scars in organs where they lodge or are deposited. Symptoms are related to the number and location of the eggs in the human host: *Schistosoma mansoni* and *S. japonicum* give rise primarily to hepatic and intestinal pathology and early signs and symptoms include diarrhea, abdominal pain and hepatosplenomegaly. *S. japonicum* can also cause CNS disease, with Jacksonian seizures. *S. haematobium* gives rise to urinary manifestations, and early signs and symptoms include dysuria, urinary frequency and hematuria at the end of urination; CNS disease has, rarely, been reported.

The WHO-recommended case definitions in endemic areas are: a) for urinary schistosomiasis: visible hematuria or positive reagent strip for hematuria, or with eggs of *S. haematobium* in urine (confirmed case); b) for intestinal schistosomiasis: non-specific abdominal symptoms, blood in stool, hepato(spleno)megaly (suspected case) or presence of eggs in stools (confirmed case).

The most important effects are the late complications that arise from chronic infection: liver fibrosis, portal hypertension and its sequelae and possibly colorectal malignancy in the intestinal forms; obstructive uropathy, superimposed bacterial infection, infertility and bladder cancer in the urinary form of schistosomiasis. Eggs can be deposited at ectopic sites, including the brain, spinal cord, skin, pelvis and vulvovaginal areas.

The larvae of certain schistosomes of birds and mammals may penetrate the human skin and cause a dermatitis, sometimes known as "swimmer's itch"; these schistosomes do not mature in humans. Such infections may be prevalent among bathers in lakes in many parts of the world. However, the clinical entity of "seabather's eruption", a pruritic dermatitis that appears principally where the bathing suit has been worn has been shown to be caused by the larval stage of some jellyfish species.

Definitive diagnosis of schistosomiasis depends on demonstration of eggs in biopsy specimens, or in the stool by direct smear or on a Kato thick smear, or in urine by the examination of a urine sediment or Nuclepore® filtration. Urine filtration is especially useful for *S. haematobium* infections. Useful immunological tests include immunoblot analysis, the circumoval precipitin test, IFA and ELISA with egg or adult worm antigen, and RIA with purified egg or adult antigens; positive results on serological antibody detection tests indicate prior infection and are not proof of current infection. More recently, various assays developed to detect schistosome antigens directly in serum or urine have proved useful in detecting current infection and in assessing cure after treatment.

2. Infectious agents—*Schistosoma mansoni, S. haematobium* and *S. japonicum* are the major species causing human disease. *S. mekongi, S. malayensis, S. mattheei* and *S. intercalatum* are of importance only in limited areas.

3. Occurrence—*S. mansoni* is found in Africa (including Madagascar), the Arabian Peninsula; Brazil, Suriname and Venezuela in South America and in some Caribbean islands. *S. haematobium* is found in Africa (including Madagascar) and the Middle East. *S. japonicum* is found in China, the Philippines and Sulawesi (Celebes) in Indonesia; no new cases have been found in Japan since 1978 after an intensive control program. *S. mekongi* is found in the Mekong River area of Cambodia and the Lao People's Democratic Republic. *S. intercalatum* occurs in parts of western Africa, including Cameroon, Chad, the Democratic Republic of the Congo, Gabon and Sao Tome. *S. malayensis* is known only from peninsular Malaysia. Human infection with the bovine parasite *S. mattheei* has been reported from southern Africa.

4. Reservoir—Humans are the principal reservoir of *S. haematobium, S. intercalatum* and *S. mansoni*, although the latter has been reported to occur in rodents. People, dogs, cats, pigs, cattle, water buffalo and wild rodents are potential hosts of *S. japonicum*; their relative epidemiological importance varies in different regions. *S. malayensis* appears to be a rodent parasite that occasionally infects humans. Epidemiological persistence of the parasite depends on the presence of an appropriate snail as intermediate host, i.e. species of the genera *Biomphalaria* for *S. mansoni*; *Bulinus* for *S. haematobium, S. intercalatum* and *S. mattheei*; *Oncomelania* for *S. japonicum*; *Neotricula* for *S. mekongi*; and *Robertsiella* for *S. malayensis*.

5. Mode of transmission—Infection is acquired from water containing free-swimming larval forms (cercariae) that have developed in snails.

The eggs of *S. haematobium* leave the mammalian body mainly in the urine, those of the other species in the feces. The eggs hatch in water and the liberated larvae (miracidia) penetrate into suitable freshwater snail hosts. After several weeks, the cercariae emerge from the snail and penetrate human skin, usually while the person is working, swimming or wading in water; they enter the bloodstream, are carried to blood vessels of the lungs, migrate to the liver, develop to maturity and then migrate to veins of the abdominal cavity.

Adult forms of *S. mansoni*, *S. japonicum*, *S. mekongi*, *S. mattheei* and *S. intercalatum* usually remain in mesenteric veins; those of *S. haematobium* usually migrate through anastomoses into the vesical plexus of the urinary bladder. Eggs are deposited in venules and escape into the lumen of the bowel or urinary bladder or end up lodging in other organs, including the liver and the lungs.

6. Incubation period—Acute systemic manifestations (Katayama fever) may occur in primary infections 2–6 weeks after exposure, immediately preceding and during initial egg deposition. Acute systemic manifestations are uncommon but can occur with *S. haematobium* infections.

7. Period of communicability—Not communicable from person to person; people with schistosomiasis may spread the infection by discharging eggs in urine and/or feces into bodies of water for as long as they excrete eggs; it is common for human infections with *S. mansoni* and *S. haematobium* to last in excess of 10 years. Infected snails will release cercariae for as long as they live, a period that may last from several weeks to about 3 months.

8. Susceptibility—Susceptibility is universal; any immunity developing as a result of infection is variable and not yet fully investigated.

9. Methods of control—

    A. Preventive measures:

        1) Treat patients in endemic areas with praziquantel to relieve suffering and prevent disease progression. Regularly treat high-risk groups such as schoolage children, women of childbearing age or special occupational groups in endemic areas. A height-measuring pole (http://whqlibdoc.who.int/trs/WHO_TRS_912.pdf) has been tested in Africa and facilitates praziquantel dosage.

        2) Educate the public in endemic areas to seek treatment early and regularly and to protect themselves.

        3) Dispose of feces and urine so that viable eggs will not reach bodies of fresh water containing intermediate snail hosts. Control of animals infected with *S. japonicum* is desirable but difficult.

4) Improve irrigation and agriculture practices; reduce snail habitats by removing vegetation, by draining and filling, or by lining canals with concrete.

5) Treat snail-breeding sites with molluscicides. Cost may limit the use of these agents.

6) Individual protection: prevent exposure to contaminated water (e.g. rubber boots). To minimize cercarial penetration after brief or accidental water exposure, vigorously and completely towel dry skin surfaces that are wet with suspected water. Apply 70% alcohol immediately to the skin to kill surface cercariae.

7) Provide water for drinking, bathing and washing clothes from sources free of cercariae or treated to kill them. Effective measures for inactivating cercariae include water treatment with iodine or chlorine. Allowing water to stand 48–72 hours before use is also effective.

8) Travellers visiting endemic areas should be advised of the risks and informed about preventive measures.

B. Control of patient, contacts and the immediate environment:

1) Report to local health authority: in selected endemic areas; in many countries, not a reportable disease, Class 3 (see Reporting).

2) Isolation: Not applicable.

3) Concurrent disinfection: Sanitary disposal of feces and urine.

4) Quarantine: Not applicable.

5) Immmunization of contacts: Not applicable.

6) Investigation of contacts and source of infection: Examine contacts for infection from a common source.

7) Specific treatment: praziquantel is the drug of choice against all species. A single oral dose of 40 mg/kg is generally sufficient for cure rates of 80–90% and dramatic reductions in egg excretion. For *S. japonicum*, the dose may be increased up to 60 mg/kg. Alternative drugs are oxamniquine for *S. mansoni* and metrifonate for *S. haematobium*.

C. Epidemic measures: Examine for schistosomiasis and treat all who are infected, but especially those with disease and/or moderate to heavy intensity of infection; pay particular attention to children. Provide clean water, warn people against contact with water potentially containing cercariae and prohibit contamination of water. Treat areas that have high snail densities with molluscicides.

D. Disaster implications: None.

E. *International measures:* WHO Collaborating Centres. Further informnation on http://www.who.int/tdr/diseases/schisto/default.htm

[D. Engels]

SEVERE ACUTE RESPIRATORY SYNDROME ICD-10 U04.9 (provisional)
SARS

1. Identification—A severe respiratory infection with associated gastrointestinal manifestations in an as yet unknown percentage of those infected, Severe Acute Respiratory Syndrome (SARS) was first recognized in February 2003. The causal agent is a coronavirus. The disease is thought to have originated in the Guandong Province of China, with emergence into human populations sometime in November 2002. By July 2003, major outbreaks had occurred at 6 sites: Canada, China (originating in Guangdong Province and spreading to major cities in other areas, including Taiwan and the Special Administrative Region of Hong Kong), Singapore and Viet Nam. The disease spread to more than 20 additional sites throughout the world, following major airline routes. The major part of the spread occurred in hospitals and among families and contacts of hospital workers.

SARS presents with malaise, myalgia and fever, quickly followed by respiratory symptoms including cough and shortness of breath. Diarrhea may occur. Symptoms may worsen for several days coinciding with maximum viraemia at 10 days after onset.

Laboratories performing SARS-specific PCR tests must adopt strict criteria to confirm positive results, especially in low prevalence areas, where positive predictive value will be lower.

Diagnostic tests include PCR, ELISA and IFA. A confirmed positive PCR for SARS requires at least 2 different clinical specimens (e.g. nasopharyngeal and stool), or the same clinical specimen collected on 2 or more days during illness (e.g. 2 or more nasopharyngeal aspirates), or 2 different assays, or repeat PCR using a new extract from the original clinical sample on each occasion of testing.

The PCR procedure must include appropriate negative and positive controls in each run. A positive PCR result must be confirmed by repeat PCR using the original sample, or testing the same sample in another laboratory. The sensitivity of PCR tests for SARS depends on specimen and time of testing during the illness. Sensitivity can be increased if multiple specimens/multiple body sites are tested. Correctly executed PCR tests have excellent specificity for SARS; technical problems (e.g. laboratory contamination) may lead to false-positive results and each positive PCR test should thus be verified. Amplifying a second genome region further increases test specificity.

An ELISA or IFA seroconversion is defined as a negative test on acute serum followed by a positive test on convalescent serum or a 4-fold or greater rise in antibody titre between acute and convalescent phase sera tested in parallel. An antibody rise between acute and convalescent phase sera tested in parallel is highly specific. Because SARS is a new infection in humans, to the SARS coronaviruses (SARS-CoV) are not found in populations that have not been exposed to the virus.

Virus isolation is done by cell culture of SARS-CoV from any specimen, plus PCR confirmation using a validated method. In the post-outbreak period, all sporadic cases and clusters should be independently tested at another SARS reference laboratory with validated methods. As of 1 October 2003 WHO surveillance case definitions include definitions for both a suspect and a probable case. The surveillance case definitions are based on available clinical and epidemiological data and are supplemented by laboratory tests. Case definitions continue to be reviewed as diagnostic tests currently used in research settings become more widely available.

A suspect case is a person presenting after 1 November 2002 with a history of: high fever (>38°C/100.4°F) and cough or breathing difficulty and one or more of the following exposures during the 10 days prior to onset of symptoms: close contact (caring for, living with or in direct contact with respiratory secretions or body fluids) with a suspect or probable case of SARS; history of travel to an area with recent local transmission of SARS; current residency in an area with recent local transmission of SARS.

A person with an unexplained acute respiratory illness resulting in death after 1 November 2002 on whom no autopsy has been performed is also considered a *suspect case* if one or more of the following occurred during the 10 days prior to symptoms onset: close contact with a suspect or probable case of SARS, history of travel to an area with recent local SARS transmission, residence in an area with recent local transmission of SARS at the time of death.

A probable case is a suspect case with X-ray evidence of infiltrates consistent with pneumonia or respiratory distress syndrome (RDS), or positive for SARS coronavirus by one or more assays, or presenting autopsy findings consistent with RDS without identifiable cause.

A case should be excluded from surveillance if an alternative diagnosis can fully explain the illness as more diagnostic tests continue to be performed and the disease evolves. Because SARS is currently a diagnosis of exclusion, the status of a reported case may change over time. A case initially classified as suspect or probable for whom an alternative diagnosis can fully explain the illness should be excluded after considering the possibility of co-infection. A suspect case who, after investigation, fulfils the probable case definition should be reclassified as "probable" and a suspect case with a normal chest X-ray should be treated as appropriate and monitored for 7 days. Cases in which recovery is inadequate should be re-evaluated by chest X-ray. A suspect case in whom recovery is adequate but where illness cannot be fully explained by an alternative diagnosis should remain as "suspect". A suspect case who dies and on whom no autopsy is conducted should remain classified as "suspect" unless identified as being part of a chain transmission of SARS, at which time the case should be reclassified as "probable". If an autopsy has been conducted and no pathological evidence of RDS found, the case should be excluded as a case of SARS.

The clinical spectrum and course of SARS vary and appear to depend on immunological factors as yet not fully understood. From a review of probable cases, dyspnoea sometimes rapidly progresses to respiratory failure requiring ventilation; about 89% of cases recover and the case fatality rate is about 11%. From data collected during outbreaks, the likelihood of death from SARS appears to depend on characteristics of those infected, including age and presence of underlying disease. Current understanding, based on limited numbers of patients, suggests that the case fatality is less than 1% in persons aged 24 years or younger, 6% in persons aged 25 to 44 years, 15% in persons aged 45 to 64 years, and above 50% in persons aged 65 years or more.

2. Infectious agent—SARS is caused by a coronavirus similar, on electron microscopy, to animal coronaviruses. It is stable in feces and urine at room temperature for at least 1–2 days, and for up to 4 days in stools from patients who manifest diarrhea. The SARS virus loses infectivity after exposure to different commonly used disinfectants and fixatives. Heat at 56°C (132.8°F) kills the SARS coronavirus at approximately 10 000 units per 15 minutes.

3. Occurrence—Major outbreaks of SARS occurred during the period November 2002 to July 2003 in Canada, China (including Hong Kong Special Administrative Region and Taiwan), Singapore and Viet Nam. The virus is known to have been transported by infected humans to over 20 additional sites in Africa, the Americas, Asia, Australia, Europe, the Middle East and the Pacific. On July 5, 2003 WHO reported that person-to-person transmission of the SARS virus had been interrupted at all outbreak sites and recommended that intensified surveillance be continued to determine whether or not the disease had become endemic and would reappear, and so that in the case of re-emergence into human populations it would be detected. An isolated event in which a laboratory worker became PCR positive for the SARS virus occurred in Singapore in early September 2003.

A similar isolated laboratory worker infection occurred 3 months later in Taipei (Taiwan, China), without secondary transmission. A third laboratory infection involving 2 workers occurred in Beijing in April 2004. One of the cases transmitted the infection to a family member and a health worker, which resulted in a small third generation outbreak and full containment activities by the Chinese health authorities.

4. Reservoir—Unknown. Initial studies in Guandong Province, China, showed similar coronaviruses in some animal species sold in markets and further study continues.

5. Mode of transmission—SARS is transmitted from person to person by close contact: caring for, living with, or direct contact with respiratory secretions or body fluids of a suspect or probable case of SARS. This is thought to be primarily spread via droplets and possibly fomites. In one instance, the virus is thought to have been transmitted from person to person through some environmental vehicle, possibly aerosolised sewerage or transport of sewerage by mechanical vectors. Retrospective studies of this particular mode of transmission continue.

6. Incubation period—From 3 to 10 days.

7. Period of communicability—Not yet completely understood. Initial studies suggest that transmission does not occur before onset of clinical signs and symptoms, and that maximum period of communicability is less than 21 days. Health workers are at great risk, especially if involved in pulmonary procedures such as intubation or nebulization, and serve as a major entry point of the disease into the community.

8. Susceptibility—Unknown but assumed to be universal. At present race and gender appear not to alter susceptibility. Because of the small numbers of cases reported among children, it has not been possible to assess the influence of age.

9. Methods of control—

A. Preventive measures:

1) Identify all suspect and probable cases using the WHO case definitions:

Persons who arrive at health care facilities and require SARS assessment must be rapidly diverted by triage nurses to a separate area to minimize transmission to other patients and from probable SARS patients, and be given a face mask, preferably one that provides filtration of expired air.

Health workers involved in the triage process should wear a face mask (N/R/P 95/99/100 or FFP 2/3 or equivalent national manufacturing standard) with eye protection, and wash hands before and after contact with any patient, after activities likely to cause contamination and after removing gloves.

Soiled gloves, stethoscopes and other equipment must be treated with care as they have potential to spread infection. Disinfectants such as fresh bleach solutions must be widely available at appropriate concentrations.

2) Isolation of probable cases:

Probable SARS cases should be isolated and accommodated as follows in descending order of preference: negative pressure rooms with door closed, single room with own bathroom facilities, cohort placement in an area with an independent air supply, exhaust system and bathroom facilities. If an independent air supply is not feasible, air conditioning should be turned off and windows opened (if away from public places) for good ventilation.

Strict universal precautions for infection control must be practised using precautions for airborne, droplet and contact transmission; all staff, including ancillary staff, must be fully trained in infection control and use personal protective equipment (PPE):

- Face mask providing appropriate respiratory protection (NRP 95/99/100 or FFP 2/3 or equivalent manufacturing standard or standard applicable to the country of manufacture)
- Single pair of gloves
- Eye protection
- Disposable gown
- Apron
- Footwear that can be decontaminated.

Disposable equipment should be used wherever possible in treatment and care of patients with SARS, and disposed of appropriately. If devices are to be reused, they must be sterilized according to manufacturers' instructions. Surfaces should be cleaned with broad spectrum disinfectants of proven antiviral activity

Movement of patients outside the isolation unit should be avoided. If moved, patients should wear a face mask. Visits should be kept to a minimum and personal preventive equipment used under supervision.

Handwashing is crucial and access to clean water essential with handwashing before and after contact with any patient, after activities likely to cause contamination, and after removing gloves. Alcohol-based skin disinfectants can be used if there is no obvious organic material contamination.

Particular attention should be paid to interventions such as use of nebulizers, chest physiotherapy, bronchoscopy or gastroscopy and other interventions that may disrupt the respiratory tract or place the healthcare worker in close proximity to the patient and to potentially infected secretions.

All sharp and cutting instruments must be handled promptly and safely; patients' linen must be prepared on site for the laundry staff and placed into biohazard bags.

3) Contract tracing: For all persons fitting the suspect or probable case definition for SARS. From current epidemiological evidence, a contact is a person who cared for, lived with, or had direct contact with the respiratory secretions, body fluids and/or excretion (e.g. feces) of a suspect or probable cases of SARS. Contact tracing must be systematic for contacts during an agreed period prior to the onset of symptoms in the suspect or probable SARS case.

B. Control of patients, contacts and the immediate environment:

1) Patient management:

Hospitalize under isolation or cohort with other suspect or probable SARS cases, keeping the 2 categories of patients separated.

Obtain samples (sputum, blood, serum and urine,) to exclude standard causes of pneumonia (including atypical causes); consider possibility of coinfection with SARS and take appropriate chest radiographs. Obtain samples to aid clinical diagnosis SARS including: white blood cell count, platelet count, creatinine phosphokinase, liver function tests, urea and electrolytes, C reactive protein and paired sera.

Use full personal protection equipment for collection of specimens and for treatment/interventions that may cause aerosolization, such as the use of nebulisers with a bronchodilator, chest physiotherapy, bronchoscopy, gastroscopy, any procedure/intervention that may disrupt the respiratory tract.

At the time of admission, prescription of antibiotics for the treatment of community-acquired pneumonia is recommended until diagnoses of treatable causes of RDS have been excluded. Numerous antibiotherapies have been tried for treatment of SARS with no clear effect. Ribavirin with or without use of steroids has been used in several patients, but its effectiveness has not been proven and there has been a high incidence of severe adverse reactions. It has been proposed that a coordinated multi-centered approach to establishing the effectiveness of ribavirin therapy and other proposed interventions be examined.

2) Contact management:

Give information on the signs and symptoms and means of transmission to each contact.

Place under active surveillance for 10 days and recommend voluntary isolation at home and record temperature daily, stressing to the contact that the most consistent first symptom that is likely to appear is fever.

Ensure contact is visited or telephoned daily by a member

of the public health care team to determine whether fever or other signs and symptoms are developing.

If the contact develops fever or other SARS signs and symptoms, follow up examination should be done at an appropriate health care facility.

If the suspect or probable SARS case has been removed from surveillance because an alternative diagnosis can fully explain the illness, contacts can also be removed from surveillance and discharged from follow up.

C. Epidemic Measures:

During the SARS outbreaks of 2003 the perception of risk of infection by the general population was far greater than the actual risk of infection. Epidemic measures therefore should clearly inform the general public.

Establish a national SARS advisory group, including all governmental sectors concerned, to oversee epidemic measures, including epidemiological, clinical and other investigations that are conducted in the quest for more information.

Educate the population about the risk of infection, defining close contact with a SARS case and the signs and symptoms of SARS, and providing clear guidance as to how to avoid contact with SARS cases through mass media and/or other means.

Establish telephone "hot line" or other means of dealing with requests from the general public, and ensure that the means of contacting this resource are clearly provided to the general public.

Ensure adequate triage facilities and clearly indicate to the general public where they are located and how they can be accessed.

D. Disaster Implications:

As with other emerging infections, severe adverse economic impact and socio-economic consequences have been shown to occur.

E. International Measures:

WHO maintains global surveillance for clinically apparent cases of SARS (probable and suspect cases). Testing of clinically well contacts of probable or suspect SARS cases and community-based serological surveys are being conducted as part of epidemiological studies—this may ultimately change our understanding of SARS transmission (persons who test as SARS CoV positive in these studies should not be notified as SARS cases to WHO at this time).

WHO provides regular information updates and evidence-based travel recommendations, effective in limiting the international spread of infection, through the revision process of the *International Health Regulations*. A global response facilitating the work and exchange of information among scientists, clinicians and public health experts has been shown to be effective in providing information and effective evidence-based policies and strategies.

[D. Heymann]

SHIGELLOSIS
ICD-9 004; ICD-10 A03
(Bacillary dysentery)

1. Identification—An acute bacterial disease involving the distal small intestine and colon, characterized by loose stools of small volume accompanied by fever, nausea and sometimes toxaemia, vomiting, cramps and tenesmus. In typical cases, the stools contain blood and mucus (dysentery) resulting from mucosal ulcerations and confluent colonic crypt microabscesses caused by the invasive organisms; many cases present with a watery diarrhea. Convulsions may be an important complication in young children. Bacteraemia is uncommon. Mild and asymptomatic infections occur; illness is usually self-limited, lasting on average 4–7 days. Severity and case-fatality rate vary with the host (age and pre-existing nutritional state) and the serotype. *Shigella dysenteriae* 1 (Shiga bacillus) spreads in epidemics and is often associated with serious disease and complications including toxic megacolon, intestinal perforation and the hemolytic-uraemic syndrome; case-fatality rates have been as high as 20% among hospitalized cases even in recent years. In contrast, many infections with *S. sonnei* result in a short clinical course and an almost negligible case fatality rate except in immunocompromised hosts. Certain strains of *S. flexneri* can cause a reactive arthropathy (Reiter syndrome), especially in persons who are genetically predisposed by having HLA-B27 antigen.

Isolation of *Shigella* from feces or rectal swabs provides the bacteriological diagnosis. Prompt laboratory processing of specimens and use of appropriate media (differential, low selectivity–MacConkey agar—together with high selectivity XLD or S/S agar) increase the likelihood of *Shigella* isolation. Isolation of *S. dysenteriae* type 1 requires special efforts, since this organism is inhibited by some selective media, including S/S agar. Outside the human body *Shigella* remains viable only for a short period, which is why stool specimens must be processed rapidly after collection. Infection is usually associated with large numbers of fecal leukocytes detected through microscopical examination of stool mucus stained with methylene blue or Gram.

2. Infectious agents—The genus *Shigella* comprises 4 species or serogroups: A, *S. dysenteriae*; B, *S. flexneri*; C, *S. boydii*; D, *S. sonnei*. Groups A, B and C are further divided into 12, 14, and 18 serotypes and subtypes, respectively, designated by arabic numbers and lower case letters (e.g. *S. flexneri* 2a). *S. sonnei* (Group D) consists of a single serotype. A specific virulence plasmid is necessary for the epithelial cell invasiveness manifested by Shigellae. The infectious dose for humans is low (10–100 bacteria have caused disease in volunteers).

3. Occurrence—Worldwide; shigellosis causes an estimated 600 000 deaths per year. Two-thirds of the cases, and most of the deaths, are in children under 10. Illness in infants under 6 months is unusual. Secondary attack rates in households can be as high as 40%. Outbreaks occur under conditions of crowding; and where personal hygiene is poor, such as in prisons, institutions for children, day care centers, mental hospitals and crowded refugee camps, as well as among men who have sex with men. Shigellosis is endemic in both tropical and temperate climates; reported cases represent only a small proportion of cases, even in developed areas. The geographical distribution of the 4 Shigella serogroups is different, as is their pathogenicity.

More than one serotype is commonly present in a community; mixed infections with other intestinal pathogens also occur. In general, *S. flexneri*, *S. boydii* and *S. dysenteriae* account for most isolates from developing countries. *S. dysenteriae* type 1 is of particular concern in developing countries and complex emergency situations where huge outbreaks can occur. *S. sonnei* is most common in industrialized countries, where the disease is generally less severe. Multidrug-resistant Shigella (including *S. dysenteriae* 1) with considerable geographical variations have appeared worldwide, in relation with the widespread use of antimicrobial agents.

4. Reservoir—The only significant reservoir is humans, although prolonged outbreaks have occurred in primate colonies.

5. Mode of transmission—Mainly by direct or indirect fecal-oral transmission from a symptomatic patient or a short-term asymptomatic carrier. Infection may occur after the ingestion of contaminated food or water as well as from person to person. The infective dose can be as low as 10–100 organisms. Individuals primarily responsible for transmission include those who fail to clean hands and under fingernails thoroughly after defecation. They may spread infection to others directly by physical contact or indirectly by contaminating food. Water and milk transmission may occur as the result of direct fecal contamination; flies can transfer organisms from latrines to uncovered food items.

6. Incubation period—Usually 1–3 days, but may range from 12 to 96 hours; up to 1 week for *S. dysenteriae* 1.

7. Period of communicability—During acute infection and until the infectious agent is no longer present in feces, usually within 4 weeks after illness. Asymptomatic carriers may transmit infection; rarely, the carrier state may persist for months or longer. Appropriate antimicrobial treatment usually reduces duration of carriage to a few days.

8. Susceptibility—Susceptibility is general, infection following ingestion of a small number of organisms; in endemic areas the disease is more severe in young children than in adults, among whom many infections may be asymptomatic. The elderly, the debilitated and the malnourished of all ages are particularly susceptible to severe disease and death. Breast-feeding is protective for infants and young children. Studies with experimental serotype-specific live oral vaccines and parenteral polysaccharide conjugate vaccines show protection of short duration (1 year) against infection with the homologous serotype.

9. Methods of control—It is not possible to provide a specific set of guidelines applicable to all situations. General measures to improve hygiene are important but often difficult to implement because of their cost. An organized effort to promote careful handwashing with soap and water is the single most important control measure to decrease transmission rates in most settings.

The potentially high case-fatality rate in infections with *S. dysenteriae* 1, coupled with antibiotic resistance, calls for measures comparable to those for typhoid fever, including the need to identify the source(s) of all infections. In contrast, an isolated infection with *S. sonnei* in a private home would not deserve such an approach. Common source foodborne or waterborne outbreaks require prompt investigation and intervention whatever the infecting species. Institutional outbreaks may require special measures, including separate housing for cases and new admissions, a vigorous program of supervised handwashing, and repeated cultures of patients and attendants. The most difficult outbreaks to control are those that involve groups of young children (not yet toilet-trained) or the mentally deficient, and those where there is an inadequate supply of water. Closure of affected day care centers may lead to placement of infected children in other centers with subsequent transmission in the latter, and is not by itself an effective control measure.

A. *Preventive measures:* Same as those listed under typhoid fever, 9A1-9A10, except that no commercial vaccine is available.

B. *Control of patient, contacts and the immediate environment:*

1) Report to local health authority: Case report obligatory in many countries, Class 2 (see Reporting). Recognition and report of outbreaks in child care centers and institutions are especially important.

2) Isolation: During acute illness, enteric precautions. Because of the small infective dose, patients with known *Shigella* infections should not be employed to handle food or to provide child or patient care until 2 successive fecal samples or rectal swabs (collected 24 or more hours apart, but not sooner than 48 hours after discontinuance of antimicrobials) are found to be *Shigella*-free. Patients must be told of the importance and effectiveness of handwashing with soap and

water after defecation as a means of curtailing transmission of *Shigella*.

3) Concurrent disinfection: Of feces and contaminated articles. In communities with an adequate sewage disposal system, feces can be discharged directly into sewers without preliminary disinfection. Terminal cleaning.

4) Quarantine: Currently evaluated from the experiences of those countries with outbreaks.

5) Management of contacts: Whenever feasible, ill contacts should be excluded from food handling and the care of children or patients until diarrhea ceases and 2 successive negative stool cultures are obtained at least 24 hours apart and at least 48 hours after discontinuation of antibiotics. Thorough handwashing after defecation and before handling food or caring for children or patients is essential if such contacts are unavoidable.

6) Investigation of contacts and source of infection: The search for unrecognized mild cases and convalescent carriers among contacts may be unproductive and seldom contributes to the control of an outbreak. Cultures of contacts should generally be confined to food handlers, attendants and children in hospitals, and other situations where the spread of infection is particularly likely.

7) Specific treatment: Fluid and electrolyte replacement is important when diarrhea is watery or there are signs of dehydration (see Cholera, 9B7). Antibiotics, selected according to the prevailing antimicrobial sensitivity pattern of where cases occur, shorten the duration and severity of illness and the duration of pathogen excretion. They should be used in individual cases if warranted by the severity of illness or to protect contacts (e.g. in day care centers or institutions) when epidemiologically indicated. During the past 50 years *Shigella* have shown a propensity to acquire resistance against newly introduced antimicrobials that were initially highly effective. Multidrug resistance to most of the low-cost antibiotics (ampicillin, trimethoprim-sufamethoxazole) is common and the choice of specific agents will depend on the antibiogram of the isolated strain or on local antimicrobial susceptibility patterns. In many areas, the high prevalence of *Shigella* resistance to trimethoprim-sufamethoxazole, ampicillin and tetracycline has resulted in a reliance on fluoroquinolones such as ciprofloxacin as first line treatment, but resistance to these has also occurred. The use of antimotility agents such as loperamide is contraindicated in children and generally discouraged in adults since these drugs may prolong illness. If administered in an attempt to alleviate the severe cramps that often accompany

shigellosis, antimotility agents should be limited to 1 or at most 2 doses and never be given without concomitant antimicrobial therapy.

C. Epidemic measures:

1) Report at once to the local health authority any group of cases of acute diarrheal disorder, even in the absence of specific identification of the causal agent.
2) Investigate water, food, and milk supplies, and use general sanitation measures.
3) Prophylactic administration of antibiotics is not recommended.
4) Publicize the importance of handwashing after defecation; provide soap and individual paper towels if otherwise not available.

D. Disaster implications: A potential problem where personal hygiene and environmental sanitation are deficient (see Typhoid fever).

E. International measures: WHO Collaborating Centres.

[C. Chaignat]

SMALLPOX   ICD-9 050; ICD-10 B03

The last naturally acquired case of smallpox in the world occurred in October 1977 in Somalia; global eradication was certified 2 years later (1979) by WHO and sanctioned by the World Health Assembly (WHA) in May 1980. Except for a laboratory-associated smallpox death at the University of Birmingham, England, in 1978, no further cases have been identified. All known variola virus stocks are held under security at CDC, Atlanta GA, USA, or the State Research Centre of Virology and Biotechnology, Koltsovo, Novosibirsk Region, the Russian Federation. In response to concerns that live variola virus may be needed for research in the event that smallpox should re-emerge as result of accidental or intentional release, the WHA in May 1999 authorized that virus be retained at the laboratories in the Russian Federation and the USA for the purposes of essential research. The WHA reaffirmed that destruction of all the remaining virus stocks is still the Organization's ultimate goal and has appointed a group of experts to determine and oversee the research that must be carried out before the virus can be destroyed. WHO has also set up a biosafety inspection program for the 2 laboratories where official stocks are kept, in order to make sure they are secure and research can be carried out safely.

Because of increasing concerns about the potential for deliberate use of clandestine supplies of variola virus, it is important that health care workers become familiar with the clinical and epidemiological features of smallpox and how it can be distinguished from chickenpox.

1. Identification—Smallpox was a systemic viral disease generally presenting with a characteristic skin eruption. Preceding the appearance of the rash was a prodrome of sudden onset, with high fever (40°C/104°F), malaise, headache, prostration, severe backache and occasional abdominal pain and vomiting; a clinical picture that resembled influenza. After 2–4 days, the fever began to fall and a deep-seated rash developed in which individual lesions containing infectious virus progressed through successive stages of macules, papules, vesicles, pustules, then crusted scabs that fell off 3–4 weeks after the appearance of the rash. The lesions first appeared on the face and extremities, including the palms and soles, and subsequently on the trunk—the so-called centrifugal rash distribution—and were at the same stage of development in a given area.

Two types of smallpox were recognized during the 20th century: *variola minor* (alastrim), which had a case fatality rate of less than 1% and *variola major* with a fatality rate among unvaccinated populations of 20–50% or more. Fatalities normally occurred between the fifth and seventh day, occasionally as late as the second week. Fewer than 3% of variola major cases experienced a fulminant course, characterized by a severe prodrome, prostration, and bleeding into the skin and mucous membranes; such hemorrhagic cases were rapidly fatal. The usual vesicular rash did not appear and the disease might have been confused with severe leukaemia, meningococcaemia or idiopathic thrombocytopenic purpura. The rash of smallpox could also be significantly modified in previously vaccinated persons, to the extent that only a few highly atypical lesions might be seen. In such cases, prodromal illness was not modified but the maturation of lesions was accelerated with crusting by the tenth day.

Smallpox was most frequently confused with chickenpox, in which skin lesions commonly occur in successive crops with several stages of maturity at the same time. The chickenpox rash is more abundant on covered than on exposed parts of the body; the rash is centripetal rather than centrifugal. Smallpox was indicated by a clear-cut prodromal illness; by the more or less simultaneous appearance of all lesions when the fever broke; by the similarity of appearance of all lesions in a given area rather than successive crops; and by more deep-seated lesions, often involving sebaceous glands and scarring of the pitted lesions (chickenpox lesions are superficial and chickenpox rash is usually pruritic). Smallpox lesions were virtually never seen at the apex of the axilla.

Outbreaks of variola minor (alastrim) occurred in the late 19th century. Although the rash was like that in ordinary smallpox, patients generally experienced less severe systemic reactions, and hemorrhagic cases were virtually unknown.

Laboratory confirmation used isolation of the virus on chorioallantoic membranes or tissue culture from the scrapings of lesions, from vesicular or pustular fluid, from crusts, and sometimes from blood during the febrile prodrome. Electron microscopy or immunodiffusion technique often permitted a rapid provisional diagnosis. Molecular methods, such as PCR, are now available for rapid diagnosis of smallpox and other orthopoxvirus infections. Should smallpox infection be suspected, immediate communication by national authorities with WHO is suggested for advice on appropriate laboratories for diagnosis.

2. **Infectious agent**—Variola virus, a species of *Orthopoxvirus*.

3. **Occurrence**—Formerly a worldwide disease; no known human cases since 1978.

4. **Reservoir**—Smallpox was exclusively a human disease, with no known animal or environmental reservoir. Currently, the virus is maintained only in designated laboratories.

5. **Mode of transmission**—Infection usually occurred via the respiratory tract (droplet spread) or skin inoculation. The conjunctivae or the placenta were occasional portals of entry.

6. **Incubation period**—From 7–19 days; commonly 10–14 days to onset of illness and 2–4 days more to onset of rash.

7. **Period of communicability**—From the time of development of the earliest lesions to disappearance of all scabs; about 3 weeks. The risk of transmission appears to have been highest at the appearance of the earliest lesions, through droplet spread from the oropharyngeal enanthem.

8. **Susceptibility**—Susceptibility among the unvaccinated is universal.

9. **Methods of control**—Control of smallpox is based on identification and isolation of cases, vaccination (vaccinia virus) of contacts and those living in the immediate vicinity (ring vaccination), surveillance of contacts (including daily monitoring of temperature) and isolation of those contacts in whom fever develops.

Because of the relatively long period of incubation for smallpox, vaccination within a 4-day period after exposure can prevent or attenuate clinical illness.

Should a non-varicella, smallpox-like case be suspected, IMMEDIATE TELEPHONIC COMMUNICATION WITH LOCAL NATIONAL HEALTH AUTHORITIES IS OBLIGATORY. THESE SHOULD IMMEDIATELY INFORM WHO. Further information on http://www.who.int/csr/disease/smallpox.

VACCINIA   ICD-9 051.0; ICD-10 B08.0

Vaccinia virus, the immunizing agent used to eradicate smallpox, has been genetically engineered into candidate recombinant vaccines (some are in clinical trials), with low potential for spread to nonimmune contacts. Vaccination with licensed smallpox vaccine is recommended for all laboratory workers at high risk of contracting infection, such as those who directly handle cultures or animals contaminated or infected with vaccinia or other orthopoxviruses that infect humans. It may be considered for other health care personnel who are at lower risk of infection, such as doctors and nurses whose contact with these viruses is limited to contaminated dressings. WHO does not recommend vaccination in the general public because the risk of death (1 per 1 000 000 doses) or serious side-effects is greater than the known risk of infection with smallpox. Vaccination is contraindicated in persons with deficient immune systems; persons with eczema or certain other dermatitis disorders; and pregnant women. Vaccine immune globulin can be obtained for laboratory workers, in the USA through CDC Drug Service (404 639-3670), and from public health agencies in other industrialized countries. Vaccination should be repeated unless a major reaction (one that is indurated and erythematous 7 days after vaccination), or "take" has developed. Booster vaccinations are recommended within 10 years in categories for which vaccine is recommended. WHO maintains a supply of the vaccine seed lot (vaccinia virus strain Lister Elstree) at the WHO Collaborating Centre for Smallpox Vaccine at the National Institute of Public Health and Environmental Protection in Bilthoven, The Netherlands. WHO also maintains a stockpile of vaccine should an outbreak occur.

MONKEYPOX   ICD-9 051.9; ICD-10 B04

Human monkeypox is a sporadic zoonotic infection first identified (1970) from remote rural villages in central and western African rainforest countries as smallpox disappeared. Clinically the disease closely resembles ordinary or modified smallpox, but lymphadenopathy is a more prominent feature in many cases and occurs in the early stage of the disease. Pleomorphism and "cropping" similar to that seen in chickenpox are observed in 20% of patients. The natural history of the disease is unclear; humans, primates and squirrels appear to be involved in the enzootic cycle. The disease affects all age groups; children under 16 have historically constituted the greatest proportion of cases. The case-fatality rate among children not vaccinated against smallpox ranges from 1% to 14%. Smallpox vaccination protects against infection in some instances and in some others mitigates clinical manifestations. Between 1970 and 1994, over 400 cases were reported from western and central Africa; the Democratic Republic of the Congo (formerly Zaire) accounted for about 95% of reported cases during a 5-year surveillance (1981–1986). Poor public health infrastructure and other factors complicated accurate case reporting. Recently, a prolonged outbreak of human monkeypox occurred in the Democratic Republic of the Congo: it has been postulated that lack of vaccination and an epizootic allowed multiple virus transmission events to humans across the species barrier.

In the 1980s about 75% of reported cases were attributable to contact with affected animals; in recent outbreaks it appears that a larger number of cases were attributable to person-to-person contact. The longest chain of person-to-person transmission was 7 reported serial cases, but serial transmission usually did not extend beyond secondary. Epidemiological data suggests a secondary attack rate of about 8%. Most cases have occurred either singly or in clusters in small remote villages, usually in tropical rainforest where the population has multiple contacts with several types of wild animals. Ecological studies in the 1980s point to squirrels (*Funisciurus* and *Heliosciurus*), abundant among the oil palms surrounding the villages, as a significant local reservoir host. Maintenance of an animal reservoir and animal contact is required to sustain the disease among humans. Thus, human infection may be controllable by education to limit contact with infected cases and potentially infected animals. A recent outbreak of human monkeypox in the USA, thought to be related to importation and sale of exotic animals from western Africa as pets, resulted in over 70 cases, mainly among children and animal handlers.

Monkeypox virus is a species of the genus *Orthopoxvirus*, with biological properties and a genome map distinct from variola virus. There is no evidence that monkeypox will become a public health threat outside of enzootic areas. Cross-protective vaccination against smallpox is not recommended by WHO. A WHO Technical Advisory Committee on monkeypox has recently recommended continued studies, in particular, intensified prospective surveillance and ecological studies.

[D. Heymann]

SPOROTRICHOSIS   ICD-9 117.1; ICD-10 B42

1. Identification—A fungal disease, usually of the skin, often of an extremity, which begins as a nodule. As the nodule grows, lymphatics draining the area become firm and cord-like and form a series of nodules, which in turn may soften and ulcerate. Osteoarticular, pulmonary and multifocal infections are rare except as regards multifocal infections for patients with HIV infection. Fatalities are uncommon.

Culture of a biopsy, pus or exudate confirms the diagnosis. Organisms are rarely visualized by direct smear. Biopsied tissue should be examined with fungal stains.

2. Infectious agent—*Sporothrix schenckii*, a dimorphic fungus.

3. Occurrence—Reported worldwide, an occupational disease of farmers, gardeners and horticulturists. The disease is characteristically sporadic and relatively uncommon. An epidemic among gold miners in South Africa involved some 3000 people; fungus was growing on mine timbers. Contact with infected cats was an exposure risk in a Brazilian outbreak in 2003.

4. Reservoir—Soil, decaying vegetation, wood, moss and hay.

5. Mode of transmission—Introduction of fungus through the skin pricks from thorns or barbs, handling of sphagnum moss or slivers from wood or lumber. Outbreaks have occurred among children playing in and adults working with baled hay. Pulmonary sporotrichosis presumably arises through inhalation of conidia. Persons handling sick cats are an occupational risk group.

6. Incubation period—The lymphatic form may develop 1 week to 3 months after injury.

7. Period of communicability—Person-to-person transmission has only rarely been documented.

8. Susceptibility—Unknown.

9. Methods of control—

    A. Preventive measures: Treat lumber with fungicides in industries where disease occurs. Wear gloves and long sleeves when working with sphagnum moss, and use personal protection when handling sick cats.

    B. Control of patient, contacts and the immediate environment:

      1) Report to local health authority: Official report not ordinarily justifiable, Class 5 (see Reporting).
      2) Isolation: Not applicable.
      3) Concurrent disinfection: Of discharges and dressings. Terminal cleaning.
      4) Quarantine: Not applicable.
      5) Immunization of contacts: Not applicable.
      6) Investigation of contacts and source of infection: Seek undiagnosed and untreated cases.
      7) Specific treatment: Orally administered saturated solution of potassium iodide (increased drop by drop from 1–2 ml to 4–6 ml), given 3 times daily, or itraconazole are effective in lymphocutaneous infection; in extracutaneous forms, amphotericin B is the drug of choice, but itraconazole is also useful.

C. Epidemic measures: Determine source to limit future exposures. In the South African epidemic, mine timbers were sprayed with a mixture of zinc sulfate and triolith in order to control the epidemic.

D. Disaster implications: None.

E. International measures: None.

[A.M. Kimball]

STAPHYLOCOCCAL DISEASES

Staphylococci produce a variety of syndromes with clinical manifestations ranging from a single pustule to sepsis and death. A pus-containing lesion (or lesions) is the primary clinical finding, abscess formation is the typical pathological manifestation; production of toxins may also lead to staphylococcal diseases, as in toxic shock syndrome. Virulence of bacterial strains varies greatly. The most important human pathogen is *Staphylococcus aureus*. Most strains ferment mannitol and are coagulase-positive. However, coagulase-negative strains are increasingly important, especially in bloodstream infections among patients with intravascular catheters or prosthetic materials, in female urinary tract infections and in nosocomial infections.

Staphylococcal disease has different clinical and epidemiological patterns in the general community, in newborns, in menstruating women and among hospitalized patients; each will be presented separately. Staphylococcal food poisoning, an intoxication and not an infection, is also discussed separately (see Foodborne intoxications, section I, Staphylococcal).

I. STAPHYLOCOCCAL DISEASE IN THE COMMUNITY

BOILS, CARBUNCLES, FURUNCLES, ABSCESSES	ICD-9 680, 041.1; ICD-10 L02; B95.6-B95.8
IMPETIGO	ICD-9 684, 041.1; ICD-10 L01
CELLULITIS	ICD-9 682.9; ICD-10 L03
STAPHYLOCOCCAL SEPSIS	ICD-9 038.1; ICD-10 A41.0-A41.2
STAPHYLOCOCCAL PNEUMONIA	ICD-9 482.4; ICD-10 J15.2
ARTHRITIS	ICD-9 711.0, 041.1; ICD-10 M00.0
OSTEOMYELITIS	ICD-9 730, 041.1; ICD-10 M86
ENDOCARDITIS	ICD-9 421.0, 041.1; ICD-10 133.0

1. **Identification**—The common bacterial skin lesions are impetigo, folliculitis, furuncles, carbuncles, abscesses and infected lacerations. The basic lesion of impetigo is described in section II, 1; a distinctive "scalded skin" syndrome is associated with certain strains of *Staphylococcus aureus*, which elaborate an epidermolytic toxin. Other skin lesions are localized and discrete. Constitutional symptoms are unusual; if lesions extend or are widespread, fever, malaise, headache and anorexia may develop. Usually, lesions are uncomplicated, but seeding of the bloodstream may lead to pneumonia, lung abscess, osteomyelitis, sepsis, endocarditis, arthritis or meningitis. In addition to primary skin lesions, staphylococcal conjunctivitis occurs in newborns and the elderly. Staphylococcal pneumonia is a well-recognized complication of influenza. Staphylococcal endocarditis and other complications of staphylococcal bacteraemia may result from parenteral use of illicit drugs or nosocomially from intravenous catheters and other devices. Embolic skin lesions are frequent complications of endocarditis and/or bacteraemia.

Coagulase-negative staphylococci may cause sepsis, meningitis, endocarditis or urinary tract infections and are increasing in frequency, usually in connection with prosthetic devices or indwelling catheters.

Diagnosis is confirmed by isolation of the organism.

2. **Infectious agent**—Various coagulase-positive strains of *Staphylococcus aureus*. Most strains of staphylococci may be characterized through molecular methods such as pulsed-field gel electrophoresis, phage type, or antibiotic resistance profile; epidemics are caused by relatively few specific strains. The majority of clinical isolates of *Staphylococcus aureus*, whether community- or hospital-acquired, are resistant to penicillin G, and multiresistant (including methicillin-resistant) strains have

become widespread. Evidence suggests that slime-producing strains of coagulase-negative staphylococci may be more pathogenic, but the data are inconclusive. *S. saprophyticus* is a common cause of urinary tract infection in young women.

3. Occurrence—Worldwide. Highest incidence in areas where hygiene conditions (especially the use of soap and water) are suboptimal and people are crowded; common among children, especially in warm weather. The disease occurs sporadically and as small epidemics in families and summer camps, various members developing recurrent illness due to the same staphylococcal strain (hidden carriers).

4. Reservoir—Humans; rarely animals.

5. Mode of transmission—The major site of colonization is the anterior nares; 20%–30% of the general population are nasal carriers of coagulase-positive staphylococci. Autoinfection is responsible for at least one-third of infections. Persons with a draining lesion or purulent discharge are the most common sources of epidemic spread. Transmission is through contact with a person who has a purulent lesion or is an asymptomatic (usually nasal) carrier of a pathogenic strain. Some carriers are more effective disseminators of infection than others. The role of contaminated objects has been overstressed; hands are the most important instrument for transmitting infection. Airborne spread is rare but has been demonstrated in patients with associated viral respiratory disease.

6. Incubation period—Variable and indefinite.

7. Period of communicability—As long as purulent lesions continue to drain or the carrier state persists. Autoinfection may continue for the period of nasal colonization or duration of active lesions.

8. Susceptibility—Immune mechanisms depend mainly on an intact opsonization/phagocytosis axis involving neutrophils. Susceptibility is greatest among the newborn and the chronically ill. Elderly and debilitated people, drug abusers, and those with diabetes mellitus, cystic fibrosis, chronic renal failure, agammaglobulinaemia, disorders of neutrophil function (e.g. agranulocytosis, chronic granulomatous disease), neoplastic disease and burns are particularly susceptible. Use of steroids and antimetabolites also increases susceptibility.

9. Methods of control—

    A. Preventive measures:

        1) Educate the public and health personnel in personal hygiene, especially handwashing and the importance of not sharing toilet articles.

        2) Treat initial cases in children and families promptly.

B. Control of patient, contacts and the immediate environment:

1) Report to local health authority: Obligatory report of outbreaks in schools, summer camps and other population groups; also any recognized concentration of cases in the community for many industrialized countries. No individual case report, Class 4 (see Reporting).

2) Isolation: Not practical in most communities; infected people should avoid contact with infants and debilitated people.

3) Concurrent disinfection: Place dressings from open lesions and discharges in disposable bags; dispose of these in a practical and safe manner.

4) Quarantine: Not applicable.

5) Immmunization of contacts: Not applicable.

6) Investigation of contacts and source of infection: Search for draining lesions; occasionally, determination of nasal carrier status of the pathogenic strain among family members or health care workers (as appropriate) is useful.

7) Specific treatment: In localized skin infections, systemic antimicrobials are not indicated unless infection spreads significantly or complications ensue; local skin cleaning followed by application of an appropriate topical antimicrobial (such as mupirocin, 4 times a day) is adequate. Avoid wet compresses, which may spread infection; hot dry compresses may help localized infections. Incise abscesses to permit drainage of pus and possible removal of foreign bodies. For severe staphylococcal infections, use penicillinase-resistant penicillin; if there is hypersensitivity to penicillin, use a cephalosporin active against staphylococci (unless there is a history of immediate hypersensitivity to penicillin) or a macrolide. In severe systemic infections, choice of antibiotics should be governed by results of susceptibility tests on isolates. Vancomycin is the treatment of choice for severe infections caused by coagulase-negative staphylococci and methicillin-resistant *S. aureus*; prompt parenteral treatment is important.

   Strains of *Staphylococcus aureus* with decreased susceptibility to vancomycin and other glycopeptide antibiotics are reported from many countries worldwide. These were recovered from patients treated with vancomycin for extended periods (months). Occasional strains with high-level vancomycin resistance have recently been detected.

C. Epidemic measures:

1) Search and treat those with clinical illness, especially with draining lesions; strict personal hygiene with emphasis on

handwashing. Culture for nasal carriers of the epidemic strain and treat locally with mupirocin and, if unsuccessful, orally administered antimicrobials.

2) Investigate unusual or abrupt prevalence increases in community staphylococcal infections for a possible common source, e.g. an unrecognized hospital epidemic.

D. Disaster implications: None.

E. International measures: WHO Collaborating Centres.

II. STAPHYLOCOCCAL DISEASE IN HOSPITAL NURSERIES

IMPETIGO
   NEONATORUM   ICD-9 684, 041.1; ICD-10 L00
STAPHYLOCOCCAL SCALDED
   SKIN SYNDROME   ICD-9 695.8
(SSSS, Ritter disease)
ABSCESS OF THE
   BREAST   ICD-9 771.5, 041.1; ICD-10 P39.0

1. Identification—Impetigo or pustulosis of the newborn and other purulent skin manifestations are the staphylococcal diseases most frequently acquired in nurseries. Characteristic skin lesions develop secondary to colonization of nose, umbilicus, circumcision site, rectum or conjunctivae. Colonization of these sites with staphylococcal strains is a normal occurrence and does not imply disease.

Lesions most commonly occur in diaper and intertriginous areas but also elsewhere on the body. They are initially vesicular, rapidly turning seropurulent, surrounded by an erythematous base; bullae may form (bullous impetigo). Rupture of pustules favors their spread. Complications are unusual, although lymphadenitis, furunculosis, breast abscess, pneumonia, sepsis, arthritis, osteomyelitis and other have been reported.

Though uncommon, staphylococcal scalded skin syndrome (SSSS or Ritter disease, pemphigus neonatorum) may occur; clinical manifestations range from diffuse scarlatiniform erythema to generalized bullous desquamation. Like bullous impetigo, it is caused by strains of *S. aureus*, usually phage type II, which produce an epidermolytic toxin.

2. Infectious agent—See Staphylococcal disease in the community (Section I, 2).

3. Occurrence—Worldwide. Problems occur mainly in hospitals, are promoted by lax aseptic techniques and are exaggerated by development of antibiotic-resistant strains (hospital strains).

4. Reservoir—See Staphylococcal disease in the community (Section I, 4).

5. Mode of transmission—Primary spread by hands of hospital personnel; rarely airborne.

6. Incubation period—Commonly 4-10 days; disease may not occur until several months after colonization.

7. Period of communicability—See Staphylococcal disease in the community (Section I, 7).

8. Susceptibility—Susceptibility of newborn appears to be general. For the duration of colonization with pathogenic strains, infants remain at risk of disease.

9. Methods of control—

   A. Preventive measures:

   1) Use aseptic techniques when necessary and wash hands before contact with each infant in nurseries.
   2) Personnel with minor lesions (pustules, boils, abscesses, paronychia, conjunctivitis, severe acne, otitis external or infected lacerations) must not be permitted to work in the nursery.
   3) Surveillance and supervision through an active hospital infection control committee; they include a regular system for investigating, reporting and reviewing hospital-acquired infections. Illness developing after discharge from hospital must also be investigated and recorded, preferably through active surveillance of all discharged newborns after about 1 month.
   4) Some advocate routine application of antibacterial substances such as gentian violet, acriflavine, chlorhexidine or bacitracin ointment to the umbilical cord stump while in the hospital.

   B. Control of patient, contacts and the immediate environment:

   1) Report to local health authority: Obligatory report of epidemics; no individual case report, Class 4 (see Reporting).
   2) Isolation: Without delay, place all known or suspected cases in the nursery on contact isolation precautions.
   3) Concurrent disinfection: See Staphylococcal disease in the community (Section I, 9B3).
   4) Quarantine: Not applicable.
   5) Immmunization of contacts: Not applicable.
   6) Investigation of contacts and source of infection: See epidemic measures in 9C.

7) Specific treatment: Localized impetigo: cleanse skin and apply topical mupirocin ointment 4 times a day; widespread lesions may be treated orally with an antistaphylococcal antimicrobial such as cephalexin or cloxacillin. Serious infections require parenteral treatment (Section I, 9B7). Nasal decontamination with mupirocin is indicated to prevent recurrence.

C. Epidemic measures:

1) The occurrence of 2 or more concurrent cases of staphylococcal disease related to a nursery or a maternity ward is presumptive evidence of an outbreak and warrants investigation. Culture all lesions to determine antibiotic resistance pattern and type of epidemic strain. The laboratory should keep clinically important isolates for 6 months before discarding them, so as to support possible epidemiological investigation using antibiotic sensitivity patterns or pulsed-field gel electrophoresis.

2) In nursery outbreaks, institute isolation precautions for cases and contacts until all have been discharged. Use a rotational system ("cohorting") where one unit (A) is filled and subsequent babies are admitted to another nursery (B) while the initial unit (A) discharges infants and is cleaned before new admissions. If facilities are present for baby in-rooming, this may reduce risk. Colonized or infected infants should be grouped in another cohort. Assignments of nursing and other ward personnel should be restricted to specific cohorts.

Before admitting new patients, wash cribs, beds and other furniture with an approved disinfectant. Autoclave instruments that enter sterile body sites, wipe mattresses and thoroughly launder bedding and diapers (or use disposable diapers).

3) Examine *all* patient care personnel for draining lesions anywhere on the body. Perform an epidemiological investigation, and if one or more personnel are associated with the disease, culture nasal specimens from them and all others in contact with infants. It may become necessary to exclude and treat all carriers of the epidemic strain until cultures are negative. Treatment of asymptomatic carriers is directed at suppressing the nasal carrier state, usually through local application of appropriate antibiotic ointments to the nasal vestibule, sometimes with concurrent systemic rifampicin for 3–9 days.

4) Investigate adequacy of nursing procedures, especially availability of handwashing facilities. Emphasize strict hand-

washing; if facilities are inaccessible or inadequate, consider use of a hand antiseptic agent (e.g. alcohol) at the bedside. Personnel assigned to infected or colonized infants should not work with noncolonized newborns.

5) Although prohibited for routine use in the USA, preparations containing 3% hexachlorophene may be used during an outbreak. Full-term infants may be bathed (diaper area only) as soon after birth as possible and daily until they are discharged. After bathing is completed, wash hexachlorophene off thoroughly because systemic absorption may result in CNS damage.

D. Disaster implications: None.

E. International measures: WHO Collaborating Centres.

III. STAPHYLOCOCCAL DISEASE ON HOSPITAL MEDICAL AND SURGICAL WARDS   ICD-9 998.5; ICD-10 T81.4

1. Identification—Lesions vary from simple furuncles or stitch abscesses to extensively infected bedsores or surgical wounds, septic phlebitis, acute or chronic osteomyelitis, pneumonia, meningitis, endocarditis or sepsis. Postoperative staphylococcal disease is a constant threat to the convalescence of the hospitalized surgical patient. The increasing complexity of surgical operations, greater organ exposure and more prolonged anaesthesia promote entry of staphylococci. Increased use of prosthetic devices and indwelling catheters accounts for increased incidence of nosocomial staphylococcal infections. A toxic state can complicate infection (toxic shock syndrome) if the strain produces toxins (this is an ever-present risk). Frequent and sometimes injudicious use of antimicrobials has increased the prevalence of antibiotic-resistant staphylococci. Verification depends on isolation of *Staphylococcus aureus*, associated with a clinical illness compatible with the bacteriological findings.

2. Infectious agent—*Staphylococcus aureus*; see section I, 2. Resistance to penicillin occurs in 95% of strains and increasing proportions are resistant to semisynthetic penicillins (e.g. methicillin), aminoglycosides (e.g. gentamicin) and quinolones.

3. Occurrence—Worldwide. Staphylococcal infection is a major form of acquired sepsis in the general wards of hospitals. Attack rates may assume epidemic proportions and community spread may occur when hospital-infected patients are discharged.

4., 5., 6. and 7. Reservoir, Mode of transmission, Incubation period and **Period of communicability**—See Staphylococcal disease in the community (Section I, 4, 5, 6 and 7).

8. Susceptibility—See section I. Widespread use of continuous intravenous treatment with indwelling catheters and parenteral injections has opened new portals of entry for infectious agents.

9. Methods of control—

A. Preventive measures:

1) Educate hospital medical staff to use common, narrow-spectrum antimicrobials for simple staphylococcal infections for short periods and reserve certain antibiotics (e.g. cephalosporins for penicillin-resistant and vancomycin for beta-lactam resistant staphylococcal infections).
2) A hospital infection control committee must enforce strict aseptic technique and provide programs to monitor nosocomial infections.
3) Change sites of IV needle infusions every 48 hours; establish a monitoring system for the examination of central venous lines.

B. Control of patient, contacts and the immediate environment:

1) Report to local health authority: Obligatory report of epidemics; no individual case report, Class 4 (see Reporting).
2) Isolation: Whenever staphylococci are known or suspected to be abundant in draining pus or the sputum of a patient with pneumonia, the patient should be placed in a private room. This is not required when wound drainage is scanty, provided an occlusive dressing is used and care is taken in changing dressings to prevent environmental contamination. Health care workers must practise appropriate hand-washing, gloving and gowning techniques.
3) Concurrent disinfection: See Staphylococcal disease in the community (Section I, 9B3).
4) Quarantine: Not applicable.
5) Immmunization of contacts: Not applicable.
6) Investigation of contacts and source of infection: Not practical for sporadic cases (see 9C).
7) Specific treatment: Appropriate antimicrobials as determined through antibiotic sensitivity tests. Life-threatening infections should be treated with vancomycin pending test results.

C. Epidemic measures:

1) The occurrence of 2 or more cases with epidemiological association is sufficient to suspect epidemic spread and to initiate investigation.
2) See section II, 9C3.

3) Review and enforce rigid aseptic techniques.

D. Disaster implications: None.

E. International measures: WHO Collaborating Centres.

IV. TOXIC SHOCK SYNDROME ICD-9 785.5; ICD-10 A48.3

Toxic shock syndrome (TSS) is a severe illness characterized by sudden onset of high fever, vomiting, profuse watery diarrhea and myalgia, followed by hypotension and, in severe cases, shock. An erythematous "sunburn-like" rash is present during the acute phase; about 1–2 weeks after onset, with desquamation of the skin, especially of palms and soles. Fever is usually >38.8°C (102°F), systolic blood pressure <90 mm Hg and 3 or more of the following organ systems are involved: GI; muscular (severe myalgia and/or creatine phosphokinase level more than twice the normal upper limit); mucous membranes (vaginal, pharyngeal and/or conjunctival hyperaemia); renal (blood urea nitrogen or creatinine more than twice normal and/or sterile pyuria); hepatic (AST or ALT more than twice normal); hematological (platelets <100 000/mm³; SI units <100 × 109/L); and CNS (disorientation or alterations in consciousness without focal neurological signs).

Blood, throat and CSF cultures are negative for pathogens; the recovery of *S. aureus* from any of these sites does not invalidate a case. Serological tests for Rocky Mountain spotted fever, leptospirosis and measles are negative.

Most cases of TSS have been associated with strains of *S. aureus* producing toxic shock syndrome toxin 1. These strains, rarely present in vaginal cultures from healthy women, are regularly recovered from women with menstrually associated TSS or in those with TSS after gynaecological surgery.

Although almost all early cases of TSS occurred in women during menstruation, and most with vaginal tampon use, only 55% of cases now reported are associated with menses. Other risk factors include use of contraceptive diaphragms and vaginal contraceptive sponges, and infection following childbirth or abortion. Instructions for sponge use advising these should not be left in place for more than 30 hours must be heeded. A growing number of cases in men and women have shown *S. aureus* isolated from focal lesions of skin, bone, respiratory tract and surgical sites. No source of infection could be found in one-third of cases, where rash is often scant or indetectable.

Menstrual TSS can be prevented by avoiding use of highly absorbent vaginal tampons; risk may be reduced by using tampons intermittently (that is, not all day and all night throughout the period) and using less absorbent tampons. Women who develop a high fever and vomiting or diarrhea during menstruation must discontinue tampon use immediately and consult a physician. It is not known when those who have had an episode of menstrual TSS can safely resume tampon use.

A syndrome virtually identical to that occurring with *S. aureus* infection occurs with infection caused by group A beta-hemolytic streptococci.

Treatment of TSS is largely supportive. Efforts should be made to eradicate potential foci of *S. aureus* infection through drainage of wounds, removal of vaginal or other foreign bodies (e.g. wound packing) and use of beta-lactam resistant antistaphylococcal drugs. Clindamycin may help reduce toxin production.

[F. Waldvogel]

STREPTOCOCCAL DISEASES CAUSED BY GROUP A (BETA HEMOLYTIC) STREPTOCOCCI
ICD-9 034, 035, 670; ICD-10 A49.1, J02.0, A38, L01.0, A46, 085
(Streptococcal sore throat, Streptococcal infection, Scarlet fever, Impetigo, Erysipelas, Puerperal fever, Rheumatic fever)

1. Identification—Group A streptococci cause a variety of diseases. The most frequently encountered conditions are streptococcal pharyngitis/tonsillitis (sore throat) (ICD-10 J02.0) and streptococcal skin infections (impetigo or pyoderma). Other diseases and infections include scarlet fever (ICD-9 034.1/ICD-10 A38), puerperal fever (ICD-9 670/ICD-10 O85), septicemia, erysipelas, cellulitis, mastoiditis, otitis media, pneumonia, peritonsillitis, wound infections and rarely, necrotizing fasciitis, rheumatic fever and a toxic shock-like syndrome. One or other form of clinical disease often predominates during outbreaks.

Symptoms may be minimal or absent; patients with streptococcal sore throat typically exhibit sudden onset of fever, exudative tonsillitis or pharyngitis (sore throat), with tender, enlarged anterior cervical lymph nodes. The pharynx, the tonsillar pillars and soft palate may be injected and oedematous; petechiae may be present against a background of diffuse redness. Coincident or subsequent otitis media or peritonsillar abscess may occur; as may acute glomerulonephritis (1–5 weeks, mean 10 days) or acute rheumatic fever (mean 19 days). Rheumatic heart (valvular) disease occurs days to weeks after acute streptococcal infection, Sydenham chorea several months following infection.

Streptococcal skin infection (pyoderma, impetigo) is usually superficial and may proceed through vesicular, pustular and encrusted stages. Scarlatiniform rash is unusual and rheumatic fever is not a sequel; however, glomerulonephritis may occur later, usually 3 weeks after the skin infection.

Scarlet fever is a form of streptococcal disease characterized by a skin rash, occurring when the infecting strain produces a pyrogenic exotoxin (erythrogenic toxin) and the patient is sensitized but not immune to the toxin. Clinical characteristics may include all symptoms associated with a streptococcal sore throat (or with a streptococcal wound, skin or puerperal infection) as well as enanthem, strawberry tongue and exanthem. The rash is usually a fine erythema, commonly punctate, blanching on pressure, often felt (like sandpaper) better than seen and appearing most often on the neck, chest, folds of the axilla, elbow, groin and inner surfaces of the thighs.

Typically, the scarlet fever rash does not involve the face, but there is flushing of the cheeks and circumoral pallor. High fever, nausea and vomiting often accompany severe infections. During convalescence, desquamation of the skin occurs at the tips of fingers and toes, less often over wide areas of trunk and limbs, including palms and soles; it is more pronounced where the exanthem was severe. The case-fatality rate in some parts of the world has occasionally been as high as 3%. Scarlet fever may be followed by the same sequelae as streptococcal sore throat.

Erysipelas is an acute cellulitis characterized by fever, constitutional symptoms, leukocytosis and a red, tender, oedematous spreading lesion of the skin, often with a definite raised border. The central point of origin tends to clear as the periphery extends. Face and legs are common sites. Recurrences are frequent. The disease is more common in women and may be especially severe, with bacteraemia, in patients suffering from debilitating disease. Case-fatality rates vary depending on the part of the body affected and whether there is an associated disease. Erysipelas due to group A streptococci is to be distinguished from erysipeloid caused by *Erysipelothrix rhusiopathiae*, a localized cutaneous infection seen primarily as an occupational disease of people handling freshwater fish or shellfish, infected swine or turkeys or their tissues or, rarely, sheep, cattle, chickens or pheasants.

Perianal cellulitis due to group A streptococci has been recognized more frequently in recent years.

Streptococcal puerperal fever is an acute disease, usually febrile, with local and general symptoms/signs of bacterial invasion of the genital tract and sometimes the bloodstream in the postpartum or postabortion patient. Case-fatality rate is low when streptococcal puerperal fever is adequately treated. Puerperal infections may be caused by organisms other than hemolytic streptococci; they are clinically similar but differ bacteriologically and epidemiologically (See Staphylococcal disease).

Toxic shock syndrome (TSS) in people with invasive group A streptococcal infection has been increasingly recognized since 1987. Predominant clinical features include hypotension and any of the following: renal impairment; thrombocytopenia; disseminated intravascular coagulation (DIC); SGOT or bilirubin elevation; adult respiratory distress syndrome; a generalized erythematous macular rash or soft-tissue necrosis (necrotizing fasciitis). TSS may occur with either systemic or focal (throat, skin, lung sites) group A streptococcal infections.

Streptococci of other groups can produce infections in humans. Beta-hemolytic organisms of group B found in the human vagina may cause neonatal sepsis and suppurative meningitis (see Group B streptococcal disease of the newborn), as well as urinary tract infections, postpartum endometritis and other systemic disease in adults, especially those with diabetes mellitus. Group D organisms (including enterococci), hemolytic or nonhemolytic, are involved in bacterial endocarditis and urinary tract infections. Groups C and G have produced outbreaks of streptococcal tonsillitis, usually foodborne; their role in sporadic cases is less well-defined. Glomerulonephritis has followed group C infections, but has very rarely been reported after group G infection; neither group causes rheumatic fever. Group C and G infections are more common in adolescents and young adults. Alpha-hemolytic streptococci are also a common cause of bacterial endocarditis.

Provisional laboratory findings for group A streptococcal disease are based on the isolation of the organisms from affected tissues on blood agar or other appropriate media, or on identification of group A streptococcal antigen in pharyngeal secretions (the rapid antigen detection test). Colony morphology and the production of clear beta-hemolysis on blood agar made with sheep's blood identify streptococci on cultures; inhibition by special antibiotic discs containing bacitracin (0.02–0.04 units) constitutes tentative identification. Specific serogrouping procedures provide definitive identification. Antigen detection tests also allow rapid identification, demonstrating a rise in serum antibody titre (antistreptolysin O, antihyaluronidase (not commercially available), anti-DNA-ase B) between acute and convalescent stages of illness; high titres may persist for several months.

In the USA, the current recommended practice is to first do a rapid antigen detection test (high specificity but low sensitivity) and, if this is positive, assume the patient has a group A streptococcal infection. If the result is negative or equivocal, a throat culture should be done to guide management and prevent superfluous antibiotherapy.

2. **Infectious agent**—*Streptococcus pyogenes*, group A streptococci of over 130 serologically distinct types that vary by geographic and time distributions. Group A streptococci producing skin infections usually differ serologically from those associated with throat infections. In scarlet fever, 3 immunologically different types of erythrogenic toxin (pyrogenic exotoxins A, B and C) have been demonstrated. In TSS, 80% of isolates produce pyrogenic exotoxin A. While beta-hemolysis is characteristic of group A streptococci, strains of groups B, C and G are often also beta-hemolytic. Phenotypically mucoid strains have been involved in recent outbreaks of rheumatic fever.

3. **Occurrence**—Streptococcal pharyngitis/tonsillitis and scarlet fever

are common in temperate zones, well recognized in semitropical areas and less frequently recognized in tropical climates. Inapparent infections are at least as common in tropical as in temperate zones. In the USA, streptococcal diseases may be endemic, epidemic or sporadic. Before the age of 2–3, streptococcal infections may occur but streptococcal pharyngitis is unusual; this peaks in age group 6–12 and declines thereafter. Cases occur year round but peak in colder seasons. Group A streptococcal infections caused by specific types of M protein (M-types), especially types 1, 3, 4, 12 and 25, have frequently been associated with the development of acute glomerulonephritis after pharyngeal infection.

Acute rheumatic fever may occur as a nonsuppurative complication following infection with group A serotypes that have the capacity to produce clinical infection of the upper respiratory tract. This complication had virtually disappeared from industrialized countries until the mid-nineteen eighties; increased numbers are being reported. Many of the reported cases have followed infections by specific group A serotypes, such as M-types 1, 3, 5, 6 and 18.

Rheumatic fever remains a great health problem in the developing world. The highest incidence, during late winter and spring, corresponds to that of pharyngitis. Age group 3–15 is most often affected, as are military and school populations. Together with reappearance of rheumatic fever, more severe streptococcal infections have also been reported; including generalized infections and toxic shock syndrome.

In the USA, of the estimated 10 000–15 000 annual cases of severe infection by group A streptococcus, 500–1500 develop necrotizing fasciitis.

The highest incidence of streptococcal impetigo occurs in young children in the latter part of the hot season in hot climates. Nephritis following skin infections is associated with a limited number of streptococcal M-types (among which types 2, 49, 55, 57, 58, 59, 60) that generally differ from those associated with nephritis following infections of the upper respiratory tract.

Geographical and seasonal distribution of erysipelas are similar to those for scarlet fever and streptococcal sore throat; erysipelas is most common in infants and those over 20. Occurrence is sporadic, even during epidemics of streptococcal infection.

Reliable morbidity data do not exist for puerperal fever. In industrialized countries, morbidity and mortality have declined, although epidemics may still occur in institutions where aseptic technique is faulty.

4. **Reservoir**—Humans.

5. **Mode of transmission**—Large respiratory droplets or direct contact with patients or carriers, rarely indirect contact through objects. Individuals with acute upper respiratory tract (especially nasal) infections are particularly likely to transmit infection. Casual contact rarely leads to infection. In populations where impetigo is prevalent, group A strepto-

cocci may be recovered from the normal skin for 1-2 weeks before skin lesions develop; the same strain may appear in the throat (without clinical evidence of throat infection) usually late in the course of the skin infection.

Anal, vaginal, skin and pharyngeal carriers have been responsible for nosocomial outbreaks of serious streptococcal infection, particularly following surgical procedures. Many such outbreaks have been traced to operating room personnel. Identification of the carrier often involves intensive epidemiological and microbiological investigation; eradication of the carrier state is often difficult and may require multiple courses of specific antibiotic regimens (see 9, B7). Dried streptococci reaching the air via contaminated items (floor dust, lint from bedclothes, handkerchiefs) may be viable but apparently do not infect mucous membranes and intact skin.

Explosive outbreaks of streptococcal sore throat may follow ingestion of contaminated food. Milk and milk products have been associated most frequently with foodborne outbreaks; egg salad and similar preparations have recently been implicated. Group B organisms that cause human and bovine disease differ biochemically, but group A streptococci may be transmitted to cattle from human carriers, then spread through raw milk from these cattle. Contamination of milk or egg products by humans appears to be the important source of foodborne episodes. Milkborne group C outbreaks have been traced to infected cows.

6. Incubation period—Short, usually 1-3 days, rarely longer.

7. Period of communicability—In untreated, uncomplicated cases, 10-21 days; in untreated conditions with purulent discharges, weeks or months. With adequate penicillin treatment, transmissibility generally ends within 24 hours. Patients with untreated streptococcal pharyngitis may carry the organism for weeks or months, usually in decreasing numbers; contagiousness for these patients decreases sharply in 2-3 weeks after onset of infection.

8. Susceptibility—Susceptibility to streptococcal pharyngitis/tonsillitis and scarlet fever is general, although many people develop either antitoxin- or type-specific antibacterial immunity, or both, through inapparent infection. Antibacterial immunity develops against the specific M-type of group A streptococcus that induced infection and may last for years. Antibiotherapy may interfere with the development of type-specific immunity. No differences in susceptibility have been defined for men and women; reported racial differences probably relate to environmental factors.

Repeated attacks of pharyngitis/tonsillitis or other disease due to different types of streptococci are relatively frequent. Immunity against erythrogenic toxin, and hence against rash, develops within a week after onset of scarlet fever and is usually permanent; second attacks of scarlet fever are rare, but may occur because of the 3 immunological forms of toxin. Some degree of passive immunity to group A streptococcal disease occurs in newborns with transplacental maternal type specific antibodies.

Patients who had one attack of rheumatic fever have a significant risk of recurrence of rheumatic fever, often with further cardiac damage following group A streptococcal infections. Individuals who had erysipelas appear predisposed to subsequent attacks. Recurrence of glomerulonephritis is unusual, perhaps because very few M-types are "nephritogenic".

9. **Methods of control—**

   A. *Preventive measures:*

   1) Educate the public and health workers about modes of transmission; about the relationship of streptococcal infection to acute rheumatic fever, Sydenham chorea, rheumatic heart disease and glomerulonephritis; and about the need for prompt diagnosis and completion of the full course of antibiotherapy prescribed for streptococcal infections.
   2) Provide easily accessible laboratory facilities for recognition of group A hemolytic streptococci.
   3) Pasteurize milk and exclude infected people from handling milk likely to become contaminated.
   4) Prepare other potentially dangerous foods just prior to serving or adequately refrigerate in small quantities at 4°C (39°F) or less.
   5) Exclude people with skin lesions from food handling.
   6) Secondary prevention of complications: To prevent streptococcal reinfection and possible recurrence of rheumatic fever, erysipelas or chorea, monthly injections of long-acting benzathine penicillin G (or daily penicillin orally in compliant patients) should be given for at least 5 years. Those who do not tolerate penicillin may be given sulfisoxazole orally or erythromycin if necessary.

   B. *Control of patient, contacts and the immediate environment:*

   1) Report to local health authority: Obligatory report of epidemics, Class 4. Acute rheumatic fever and/or streptococcal TSS reportable in some localities, Class 3 (see Reporting).
   2) Isolation: Drainage and secretion precautions may be terminated after 24 hours' effective antibiotherapy; antibiotherapy should be continued for 10 days to avoid development of rheumatic heart disease.
   3) Concurrent disinfection: Of purulent discharges and all articles soiled therewith. Terminal cleaning.
   4) Quarantine: Not applicable.

5) Immmunization of contacts: Not applicable; a readily available vaccine against streptococcus A is unlikely in the immediate future.

6) Investigation of contacts and source of infection: Culture symptomatic contacts. Search for and treat carriers in well-documented epidemics of streptococcal infection and in high risk situations (e.g. evidence of streptococcal infection in families with multiple cases of rheumatic fever or streptococcal TSS, occurrence of cases of rheumatic fever or acute nephritis in a population group such as a school, outbreaks of postoperative wound infections).

7) Specific treatment: Penicillin; several forms: benzathine penicillin G, IM (treatment of choice), or oral penicillin G or penicillin V (which is more absorbable). There has never been a documented penicillin-resistant strain of group A beta-hemolytic streptococci. Treatment must provide adequate penicillin levels for 10 days. While antibiotherapy may shorten clinical illness somewhat, it is also recognized that patients with streptococcal pharyngitis improve in 3-4 days without antibiotherapy. Appropriate antibiotherapy reduces the frequency of suppurative complications and prevents the development of most cases of acute rheumatic fever. It may also reduce the risk of acute glomerulonephritis after pharyngeal infection (not confirmed for acute nephritis after skin infections) and prevent further spread of the organism in the community. Erythromycin is the preferred treatment for penicillin sensitive patients, but strains resistant to this antibiotic have been reported (up to 38%), most notably in Asia and Europe. Clindamycin or a cephalosporin can be used when penicillin and erythromycin are contraindicated, e.g. because of allergy or resistance. Sulfonamides do not eliminate streptococci from the throat nor do they prevent nonsuppurative complications. Many group A streptococcal strains are resistant to the tetracyclines and these should not be used against streptococcal pharyngitis.

C. Epidemic measures:

1) Determine source and manner of spread (person-to-person, milk, food). Outbreaks can often be traced to an individual with an acute or persistent streptococcal infection or bearing streptococci (nose, throat, skin, vagina or perianal area) through identification of the M-type of the streptococcus.

2) Investigate promptly any unusual grouping of cases to identify possible common sources, such as contaminated milk or foods.

3) For outbreaks in special close contact groups (e.g. the military, day care centers, schools, nursing homes), it may be necessary to administer penicillin to the entire group to terminate spread.

D. **Disaster implications:** Patients with thermal burns or wounds are highly susceptible to streptococcal infections of the affected area.

E. **International measures:** WHO Collaborating Centres.

[E. Kaplan]

GROUP B STREPTOCOCCAL SEPSIS OF THE NEWBORN   ICD-9 771.8; ICD-10 P36.0

Human subtypes of group B streptococci (*S. agalactiae*) produce invasive disease in the newborn under 2 distinct forms. Early onset disease (from 1–7 days), with sepsis, pneumonia and less frequently meningitis, osteomyelitis or septic arthritis, is acquired in utero or during delivery. Late onset disease (7 days to several months) is acquired in about half the cases through person-to-person contact and presents mostly as meningitis or sepsis. Premature babies are more susceptible to Group B streptococci infection than full-term babies, but most babies who get disease from these streptococci (75%) are full term. Advances in neonatal care has led to a fall in the case fatality rate from 50% to 4%. Survivors may have speech, hearing or visual problems, psychomotor retardation or seizure disorders if there has been meningeal involvement.

About 10%–30% of pregnant women harbour group B streptococci in the genital tract, and about 1% of their offspring may develop symptomatic infection. Group B streptococci found in bovine mastitis are not a cause of this disease. Two prevention methods have been used successfully. The risk-based method identifies candidates for intrapartum chemoprophylaxis according to the presence of any of the following intrapartum risk factors for early-onset disease: delivery at <37 weeks, intrapartum temperature >38.0°C (>100.4°F), or rupture of membranes for 18 hours or more. The screening-based method recommends screening all pregnant women for vaginal and rectal GBS colonization between 35 and 37 weeks' gestation and offering women with colonization intrapartum antibiotics during labour. In both cases, women with GBS bacteriuria during the current pregnancy, or who previously gave birth to an infant with early-onset GBS disease are candidates for intrapartum antibiotic prophylaxis.

Compelling evidence for a strong protective effect of the screening-based strategy relative to the risk-based strategy led to the current recommendation of prenatal screening by vaginal-rectal culture for group B streptococcus colonization at 35–37 weeks' gestation and chemoprophylaxis for all pregnant women identified as GBS carriers at the time of labour or rupture of membranes. Women whose culture results are unknown at the time of delivery should be managed according to the risk-based approach mentioned earlier.

The administration to women colonized with group B streptococci of intravenous penicillin or ampicillin at the onset and throughout labour interrupts transmission to newborn infants, decreasing infection and mortality. Penicillin is the preferred agent in women without penicillin allergy. No GBS isolates with confirmed resistance to penicillin or ampicillin have been observed to date. Alternative regimens for allergic women include clindamycin, erytromycin and cefazolin. Routine use of antimicrobial prophylaxis for newborns whose mothers received intrapartum chemoprophylaxis for GBS infection is not recommended, although therapeutic use of these agents is appropriate for infants with clinically suspected sepsis. A vaccine for pregnant women to stimulate antibody production against invasive disease in newborns is under development.

[O. Lincetto]

DENTAL CARIES OF EARLY CHILDHOOD, STREPTOCOCCAL ICD-9 521.0; ICD-10 K02
(Nursing bottle caries, Baby bottle tooth decay)

While the cause of dental caries in young children is multifactorial, the subject is included in this section because of the involvement of a streptococcal species.

In early childhood a characteristic pattern of dental caries occurs, in which maxillary primary incisors are routinely affected with carious lesions, but mandibular primary incisors are rarely involved; involvement of other primary teeth varies. Because of the association of this pattern with a specific feeding habit, the process was called nursing bottle caries or baby bottle tooth decay, but it also occurs in children using feeding cups.

Streptococcus mutans is present in these carious lesions. These Gram-positive facultative anaerobes produce caries in young experimental animals in the presence of dietary sugar. They are members of the *viridans* group of streptococci; hemolysis of blood agar is usually alpha or gamma. They require a nonshedding oral surface for colonization and are common residents of dental plaque.

Early childhood caries occurs worldwide, with highest prevalence in developing countries. Disadvantaged children, regardless of ethnicity or culture, and those with low birthweight, are most frequently involved; enamel hypoplasia, which may occur because of compromised nutritional status during formative stages of primary dentition, is often associated. The main reservoir from which infants acquire *mutans* streptococci is the mother; strains isolated from mothers and their babies show similar or identical bacteriocin profiles and identical plasmid or chromosomal DNA patterns.

Mother-to-child transmission occurs through transfer of infected saliva by kissing the baby on the mouth or, more likely, by moistening the nipple or pacifier or by tasting food on the baby's spoon before serving it. Colonization by maternal organisms largely depends on inoculum size; mothers with extensive dental caries usually have high levels of *mutans* streptococci in their saliva.

To prevent dental caries of early childhood, promote good oral hygiene in mothers and encourage early weaning from the bottle. Counsel parents and caretakers about the dangers of dental caries from feeding children milk and other beverages containing sugar and of transferring saliva to a baby's mouth when mothers and other caretakers have untreated carious teeth.

[P. Petersen]

STRONGYLOIDIASIS ICD-9 127.2; ICD-10 B78

1. Identification—An often asymptomatic helminthic infection of the duodenum and upper jejunum. Clinical manifestations include transient dermatitis when larvae of the parasite penetrate the skin on initial infection; cough, rales and sometimes demonstrable pneumonitis when larvae pass through the lungs; or abdominal symptoms caused by the adult female worm in the intestinal mucosa. Symptoms of chronic infection may be mild or severe, depending on the intensity of infection.

Classic symptoms include abdominal pain (usually epigastric, often suggesting peptic ulcer), diarrhea and urticaria; sometimes also nausea, weight loss, vomiting, weakness and constipation. Intensely pruritic dermatitis (larva currens) radiating from the anus may occur; as can stationary wheals lasting 1–2 days as well as a migrating serpiginous rash moving several centimeters per hour across the trunk. Rarely, intestinal autoinfection with increasing worm burden may lead to disseminated strongyloidiasis with wasting, pulmonary involvement and death, particularly but not exclusively in the immunocompromised host. In these cases, secondary Gram-negative sepsis is common. Eosinophilia is usually moderate (10%–25%) in the chronic stage and in those with intercurrent infections, especially persons infected with human T-cell lymphotrophic virus (HTLV-1) and those receiving chemotherapy for malignancies, but may be normal or low with dissemination.

Diagnosis entails identifying larvae in concentrated stool specimens (motile in freshly passed feces), in the agar plate method, in duodenal aspirates or, occasionally, in sputum. Ruling out the diagnosis may require repeat examinations. Held at room temperature for 24 hours or more, feces may show developing stages of the parasite, including rhabditiform (noninfective) larvae and filariform (infective) larvae (these must be distinguished from larvae of hookworm species) and free-living adults. Serological tests based on larval stage antigens are positive in 80%–85% of infected patients.

2. Infectious agents—*Strongyloides stercoralis* and *S. fulleborni*, nematodes.

3. Occurrence—Throughout tropical and temperate areas; more common in warm, wet regions. Prevalence in endemic areas not accurately known. May be prevalent in residents of institutions where personal hygiene is poor. *S. fulleborni* has been reported only in Africa and in Papua New Guinea.

4. Reservoir—Humans are the principal reservoir of *S. stercoralis*, with occasional transmission of dog and cat strains to humans. Nonhuman primates are the reservoir of *S. fulleborni* in Africa. Person-to-person transmission may also occur.

5. Mode of transmission—Infective (filariform) larvae develop in feces or moist soil contaminated with feces, penetrate the skin, enter the venous circulation and are carried to the lungs. They penetrate capillary walls, enter the alveoli, ascend the trachea to the epiglottis and descend into the digestive tract to reach the upper part of the small intestine, where development of the adult female is completed.

The adult worm, a parthenogenetic female, lives embedded in the mucosal epithelium of the intestine, especially the duodenum, where eggs are deposited. These hatch and liberate rhabditiform (noninfective) larvae that migrate into the intestinal lumen, exit in feces and develop after reaching the soil into either infective filariform larvae (which may infect the same or a new host) or free-living male and female adults. The free-living fertilized females produce eggs that hatch and liberate rhabditiform larvae, which may become filariform larvae within 24–36 hours. In some individuals, rhabditiform larvae may develop to the infective stage before leaving the body and penetrate through the intestinal mucosa or perianal skin; the resulting autoinfection can cause persistent infection for many years.

6. Incubation period—From penetration of the skin by filariform larvae until rhabditiform larvae appear in the feces takes 2–4 weeks; the period until symptoms appear is indefinite and variable.

7. Period of communicability—As long as living worms remain in the intestine; up to 35 years in cases of autoinfection.

8. Susceptibility—Susceptibility is universal. Acquired immunity has been demonstrated in laboratory animals but not in humans. HIV-infected patients with AIDS, with malignant disease or on immunosuppressive medication are at risk of dissemination.

9. **Methods of control—**

   A. *Preventive measures:*

   1) Dispose of human feces in a safe manner.
   2) Pay strict attention to hygienic habits, including use of footwear in endemic areas.
   3) Rule out strongyloidiasis before initiating immunosuppressive treatment.
   4) Examine and treat infected dogs, cats and monkeys in contact with people.

   B. *Control of patient, contacts and the immediate environment:*

   1) Report to local health authority: Official report not ordinarily justifiable, Class 5 (see Reporting).
   2) Isolation: Not applicable.
   3) Concurrent disinfection: Safe disposal of feces.
   4) Quarantine: Not applicable.
   5) Immmunization of contacts: Not applicable.
   6) Investigation of contacts and source of infection: Members of the same household or institution should be examined for evidence of infection.
   7) Specific treatment: Because of the potential for autoinfection and dissemination, all infections, regardless of worm burden, should be treated. Ivermectin is the drug of choice; thiabendazole or albendazole are less efficient alternatives. Repeated courses of treatment may be required.

   C. *Epidemic measures:* Not applicable; a sporadic disease.

   D. *Disaster implications:* None.

   E. *International measures:* None.

   [L. Savioli]

SYPHILIS
I. VENEREAL SYPHILIS   ICD-9 090-096; ICD-10 A50-A52
(Lues)

1. Identification—An acute and chronic treponemal disease characterized clinically by a primary lesion, a secondary eruption involving skin and mucous membranes, long periods of latency, and late lesions of skin, bone, viscera, the CNS and cardiovascular system. The primary lesion (chancre) usually appears about 3 weeks after exposure as an indurated, painless ulcer with a serous exudate at the site of initial invasion. Invasion of the bloodstream precedes the initial lesion; a firm, nonfluctuant, painless satellite lymph node (bubo) commonly follows.

Infection may occur without a clinically evident external chancre; e.g. in the rectum or on the cervix. After 4-6 weeks, even without specific treatment, the chancre begins to involute and, in most cases, a generalized secondary eruption appears, often accompanied by mild constitutional symptoms. A symmetrical maculopapular rash involving the palms and soles, with associated lymphadenopathy, is classic. There is some evidence that HIV immunosupressed patients may have less defence against CNS infection. Secondary manifestations resolve spontaneously within weeks to 12 months; all untreated cases will go on to latent infection for weeks to years, and one-third will exhibit tertiary syphilis signs and symptoms. In the early years of latency, there may be recurrence of infectious lesions of the skin and mucous membranes.

CNS disease, manifested as acute syphilitic meningitis, may occur at any time in secondary or early latent syphilis, later as meningovascular syphilis, and finally as paresis or tabes dorsalis. Latency sometimes continues through life. In other instances, and unpredictably, 5-20 years after initial infection, disabling lesions occur in the aorta (cardiovascular syphilis) or gummas may occur in the skin, viscera, bone and/or mucosal surfaces. Death or serious disability rarely occurs during early stages; late manifestations shorten life, impair health and limit occupational efficiency. The widespread use of antimicrobials has decreased the frequency of late manifestations. Concurrent HIV infection may increase the risk of CNS syphilis; neurosyphilis must be considered in the differential diagnosis of HIV-infected individuals with CNS symptoms.

Fetal infection results in congenital syphilis and occurs with high frequency in untreated early infections of pregnant women. It frequently causes abortion or stillbirth and may cause infant death through preterm delivery of low birthweight infants or from generalized systemic disease. Congenital infection may result in late manifestations that include involvement of the CNS with occasional stigmata such as Hutchinson teeth (small, wide-spaced, greyish incisors), saddlenose, sabre shins (periostitis), interstitial keratitis and deafness. Congenital syphilis can be asymptomatic, especially in the first weeks of life.

The laboratory diagnosis of syphilis is usually made through serological testing of blood (and CSF when indicated). Reactive tests with nontreponemal antigens (e.g. RPR [rapid plasma reagin] or VDRL [Venereal Disease Research Laboratory]) must be confirmed by tests using treponemal antigens (i.a., FTA-Abs [fluorescent treponemal antibody absorbed] or TPHA [*T. pallidum* hemagglutinating antibody]), when available, to aid in excluding biological false-positive reactions. For screening newborns, serum is preferred over cord blood, which produces more false-positive reactions. Primary and secondary syphilis can be confirmed through darkfield or phase-contrast examination or FA antibody staining of exudates from lesions or aspirates from lymph nodes if no antibiotic has been administered. Serological tests are usually nonreactive during the early primary stage while the chancre is still present; a darkfield examination of all genital ulcerative lesions can be useful, particularly in suspected early seronegative primary syphilis.

2. Infectious agent—*Treponema pallidum*, subsp. *pallidum*, a spirochaete.

3. Occurrence—Widespread; in industrialized countries sexually active young people between 20 and 29 are primarily involved. Racial differences in incidence reflect social rather than biological factors. Syphilis is usually more prevalent in urban than rural areas, and in some cultures, in males more than in females. After some decline in the late 1970s and early 1980s, incidence has increased again in recent years, notably in western Europe and the USA; in Eastern Europe, contributing factors include a decline in the economy, a breakdown of health systems and an increase in main city sex trade.

4. Reservoir—Humans.

5. Mode of transmission—Direct contact with infectious exudates from obvious or concealed, moist, early lesions of skin and mucous membranes of infected people during sexual contact; exposure nearly always occurs during oral, anal or vaginal intercourse. Transmission by kissing or fondling children with early congenital disease occurs rarely. Transplacental infection of the fetus occurs during the pregnancy of an infected woman.

Transmission can occur through blood transfusion if the donor is in the early stages of disease. Infection through contact with contaminated articles may be theoretically possible but is extraordinarily rare. Health professionals have developed primary lesions on the hands following unprotected clinical examination of infectious lesions.

6. Incubation period—10 days to 3 months, usually 3 weeks.

7. Period of communicability—Communicability exists when moist mucocutaneous lesions of primary and secondary syphilis are present. The distinction between the infectious primary and secondary stages and the noninfectious early latent stage of syphilis is somewhat arbitrary with regard to communicability, since primary and secondary stage lesions may not be apparent to the infected individual. Lesions of secondary syphilis may recur with decreasing frequency up to 4 years after infection, but transmission of infection is rare after the first year. In the USA infectious early syphilis is usually defined as ending after the first year of infection.

Transmission of syphilis from mother to fetus is most probable during early maternal syphilis but can occur throughout the latent period. Infected infants may have moist mucocutaneous lesions that are more widespread than in adult syphilis and are a potential source of infection.

8. Susceptibility—Susceptibility is universal, though only approximately 30% of exposures result in infection. Infection leads to gradual development of immunity against *T. pallidum* and, to some extent, against heterologous treponemes; immunity often fails to develop because of early treatment in the primary and secondary stages. Concurrent HIV infection may reduce the normal host response to *T. pallidum*.

9. Methods of control—

    A. *Preventive measures:* (applicable to all STDs). Emphasis on early detection and effective treatment of patients with transmissible syphilis and their contacts should not preclude search for people with latent syphilis to prevent relapse and disability due to late manifestations.

        1) Educate the community in general health promotion measures; provide health and sex instruction that teaches the value of delaying sexual activity until the onset of sexual maturity as well as the importance of establishing mutually monogamous relationships and reducing the numbers of sexual partners. Syphilis serology must be included in the workup of all cases of STD and should be a routine part of prenatal examination. Congenital syphilis is prevented through serological examination in early pregnancy and again in late pregnancy and at delivery in high prevalence populations; treat those who are reactive.

        2) Protect the community by preventing and controlling STDs in sex workers and their clients and by discouraging multiple sexual partners and anonymous or casual sexual activity. Teach methods of personal prophylaxis applicable before, during and after exposure, especially the correct and consistent use of condoms.

        3) Provide health care facilities for early diagnosis and treatment of STIs; encourage their use through education of the public about symptoms of STIs and modes of spread; make these services culturally appropriate and readily accessible and acceptable, regardless of economic status. Establish intensive case-finding programs that include interviewing patients and partner notification; for syphilis, repeated serological screening within special populations with known high incidence of STIs. Follow cases serologically to exclude other STI infections such as HIV.

    B. *Control of patient, contacts and the immediate environment:*

        1) Report to local health authority: Case report of early infectious syphilis and congenital syphilis is required in most countries, Class 2 (see Reporting); laboratories must report

reactive serology and positive darkfield examinations in many areas. Confidentiality of the individual must be safeguarded.

2) Isolation: For hospitalized patients, universal precautions for blood and body secretions. Patients should refrain from sexual intercourse until treatment is completed and lesions disappear; to avoid reinfection, they should refrain from sexual activity with previous partners until the latter have been examined and treated.

3) Concurrent disinfection: Not applicable in adequately treated cases; avoid contact with discharges from open lesions and articles soiled therewith.

4) Quarantine: Not applicable.

5) Immunization of contacts: Not applicable.

6) Investigation of contacts and source of infection: A fundamental feature of programs for syphilis control is the interviewing of patients to identify sexual contacts from whom infection was acquired in addition to those whom the patient may have infected. Trained interviewers obtain best results. The stage of disease determines the criteria for partner notification: a) for primary syphilis, all sexual contacts during the 3 months preceding onset of symptoms; b) for secondary syphilis, contacts during the preceding 6 months; c) for early latent syphilis, those of the preceding year, if time of primary and secondary lesions cannot be established; d) for late and late latent syphilis, marital partners, and children of infected mothers; and e) for congenital syphilis, all members of the immediate family. All identified sexual contacts of confirmed cases of early syphilis exposed within 90 days of examination should receive treatment. Patients and their partners must be encouraged to obtain HIV counselling and testing.

If adequate and appropriate treatment of the mother prior to the last month of pregnancy cannot be established, all infants born to seroreactive mothers should be treated with penicillin.

7) Specific treatment: Long-acting penicillin G (benzathine penicillin), 2.4 million units in a single IM dose on the day that primary, secondary or early latent syphilis is diagnosed; this assures effective treatment even if the patient fails to return. Alternative treatment for nonpregnant patients allergic to penicillin: either doxycycline PO, 100 mg twice/day for 14 days, or tetracycline PO, 500 mg 4 times/day for 14 days.

Serological testing is important to ensure adequate treatment; tests are repeated at 3 and 6 months after treatment and later as needed. In HIV-infected patients, testing to be repeated at 1, 2 and 3 months, and at 3-month intervals thereafter. A 4-fold titre rise indicates a need for retreatment.

In a small percentage of patients treated for primary or secondary syphilis, nontreponemal tests may remain positive despite repeated treatment. Failure of nontreponemal tests to decline 4-fold by 3 months after treatment for primary or secondary syphilis identifies those at risk of treatment failure. Careful evaluation of prior treatment and additional evaluation may be required. CSF analysis should be considered (increased risk of neurosyphilis) in case of treatment failure, infection with HIV, presence of neurological findings.

Increased dosages and longer periods of treatment (benzathine penicillin G 7.2 million units total, as 3 doses of 2.4 million units IM at 1-week intervals) are indicated for late stages of syphilis. For neurosyphilis, aqueous crystalline penicillin G 18–24 million units a day administered as 3–4 million units IV every 4 hours for 10–14 days. An alternative treatment is procaine penicillin 2–4 million units IM daily, plus probenecid PO, 500 mg, 4 times/day, both for 10–14 days. Success in treatment must be verified by following serological titres and appropriate CSF examinations every 6 months until CSF cell count is normal.

Penicillin-sensitive pregnant women should have their allergy confirmed with skin tests (major and minor penicillin determinants) if test antigens are available. Patients with confirmed penicillin allergy can be desensitized and given the appropriate dose of penicillin.

For early congenital syphilis, aqueous crystalline penicillin G, 50 000 units/kg/dose, given IV or IM every 12 hours during the first 7 days of life, and every 8 hours thereafter for 10–14 days. For late congenital syphilis, if the CSF is normal without neurological involvement, children can be treated as for latent syphilis. If the CSF is abnormal, treatment for neurosyphilis is required: 200 000 units/kg/day of aqueous crystalline penicillin G at 50 000 units/kg/dose every 4 hours for 10–14 days.

C. *Epidemic measures:* Intensification of measures outlined under 9A and 9B. In protracted epidemics in selected populations (e.g. commercial sex workers) that remain refractory to standard interventions, mass treatment of the at-risk population may be considered.

D. *Disaster implications:* None.

E. *International measures:*

1) Examine groups of adolescents and young adults who move from areas of high prevalence for treponemal infections.

2) Adhere to agreements among nations as to records, provision of diagnostic and treatment facilities and contact interviews at seaports for foreign merchant seamen (e.g. Brussels Agreement).
3) Provide for rapid international exchange of information on contacts.
4) WHO Collaborating Centres.

[F. Ndowa]

SYPHILIS
II. NONVENEREAL ENDEMIC SYPHILIS
ICD-9 104.0; ICD-10 A65
(Bejel, Njovera)

1. Identification—An acute disease of limited geographic distribution, characterized clinically by an eruption of skin and mucous membranes, usually without an evident primary sore. Mucous patches of the mouth are often the first lesions, soon followed by moist papules in skinfolds and by drier lesions of the trunk and extremities. Other early skin lesions are macular or papular, often hypertrophic, and frequently circinate; lesions resemble those of venereal syphilis. Plantar and palmar hyperkeratoses occur frequently, often with painful fissuring; patchy depigmentation/hyperpigmentation of the skin and alopecia are common. Inflammatory or destructive lesions of skin, long bones and nasopharynx are late manifestations. Unlike venereal syphilis, bejel now rarely shows neurological or cardiovascular involvement. The case-fatality rate is low.

Darkfield examination can demonstrate organisms in lesions during early disease. Serological tests for syphilis are reactive in the early stages and remain so for many years then gradually tend toward reversal; response to treatment as in venereal syphilis.

2. Infectious agent—*Treponema pallidum*, subsp. *endemicum*, a spirochete indistinguishable from that of syphilis except through molecular testing.

3. Occurrence—A common disease of childhood in localized areas with poor socioeconomic conditions and primitive sanitary and dwelling arrangements. Low level transmission in a few foci in the eastern Mediterranean including the Middle East; major foci exist in the Sahel region of Africa.

4. Reservoir—Humans.

5. Mode of transmission—Direct or indirect contact with infectious early lesions of skin and mucous membranes; the shared use of eating and drinking utensils and generally unsatisfactory hygienic conditions favor the latter. Congenital transmission does not occur.

6. Incubation period—From 2 weeks to 3 months.

7. Period of communicability—Until moist eruptions of skin and mucous patches disappear; sometimes several weeks or months.

8. Susceptibility—Similar to that for venereal syphilis.

9. Methods of control—

 A. *Preventive measures:* See Yaws, 9A.

 B. *Control of patient, contacts and the immediate environment:*

    1) Report to local health authority: In selected endemic areas; in most countries not a reportable disease, Class 3 (see Reporting).
    2), 3), 4), 5), 6) and 7) Isolation, Concurrent disinfection, Quarantine, Immunization of contacts, Investigation of contacts and source of infection, and Specific treatment: See Yaws, 9B, applicable to all nonvenereal treponematoses.

 C. *Epidemic measures:* Intensification of preventive and control activities.

 D. *Disaster implications:* None.

 E. *International measures:* See Yaws, 9E. WHO Collaborating Centres.

[G.M. Antal]

TAENIASIS   ICD-9 123; ICD-10 B68

TAENIA SOLIUM TAENIASIS
   INTESTINAL FORM   ICD-9 123.0; ICD-10 B68.0
(Pork tapeworm)
TAENIA SAGINATA
   TAENIASIS   ICD-9 123.2; ICD-10 B68.1
(Beef tapeworm)
CYSTICERCOSIS   ICD-9 123.l; ICD-10 B69
(Cysticerciasis, *Taenia solium* cysticercosis)

1. Identification—Taeniasis is an intestinal infection with the adult stage of large tapeworms; cysticercosis is a tissue infection with the larval stage of one species, *Taenia solium*. Clinical manifestations of infection with the adult worm, if present, are variable and may include nervousness,

insomnia, anorexia, weight loss, abdominal pain and digestive disturbances. Except for the annoyance of having segments of worms emerging
from the anus, many infections are asymptomatic. Taeniasis is usually a
nonfatal infection, but the larval stage of *T. solium* may cause fatal
cysticercosis.

Larval infection of humans with the pork tapeworm, cysticercosis, may
produce serious somatic disease, usually involving the CNS. When eggs or
proglottids of the pork tapeworm are swallowed by people, the eggs hatch
in the small intestine and the larvae migrate to the subcutaneous tissues,
striated muscles, and other tissues and vital organs of the body, where they
form cysticerci. Consequences may be grave when larvae localize in the
eye, CNS or heart. In the presence of somatic cysticercosis, epileptiform
seizures, headache, signs of intracranial hypertension or psychiatric
disturbances strongly suggest cerebral involvement. Neurocysticercosis
may cause serious disability but with a relatively low case-fatality rate.

Infection with an adult tapeworm is diagnosed by identification of
proglottids (segments), eggs or antigens of the worm in the feces or on
anal swabs. Eggs of *T. solium* and *T. saginata* cannot be differentiated
morphologically. Specific diagnosis is based on the morphology of the
scolex (head) and/or gravid proglottids.

Specific serological tests should support the clinical diagnosis of cysticercosis. Subcutaneous cysticerci may be visible or palpable; microscopic
examination of an excised cysticercus confirms the diagnosis. Cysticercosis in intracerebral and other tissues may be recognized by CAT scan or
MRI, or by X-ray when the cysticerci are calcified.

2. Infectious agents—*Taenia solium*, the pork tapeworm, causes
both intestinal infection with the adult worm and extraintestinal infection
with the larvae (cysticerci). *T. saginata*, the beef tapeworm, only causes
intestinal infection with the adult worm in humans.

3. Occurrence—Worldwide; particularly frequent wherever beef or
pork is eaten raw or insufficiently cooked and where sanitary conditions
allow pigs and cattle to have access to human feces. Prevalence is highest
in parts of Latin America, Africa, south and southeastern Asia and eastern
Europe, and infection is common in immigrants from these areas. Transmission of *T. solium* is rare in Canada, the USA, western Europe and most
parts of Asia and the Pacific. Although fecal-oral transmission related to
immigrants with imported *T. solium* infections has been reported with
increasing frequency in the USA, these immigrants are unlikely to spread
infection significantly in countries with good sanitation.

4. Reservoir—Humans are the definitive host of both species of
taenia; cattle are the intermediate hosts for *T. saginata* and pigs for *T.
solium*.

5. Mode of transmission—Eggs of *T. saginata* passed in the stool of
an infected person are infectious only to cattle, in the flesh of which the

parasites develop into cysticercus bovis, the larval stage of *T. saginata*. In humans, infection follows ingestion of raw or undercooked beef containing cysticerci; in the intestine, the adult worm develops attached to the jejunal mucosa.

Intestinal infection due to *T. solium* in humans follows ingestion of raw or undercooked infected pork ("measly pork"), with subsequent development of the adult worm in the intestine. Human cysticercosis occurs either by direct transfer of *T. solium* eggs from the feces of people harbouring an adult worm to their own mouth (autoinfection) or another's or indirectly by ingestion of food or water contaminated with eggs. When humans or pigs ingest eggs of *T. solium*, the embryos escape from the shells, penetrate the intestinal wall into lymphatics or blood vessels and hence to the various tissues, where they develop to produce cysticercosis.

6. Incubation period—Symptoms of cysticercosis may appear from weeks to 10 years or more after infection. Eggs appear in the stool 8–12 weeks after infection with the adult *T. solium* tapeworm, 10–14 weeks with *T. saginata*.

7. Period of communicability—*T. saginata* is not directly transmitted from person to person, but *T. solium* may be. Eggs of both species are disseminated into the environment as long as the worm remains in the intestine, sometimes more than 30 years; eggs may remain viable in the environment for months.

8. Susceptibility—Susceptibility is general. No apparent resistance follows infection; the presence of more than one tapeworm in a person has rarely been reported.

9. Methods of control—

   A. Preventive measures:

   1) Educate the public to prevent fecal contamination of soil, water, and human and animal food; to avoid use of sewage effluents for pasture irrigation; and to cook beef and pork thoroughly.

   2) Identification and immediate treatment or institution of enteric precautions for people harbouring adult *T. solium* is essential to prevent human cysticercosis. *T. solium* eggs are infective immediately on leaving the host and may produce severe human illness. Appropriate measures to protect patients from themselves and their contacts are necessary.

   3) Freezing pork or beef at a temperature below -5°C (23°F) for more than 4 days kills the cysticerci effectively. Irradiation is very effective at 1 kGy.

   4) Inspection of the carcases of cattle and swine will detect only a proportion of infected carcases; these should be condemned, irradiated or processed into cooked products.

    5) Prevent swine access to latrines and human feces.

B. Control of patient, contacts and the immediate environment:

    1) Report to local health authority: Selectively reportable, Class 3 (see Reporting).

    2) Isolation: Not applicable. Stools of patients with untreated taeniasis due to *T. solium* may be infective (see 9A2).

    3) Concurrent disinfection: Dispose of feces in a sanitary manner; emphasize strict sanitation, with handwashing after defecating and before eating, especially for *T. solium*.

    4) Quarantine: Not applicable.

    5) Immmunization of contacts: Not applicable.

    6) Investigation of contacts and source of infection: Evaluate symptomatic contacts.

    7) Specific treatment: Praziquantel is effective in the treatment of *T. saginata* and *T. solium* intestinal infections. Niclosamide, no longer widely available, is an alternative. Patients with active CNS cysticercosis may benefit from treatment with praziquantel or albendazole under hospitalization; a short course of corticosteroids is usually given to control cerebral oedema due to dying cysticerci. Where cysticidal treatment is not indicated, symptomatic treatment, such as with anti-epileptic drugs, may bring relief. In some cases surgical intervention may be needed to relieve symptoms.

C. Epidemic measures: Not applicable.

D. Disaster implications: None.

E. International measures: Collaborating Centres, FAO and WHO.

ASIAN TAENIASIS

    Human infections have been reported from Taiwan (China), Indonesia, the Republic of Korea, the Philippines and Thailand with a *T. saginata*-like tapeworm acquired by eating uncooked liver and other viscera of pigs; in experimental studies this organism produced cysticerci only in the livers of pigs, cattle, goats and monkeys. This organism is now classified as a subspecies of *T. saginata*.

[D. Engels/J. Schlundt]

TETANUS   ICD-9 037; ICD-10 A35
(Lockjaw)
(Obstetrical tetanus: ICD-10 A34)

    1. Identification—An acute disease induced by an exotoxin of the tetanus bacillus, which grows anaerobically at the site of an injury. The disease is characterized by painful muscular contractions, primarily of the masseter and neck muscles, secondarily of trunk muscles. A common first sign suggestive of tetanus in older children and adults is abdominal rigidity, though rigidity is sometimes confined to the region of injury. Generalized spasms occur, frequently induced by sensory stimuli; typical features of the tetanic spasm are the position of opisthotonos and the facial expression known as "risus sardonicus." History of an injury or apparent portal of entry may be lacking. The case-fatality rate ranges from 10% to over 80%, it is highest in infants and the elderly, and varies inversely with the length of the incubation period and the availability of experienced intensive care unit personnel and resources.

Attempts at laboratory confirmation are of little help. The organism is rarely recovered from the site of infection, and usually there is no detectable antibody response.

2. Infectious agent—*Clostridium tetani*, the tetanus bacillus.

3. Occurrence—Worldwide. The disease is more common in agricultural regions and in areas where contact with animal excreta is more likely and immunization is inadequate. Parenteral use of drugs by addicts, particularly intramuscular or subcutaneous use, can result in individual cases and occasional circumscribed outbreaks. In 2001, an estimated 282 000 people worldwide died of tetanus, most of them in Asia, Africa and South America. In rural and tropical areas people are especially at risk, and tetanus neonatorum is common (see below). There is some inconclusive evidence that at high altitude the risk for tetanus could be lower. The disease is sporadic and relatively uncommon in most industrial countries.

4. Reservoir—Intestines of horses and other animals, including humans, in which the organism is a harmless normal inhabitant. Soil or fomites contaminated with animal and human feces. Tetanus spores, ubiquitous in the environment, can contaminate wounds of all types.

5. Mode of transmission—Tetanus spores are usually introduced into the body through a puncture wound contaminated with soil, street dust or animal or human feces; through lacerations, burns and trivial or unnoticed wounds; or by injected contaminated drugs (e.g. street drugs). Tetanus occasionally follows surgical procedures, which include circumcision and abortions performed under unhygienic conditions. The presence of necrotic tissue and/or foreign bodies favors growth of the anaerobic pathogen. Cases have followed injuries considered too trivial for medical consultation.

6. Incubation period—Usually 3–21 days, although it may range from 1 day to several months, depending on the character, extent and location of the wound; average 10 days. Most cases occur within 14 days. In general, shorter incubation periods are associated with more heavily contaminated wounds, more severe disease and a worse prognosis.

7. Period of communicability—No direct person-to-person transmission.

8. Susceptibility and resistance—Susceptibility is general. Active immunity is induced by tetanus toxoid and persists for at least 10 years after full immunization; transient passive immunity follows injection of tetanus immune globulin (TIG) or tetanus antitoxin (equine origin). Infants of actively immunized mothers acquire passive immunity that protects them from neonatal tetanus. Recovery from tetanus may not result in immunity; second attacks can occur and primary immunization is indicated after recovery.

9. Methods of control—

    A. Preventive measures:

        1) Educate the public on the necessity for complete immunization with tetanus toxoid, the hazards of puncture wounds and closed injuries that are particularly liable to be complicated by tetanus, and the potential need after injury for active and/or passive prophylaxis.

        2) Universal active immunization with adsorbed tetanus toxoid (TT), which gives durable protection for at least 10 years; after the initial basic series has been completed, single booster doses elicit high levels of immunity. In children under 7, the toxoid is generally administered together with diphtheria toxoid and pertussis vaccine as a triple (DTP or DTaP) antigen, or as double (DT) antigen when contraindications to pertussis vaccine exist. Preparations that include other antigens including *Haemophilus influenzae* type b conjugate vaccines (DTP-Hib), Hepatitis B vaccine (DTP-HB), and/or inactivated polio vaccine are also available in some countries. Td is used for those older than age 7. In countries with incomplete immunization programs for children, all pregnant women should receive 2 doses of tetanus toxoid in the first pregnancy, with an interval of at least 1 month, and with the second dose at least 2 weeks prior to childbirth. Booster doses may be necessary to ensure ongoing protection (see below). Nonadsorbed ("plain") preparations are less immunogenic for primary immunization or booster shots. Minor local reactions following tetanus toxoid injections are relatively frequent; severe local and systemic reactions are infrequent but do occur, particularly after excessive numbers of prior doses have been given.

           a) The schedule recommended for tetanus immunization in childhood is the same as for diphtheria (see Diphtheria, 9A).

           b) While tetanus toxoid is recommended for universal use regardless of age, it is especially important for workers in contact with soil, sewage and domestic animals; members of the military forces; policemen and others with greater than usual risk of traumatic injury; and older adults who are currently at highest risk for tetanus and tetanus-related mortality. Vaccine-induced maternal immunity is important in preventing maternal and neonatal tetanus.

c) Active protection should be maintained by administering booster doses of Td every 10 years.

d) For children and adults who are severely immunocompromised or infected with HIV, tetanus toxoid is indicated in the same schedule and dose as for immunocompetent persons even though the immune response may be suboptimal.

3) Prophylaxis in wound management: Tetanus prophylaxis in patients with wounds is based on careful assessment of whether the wound is clean or contaminated, the immunization status of the patient, proper use of tetanus toxoid and/or TIG (see table below), wound cleaning and, where required, surgical debridement and the proper use of antibiotics.

a) Those who have been completely immunized and who sustain minor and uncontaminated wounds require a booster dose of toxoid only if more than 10 years have elapsed since the last dose was given. For major and/or contaminated wounds, a single booster injection of tetanus toxoid (preferably Td) should be administered promptly on the day of injury if the patient has not received tetanus toxoid within the preceding 5 years.

b) Persons who have not completed a full primary series of tetanus toxoid require a dose of toxoid as soon as possible following the wound and may require passive immunization with human TIG if the wound is a major one and/or if it is contaminated with soil containing animal excreta. DTP/DTaP, DT or Td, as determined by the age of the patient and previous immunization history, should be used at the time of the wound, and ultimately to complete the primary series.

Passive immunization with at least 250 IU of TIG IM (or 1500 to 5000 IU of antitoxin of animal origin if globulin is not available), regardless of the patient's age, is indicated for patients with other than clean, minor wounds and a history of no, unknown or fewer than 3 previous tetanus toxoid doses. When tetanus toxoid and TIG or antitoxin are given concurrently, separate syringes and separate sites must be used.

When antitoxin of animal origin is given, it is essential

to avoid anaphylaxis by first injecting 0.02 ml of a 1:100 dilution in physiologic saline intradermally, with a syringe containing adrenaline on hand. Pretest with a 1:1000 dilution if there has been prior animal serum exposure, together with a similar injection of physiologic saline as a negative control. If after 15–20 minutes there is a wheal with surrounding erythema at least 3 mm larger than the negative control, it is necessary to desensitize the individual. Antibiotics may theoretically prevent the multiplication of *C. tetani* in the wound and thus reduce production of toxin, but this does not obviate the need for prompt treatment of the wound together with appropriate immunization.

Summary Guide to Tetanus Prophylaxis in Routine Wound Management[1]

History of tetanus immunization (doses)	Clean, minor wounds		All other wounds	
	Td[2]	TIG	Td[2]	TIG
Uncertain or <3	Yes	No	Yes	Yes
3 or more	No[3]	No	No[4]	No

[1]Important details in the text.

[2]For children under 7, DTaP or DTP (DT, if pertussis vaccine contraindicated) preferred to tetanus toxoid alone. For persons 7 or older, Td preferred to tetanus toxoid alone.

[3]Yes, if more than 10 years since last dose.

[4]Yes, if more than 5 years since last dose. More frequent boosters are not needed and can accentuate side-effects.

B. Control of patient, contacts and the immediate environment:

1) Report to local health authority: Case report required in most countries, Class 2 (see Reporting).
2) Isolation: Not applicable.
3) Concurrent disinfection: Not applicable.
4) Quarantine: Not applicable.
5) Immmunization of contacts: Not applicable.
6) Investigation of contacts and source of infection: Case investigation to determine circumstances of injury.
7) Specific treatment: TIG IM in doses of 3000–6000 IU. If immunoglobulin not available, tetanus antitoxin (equine origin) in a single large dose should be given IV following appropriate testing for hypersensitivity. Metronidazole, the most appropriate antibiotic in terms of recovery time and case-fatality, should be given for 7–14 days in large doses; this also allows for a reduction in the amount of muscle relaxants

and sedatives required. The wound should be debrided widely and excised if possible. Wide debridement of the umbilical stump in neonates is not indicated. Maintain an adequate airway and employ sedation as indicated; muscle relaxant drugs together with tracheostomy or nasotracheal intubation and mechanically assisted respiration may be lifesaving. Active immunization should be initiated concurrently with treatment.

C. Epidemic measures: In the rare outbreak, search for contaminated street drugs or other common-use injections.

D. Disaster implications: Social upheaval (military conflicts, riots) and natural disasters (floods, hurricanes, earthquakes) that cause many traumatic injuries in nonimmunized populations will result in an increased need for TIG or tetanus antitoxin and toxoid for injured patients.

E. International measures: Up-to-date immunization against tetanus is advised for international travellers.

TETANUS NEONATORUM   ICD-9 771.3; ICD-10 A33

Tetanus neonatorum is a serious health problem in many developing countries where maternity care services are limited and immunization against tetanus is inadequate. In the past 10 years the incidence of tetanus neonatorum has declined considerably in many developing countries thanks to improved training of birth attendants and to immunization with tetanus toxoid for women of childbearing age. Despite this decline, WHO estimates that tetanus neonatorum still causes about 200 000 deaths each year, mainly in the developing world. Most newborn infants with tetanus have been born to nonimmunized mothers delivered by an untrained birth attendant outside a hospital.

The disease usually occurs through introduction via the umbilical cord of tetanus spores during delivery through the use of an unclean instrument to cut the cord, or after delivery by 'dressing' the umbilical stump with substances heavily contaminated with tetanus spores, frequently as part of natal rituals.

In neonates, inability to nurse is the most common presenting sign. Tetanus neonatorum is typified by a newborn infant who sucks and cries well for the first few days after birth but subsequently develops progressive difficulty and then inability to feed because of trismus, generalized stiffness with spasms or convulsions and opisthotonos. The average incubation period is about 6 days, with a range from 3 to 28 days. Overall, case-fatality rates for neonatal tetanus are very high, exceeding 80% among cases with short incubation periods. Neurological sequelae including mild retardation occur in 5% to over 20% of those children who survive.

Prevention of tetanus neonatorum can be achieved through a combination of 2 approaches: a) improving maternity care with emphasis on increasing the tetanus toxoid immunization coverage of women of childbearing age (especially pregnant women), and b) increasing the proportion of deliveries attended by trained attendants.

Important control measures include licensing of midwives; providing professional supervision and education as to methods, equipment and techniques of asepsis in childbirth; and educating mothers, relatives and attendants in the practice of strict asepsis of the umbilical stump of newborn infants. The latter is especially important in many areas where strips of bamboo are used to sever the umbilical cord or where ashes, cow dung poultices or other contaminated substances are traditionally applied to the umbilicus. In those areas, any woman of childbearing age visiting a health facility should be screened and offered immunization, no matter what the reason for the visit.

Nonimmunized women should receive at least 2 doses of tetanus toxoid according to the following schedule: the first dose at initial contact or as early as possible during pregnancy, the second dose 4 weeks after the first and preferably at least 2 weeks before delivery. A third dose could be given 6–12 months after the second, or during the next pregnancy. An additional 2 doses should be given at annual intervals when the mother is in contact with the health service or during her subsequent pregnancies. A total of 5 doses protects the previously unimmunized woman throughout the entire childbearing period. Women whose infants have a risk of neonatal tetanus but who themselves have received 3 or 4 doses of DTP/DTaP as children need only receive 2 doses of tetanus toxoid during each of their first 2 pregnancies.

[J. Vandelaer]

TOXOCARIASIS   ICD-9 128.0; ICD-10 B83.0
(Visceral larva migrans, Larva migrans visceralis, Ocular larva migrans, *Toxocara [canis] [cati]* infection)

   1. **Identification**—A chronic infection and usually mild disease, predominantly of young children but increasingly recognized in adults, caused by migration of larval forms of toxocara species in the organs and tissues. It is characterized by eosinophilia of variable duration, hepatomegaly, hyperglobulinaemia, pulmonary symptoms and fever. With an acute and heavy infection, the WBC count may reach 100 000/mm³ or more (SI units more than $100 \times 10^9/L$), with 50%–90% eosinophils. Symptoms may persist for a year or longer; symptomatology is related to total parasite load. Pneumonitis, chronic abdominal pain, a generalized rash and focal neurological disturbances may occur, as may endophthalmitis (caused by

larvae entering the eye), usually in older children; this can result in loss of vision in the affected eye (ocular larva migrans). Retinal lesions must be differentiated from retinoblastoma and other retinal masses. The disease is rarely fatal.

ELISA testing with larval-stage antigens is 75%–90% sensitive in visceral larva migrans and in ocular infections. Western blotting procedures can be used to increase specificity of the ELISA screening test.

2. Infectious agents—*Toxocara canis* and *T. cati*, predominantly the former.

3. Occurrence—Worldwide. Severe disease occurs sporadically and affects mainly children aged 14–40 months, but also in older age groups. Siblings often have eosinophilia or other evidence of light or residual infection. Serological studies in asymptomatic children have shown a wide range in different populations. Internationally, seroprevalence ranges from lows of 0%–4% in Germany and urban Spain (Madrid) to 83% in some Caribbean subpopulations. Adults are less often acutely infected.

4. Reservoir—For dogs and cats, *T. canis* and *T. cati*, respectively. Puppies are infected by transplacental and transmammary migration of larvae and pass eggs in their stools by the time they are 3 weeks old. Infection among bitches may end or become dormant with sexual maturity; with pregnancy, however, *T. canis* larvae become active and infect the fetuses, and also newborn pups through milk. Similar though less marked differences apply for cats; older animals are less susceptible than young.

5. Mode of transmission—For most infections in children, by direct or indirect transmission of infective toxocara eggs from contaminated soil to the mouth, directly by contact with infected soil or indirectly by eating unwashed raw vegetables. Some infections may occur through ingestion of larvae in raw liver from infected chickens, cattle and sheep.

Eggs are shed in feces of infected dogs and cats; up to 30% of soil samples from certain parks in the United Kingdom and the USA contained eggs; in certain parks in Japan, up to 75% of sandboxes contained eggs. Eggs require 1–3 weeks' incubation to become infective, but remain viable and infective in soil for many months; they are adversely affected by desiccation.

After ingestion, embryonated eggs hatch in the intestine; larvae penetrate the wall and migrate to the liver and other tissues via the lymphatic and circulatory systems. From the liver, larvae spread to other tissues, particularly the lungs and abdominal organs (visceral larva migrans) or the eyes (ocular larva migrans), and induce granulomatous lesions. The parasites cannot replicate in the human or other end-stage hosts; viable larvae may remain in tissues for years, usually in the absence of symptomatic disease. When the tissues of end-stage hosts are eaten, the larvae may be infective for the new host.

6. Incubation period—In children, weeks or months, depending on intensity of infection, reinfection and sensitivity of the patient. Ocular manifestations may occur as late as 4–10 years after initial infection. In infections through ingestion of raw liver, very short incubation periods (hours or days) have been reported.

7. Period of communicability—No direct person-to-person transmission.

8. Susceptibility—Lower incidence in older children and adults relating mainly to lesser exposure. Reinfection can occur.

9. Methods of control—

  A. Preventive measures:

  1) Educate the public, especially pet owners, concerning sources and origin of the infection, particularly the danger of pica, of exposure to areas contaminated with feces of untreated puppies and of ingestion of raw or undercooked liver of animals exposed to dogs or cats. Parents of toddlers should be made aware of the risk associated with pets in the household and how to minimize them.
  2) Prevent contamination of soil by dog and cat feces in areas immediately adjacent to houses and children's play areas, especially in urban areas and multiple housing projects. Encourage cat and dog owners to practice responsible pet ownership, including prompt removal of pets' feces from areas of public access. Control stray dogs and cats.
  3) Require removal of canine and feline feces passed in play areas. Children's sandboxes offer an attractive site for defecating cats; cover when not in use.
  4) Deworm dogs and cats beginning at 3 weeks of age, repeated 3 times at 2-week intervals, and every 6 months thereafter. Also treat lactating bitches. Dispose of feces passed as a result of treatment, as well as other stools, in a sanitary manner.
  5) Always wash hands after handling soil and before eating.
  6) Teach children not to put dirty objects into their mouths.

  B. Control of patient, contacts and the immediate environment:

  1) Report to local health authority: Official report not ordinarily justifiable, Class 5 (see Reporting).
  2) Isolation: Not applicable.
  3) Concurrent disinfection: Not applicable.
  4) Quarantine: Not applicable.
  5) Immmunization of contacts: Not applicable.

6) Investigation of contacts and source of infection: Search for site of infection of index case; identify others exposed. Intensify preventive measures (see 9A). Treatment of asymptomatic, ELISA positive individuals is not indicated; one may consider treatment for those with hypereosinophilia.

7) Specific treatment: Mebendazole or albendazole is the anthelminthic of choice because of relative safety. Diethylcarbamazine and thiabendazole have been used; effectiveness of anthelminthics is questionable at best.

C. Epidemic measures: Not applicable.

D. Disaster implications: None.

E. International measures: None.

GNATHOSTOMIASIS   ICD-9 128.1; ICD-10 B83.1

Another visceral larva migrans, common in Thailand and elsewhere in southeastern Asia, is caused by *Gnathostoma spinigerum*, a nematode parasite of dogs and cats. Following ingestion of undercooked fish and poultry containing third stage larvae, the parasites migrate through the tissue of humans or animals, forming transient inflammatory lesions or abscesses in various parts of the body. Larvae may invade the brain, producing focal cerebral lesions associated with eosinophilic pleocytosis. Anthelminthic drugs, including albendazole and mebendazole, are of questionable value, and these drugs are considered investigational.

CUTANEOUS LARVA
  MIGRANS   ICD-9 126; ICD-10 B76.9
DUE TO *ANCYLOSTOMA*
  BRAZILIENSE   ICD-9 126.2; ICD-10 B76.0
DUE TO *ANCYLOSTOMA*
  CANINUM   ICD-9 126.8; ICD-10 B76.0
(Creeping eruption)

Infective larvae of dog and cat hookworms, *Ancylostoma braziliense* and *A. caninum*, cause a dermatitis called "creeping eruption", that affects utility workers, gardeners, children, seabathers and others who come in contact with damp sandy soil contaminated with dog and cat feces; in the USA, most prevalent in the southeastern areas. The larvae enter the skin and migrate intracutaneously for long periods; eventually they may penetrate to deeper tissues. Each larva causes a serpiginous track, advancing several millimeters to a few centimeters a day, with intense itching especially at night. The cutaneous disease is self-limited, with spontaneous cure after weeks or months. Freezing the area with ethyl chloride spray can kill individual larvae. Thiabendazole is effective as a topical ointment; albendazole or ivermectin is effective systemically. *A. caninum* larvae may migrate to the small intestine where they cause eosinophilic enteritis; these zoonotic infections respond to treatment with pyrantel pamoate, mebendazole or albendazole.

[A. Montresor]

TOXOPLASMOSIS	ICD-9 130; ICD-10 B58
CONGENITAL	
TOXOPLASMOSIS	ICD-9 771.2; ICD-10 P37.1

1. **Identification**—A systemic coccidian protozoan disease; infections are frequently asymptomatic, or present as acute disease with lymphadenopathy only, or resemble infectious mononucleosis, with fever, lymphadenopathy and lymphocytosis persisting for days or weeks. Development of an immune response decreases parasitaemia, but *Toxoplasma* cysts remaining in the tissues contain viable organisms. These cysts may reactivate if the immune system becomes compromised. Among immunodeficient individuals, including HIV-infected patients, primary or reactivated infection may cause a maculopapular rash, generalized skeletal muscle involvement, cerebritis, chorioretinitis, pneumonia, myocarditis and/or death. Cerebral toxoplasmosis is a frequent component of AIDS.

A primary infection during early pregnancy may lead to fetal infection with death of the fetus or manifestations such as chorioretinitis, brain damage with intracerebral calcification, hydrocephaly, microcephaly, fever, jaundice, rash, hepatosplenomegaly, xanthochromic CSF and convulsions evident at birth or shortly thereafter. Later in pregnancy, maternal infection results in mild or subclinical fetal disease with delayed manifestations such as recurrent or chronic chorioretinitis. In immunosuppressed pregnant women who are *Toxoplasma*-seropositive, a reactivation of latent infection may rarely result in congenital toxoplasmosis.

Diagnosis is based on clinical signs and supportive serological results, demonstration of the agent in body tissues or fluids by biopsy or necropsy, or isolation in animals or cell culture. Rising antibody titres are corroborative of active infection; the presence of specific IgM and/or rising IgG titres in sequential sera of newborns is conclusive evidence of congenital infection. High IgG antibody levels may persist for years with no relation to active disease.

2. **Infectious agent**—*Toxoplasma gondii*, an intracellular coccidian protozoan of cats, belonging to the family Sarcocystidae, in the class Sporozoa.

3. **Occurrence**—Worldwide in mammals and birds. Infection in humans is common.

4. **Reservoir**—The definitive hosts of *T. gondii* are cats and other

felines, which acquire infection mainly from eating infected mammals (especially rodents) or birds, probably also from oocysts acquired during natural licking/grooming. Felines alone harbour parasites in the intestinal tract, where the sexual stage of life cycle occurs, resulting in excretion of oocysts in feces for 10-20 days, rarely longer.

The intermediate hosts of *T. gondii* include sheep, goats, rodents, swine, cattle, chickens and birds; all may carry an infective stage of *T. gondii* encysted in tissue, especially muscle and brain. Tissue cysts remain viable for long periods, perhaps lifelong. Cattle seem able to cope with natural *Toxoplasma* infection.

5. Mode of transmission—Transplacental infection occurs in humans when a pregnant woman has rapidly dividing cells (tachyzoites) circulating in the bloodstream, usually during primary infection. Children may become infected by ingesting infective oocysts from dirt in sandboxes, playgrounds and yards in which cats have defecated. Infections arise from eating raw or undercooked infected meat (pork or mutton, very rarely beef) containing tissue cysts, or through ingestion of infective oocysts in food or water contaminated with feline feces. Inhalation of sporulated oocysts was associated with one outbreak; another was associated epidemiologically with consumption of raw goat milk. Infection may occur through blood transfusion or organ transplantation from an infected donor.

6. Incubation period—From 10 to 23 days in one common source outbreak from ingestion of undercooked meat; 5-20 days in another outbreak associated with cats.

7. Period of communicability—No direct person-to-person transmission except in utero. Oocysts shed by cats sporulate and become infective 1-5 days later and may remain infective in water or moist soil for over a year. Cysts in the flesh of infected animals remain infective as long as the meat is edible and uncooked.

8. Susceptibility—Susceptibility to infection is general, but immunity is readily acquired and most infections are asymptomatic. Duration and degree of immunity are unknown but they are assumed to be long-lasting or permanent; antibodies persist for years, probably for life. Patients undergoing cytotoxic or immunosuppressive treatment or HIV-infected patients are at high risk of developing illness from reactivated infection.

9. Methods of control—

    A. Preventive measures:

        1) Educate pregnant women about preventive measures:

            a) Use irradiated meats or cook them to 66°C (150°F) before eating. Freezing meat down to -20°C (-4°F) for 24 hours is a good alternative.

b) Unless they are known to have antibodies to *T. gondii*, pregnant women must avoid cleaning litter pans and avoid contact with cats of unknown feeding history. They must wear gloves during gardening and wash hands thoroughly after work and before eating.

2) Feed cats dry, canned or boiled food and discourage hunting (i.e. keep them as indoor pets only).

3) Dispose of cat feces and litter daily (before sporocysts become infective). Faeces can be flushed down the toilet, burned or deeply buried. Disinfect litter pans daily by scalding; wear gloves or wash hands thoroughly after handling potentially infective material. Dispose of dried litter without shaking, to avoid aerial dispersal of oocysts.

4) Wash hands thoroughly before eating and after handling raw meat or after contact with soil possibly contaminated with cat feces.

5) Control stray cats and prevent their access to sandboxes and sand piles used by children for play. Keep sandboxes covered when not in use.

6) Patients with AIDS who experience symptomatic toxoplasmosis must receive prophylactic treatment throughout life with pyrimethamine, sulfadiazine and folinic acid.

B. Control of patient, contacts and the immediate environment:

1) Report to local health authority: Not ordinarily required, but reportable in some countries to facilitate further epidemiological understanding of the disease, Class 3 (see Reporting).

2) Isolation: Not applicable.

3) Concurrent disinfection: Not applicable.

4) Quarantine: Not applicable.

5) Immmunization of contacts: Not applicable.

6) Investigation of contacts and source of infection: In congenital cases, determine antibody titres in mother; in acquired cases, determine antibody titres in members of the household and common exposure to cat feces, soil, raw meat or unwashed vegetables.

7) Specific treatment: Treatment not routinely indicated for a healthy immunocompetent host, except for initial infection during pregnancy or presence of active chorioretinitis, myocarditis or other organ involvement. Pyrimethamine combined with sulfadiazine and folinic acid (to avoid bone marrow depression) for 4 weeks is the preferred treatment for those with severe symptomatic disease. Clindamycin has been used in addition to these agents to treat ocular toxoplasmosis. In ocular disease, systemic corticosteroids

are indicated when irreversible loss of vision can occur from lesions of the macula, papillomacular bundle or optic nerve.

Treatment of pregnant women is problematic. Spiramycin is commonly used to prevent placental infection; pyrimethamine and sulfadiazine should be considered if ultrasound or other investigations indicate that fetal infection has occurred. Because of concerns about possible teratogenicity, pyrimethamine should not be given during the first 16 weeks of pregnancy; sulfadiazine may be administered alone in this case. Infants whose mothers had primary infections or were HIV positive during pregnancy should be treated with pyrimethamine-sulfadiazine-folinic acid during their 1st year of life or until congenital infection is ruled out, in order to prevent chorioretinitis and other sequelae. There are no clear guidelines yet for the management of infants born to HIV infected mothers who are seropositive for *Toxoplasma*.

C. Epidemic measures: None.

D. Disaster implications: None.

E. International measures: The EU zoonosis directive (92/117 EEG) mentions toxoplasmosis under category B (collection of data in Member States when available). WHO Collaborating Centres.

[F. van Knapen]

TRACHOMA   ICD-9 076; ICD-10 A71

1. Identification—A chlamydial conjunctivitis of insidious or abrupt onset; the infection may persist for a few years if untreated, but the characteristic lifetime duration of active disease in hyperendemic areas is the result of frequent reinfection. The disease is characterized by the presence of lymphoid follicles and diffuse conjunctival inflammation (papillary hypertrophy), particularly on the tarsal conjunctiva lining the upper eyelid. The inflammation produces superficial vascularization of the cornea (pannus) and scarring of the conjunctiva, which increases with the severity and duration of inflammatory disease.

The marked conjunctival scarring causes in-turning of eyelashes and lid deformities (trichiasis and entropion) that in turn cause chronic abrasion of the cornea and scarring with visual impairment and blindness later in adult life. Secondary bacterial infections frequently occur in populations with endemic trachoma and contribute to the communicability and severity of the disease.

Early trachoma in some developing countries is an endemic childhood disease. Early stages of trachoma may be indistinguishable from conjunctivitis caused by other bacteria (including genital strains of *Chlamydia trachomatis*). Differential diagnosis includes molluscum contagiosum nodules of the eyelids, toxic reactions to chronically administered eye drops and chronic staphylococcal lid-margin infection. An allergic reaction to contact lenses (giant papillary conjunctivitis) may produce a trachoma-like syndrome with tarsal nodules (giant papillae), conjunctival scarring and corneal pannus.

Laboratory diagnosis is made through Giemsa-stained smears for the detection of intracellular chlamydial elementary bodies in epithelial cells of conjunctival scrapings; IF after methanol fixation of the smear; detection of chlamydial antigen by EIA or DNA by probe; or isolation of the agent in special cell culture.

2. Infectious agent—*Chlamydia trachomatis* serovars A, B, Ba and C. Some strains are indistinguishable from those of chlamydial conjunctivitis; serovars B, Ba and C have been isolated from genital chlamydial infections.

3. Occurrence—Worldwide, as an endemic disease most often of poor rural communities in developing countries. In endemic areas, trachoma presents in childhood, then subsides in adolescence, leaving varying degrees of potentially disabling scarring. Blinding trachoma is still widespread in the Middle East, northern and sub-Saharan Africa, parts of the Indian subcontinent, southeastern Asia and China. Pockets of blinding trachoma also occur in Latin America, Australia (among Aboriginals) and the Pacific islands.

The disease occurs among population groups with poor hygiene, poverty and crowded living conditions, particularly in dry dusty regions. The late complications of trachoma (in-turned lids and corneal scarring) occur in older people who had infectious trachoma in childhood; these people are rarely infectious.

4. Reservoir—Humans.

5. Mode of transmission—Through direct contact with infectious ocular or nasopharyngeal discharges on fingers or indirect contact with contaminated fomites such as towels, clothes and nasopharyngeal discharges from infected people and materials soiled therewith. Flies, especially *Musca sorbens* in Africa and the Middle East, contribute to the spread of the disease. In children with active trachoma, *Chlamydia* can be recovered from the nasopharynx and rectum, but the trachoma serovars do not appear to have a genital reservoir in endemic communities.

6. Incubation period—From 5 to 12 days (based on volunteer studies).

7. Period of communicability—As long as active lesions are present in the conjunctivae and adnexal mucous membranes; this may last a few years. Concentration of the agent in the tissues is greatly reduced with cicatrization, but increases again with reactivation and recurrence of infective discharges. Infectivity ceases within 2–3 days of the start of antibiotherapy, long before clinical improvement.

8. Susceptibility—Susceptibility is general; while there is no absolute immunity conferred by infection, the severity of active disease due to reinfection gradually decreases over the childhood years and active infection is no longer seen in older children or young adults. In endemic areas, children have active disease more frequently than adults. The severity of disease is often related to living conditions, particularly poor hygiene; exposure to dry winds, dust and fine sand may also contribute. Although studies have shown that vaccines could prevent infection and reduce severity of infection, considerations of cost and time-limited effectiveness preclude their use.

9. Methods of control—

A. Preventive measures:

1) Educate the public on the need for personal hygiene, especially the risk of common-use towels.
2) Improve basic sanitation, including availability and use of soap and water; encourage washing the face; avoid common-use towels.
3) Provide adequate case-finding and treatment facilities, with emphasis on preschool children.
4) Conduct epidemiological investigations to determine important factors in the occurrence of the disease for specific situations.

B. Control of patient, contacts and the immediate environment:

1) Report to local health authority: Case report required in some countries of low endemicity, Class 2 (see Reporting).
2) Isolation: Not practical in most areas where the disease occurs. For hospitalized patients, drainage and secretion precautions.
3) Concurrent disinfection: Of eye and nasal discharges and contaminated articles.
4) Quarantine: Not applicable.
5) Immmunization of contacts: Not applicable.
6) Investigation of contacts and source of infection: Members of family, playmates and schoolmates.
7) Specific treatment: In areas where the disease is severe and highly prevalent, mass treatment of the whole population, especially children, with oral azithromycin (20 mg/kg up to

1 gram, once or twice a year) or topical tetracycline ointment (twice daily for 6 weeks).

C. *Epidemic measures:* In regions of hyperendemic prevalence, mass treatment campaigns have been successful in reducing severity and frequency when associated with education in personal hygiene, especially cleanliness of the face, and improvement of the sanitary environment, particularly a good water supply.

D. *Disaster implications:* None.

E. *International measures:* WHO Collaborating Centres. WHO/ Alliance for the Global Elimination of blinding Trachoma.

[S. Resnikoff]

TRENCH FEVER
(Quintana fever)

ICD-9 083.1; ICD-10 A79.0

1. Identification—A typically nonfatal, febrile bacterial septicemic disease varying in manifestations and severity, characterized by headache, malaise, pain and tenderness, especially on the shins. Onset is either sudden or slow, with a fever that may be relapsing (usually with a 5-day periodicity), typhoid-like or limited to a single febrile episode lasting several days. Splenomegaly is common; a transient macular rash may occur. Symptoms may continue to recur many years after the primary infection, which may be subclinical with organisms circulating in the blood for months, with or without recurrence of symptoms. Bacteraemia, osteomyelitis and bacillary angiomatosis can occur in immunocompromised patients, especially those with HIV infection. Endocarditis has been associated with trench fever infections especially among homeless or alcoholic individuals.

Laboratory diagnosis is made by culture of patient blood on blood or chocolate agar under 5% CO_2. Microcolonies are visible after 8–21 days incubation at 37°C (98.6°F). Infection evokes genus-specific antibodies detectable by serological tests. ELISA tests are highly sensitive and an IFA test, are commercially available.

2. Infectious agent—*Bartonella quintana* (formerly *Rochalimaea quintana*).

3. Occurrence—Epidemics occurred in Europe during World Wars I and II among those living in crowded, unhygienic conditions; the disease is encountered especially among the homeless and persons infested with lice. Endemic foci have been detected in Burundi, Ethiopia, France,

Mexico, Peru, Poland, the former Soviet Union, USA and North Africa. Two forms of infection have been documented during the 1990s in France and USA: an opportunistic febrile infection in patients with HIV infection (sometimes presenting as bacillary angiomatosis, see Cat scratch disease); and a louse-borne febrile disease in homeless or alcoholic individuals, the so-called "urban trench fever" which may be associated with endocarditis.

4. **Reservoir**—Humans. The intermediate host and vector is the body louse, *Pediculus humanus corporis*. The organism multiplies extracellularly in the gut lumen for the duration of the insect's life, which is approximately 5 weeks after hatching. No transovarial transmission occurs. Cat fleas and ticks may be also infected.

5. **Mode of transmission**—Not directly transmitted from person to person. People are infected by inoculation of the organism in louse feces through a break in the skin. Infected lice begin to excrete infectious feces 5–12 days after ingesting infective blood; this continues for the remainder of their life span. The disease spreads when lice leave abnormally hot (febrile) or cold (dead) bodies in search of a normothermic host.

6. **Incubation period**—Generally 7–30 days.

7. **Period of communicability**—Organisms may circulate in the blood (thus infecting lice) for weeks, months or years and may recur with or without symptoms. A history of trench fever is a permanent contraindication to blood donation.

8. **Susceptibility**—Susceptibility is general. The degree of postinfection immunity to either reinfection or disease is unknown.

9. **Methods of control—**

A. *Preventive measures:* Delousing procedures: Dust clothing and body with an effective insecticide.

B. *Control of patient, contacts and the immediate environment:*

   1) Report to local health authority so that an evaluation of louse infestation in the population may be made and appropriate measures taken; Class 3 (see Reporting).
   2) Isolation: None after delousing.
   3) Concurrent disinfection: Treat louse-infested clothing to kill the lice.
   4) Quarantine: Not applicable.
   5) Immmunization of contacts: Not applicable.
   6) Investigation of contacts and source of infection: Search bodies and clothing of people at risk for the presence of lice; delouse if indicated.
   7) Specific treatment: tetracyclines for 2–4 weeks. Patients should first be carefully evaluated for endocarditis, as this will

change the duration and follow-up of antibiotherapy. Relapse may occur, despite antibiotherapy, in both immunocompromised and immunocompetent patients.

C. *Epidemic measures:* Systematic application of residual insecticide to clothing of all people in affected population (see 9A).

D. *Disaster implications:* Risk is increased when louse infested people are forced to live in crowded, unhygienic shelters (see 9B1).

E. *International measures:* WHO Collaborating Centres.

[D. Raoult]

TRICHINELLOSIS   ICD-9 124; ICD-10 B75
(Trichiniasis, Trichinosis)

1. Identification—A disease caused by an intestinal roundworm whose larvae (trichinae) migrate to and become encapsulated in the muscles. Clinical illness in humans is highly variable and can range from inapparent infection to a fulminating, fatal disease, depending on the number of larvae ingested. Sudden appearance of muscle soreness and pain together with oedema of the upper eyelids and fever are early characteristic signs. These are sometimes followed by subconjunctival, subungual and retinal hemorrhages, pain and photophobia. Thirst, profuse sweating, chills, weakness, prostration and rapidly increasing eosinophilia may follow shortly after the ocular signs.

Gastrointestinal symptoms, such as diarrhea, due to the intraintestinal activity of the adult worms, may precede the ocular manifestations. Remittent fever is usual, sometimes as high as 40°C (104°F); the fever terminates after 1–6 weeks, depending on intensity of infection. Cardiac and neurological complications may appear in the third to sixth week; in the most severe cases, death due to myocardial failure may occur in either the first to second week or between the fourth and eighth weeks.

Serological tests and marked eosinophilia may aid in diagnosis. Biopsy of skeletal muscle, taken more than 10 days after infection (most often positive after the fourth or fifth week of infection), frequently provides conclusive evidence of infection by demonstrating the uncalcified parasite cyst.

2. Infectious agent—*Trichinella spiralis*, an intestinal nematode. Separate taxonomic designations have been accepted for isolates found in the Arctic (*T. nativa*), Palaearctic (*T. britovi*, present in carnivore mammals and sometimes wild boar and domestic pigs in Europe and Asia), in Africa (*T. nelsoni*) and in several regions of the world (*T. pseudospiralis*).

3. Occurrence—Worldwide, but variable in incidence, depending in part on practices of eating and preparing pork or wild animal meat and the extent to which the disease is recognized and reported. Cases usually are sporadic and outbreaks localized, often resulting from eating sausage and other meat products using pork or shared meat from Arctic mammals. Several outbreaks been reported in France and Italy through infected horse meat.

4. Reservoir—Swine, dogs, cats, horses, rats and many wild animals, including fox, wolf, bear, polar bear, wild boar and marine mammals in the Arctic, and hyaena, jackal, lion and leopard in the tropics. A new species (*T. zimbabwensis*) has been found in farmed crocodiles; health risks for humans consuming crocodile meat are unknown.

5. Mode of transmission—Consumption of raw or insufficiently cooked flesh of animals containing viable encysted larvae, chiefly pork and pork products, and beef products, such as hamburger adulterated intentionally or inadvertently with raw pork. In the epithelium of the small intestine, larvae develop into adults. Gravid female worms then produce larvae, which penetrate the lymphatics or venules and are disseminated via the bloodstream throughout the body. The larvae become encapsulated in skeletal muscle.

6. Incubation period—Systemic symptoms usually appear about 8–15 days after ingestion of infected meat; this varies from 5 to 45 days depending on the number of parasites involved. GI symptoms may appear within a few days.

7. Period of communicability—Not transmitted directly from person to person. Animal hosts remain infective for months, and their meat stays infective for appreciable periods unless cooked, frozen or irradiated to kill the larvae (see 9A).

8. Susceptibility—Susceptibility is universal. Infection results in partial immunity.

9. Methods of control—

A. Preventive measures:

1) Educate the public on the need to cook all fresh pork and pork products and meat from wild animals at a temperature and for a time sufficient to allow all parts to reach at least 71°C (160°F), or until meat changes from pink to grey, which allows a sufficient margin of safety. This should be done unless it has been established that these meat products have

been processed either by heating, curing, freezing or irradiation adequate to kill trichinae.

2) Grind pork in a separate grinder or clean the grinder thoroughly before and after processing other meats.

3) Adopt regulations to encourage commercial irradiation processing of pork products. Testing carcases for infection with a digestion technique and immunodiagnosis of pigs with an approved ELISA test are both useful.

4) Adopt and enforce regulations that allow only certified trichinae-free pork to be used in raw pork products that have a cooked appearance or in products that traditionally are not heated sufficiently to kill trichinae during final preparation.

5) Adopt laws and regulations to require and enforce the cooking of garbage and offal before feeding to swine.

6) Educate hunters to cook the meat of walrus, seal, wild boar, bear and other wild animals thoroughly.

7) Freezing temperatures maintained throughout the mass of the infected meat are effective in inactivating trichinae; holding pieces of pork up to 15 cm thick at a temperature of −15°C (5°F) for 30 days or −25°C (−13°F) or lower for 10 days will effectively destroy all common types of trichinae cysts. Hold thicker pieces at the lower temperature for at least 20 days. These temperatures will not inactivate the cold-resistant Arctic strains (*T. nativa* and possibly *T. britovi*) found in walrus and bear meat and rarely in swine. For *T. nativa*, meat must be heated at more than 60°C (140°F) for a duration related to the thickness of the meat.

8) Exposure of pork cuts or carcases to low-level gamma irradiation effectively sterilizes and, at higher doses, kills encysted trichinae.

B. *Control of patient, contacts and the immediate environment:*

1) Report to local health authority: Case report required in most countries, Class 2 (see Reporting).

2) Isolation: Not applicable.

3) Concurrent disinfection: Not applicable.

4) Quarantine: Not applicable.

5) Immmunization of contacts: Not applicable.

6) Investigation of contacts and source of infection: Check family members and persons who have eaten meat suspected as the source of infection. Dispose of any remaining suspected food.

7) Specific treatment: Albendazole or mebendazole are effective in the intestinal stage and in the muscular stage. Corticosteroids are indicated only in severe cases to alleviate symptoms of inflammatory reaction when the CNS or heart is involved;

however, they delay elimination of adult worms from the intestine. In rare situations where infected meat is known to have been consumed, prompt administration of anthelminthic treatment may prevent development of symptoms.

C. *Epidemic measures:* Epidemiological study to determine the common food involved. Confiscate remainder of suspected food and correct faulty practices. Eliminate infected herds of swine.

D. *Disaster implications:* None.

E. *International measures:* WHO Collaborating Centres.

[D. Engels]

TRICHOMONIASIS ICD-9 131; ICD-10 A59

1. Identification—A common and persistent protozoan disease of the genitourinary tract, characterized in women by vaginitis, with small petechial or sometimes punctate red "strawberry" spots and a profuse, thin, foamy, greenish-yellow discharge with foul odor. The disease may cause urethritis or cystitis but is frequently asymptomatic; it may also cause obstetric complications and may facilitate HIV infection. In men, the infectious agent invades the prostate, urethra or seminal vesicles; it often causes only mild symptoms but may cause as much as 5%-10% of nongonococcal urethritis in some areas.

Trichomoniasis often coexists with gonorrhoea, in some studies up to 40% of persons with gonorrhoea have concurrent trichomoniasis, and the majority of women with trichomoniasis also have bacterial vaginosis; a full assessment for STI pathogens ("STI check") must be carried out when trichomoniasis is diagnosed.

Diagnosis is through identification of the motile parasite, either by microscopic examination of discharges or by culture, which is more sensitive. The organisms can be seen on a Papanicolaou smear. PCR testing is available but is insufficiently reliable for routine use.

2. Infectious agent—*Trichomonas vaginalis*, a flagellate protozoan.

3. Occurrence—Widespread; a frequent disease, primarily of adults, with the highest incidence among females 16–35 years. Overall, about 20% of females may become infected during their reproductive years.

4. Reservoir—Humans.

5. Mode of transmission—Through contact with vaginal and urethral discharges of infected people during sexual intercourse.

6. Incubation period—4-20 days, average 7 days; many are symptom-free carriers for years.

7. Period of communicability—For the duration of the persistent infection, which may last years.

8. Susceptibility—Susceptibility to infection is general, but clinical disease is seen mainly in females.

9. Methods of control—

A. **Preventive measures:** Educate the public to seek medical advice whenever there is an abnormal discharge from the genitalia and to refrain from sexual intercourse until investigation and treatment of self and partner(s) are completed. Promotion of "safer sex" behaviour, including condom use, is recommended for all sexual contacts where mutual monogamy is not the case.

B. **Control of patient, contacts and the immediate environment:**

1) Report to local health authority: Official report not ordinarily justifiable, Class 5 (see Reporting).
2) Isolation: Avoid sexual relations during period of infection and treatment.
3) Concurrent disinfection: Not applicable; the organism does not withstand drying.
4) Quarantine: Not applicable.
5) Immmunization of contacts: Not applicable.
6) Investigation of contacts and source of infection: Evaluate sexual partners for other STDs and treat concurrently.
7) Specific treatment: oral metronidazole, tinidazole or ornidazole is effective in both male and female patients; contraindicated during the first trimester of pregnancy. Clotrimazole, produces symptomatic relief and may cure up to 50% of patients. Concurrently treat sexual partner(s) to prevent reinfection. Cases of metronidazole resistance have been reported and should be treated with topical intravaginal paromomycin.

C. **Epidemic measures:** None.

D. **Disaster implications:** None.

E. **International measures:** None.

[L. Savioli]

TRICHURIASIS   ICD-9 127.3; ICD-10 B79
(Trichocephaliasis, Whipworm disease)

1. Identification—A nematode infection of the large intestine, usually asymptomatic. Heavy infections may cause bloody, mucoid stools and diarrhea. Rectal prolapse, clubbing of fingers, hypoproteinemia, anemia and growth retardation may occur in heavily infected children.

Diagnosis is made through demonstration of eggs in feces or sigmoidoscopic observation of worms attached to the wall of the lower colon in heavy infections. Eggs must be differentiated from those of *Capillaria* species.

2. Infectious agent—*Trichuris trichiura (Trichocephalus trichiurus)* or human whipworm, a nematode.

3. Occurrence—Worldwide, especially in warm, moist regions.

4. Reservoir—Humans. Animal whipworms do not infect humans.

5. Mode of transmission—Indirect, particularly through pica or ingestion of contaminated vegetables; no immediate person-to-person transmission. Eggs passed in feces require a minimum of 10-14 days in warm moist soil to become infective. Hatching of larvae follows ingestion of infective eggs from contaminated soil, attachment to the mucosa of the caecum and proximal colon, and development into mature worms. Eggs appear in the feces 70-90 days after ingestion of embryonated eggs; symptoms may appear much earlier.

6. Incubation period—Indefinite.

7. Period of communicability—Several years in untreated carriers.

8. Susceptibility—Susceptibility is universal.

9. Methods of control—

A. Preventive measures:

1) Educate all members of the family, particularly children, in the use of toilet facilities.
2) Provide adequate facilities for feces disposal.
3) Encourage satisfactory hygienic habits, especially handwashing before food handling; avoid ingestion of soil by thorough washing of vegetables and other foods contaminated with soil.
4) WHO recommends a strategy focused on high-risk groups for the control of morbidity due to soil-transmitted helminths,

including community treatment, differentiated according to prevalence and severity of infections: i) universal medication of women (once a year, including pregnant women) and preschool children 1 year or more (twice or thrice a year) if 10 000 schoolchildren show 10% or more of heavy infections (10 000+ *Trichuris* eggs per gram of feces) whatever the prevalence; ii) yearly community medication targeted to risk groups (including pregnant women) if prevalence >50% and schoolchildren show <10% of heavy infections; iii) individual case management if prevalence <50% and schoolchildren show <10% of heavy infections. Extensive monitoring has shown no significant ill effects of administration to pregnant women under these circumstances.

B. Control of patient, contacts and the immediate environment:

1) Report to local health authority: Official report not ordinarily justifiable, Class 5 (see Reporting). Advise school health authorities of unusual frequency in school populations.
2) Isolation: Not applicable.
3) Concurrent disinfection: Sanitary disposal of feces.
4) Quarantine: Not applicable.
5) Immmunization of contacts: Not applicable.
6) Investigation of contacts and source of infection: Examine feces of all symptomatic members of the family group, especially children and playmates.
7) Specific treatment: Mebendazole is the drug of choice. Albendazole (half dose for children 12–24 months), oxantel (not available in the USA) and pyrantel are alternative drugs. On theoretical grounds, pregnant women should not be treated in the first trimester unless there are specific medical or public health indications.

C. Epidemic measures: Not applicable.

D. Disaster implications: None.

E. International measures: None.

[L. Savioli]

TRYPANOSOMIASIS   ICD-9 086; ICD-10 B56-B57

I. AFRICAN
TRYPANOSOMIASIS ICD-9 086.3-086.5; ICD-10 B56
(Sleeping sickness)

1. Identification—A systemic protozoal disease. In the early stage, a painful chancre, originating as a papule and evolving into a nodule, may be found at the primary tsetse fly bite site; there may also be fever, intense headache, insomnia, painless enlarged lymph nodes, local oedema and rash. In the late stage, after the parasite crosses the blood-brain barrier, neurological signs such as disturbances of circadian rhythm, sensory disturbances, endocrine dysfunction, disorders of tonus and mobility, abnormal movements, mental changes or psychiatric disorders are correlated to the localisation of trypanosomes in the CNS; cardiac symptoms may occur in both gambiense and rhodesiense forms.

Disease due to *Trypanosoma brucei gambiense* (ICD-9 086.3; ICD-10 B56.0) may run a course of several years; the *T. b. rhodesiense* disease (ICD-9 086.4; ICD-10 B56.1) is lethal within weeks or months without treatment. Both are always fatal without treatment.

Diagnosis, which cannot be based on clinical symptoms only, depends on finding trypanosomes in blood, lymph or eventually CSF; so does staging of the disease. Parasite-concentration techniques (capillary tube centrifugation, or minianion exchange centrifugation) are almost always required in gambiense and less often in rhodesiense disease. Inoculation on laboratory rats or mice is sometimes useful in rhodesiense disease. Standard bioclinical parameters such as anemia and thrombocytopenia may provide indirect diagnostic evidence for trypanosomiasis. High IgM in blood point to the need for specific examinations. IgM concentrations in *T. b. gambiense* patients can be increased up to 16 times as a result of polyclonal, non-specific B-cell activation. The accompanying poly-specific immune response leads to production of non-trypanosome specific antibodies and auto-antibodies e.g. against fibrin, fibrinogen, DNA, red blood cells, thymocyte antigens and CNS components such as myelin, galacto-cerebrosides and neurofilament. *T. b. gambiense*-specific IgG and IgM antibodies are present in high concentrations and are mainly directed against the immunodominant surface glycoprotein antigens of the parasite. They are detectable by ELISA or immunofluorescence, using purified trypanosomal glycoproteins or whole trypanosomes of selected antigen types. The screening test of choice for *T. b. gambiense* is the card agglutination test for trypanosomiasis (CATT), a simple 5-minute test based on the agglutination of whole, fixed and stained trypanosomes in the presence of specific antibodies. Almost every control program in

T. b. gambiense endemic areas uses it for seroscreening of at-risk populations.

2. Infectious agents—*Trypanosoma brucei gambiense* and *T. b. rhodesiense*, hemoflagellates. Criteria for species differentiation are not absolute; isolates from cases of virulent, rapidly progressive disease are considered to be *T. b. rhodesiense,* especially if contracted in eastern Africa; western and central African cases are usually more chronic and considered to be due to *T. b. gambiense.*

3. Occurrence—The disease is confined to tropical Africa between 15°N and 20°S latitude, corresponding to the distribution of the tsetse fly. WHO estimates some 300 000 to 500 000 people are currently infected, with up to 60 million people in 36 countries at risk of contracting the disease. Sleeping sickness, which occurs at over 250 foci in the poorest areas of some of the least industrialized countries, ranks high in terms of disability-adjusted life years (DALY).

Outbreaks can occur when human-fly contact is intensified, or when movement of infected flies or reservoir hosts introduces virulent trypanosome strains into a tsetse-infested area or populations are displaced into endemic areas.

4. Reservoir—In *T. b. gambiense* infection, humans are the major reservoir; however, the role of domestic and wild animals is not clear. Wild animals, especially bushbucks and antelopes, and domestic cattle are the chief animal reservoirs for *T. b. rhodesiense.*

5. Mode of transmission—Through the bite of infective *Glossina*, the tsetse fly. Six species are the main vectors in nature: *G. palpalis*, *G. tachinoides*, *G. morsitans*, *G. pallidipes*, *G. swynnertoni* and *G. fuscipes*. The fly is infected by ingesting blood of a human or animal that carries trypanosomes. The parasite multiplies in the fly for 12–30 days, depending on temperature and other factors, until infective forms develop in the salivary glands. Once infected, a tsetse fly remains infective for life (average 3 months but as long as 10 months); infection is not passed from generation to generation in flies. Congenital transmission can occur in humans. Direct mechanical transmission by blood on the proboscis of *Glossina* and other biting insects, such as horseflies, or in laboratory accidents, is possible.

6. Incubation period—In *T. b. rhodesiense* infections, usually 3 days to a few weeks; *T. b. gambiense* infection has a longer incubation period of up to several months or even years.

7. Period of communicability—Communicable to the tsetse fly as long as the parasite is present in the blood of the infected person or animal. Parasitemia in humans occurs in waves of varying intensity in untreated cases and occurs at all stages of the disease.

8. **Susceptibility**—Susceptibility is general. Occasional inapparent or asymptomatic infections have been documented with both *T. b. gambiense* and *T. b. rhodesiense*. Spontaneous recovery in cases with the gambiense form without CNS involvement has been claimed, but has not been confirmed.

9. **Methods of control**—

A. *Preventive measures:* Selection of appropriate prevention methods must be based on knowledge of the local ecology of vectors and infectious agents. In a given geographic area, priority must be given to one or more of the following:

   1) Educate the public on personal protective measures against tsetse fly bites—this has limited impact because tsetse flies bite during the day at the workplace. Bednets are not useful.
   2) Reduce the parasite population by screening and diagnosing exposed populations and treating those infected. This is mainly effective for *T. b. gambiense*, where humans are the main reservoir.
   3) Destroy vector tsetse fly habitats if necessary; indiscriminate destruction of vegetation is not recommended.
   4) Reduce the tsetse fly population by appropriate use of traps and screens preferably but not necessarily impregnated with deltamethrine and by local use of residual insecticides. Aerosol insecticides sprayed by helicopter and fixed wing aircraft are usually not recommended in *T. b. gambiense* areas (forests).
   5) Prohibit blood donation from those that have visited or lived in endemic areas in Africa.

B. *Control of patient, contacts and the immediate environment:*

   1) Systematic screening of exposed populations in each *T. b. gambiense* focus, aimed at identifying asymptomatic infections at an early stage. Early diagnosis reduces both the risk of sequelae and the drug-related risks, and helps stop transmission.
      Regular surveillance in local health centers and villages for both rhodesiense and gambiense areas.
      Report to local health authority: In selected endemic areas, establish records of prevalence and encourage control measures; not a reportable disease in most countries, Class 3 (see Reporting).
   2) Isolation: Not recommended. Prevent tsetse flies from feeding on patients with trypanosomes in their blood.
   3) Concurrent disinfection: Not applicable.
   4) Quarantine: Not applicable.

5) Immmunization of contacts: Not applicable.
6) Investigation of contacts and source of infection: If the case is a member of a tour group, others in the group should be alerted and investigated.
7) Specific treatment:
Treatment differs according to form and phase of the disease. If diagnosis occurs early in the initial phase, chances of cure are high. Treatment of the neurological phase requires a drug that can cross the blood-brain barrier. If started too late, treatment cannot prevent irreversible neurological damage. Early diagnosis, allowing low-risk treatment on an outpatient basis, should be attempted in remote rural settings where the disease takes its heaviest toll. Until recently, treatment prospects have been bleak. The disease is notoriously difficult to treat, particularly in the neurological stage. Available medicines are expensive to manufacture and difficult to administer. While some are well tolerated, in others— used in the neurological phase—fatal complications are common. Problems of drug resistance have increasingly been reported in several countries.

The treatment of sleeping sickness depends on 5 key drugs needed for the different forms and stages of the disease. These drugs are available through WHO, the only provider. They are free of charge and 3 of them—pentamidine, melarsoprol, eflornithine—have at the time of writing been donated to WHO in amounts currently sufficient to meet needs until June 2006. Suramin is now donated to WHO and development work is being considered for nifurtimox— currently registered for American trypanosomiasis (q.v.)—to support "label extension" towards African trypanosomiasis.

Pentamidine (IM. 4mg/kg/d for 7 days) is used for early stages of *T. b. gambiense* and Suramin (IM. 20mg/Kg/week for 5 weeks) for early stages of *T. b. rhodesiense* infections.

Melarsoprol (IV, 2.2 mg/Kg/d for 10 days) is used to treat both forms at the neurological stage. The main adverse effect of melarsoprol—reactive encephalopathy—is often fatal. This drug must be administered in hospital and if possible in the intensive care unit.

Eflornithine (slow IV perfusion 100 mg/kg/6 hours for 14 days) is used for late-stage *T. b. gambiense* infection. This drug is difficult to administer under field conditions; it can have fatal complications but is safer than melarsoprol.

Patients treated must be re-examined for at least one and preferably 2 years for possible relapses

C. **Epidemic measures:** Mainly for *T. b. rhodesiense*: Mass surveys, urgent treatment for identified infections and tsetse fly control. If epidemics recur despite initial control measures, the measures recommended in 9A must be pursued more vigorously.

D. Disaster implications: None.

E. International measures: Promote cooperative efforts of governments in endemic areas (information, availability of diagnostic tests and means of vector control, distribution of reagents and drugs, training). WHO Collaborating Centres are available for technical and laboratory support. Further information at http://www.who.int/tdr/diseases/tryp/default.htm

[J. Jannin]

II. AMERICAN
TRYPANOSOMIASIS   ICD-9 086.2; ICD-10 B57
(Chagas disease)

1. Identification—The acute disease, with variable fever, lymphadenopathy, malaise, and hepatosplenomegaly generally occurs in children; although the majority of infections are asymptomatic or paucisymptomatic. In 20%–30% of infections, irreversible chronic manifestations generally appear later in life. An inflammatory response at the site of infection (chagoma) may last up to 8 weeks. Unilateral bipalpebral-oedema (Romana sign) occurs in a small percentage of acute cases. Life-threatening or fatal manifestations include myocarditis and meningoencephalitis.

Chronic irreversible sequelae include myocardial damage with cardiac dilatation, arrhythmias and major conduction abnormalities, and intestinal tract involvement with megaoesophagus and megacolon. Megavisceral manifestations occur mainly in central Brazil. The prevalence of megaviscera and cardiac involvement varies according to regions; the latter is not as common north of Ecuador as in southern areas. In AIDS patients, acute myocarditis and severe multifocal or diffuse meningoencephalitis with necrosis and hemorrhage occur as relapses of chronic infection. This has also been reported in cases of chronic Chagas disease with non-AIDS immunosuppression.

Infection with *Trypanosoma rangeli* occurs in foci of endemic Chagas disease extending from Central America to Colombia and Venezuela; prolonged parasitaemia occurs, sometimes coexisting with *T. cruzi* flagellates (with which *T. rangeli* shares reservoir hosts)—no clinical manifestations attributable to *T. rangeli* have been noted.

Diagnosis of Chagas disease in the acute phase is established through demonstration of the organism in blood (rarely, in a lymph node or skeletal muscle) by direct examination or after hemoconcentration, culture or xenodiagnosis (feeding noninfected triatomid bugs on the patient and finding the parasite in the bugs' feces several weeks later).

Parasitemia is most intense during febrile episodes early in the course of infection. In the chronic phase, xenodiagnosis and blood culture on diphasic media may be positive, but other methods rarely reveal parasites. Parasites are differentiated from those of *T. rangeli* by their shorter length (20 micrometers *vs* 36 micrometers) and larger kinetoplast. Serologic tests are valuable for individual diagnosis as well as for screening purposes.

2. Infectious agent—*Trypanosoma cruzi* (*Schizotrypanum cruzi*), a protozoan that occurs in humans as a hemoflagellate (trypomastigote) and as an intracellular parasite (amastigote) without an external flagellum.

3. Occurrence—The disease is confined to the Western Hemisphere, with wide geographic distribution in rural Mexico and central and South America; highly endemic in some areas. Reactivated infection in AIDS patients may cause meningoencephalitis. In addition to 5 reported acute vector-borne human infections acquired within the USA, 3 infections were acquired by blood transfusion.

Serological studies suggest the possible occurrence of other asymptomatic cases. *T. cruzi* is reported from small mammals in parts of the USA. Recent studies found serological evidence of infection in 4.9% of migrants from central America living in the Washington D.C. area.

4. Reservoir—Humans and over 150 domestic and wild mammals species, including dogs, cats, rats, mice, marsupials, edentates, rodents, chiroptera, carnivores, primates and other.

5. Mode of transmission—Infected vectors, i.e. blood-sucking species of Reduviidae (cone-nosed bugs or kissing bugs), especially various species from the genera *Triatoma*, *Rhodnius* and *Panstrongylus* have the trypanosomes in their feces. Defecation occurs during feeding; infection of humans and other mammals occurs when the freshly excreted bug feces contaminate conjunctivae, mucous membranes, abrasions or skin wounds (including the bite wound). The bugs become infected when they feed on a parasitaemic animal; the parasites multiply in the bug's gut.

Transmission may also occur by blood transfusion: there are increasing numbers of infected donors in cities because of migration from rural areas. Organisms may also cross the placenta to cause congenital infection (in 2% to 8% of pregnancies for those infected); transmission through breastfeeding seems highly unlikely, so there is currently no reason to restrict breastfeeding by chagasic mothers. Accidental laboratory infections occur occasionally; transplantation of organs from chagasic donors presents a growing risk of *T. cruzi* transmission.

6. Incubation period—About 5-14 days after bite of insect vector; 30-40 days if infected through blood transfusion.

7. Period of communicability—Organisms are regularly present in the blood during the acute period and may persist in very small numbers throughout life in symptomatic and asymptomatic people. The vector becomes infective 10-30 days after biting an infected host; gut infection in the bug persists for life (as long as 2 years).

8. Susceptibility—All ages are susceptible, but the disease is usually more severe in younger people. Immunosuppressed people, especially those with AIDS, are at risk of serious infections and complications.

9. Methods of control—

A. *Preventive measures:*

1) Educate the public on mode of spread and methods of prevention.
2) Systematically attack vectors infesting poorly constructed houses and houses with thatched roofs, using effective insecticides with residual action (spraying or use of insecticidal paints or fumigant canisters).
3) Construct or repair living areas to eliminate lodging places for insect vectors and shelter for domestic and wild reservoir animals. In certain areas, palm trees close to houses often harbour infested bugs and can be considered a risk factor.
4) Use bednets (preferably insecticide-impregnated) in houses infested by the vector.
5) Screen blood and organ donors living in or coming from endemic areas by appropriate serological tests to prevent infection by transfusion or transplants, as required by law in most countries in the Americas.

B. *Control of patient, contacts and the immediate environment:*

1) Report to local health authority: In selected endemic areas; not a reportable disease in most countries, Class 3 (see Reporting).
2) Isolation: Not generally practical. Blood and body fluid precautions for hospitalized patients.
3) Concurrent disinfection: Not applicable.
4) Quarantine: Not applicable.
5) Immmunization of contacts: Not applicable.
6) Investigation of contacts and source of infection: Search thatched roofs, bedding and rooms for vectors. All family members of a case should be examined. Serological tests and blood examinations on all blood and organ donors implicated as possible sources of transfusion- or transplant-acquired infection.
7) Specific treatment: Benznidazole, a 2-nitroimidazole derivative, has proven effective in acute cases. Nifurtimox, a nitrofurfurylidene derivative, available from the CDC Drug Service on an investigational basis and from major hospitals in endemic areas, is also useful in treatment of acute cases. Randomized controlled trials show that benznidazole substantially and significantly modifies parasite-related outcomes

compared to placebo; the same applies for chronic asymptomatic *T. cruzi* infection. The potential of trypanocidal treatment in Chagas disease among asymptomatic, chronically infected subjects is promising, but remains to be evaluated.

C. Epidemic measures: In areas of high incidence, field survey to determine distribution and density of vectors and animal hosts.

D. Disaster implications: None.

E. International measures: Control programs created in the 1960s and 1970s, based on application of residual insecticides, restarted with the Initiative for the Southern Cone Countries (ISCC: Argentina, Brazil, Bolivia, Chile, Paraguay, Uruguay) in 1991. The vector in these countries is mainly domiciliated and an ideal target for residual household spraying. Progress has been made in this region and since 1999 some countries have been declared free of vectorial transmission (e.g. Chile and Uruguay). Further research and implementation efforts are necessary in the Amazon, Andean and Central American regions, where transmission occurs through both domiciliated and non-domiciliated vectors. These regions are covered by the Andean Countries Initiative (ACI – Colombia, Ecuador, Northern Peru, Venezuela) and the Central America Countries Initiative (CACI – Belize, Costa Rica, El Salvador, Guatemala, Honduras, Nicaragua, Panama).

Further information at http://www.who.int/tdr/diseases/chagas/default.htm

[R. Salvatella Agrelo]

TUBERCULOSIS   ICD-9 010-018; ICD-10 A15-A19
(TB, TB disease)

1. Identification—A mycobacterial disease that is a major cause of disability and death in most of the world, especially developing countries. The initial infection usually goes unnoticed; tuberculin skin test sensitivity appears within 2–10 weeks. Early lung lesions commonly heal, leaving no residual changes except occasional pulmonary or tracheobronchial lymph node calcifications. About 10% of those initially infected will eventually develop active disease, half of them during the first 2 years following infection; 90% of untreated infected individuals will never develop active TB. Appropriate completion of treatment for latent TB infection (LTBI) can considerably reduce the lifetime risk of clinical tuberculosis (TB disease) and is effective in persons with HIV infection.

In some individuals, initial infection may progress rapidly to active tuberculosis. This is more common among infants, where the disease is often disseminated (e.g. miliary) or meningeal, and in the immunosuppressed, such as HIV-positive individuals.

Extrapulmonary TB occurs less commonly (30%) than pulmonary TB (70%). Children and persons with immunodeficiencies, such as HIV infection, have a higher risk of extrapulmonary TB, but pulmonary disease remains the most common type worldwide, even in these more susceptible groups. TB disease may affect any organ or tissue; in order of frequency: lymph nodes, pleura, pericardium, kidneys, bones and joints, larynx, middle ear, skin, intestines, peritoneum, eyes.

Pulmonary TB may arise from exogenous reinfection or endogenous reactivation of a latent focus originating from the initial sub-clinical infection. If untreated, about 65% of patients with sputum smear-positive pulmonary tuberculosis die within 5 years, most of these within 2 years. The classification of TB for treatment purposes is based mainly on the presence or absence of tubercle bacilli in the sputum. A smear positive for acid-fast bacilli (AFB) is indicative of high infectiousness. Fatigue, fever, night sweats and weight loss may occur early or late; localizing symptoms of cough, chest pain, hemoptysis and hoarseness become prominent in advanced stages. Radiography of the chest reveals pulmonary infiltrates, cavitations and, later, fibrotic changes with volume loss, all most commonly in the upper segments of the lobes.

Immunocompetent people who are or have been infected with *Mycobacterium tuberculosis*, *M. africanum* or *M. bovis* usually react to an intermediate strength tuberculin skin test equivalent to 5 IUs of the International Standard of Purified Protein Derivative-Standard (PPD-S). A positive reaction is defined as a 5, 10, or 15 mm induration according to the risk of exposure or disease. Among persons with active TB disease 10%–20% may have no reaction to PPD—a negative skin test does not therefore rule out active TB disease. Interpreting the PPD skin test induration size is important to define positivity and the need to start treatment of latent TB infection (previously termed chemoprophylaxis or preventive chemotherapy). An induration of 5 mm or more is considered positive among HIV-infected persons, persons on highly potent immunosuppressive treatment, persons showing fibrotic lesions on chest X-rays, and recent close contacts of infectious TB patients. A diameter of 10 mm or more is considered positive among persons infected for less than 2 years and those with high-risk conditions (e.g. diabetes mellitus, hematological disorders, injection drug use, end-stage renal disease, rapid weight loss). Any reaction of 15 mm or more should be considered positive among low-risk persons.

Skin tests for anergy are no longer recommended, even for high-risk patients. In many industrialized countries, including the USA, routine skin testing of all children is no longer recommended; children to be tested include those suspected of having active TB disease and those exposed to an infectious case; immigrants from an endemic country may also be tested. Incarcerated individuals and persons with HIV infection or children residing in a household with an HIV-infected person should be tested annually. Children should be tested every 2–3 years if exposed to persons at high risk of disease. Testing at 4–6 and 11–12 is indicated if the parents immigrated from a high-risk area or if the children reside in high-risk communities, as defined by local public health authorities.

In some persons with TB infection, delayed type hypersensitivity to tuberculin may wane with time. When skin-tested many years after initial infection, they may show a negative reaction, but the skin test may boost their ability to react to tuberculin and cause a positive reaction to subsequent tests. This "boosted" reaction may be mistaken for a new infection; it can persist for 1 to 2 years. Boosting has also been reported in persons who have received BCG. A 2-step testing procedure distinguishes boosted reactions and reactions due to new infection. If the reaction to the first test is classified as negative, a positive reaction to a second test 1–3 weeks later probably represents a boosted reaction. On the basis of this second result, the person should be classified as previously infected and managed accordingly. If the second test is also negative, the person should be classified as uninfected. Two-step testing should be used for initial skin testing of adults who will be retested periodically (e.g. health care workers), who are not known to have a prior positive skin test and have not had a tuberculin test during the previous year or so.

Demonstration of acid-fast bacilli in stained smears from sputum or other body fluids in a clinical and epidemiological situation suggestive of TB is a presumptive diagnosis of active TB disease and usually justifies initiation of antituberculosis treatment. Where resources permit, isolation of organisms of the *Mycobacterium tuberculosis* complex on culture confirms the diagnosis and also permits determination of drug susceptibility for the infecting organism. In the absence of bacteriological confirmation, active disease can be presumed if clinical, histological or radiological evidence is suggestive of TB and other likely disease processes can be ruled out.

2. Infectious agents—*Mycobacterium tuberculosis* complex. This includes *M. tuberculosis, M. africanum*, *M. canettii* (the latter two responsible for a small number of cases in Africa), all primarily from humans, and *M. bovis* primarily from cattle. Other mycobacteria occasionally produce disease clinically indistinguishable from tuberculosis; the causal agents can be identified only through culture. Genetic sequence analyses using PCR offers potential for noncultural identification.

3. Occurrence—Worldwide; industrialized countries showed downward trends of mortality and morbidity for many years, but in the mid-1980s reported cases reached a plateau; areas and population groups with a high prevalence of HIV infection or with large numbers of persons from areas with a high prevalence of tuberculosis have since increased. In regions with declining TB incidence, TB mortality and morbidity rates increase with age, and in older people rates are higher in males than in females. In regions and groups with high rates of new transmission and rising incidence, morbidity is highest among working-age adults. TB morbidity rates are higher among disadvantaged populations, and usually higher in cities than in rural areas.

In the low incidence areas of USA and many other industrialized countries, most TB disease in adults results from reactivation of latent foci remaining from an initial infection. In some large urban areas about one-third of TB disease cases may result from recent infection. Long exposure of some contacts, notably household associates, may lead to a 30% lifetime risk of becoming infected. For infected children, the lifetime risk of developing disease may approach 10%. For people infected with HIV, the annual risk has been estimated at 2%–13%, depending upon he CD4+ cell count, and the cumulative risk at up to 50%. Epidemics have been reported in enclosed spaces, such as nursing homes, shelters for the homeless, hospitals, schools, prisons, and during long-haul-flights. From 1989 to the early 1990s, extensive outbreaks of multidrug-resistant TB (MDR-TB), defined as resistance to at least isoniazid and rifampicin, have been recognized in US settings where many HIV-infected persons are congregated (hospitals, prisons, drug treatment clinics and HIV residences). These outbreaks are associated with high fatality rates and transmission of *M. tuberculosis* to health care workers. Strict enforcement of infection control guidelines, pro-active case-finding, contact investigations, and measures to ensure completion of appropriate treatment regimens have been effective in combating and preventing these outbreaks. Worldwide, 1%–2% of all TB cases at most are due to multidrug resistant strains; in some countries; e.g. parts of China, India, the former USSR, MDR-TB is a major problem.

The prevalence of TB infection detected by tuberculin testing increases with age. The incidence of infection in industrialized countries has declined rapidly in recent decades; in the USA, the annual risk of new infection is estimated to average about 10/100 000 people at most, although there probably are areas in the USA with a relatively high annual risk of new infection. In areas where human infection with mycobacteria other than tubercle bacilli is prevalent, cross-reactions complicate interpretation of the tuberculin reaction.

Human infection with *M. bovis*, the bovine tubercle bacillus, is still a problem in areas where the disease in cattle has not been controlled and milk and milk products are consumed raw.

4. Reservoir—Primarily humans, rarely primates; in some areas, diseased cattle, badgers, swine and other mammals are infected.

5. Mode of transmission—Exposure to tubercle bacilli in airborne droplet nuclei, 1 to 5 microns in diameter, produced by people with pulmonary or respiratory tract tuberculosis during expiratory efforts (coughing, singing or sneezing), and inhaled by a vulnerable contact into the pulmonary alveolae, where they are taken up by alveolar macrophages, initiating a new infection. Health care workers are exposed during procedures such as bronchoscopy or intubation and at autopsy. Laryngeal tuberculosis is highly contagious but rare. Prolonged or repeated close exposure to an infectious case may lead to infection of contacts. Direct invasion through mucous membranes or breaks in the skin may occur but is rare. Bovine tuberculosis, a rare event, results from exposure to tuberculous cattle, usually through ingestion of unpasteurized milk or dairy products, and sometimes through airborne spread to farmers and animal handlers. Except for rare situations where there is a draining sinus, extrapulmonary tuberculosis (other than laryngeal) is generally not communicable.

6. **Incubation period**—From infection to demonstrable primary lesion or significant tuberculin reaction, about 2-10 weeks. While the subsequent risk of progressive pulmonary or extrapulmonary TB is greatest within the first year or two after infection, latent infection may persist for a lifetime. Tuberculin reactivity also persists regardless of treatment. HIV infection increases the risk and shortens the interval for the development of TB disease following infection.

7. **Period of communicability**—Theoretically, as long as viable tubercle bacilli are discharged in the sputum. Some untreated or inadequately treated patients may be intermittently sputum-positive for years. The degree of communicability depends on number of bacilli discharged, virulence of the bacilli, adequacy of ventilation, exposure of bacilli to sun or UV light, and opportunities for aerosolization through coughing, sneezing, talking or singing, or during procedures such as intubations or bronchoscopies and at autopsies. Effective antimicrobial chemotherapy usually eliminates communicability within 2-4 weeks, at least in household settings, even though TB bacteria may still grow from expectorated sputum. Children with primary tuberculosis are generally not infectious.

8. **Susceptibility**—The risk of infection with the tubercle bacillus is directly related to the degree of exposure and does not appear related to genetic or other host factors. The first 12-24 months after infection constitute the most hazardous period for the development of clinical disease. The risk of developing disease is highest in children under 3, lowest in later childhood, and high again among young adults, the very old and the immunosuppressed. Population groups not previously touched by tuberculosis appear to have greater susceptibility to new infection and disease. Reactivation of long-latent infections accounts for a large proportion of TB disease cases in older people. For infected persons, susceptibility to TB disease is markedly increased by HIV infection and other forms of immunosuppression, and among the underweight or undernourished,

people with a debilitating disorder (e.g. chronic renal failure, some forms of cancer, silicosis, diabetes or gastrectomy), or substance users.

For adults with latent TB infection also infected with HIV, the lifetime risk of developing TB disease rises from an estimated 10% to up to 50%. This has resulted in a parallel pandemic of TB disease: in some urban sub-Saharan African areas, where 10–15% of the adult population are co-infected with both HIV and TB; annual TB disease rates have increased 5- to 10-fold between the 1980s and today. Under such conditions, the risk of multi-drug-resistant (MDR) TB is high where TB control is inadequate.

9. Methods of control—

A. Preventive measures:

1) Promptly identify, diagnose and treat potentially infectious patients with TB disease. Establish case-finding and treatment facilities for infectious cases to reduce transmission.

2) Ensure medical, laboratory and X-ray facilities for prompt examination of patients, contacts and suspects; ensure provision of drugs and facilities for early and complete treatment of cases and people at high risk of infection; and of beds for those needing hospitalization.

    In high incidence areas, direct microscopy examination of sputum for those presenting because of chest symptoms (with culture confirmation when possible) may give a high yield of infectious tuberculosis. In most situations, direct microscopy is the most cost-effective method of case-finding and is the first priority in developing countries. Because of serious outbreaks of MDR-TB in the 1990s, all initial isolates in the USA and many other countries must be submitted to drug susceptibility testing. In countries with limited resources/laboratory capacity, drug susceptibility testing may be restricted to re-treatment cases, such as treatment failures and defaulters of previous treatment.

3) Educate the public in mode of spread and methods of control and regarding the importance of early diagnosis and continued adherence to treatment.

4) Reduce or eliminate those social conditions that increase the risk of infection.

5) Set up TB prevention and control programs in institutional settings where health care is provided and/or where immunocompromised patients such as HIV-infected persons congregate (e.g. hospitals, drug treatment programs, prisons, nursing homes and homeless shelters).

6) Preventive chemotherapy with isoniazid for 6–12 months has been effective in preventing the progression of latent TB infection to TB disease in up to 90% of compliant individuals. Studies in adults with HIV infection have shown

the effectiveness of alternative regimens including shorter courses (2 months) of rifampicin and pyrazinamide. Since this regimen has been associated with severe hepatotoxicity it is not currently recommended for general use. It is important to rule out active TB disease before starting treatment for latent TB infection, especially in immunocompromised persons such as HIV-infected individuals, in order to avoid inadvertently treating active disease with a 1- or 2-drug regimen that would encourage the development of drug resistance. Because of the risk of isoniazid-associated hepatitis, isoniazid is not routinely advised for persons with active liver disease.

Persons started on treatment for latent TB infection must be informed of possible adverse effects (e.g. hepatitis, drug fever or severe rash), reminded of these possibilities and checked for symptoms monthly, prior to prescription refills; they should be advised to discontinue treatment and seek medical advice if suggestive symptoms develop. Baseline liver function tests are important in patients with signs, symptoms or history of liver disease and in those who abuse alcohol. Avoiding or discontinuing isoniazid generally is advised for persons with transaminase levels more than 5 times the upper limit of normal values (3 times if symptoms suggest hepatic dysfunction). Directly observed supervised treatment should be used when possible (e.g. prisons, drug treatment programs, schools) and can be administered twice weekly, adjusting dosage upwards to compensate for the reduction in frequency. Not more than 1 month's supply of medication should be given at any one time, and patients should be queried at least monthly about adverse effects. Routine biochemical monitoring for hepatitis is not necessary but monitoring is mandatory if symptoms or signs of hepatitis occur.

During pregnancy, it may be wise to postpone treatment for latent TB infection until after delivery except in high-risk individuals, and then it should be administered with caution.

Mass treatment for latent TB infection is unrealistic and unsuitable in most communities unless there is a well-organized program to supervise and encourage adherence to treatment and unless a high rate of cure can be achieved among patients with active TB disease. Persons with HIV infection and a positive PPD who do not have active TB disease should receive treatment for latent TB infection.

7) Provide public health nursing and outreach services for support to patients; ensure supervision of treatment and

arrange for examination and treatment for latent TB infection among contacts.

8) Persons infected with HIV should be skin-tested with intermediate strength PPD at the time their HIV infection is identified; they should start treatment for latent TB infection if they are PPD-positive (5 mm or more induration) and if active TB disease has been ruled out. Conversely, all people with evidence of TB disease should be considered for counselling and tested for HIV infection if appropriate counselling is available.

9) In industrialized countries where BCG immunization is not routinely carried out, selective tuberculin-testing and treatment for latent TB infection may be considered for groups at high risk of TB infection and/or HIV infection, including health care workers and groups such as prison inmates and injecting drug users; this may also be considered for foreign-born persons from areas of high tuberculosis prevalence, and possibly for travellers to and from high-prevalence areas. In population groups where disease still occurs, systematic tuberculin test surveys may help monitor the incidence of infection. Prior BCG immunization may complicate interpretation of a positive skin test in a child or recently immunized adult. Since skin test reactions from BCG wane over time, strongly positive reactions or significant increases in reactivity should be considered indicative of TB infection. In the USA, targeted testing, standard interpretation of tuberculin skin tests, and treatment for latent TB infection are recommended regardless of prior history of BCG vaccination.

10) BCG immunization of uninfected (tuberculin-negative) people induces tuberculin reactivity in approximately half of vaccinees. Tuberculin reactivity and protection vary markedly in different field trials, and are perhaps related to immunological characteristics of population, quality of vaccine, or BCG strain. Some controlled trials indicate that protection may persist for as long as 20 years in high-incidence situations; others have shown no protection at all. Meta-analyses on BCG effectiveness provide conflicting results. Ongoing efforts to develop a vaccine more effective than BCG have identified candidate vaccines that are currently undergoing testing in humans for safety and immunogenicity.

Case-control and contact studies consistently show protection against TB meningitis and disseminated disease in children under 5. Because the risk of infection is low in many industrialized countries, BCG may not be used routinely; it may be considered for children with a negative

PPD skin test who cannot be placed on preventive therapy but have continuous exposure to people with untreated or ineffectively treated active disease, or are continuously and irremovably exposed to patients infected by organisms resistant to isoniazid and rifampicin. BCG is contraindicated for people with immunodeficiency diseases including symptomatic HIV infection; WHO recommends BCG for routine immunization programs in developing countries, including asymptomatic HIV-infected children and those at high risk of acquiring HIV infection.

11) Eliminate bovine tuberculosis among dairy cattle through tuberculin testing and slaughtering of reactors; pasteurize or boil milk.

12) Take measures to prevent silicosis among those working in industrial plants and mines.

B. Control of patient, contacts and the immediate environment:

1) Report to local health authority when diagnosis is suspected: Obligatory case report in most countries, Class 2 (see Reporting). Case report must state if the case is bacteriologically positive or based on clinical and/or X-ray findings. Health departments must maintain a register of cases requiring treatment and be actively involved with planning and monitoring the course of treatment.

2) Isolation: For pulmonary tuberculosis, control of infectivity is best achieved through prompt specific drug treatment, usually leading to sputum conversion within 4–8 weeks. Hospitalization is necessary only for patients with severe illness requiring hospital-level care and for those whose medical or social circumstances make home-treatment impossible. If practicable and possible, consider placing adult patients who reside in a congregate setting with sputum-positive pulmonary tuberculosis in a private room with negative pressure ventilation. Patients should be taught to cover both mouth and nose when coughing or sneezing. Persons entering the room should preferably wear personal respiratory protective devices capable of filtering submicron particles. Patients whose sputum is bacteriologically negative, who do not cough and who are known to be on adequate chemotherapy (known or probable drug susceptibility and clear clinical response to treatment) do not require isolation, nor do children with active TB disease with negative sputum smears and no cough—they are not contagious. Adolescents should be managed as adults. The need to adhere to the prescribed chemotherapeutic regimen must be emphasized repeatedly to all patients. Proper patient support ensuring that drugs are

taken as prescribed, including DOTS (the internationally recommended strategy for TB control), is essential, especially for persons with suspected drug resistance, a previous history of poor compliance to treatment, or who live in conditions where relapse would result in exposure of many other persons.

3) Concurrent disinfection: Handwashing and good housekeeping practices must be maintained according to policy. No special precautions necessary for handling fomites. Decontamination of air may be achieved by ventilation; this may be supplemented by ultraviolet light.

4) Quarantine: Not applicable.

5) Management of contacts: In countries where BCG vaccination is not routinely undertaken, preventive chemotherapy (also referred to as chemoprophylaxis or treatment of latent TB infection—TLTBI) is usually recommended for persons who are or have been in contact with TB infection and in whom TB disease has been ruled out. Treatment is also recommended for highest-risk persons—HIV-infected and those younger than 5 years old—even though a skin test is negative, once TB disease has been ruled out. Persons with an initial negative skin test are also offered a repeat skin test about 3 months after the contact has been "broken" (which may mean the day the source case starts treatment). Small children with negative skin tests at 3 months can be taken off TLTBI at that time. HIV-infected contacts usually are advised to complete a course of TLTBI whatever the 3-month skin test result. BCG immunization of tuberculin-negative household contacts may be warranted under special circumstances (see above).

6) In the USA and many other countries, investigation of contacts and source of infection: PPD testing of all members of the household and other close contacts is recommended. If negative, a repeat skin test should be performed 2–3 months after exposure has ended. Chest X-rays should be obtained for positive reactors (at least 5 mm induration) when identified. TLTBI is indicated (see 9A6) for contacts who are positive reactors and for some initially negative reactors at high risk of developing active disease, especially young (5 or younger) and HIV-infected close contacts, at least until the repeat skin test is shown to remain negative. In many developing countries, investigation of household contacts is limited to sputum microscopy of those contacts who have symptoms suggestive of TB disease.

7) Specific treatment: Adequate patient support ensuring that drugs are taken as prescribed, including directly observed treatment, is highly effective in achieving cure and is recommended for treatment of TB disease worldwide. Patients with

TB disease must be given prompt treatment with an appropriate combination of antimicrobial drugs and sputum smears must be monitored at regular intervals. For most cases of drug-susceptible disease, a 6-month regimen is recommended, including isoniazid (INH), rifampicin (RIF), pyrazinamide (PZA) and ethambutol (EMB) for the first 2 months, followed by INH and RIF for 4 months. After drug susceptibility results become available, a specific drug regimen can be selected if drug resistant strains are present (e.g. to isoniazid and rifampicin).

As regards HIV-associated TB, interactions between drugs must be borne in mind. Rifampicin lowers serum levels of many protease inhibitors and some nucleoside reverse transcriptase inhibitors and its replacement by rifabutin can be considered when antiretrovirals are started simultaneously with anti-TB drugs, although with some loss of effectiveness for the latter. Patients on rifampicin with advanced immunosuppression must receive TB treatment at least thrice weekly or even daily. Co-trimoxazole prophylaxis against opportunistic infections may reduce mortality and mortality in HIV-infected TB patients; post-treatment isoniazid prophylaxis can decrease the risk of TB recurrence but does not affect overall survival.

If sputum fails to become negative after 2 months of regular treatment or reverts to positive after a series of negative results, or if clinical response is poor, examination for drug compliance and for bacterial drug resistance is indicated. Treatment failure (sputum smear positivity at 5 months from start of treatment) can be due to irregular drug-taking or to the presence of drug-resistant bacilli. A change in supervision practices may be required if a favorable clinical response is not observed. If drug susceptibility testing is available, at least 2 drugs to which the organisms are susceptible should be included in the regimen; a single new drug should never be added to a failing regimen. If INH or RIF cannot be included, treatment should continue for at least 18 months after cultures have become negative.

For newly diagnosed smear-positive patients in developing countries, WHO recommends that treatment include 2 months of daily doses of INH, RIF, PZA and EMB, followed by 4 months of daily or intermittent INH and RIF. All treatment should be supervised or directly observed; if treatment cannot be directly observed in the subsequent phase, 6 months of INH and EMB may be substituted.

Children receive the same regimens as adults with some modifications; susceptibility of the causal organism can often be inferred from testing isolates of the adult source case.

Children with pulmonary or extrapulmonary TB can be treated with INH, RIF, PZA for 2 months followed by INH and RIF for 4 months. EMB generally is not used until the child is old enough for color vision to be checked (usually 5 years or older), although it is usually added to the regimen of children with severe disease. Children with meningitis, miliary disease, bone/joint disease or HIV infection should be treated for 9 to 12 months.

All drugs occasionally cause adverse reactions. Thoracic surgery is rarely indicated, usually in multidrug resistant cases. For details of case management (including MDR- and HIV-associated TB) see *Treatment of tuberculosis: Guidelines for national programmes* (WHO/CDS/TB/2003.313 http://whqlibdoc.who.int/hq/2003/WHO_CDS_TB_2003.313.pdf)

Monitoring of treatment response calls for symptom evaluation and sputum smear microscopy and culture monthly, or at least after 1, 2, 5 and 6 months, as in most developing countries where only smear microscopy is readily available. Radiological abnormalities may persist for months after a bacteriological response, often with permanent scarring, and monitoring by serial chest radiographs is thus not recommended. An end-of-treatment chest X-ray in patients with pulmonary or pleural TB may help show new baseline anatomy.

WHO strongly recommends that cohort analysis of treatment outcomes include all patients registered for treatment. The 6 mutually exclusive categories of treatment results are: bacteriologically proven cure; treatment completion (without bacteriological evidence of cure); failure (smear positive at month 5); default; death; and transfer to other administrative units. Cohort analysis allows proper evaluation of treatment program performance and prompts corrective measures in case of unacceptable levels of treatment failures, deaths, and defaulting.

C. *Epidemic measures:* Recognition and treatment of aggregates of new infections and secondary cases of disease resulting from contact with an unrecognized infectious case; intensive search for and treatment of the source of infection.

D. *Disaster implications:* None.

E. *International measures:* In industrialized countries, a high proportion of new disease cases arises among foreign-born persons, especially those from high prevalence areas. In the USA the annual proportion of new cases born abroad has been growing steadily and exceeded 50% for the first time in 2002. Surveillance allows the identification of those at excess risk and, among that population, screening allows individuals to benefit from curative and preventive interventions. These include: i) adequate notification systems (physician and laboratory reports) to identify populations at risk; ii) chest radiograph, PPD, smears and culture with curative/preventive interventions for symptomatic persons among the entering foreign-born population; iii) provision of comprehensive curative and preventive services against tuberculosis; iv) provision of culturally and socially sensitive services and follow-up of interventions; v) ongoing evaluation of interventions (efficiency/efficacy).

Further information on http://www.who.int/gtb/ and http://www.stoptb.org

DISEASES DUE TO OTHER MYCOBACTERIA ICD-9 031; ICD-10 A31
(Mycobacterioses, Nontuberculous mycobacterial disease)

Mycobacteria other than *M. tuberculosis*, *M. africanum*, *M. bovis* and *M. leprae* are ubiquitous and may produce disease in humans. These acid-fast bacilli have in the past been variously termed atypical, unclassified mycobacteria, nontuberculous mycobacteria (NTM), or mycobacteria other than tuberculosis (MOTT). Of the identified species only about 15 are recognized as pathogenic to people.

Clinical syndromes associated with the pathogenic species of mycobacteria can be classified broadly as follows:

1) Disseminated disease—(in the presence of severe immunodeficiency as in AIDS)–*M. avium* complex, *M. kansasii*, *M. haemophilum*, *M. chelonae*;

2) Pulmonary disease resembling tuberculosis—*M. kansasii*, *M. avium* complex, *M. absessus*, *M. xenopi*, *M. simiae*;

3) Lymphadenitis (primarily cervical)—*M. avium* complex, *M. scrofulaceum*, *M. kansasii*;

4) Skin ulcers—*M. ulcerans* (see Buruli ulcer), *M. marinum*;

5) Post-traumatic wound infections—*M. fortuitum*, *M. chelonae*, *M. absessus*, *M. marinum*, *M. avium* complex;

6) Nosocomial disease: surgical wound infections (following cardiac surgery, mammoplasty wounds), catheter-related infections (bacteraemia, peritonitis, post-injection abscesses)—*M. fortuitum*, *M. chelonae*, *M. absessus*;

7) Crohn disease—*M. paratuberculosis* has been suggested as the causative agent in some cases of regional enteritis; incorrect diagnosis of inflammatory bowel disease may delay diagnosis and treatment of TB disease of the bowel, and worsening of disease if immunosuppressive drugs are used inadvertently.

The epidemiology of the diseases attributable to these organisms has not been well delineated, but the organisms have been found in soil, milk and water; other factors, such as host tissue damage and immunodeficiency, may predispose to infection. With the exception of organisms causing skin lesions, there is no evidence of person-to-person transmission. A single isolation from sputum or gastric washings can occur in the absence of signs or symptoms of clinical disease. Multiple isolations of MOTT from respiratory specimens, in the absence of illness or other specific pathology, may be evidence of commensal colonization, with no clinical significance. A single positive culture from a wound or tissue is generally considered diagnostic.

In general, the diagnosis of disease requiring treatment is based on repeated isolations of many colonies from symptomatic patients with progressive illness. Where human infections with nontuberculous mycobacteria are prevalent, cross-reactions may interfere with the interpretation of skin tests for *M. tuberculosis* infection. Chemotherapy is relatively effective against *M. kansasii* and *M. marinum* disease, but traditional antituberculosis drugs (especially PZA) may not be effective for other mycobacterioses. Some cases of failure of TB treatment, in settings with limited facilities for culture and sensitivity testing, may in fact be cases of disease with MOTT, which commonly are resistant to standard TB drugs. Drug susceptibility tests on the isolated organism will help select an efficient drug combination. Surgery should be given more consideration than in TB disease, especially when the disease is limited, as in localized pulmonary disease, cervical lymphadenitis or subcutaneous abscess.

Disseminated *Mycobacterium avium* complex (MAC) infection is a major problem in HIV-infected persons; until recently it was considered poorly amenable to treatment. Drug regimens containing rifabutin and clarithromycin have shown therapeutic potential. Rifabutin has been approved for MAC prophylaxis in HIV-infected patients with CD4+ counts below 100.

Further information on http://www.who.int/tdr/disease/tb/default.htm
[M. Raviglione]

TULAREMIA   ICD-9 021; ICD-10 A21
(Rabbit fever, Deer-fly fever, Ohara disease, Francis disease)

1. Identification—A zoonotic bacterial disease with diverse clinical manifestations related to route of introduction and virulence of the disease agent. The onset of disease is typically sudden and influenza-like, with high fever, chills, fatigue, general body aches, headache, and nausea. Most often it presents as an indolent skin ulcer at the site of introduction of the organism, together with swelling of the regional lymph nodes (ulceroglandular type). There may be no apparent primary ulcer, but one or more enlarged and painful lymph nodes that may suppurate (glandular type). Ingestion of organisms in contaminated food or water may produce a painful pharyngitis (with or without ulceration), abdominal pain, diarrhea and vomiting (oropharyngeal type). Inhalation of infectious material may be followed by respiratory involvement or a primary septicemic syndrome; bloodborne organisms may localize in the lung and pleural spaces. The conjunctival sac is a rare route of introduction that results in a clinical disease of painful purulent conjunctivitis with regional lymphadenitis (oculoglandular type). Pneumonia may complicate all clinical types and requires prompt identification and specific treatment to prevent development of serious symptoms.

Two subspecies with differing pathogenicity cause human disease. Isolates of *Francisella tularensis* subsp. *tularensis* (Jellison type A) are highly virulent, with a case-fatality rate of 5%–15% primarily due to untreated respiratory forms. With appropriate antibiotherapy, the case-fatality rate is low. Isolates of *F. tularensis* subsp. *holarctica* (Jellison type B) are less virulent and, even without treatment, produce few fatalities. Clinically, because of buboes and/or severe pneumonia, tularaemia may be confused with plague, as well as other infectious diseases including staphylococcal and streptococcal infections, cat-scratch fever and tuberculosis.

Diagnosis is most commonly clinical and confirmed by a titer rise in specific serum antibodies that usually appear during the second week of the disease. Using tube-agglutination, cross-reactions occur with *Brucella* species whereas ELISA-based serological testing for reactivity to *F. tularensis* is highly specific. Examination of ulcer exudate, lymph node aspirates and other clinical specimens by FA test or identification of bacterial DNA by polymerase chain reaction may provide rapid diagnosis. Diagnostic biopsy of acutely infected lymph nodes should be done only under the cover of specific antibiotherapy since it will often induce bacteraemia. The causative bacteria can be cultured on special media such as cysteine-glucose blood agar supplemented with iron or through inoculation of laboratory animals with material from lesions, blood or sputum. The subspecies are differentiated by their chemical reactions: type A organisms ferment glycerol and convert citrulline to ornithine. Extreme care must be exercised to avoid laboratory transmission of highly infectious aerosolized organisms; culture identification is performed only in reference laboratories and most cases are diagnosed serologically.

2. Infectious agent—*Francisella tularensis* (formerly *Pasteurella tularensis*), a small, Gram-negative nonmotile coccobacillus. All isolates are serologically homogeneous but are differentiated epidemiologically and biochemically into *F. tularensis* subsp. *tularensis* (Jellison type A), with an LD_{50} in rabbits of fewer than 10 bacteria, or *F. tularensis* subsp. *holarctica* (Jellison type B) with an LD_{50} greater than 10^6 bacteria in rabbits.

3. Occurrence—Tularaemia occurs throughout North America and in many parts of continental Europe, the former Soviet Union, China and Japan. In North America, most cases occur from May through August but cases are reported throughout the year. *F. tularensis* subsp. *tularensis* organisms, restricted to North America, are common in rabbits and are frequently transmitted by tick bite. *F. tularensis* subsp. *holarctica* strains commonly occur in mammals other than rabbits in North America; strains are found in voles, muskrats and water rats in Eurasia, and in rabbits in Japan.

4. Reservoir—Wild animals, especially rabbits, hares, voles, muskrats, beavers and some domestic animals; also various hard ticks. A rodent-mosquito cycle has been described for *F. tularensis* subsp. *holarctica* in the Baltic and Scandinavian countries and the Russian Federation.

5. Mode of transmission—Arthropod bites, including the wood tick *Dermacentor andersoni*, the dog tick *D. variabilis*, the lone star tick *Amblyomma americanum*, less commonly the deer fly *Chrysops discalis* and, in the Russian Federation and Sweden, various mosquito species; through inoculation of skin, conjunctival sac or oropharyngeal mucosa with contaminated water, blood or tissue while handling infected carcasses (e.g. skinning, dressing or performing necropsies); by handling or ingesting insufficiently cooked meat of infected animals; by drinking contaminated water; by inhalation of dust from contaminated soil, grain or hay; and from contaminated animal pelts and paws. Laboratory infections frequently present as respiratory tularaemia.

6. Incubation period—Related to size of inoculum; usually 3–5 days (range 1–14 days).

7. Period of communicability—No direct person-to-person transmission. The infectious agent may be found in the blood of untreated patients during the first 2 weeks of disease and in lesions for a month or more. Flies can be infective for 14 days and ticks throughout their lifetime (about 2 years). Rabbit meat frozen at -15°C (5°F) has remained infective for over 3 years.

8. Susceptibility—All ages are susceptible, and long-term immunity follows recovery; reinfection is extremely rare and has been reported only in laboratory staff.

9. Methods of control—

A. *Preventive measures:*

1) Educate the public to avoid bites of ticks, flies and mosquitoes and to avoid contact with untreated water where infection prevails among wild animals.
2) Use impervious gloves when skinning or handling animals, especially rabbits. Cook the meat of wild rabbits and rodents thoroughly. Avoid handling such meat together with vegetables.
3) Prohibit interzonal shipment of infected animals or their carcases.

4) Live attenuated vaccines applied intradermally by scarification are used extensively in the former Soviet Union, and to a limited extent for occupational risk groups in some industrialized countries.

5) Wear facemasks, gowns and impervious gloves and use negative pressure microbiological cabinets when working with cultures of *F. tularensis*.

B. **Control of patient, contacts and the immediate environment:**

1) Report to local health authority: In selected endemic areas; in many countries not a reportable disease, Class 3 (see Reporting).

2) Isolation: Drainage and secretion precautions for open lesions.

3) Concurrent disinfection: Of discharges from ulcers, lymph nodes or conjunctival sacs.

4) Quarantine: Not applicable.

5) Immunization of contacts: Not indicated.

6) Investigation of contacts and source of infection: Important in each case, with search for the origin of infection.

7) Specific treatment: Aminoglycosides (gentamicin or streptomycin) are the drugs of choice. Recent experience of treatment with ciprofloxacin has shown excellent efficacy. Tetracyclines, also effective, are associated with higher relapse rates. Many antibiotics including all beta-lactam antibiotics and modern cephalosporines are ineffective for treatment and many isolates show resistance to macrolides. Treatment with aminoglycosides or ciprofloxacin should last 10–14 days, with tetracyclines 21 days.

C. **Epidemic measures:** Search for sources of infection related to arthropods, animal hosts, water, soil and crops. Control measures as indicated in 9A.

D. **Disaster implications:** None.

E. **International measures:** None.

F. **Measures in the case of deliberate use:** Tularemia is considered to be a potential agent for deliberate use, particularly if used as an aerosol threat. As is true of plague, cases acquired by inhalation present as primary pneumonia. Such cases require prompt identification and specific treatment to prevent a fatal outcome. All diagnosed cases and especially clusters of pneumonia due to *F. tularensis* must be reported immediately to the local security and health department for appropriate investigation.

[A. Sjöstedt]

TYPHOID FEVER   ICD-9 002.0; ICD-10 A01.0
(Enteric fever, Typhus abdominalis)

PARATYPHOID
FEVER   ICD-9 002.1-002.9; ICD-10 A01.1-A01.4

1. **Identification**—A systemic bacterial disease with insidious onset of sustained fever, marked headache, malaise, anorexia, relative bradycardia, splenomegaly, nonproductive cough in the early stage of the illness, rose spots on the trunk in 25% of white-skinned patients and constipation more often than diarrhea in adults. The clinical picture varies from mild illness with low-grade fever to severe clinical disease with abdominal discomfort and multiple complications. Factors such as strain virulence, quantity of inoculum ingested, duration of illness before adequate treatment, age and previous exposure to vaccination influence severity.

Inapparent or mild illnesses occur, especially in endemic areas; 60%-90% of patients with typhoid fever do not receive medical attention or are treated as outpatients. Mild cases show no systemic involvement; the clinical picture is that of a gastroenteritis (see Salmonellosis). Nonsweating fevers, mental dullness, slight deafness and parotitis may occur. Peyer patches in the ileum can ulcerate, with intestinal hemorrhage or perforation (about 1% of cases), especially late in untreated cases. Severe forms with altered mental status have been associated with high case-fatality rates. The case-fatality rate of 10%-20% observed in the pre-antibiotic era can fall below 1% with prompt antibiotherapy. Depending on the antimicrobials used, 15%-20% of patients may experience relapses (generally milder than the initial clinical illness).

Paratyphoid fever caused by *Salmonella enterica* subsp. *enterica serovar* Paratyphi var. A and B (commonly *S.* Paratyphi A and B) presents a similar clinical picture, but tends to be milder, and the case-fatality rate is much lower. The ratio of disease caused by *Salmonella enterica* subsp. *enterica serovar* Typhi (commonly *S.* Typhi, the latter not italicized) to that caused by *S.* Paratyphi A and B is about 10:1. Relapses occur in approximately 3%-4% of cases.

The causal organisms can be isolated from blood early in the disease and from urine and feces after the first week. Blood culture is the diagnostic mainstay for typhoid fever, but bone marrow culture provides the best bacteriological confirmation even in patients who have already received antimicrobials. Because of limited sensitivity and specificity, serological tests based on agglutinating antibodies (Widal) are generally of little diagnostic value. New rapid diagnostic tests based upon the detection of specific antibodies appear very promising; they must be evaluated further with regard to sensitivity and specificity.

2. Infectious agents—In the recently proposed nomenclature for *Salmonella* the agent formerly known as *S. typhi* is called *S. enterica* subsp. *enterica* serovar Typhi (commonly *S.* Typhi). For paratyphoid fever, mainly *S.* Paratyphi A and Paratyphi B.

3. Occurrence—Worldwide; the annual estimated incidence of typhoid fever is about 17 million cases with approximately 600 000 deaths. Most of the burden of the disease occurs in the developing world. Fewer than 500 sporadic cases occur annually in the USA and the burden is similar in other industrialized countries; currently most cases in the industrialized world are imported from endemic areas. Strains resistant to chloramphenicol and other recommended antimicrobials have become prevalent in several areas of the world. Most isolates from southern and southeastern Asia, the Middle East and northeastern Africa in the 1990s carry an R factor plasmid encoding resistance to those multiple antimicrobial agents that were previously the mainstay of oral treatment including chloramphenicol, amoxicillin and trimethoprim/sulfamethoxazole.

Paratyphoid fever occurs sporadically or in limited outbreaks, probably more frequently than reports suggest. Of the 3 serotypes, paratyphoid B is most common, A less frequent and C caused by *S.* Paratyphi C) extremely rare. In China and Pakistan more cases have been reported as caused by *S.* Paratyphi than by *S.* Typhi.

4. Reservoir—Humans for both typhoid and paratyphoid; rarely, domestic animals for paratyphoid. Family contacts may be transient or permanent carriers. A carrier state may follow acute illness or mild or even subclinical infections. In most parts of the world, short-term fecal carriers are more common than urinary carriers. The chronic carrier state is most common (2%–5%) among persons infected during middle age, especially women; carriers frequently have biliary tract abnormalities including gallstones, with *S.* Typhi located in the gallbladder. The chronic urinary carrier state may occur with schistosome infections. In one outbreak of paratyphoid fever in England, dairy cows excreted *S.* Paratyphi B organisms in milk and feces.

5. Mode of transmission—Ingestion of food and water contaminated by feces and urine of patients and carriers. Important vehicles in some countries include shellfish (particularly oysters) from sewage-contaminated beds, raw fruit, vegetables fertilized by night soil and eaten raw, contaminated milk/milk products (usually through hands of carriers) and missed cases. Flies may infect foods in which the organism then multiplies to infective doses (those are lower for typhoid than for paratyphoid bacteria). Epidemiological data suggest that, while waterborne transmission of *S.* Typhi usually involves small inocula, foodborne transmission is associated with large inocula and high attack rates over short periods.

6. Incubation period—Depends on inoculum size and on host factors; from 3 days to over 60 days—usual range 8-14 days; the incubation period for paratyphoid is 1-10 days.

7. Period of communicability—As long as bacilli appear in excreta, usually from the first week throughout convalescence; variable thereafter (commonly 1-2 weeks for paratyphoid). About 10% of untreated typhoid fever patients discharge bacilli for 3 months after onset of symptoms; 2%-5% become permanent carriers. Fewer persons infected with paratyphoid organisms may become permanent gallbladder carriers.

8. Susceptibility—Susceptibility is general and is increased in individuals with gastric achlorhydria and possibly in those who are HIV-positive. Relative specific immunity follows recovery from clinical disease, inapparent infection and active immunization. In endemic areas, typhoid fever is most common in preschool children and children 5-19.

9. Methods of control—

    A. Preventive measures: Prevention is based on access to safe water and proper sanitation as well as adhesion to safe food-handling practices.

        1) Educate the public regarding the importance of handwashing. Provide suitable handwashing facilities, particularly for food handlers and attendants involved in the care of patients and children.

        2) Dispose of human feces safely and maintain fly-proof latrines. Where culturally appropriate encourage use of sufficient toilet paper to minimize finger contamination. Under field conditions, dispose of feces by burial at a site distant and downstream from the source of drinking-water.

        3) Protect, purify and chlorinate public water supplies, provide safe private supplies, and avoid possible backflow connections between water and sewer systems. For individual and small group protection, and during travel or in the field, treat water chemically or by boiling.

        4) Control flies by screening and use of insecticidal baits and traps or, where appropriate, spraying with insecticides. Control fly-breeding through frequent garbage collection and disposal and through fly control measures in latrine construction and maintenance.

        5) Use scrupulous cleanliness in food preparation and handling; refrigerate as appropriate. Pay particular attention to the storage of salads and other foods served cold. These provisions apply to home and public eating places. If uncertain about sanitary practices, select foods that are cooked and served hot, and fruit peeled by the consumer.

6) Pasteurize or boil all milk and dairy products. Supervise the sanitary aspects of commercial milk production, storage and delivery.

7) Enforce suitable quality-control procedures in industries that prepare food and drink for human consumption. Use chlorinated water for cooling during canned food processing.

8) Limit the collection and marketing of shellfish to supplies from approved sources. Boil or steam (for at least 10 minutes) before serving.

9) Instruct the community, patients, convalescents and carriers in personal hygiene. Emphasize handwashing as a routine practice after defecation and before preparing, serving or eating food.

10) Encourage breast-feeding throughout infancy; boil all milk and water used for infant feeding.

11) Typhoid carriers should be excluded from handling food and from providing patient care. Identify and supervise typhoid carriers; culture of sewage may help in locating them. Chronic carriers should not be released from supervision and restriction of occupation until local or state regulations are met, often not until 3 consecutive negative cultures are obtained from authenticated fecal specimens (and urine in areas endemic for schistosomiasis) at least 1 month apart and at least 48 hours after antimicrobial therapy has stopped. Fresh stool specimens are preferred to rectal swabs; at least 1 of the 3 consecutive negative stool specimens should be obtained by purging.

Administration of 750 mg of ciprofloxacine or 400 mg of norfloxacine twice daily for 28 days provides successful treatment of carriers in 80% of cases. Follow-up cultures are necessary to confirm cure.

12) Immunization for typhoid fever is not routinely recommended in non-endemic areas except for those subject to unusual occupational exposure to enteric infections (e.g. clinical microbiology technicians) and household members of known carriers. WHO recommends vaccination for people travelling to endemic high risk areas and school-age children living in endemic areas where typhoid fever control is a priority. Vaccination of high-risk populations is considered the most promising strategy for the control of typhoid fever.

An oral, live vaccine using *S.* Typhi strain Ty21a (requiring 3 or 4 doses, 2 days apart) and a parenteral vaccine containing the single dose polysaccharide Vi antigen are available, as protective as the whole cell bacteria vaccine and much less reactogenic; use of the old inactivated whole cell vaccine is strongly discouraged. However, Ty21a should not be used in patients receiving antibiotics or the antimalarial mefloquine. Booster doses every 2 to 5 years according to vaccine type are desirable for those at continuing risk of infection.

In field trials, oral Ty21a conferred partial protection against paratyphoid B but not as well as it protected against typhoid.

B. Control of patient, contacts and the immediate environment:

1) Report to local health authority: Obligatory case report in most countries, Class 2 (see Reporting).
2) Isolation: Enteric precautions while ill; hospital care is desirable during acute illness. Release from supervision by local health authority based on not fewer than 3 consecutive negative cultures of feces (and urine in patients with schistosomiasis) at least 24 hours apart and at least 48 hours after any antimicrobials, and not earlier than 1 month after onset. If any of these is positive, repeat cultures at monthly intervals during the 12 months following onset until at least 3 consecutive negative cultures are obtained.
3) Concurrent disinfection: Of feces, urine and articles soiled therewith. In communities with adequate sewage disposal systems, feces and urine can be disposed of directly into sewers without preliminary disinfection. Terminal cleaning.
4) Quarantine: Not applicable.
5) Immunization of contacts: Routine administration of typhoid vaccine is of limited value for family, household and nursing contacts who have been or may be exposed to active cases; it should be considered for those who may be exposed to carriers. No effective immunization for paratyphoid fever.
6) Investigation of contacts and source of infection: Determine actual or probable source of infection of every case through search for unreported cases, carriers or contaminated food, water, milk or shellfish. All members of travel groups in which a case has been identified should be followed.

The presence of elevated antibody titres to purified Vi polysaccharide is highly suggestive of the typhoid carrier state. Identification of the same phage type or molecular subtype in the carrier and in organisms isolated from patients suggests a possible chain of transmission.

Household and close contacts should not be employed in sensitive occupations (e.g. food handlers) until at least 2 negative feces and urine cultures, taken at least 24 hours apart, have been obtained.
7) Specific treatment: Evidence suggests that fluoroquinolones are the drug of choice in adults. However, recent emergence of resistance to fluoroquinolones restricts widespread and indiscriminate use in primary care facilities. If local strains are

known to be sensitive to traditional first-line antibiotics, oral chloramphenicol, amoxicillin or trimethoprim-sufoxazole (particularly in children) should be used according in accordance with local antimicrobial sensitivity patterns. Ceftriaxone, a parenteral once-daily antibiotic, is useful in patients with dulled perceptions or those with complications such that oral antibiotics cannot be used. Short-term, high dose corticosteroid treatment, combined with specific antibiotics and supportive care, reduces mortality in critically ill patients. (See 9A11 for treatment of carrier state.) Patients with concurrent schistosomiasis must also be treated with praziquantel to eliminate possible schistosome carriage of S. Typhi. Patients with confirmed intestinal perforation need intensive care as well as surgical intervention. Early intervention is crucial as morbidity rates increase with delayed surgery after perforation.

C. Epidemic measures:

1) Search intensively for the case/carrier who is the source of infection and for the vehicle (water or food) through which infection was transmitted.
2) Selectively eliminate suspected contaminated food. Pasteurize or boil milk, or exclude milk supplies and other foods suspected on epidemiological evidence, until safety is ensured.
3) Chlorinate suspected water supplies adequately under competent supervision or avoid use. All drinking-water must be chlorinated, treated with iodine or boiled before use.
4) Use of vaccine should be considered before or during an outbreak; a protective efficacy of 72% was recently obtained in an immunized community during an outbreak in Tajikistan.

D. Disaster implications:
With disruption of usual water supply and sewage disposal, and of controls on food and water, transmission of typhoid fever may occur if there are active cases or carriers in a displaced population. Efforts are advised to restore safe drinking-water supplies and excreta disposal facilities. Selective immunization of stabilized groups such as school children, prisoners and utility, municipal or hospital personnel may be helpful.

E. International measures:

1) For typhoid fever: Immunization is advised for international travellers to endemic areas, especially if travel is likely to involve exposure to unsafe food and water, or close contact

in rural areas to indigenous populations. Immunization is not a legal requirement for entry into any country.

2) WHO Collaborating Centres.

[C. Chaignat]

TYPHUS FEVER   ICD-10 A75

I. EPIDEMIC LOUSE-BORNE
   TYPHUS FEVER   ICD-9 080; ICD-10 A75
(Louse-borne typhus, Typhus exanthematicus, Classic typhus fever)

1. Identification—A rickettsial disease with variable onset; often sudden and marked by headache, chills, prostration, fever and general pains. A macular eruption appears on the 5th to 6th day, initially on the upper trunk, followed by spread to the entire body, but usually not to the face, palms or soles. The eruption is often difficult to observe on black skin. Toxaemia is usually pronounced, and the disease terminates by rapid defervescence after about 2 weeks of fever. The case-fatality rate increases with age and varies from 10% to 40% in the absence of specific treatment. Mild infections may occur without eruption, especially in children and people partially protected by prior immunization. The disease may recrudesce years after the primary attack (Brill-Zinsser disease, ICD-9 081.1; ICD-10 A75.1); this form of disease is milder, has fewer complications, and has a lower case-fatality rate.

The IF test is most commonly used for laboratory confirmation, but it does not discriminate between louse-borne and murine typhus (ICD-9 081.0; ICD-10 A75.2) unless the sera are differentially absorbed with the respective rickettsial antigen prior to testing. Blood can be collected on filter paper that are forwarded to a reference laboratory. Other diagnostic methods are EIA, PCR, immunohistochemical staining of tissues, CF with group specific or washed type-specific rickettsial antigens, and the toxin-neutralization test. Sending lice to a reference laboratory for PCR testing may help detect an outbreak. Antibody tests usually become positive in the second week.

2. Infectious agent—*Rickettsia prowazekii*.

3. Occurrence—In colder areas where people may live under unhygienic conditions and are infested with lice; explosive epidemics may occur during war and famine. Endemic foci exist in the mountainous regions of Mexico, in Central and South America, in central and eastern Africa and numerous countries of Asia. Recent outbreaks have been observed in Burundi and Rwanda. This rickettsia exists as a zoonosis of flying squirrels (*Glaucomys volans*) in the USA and there is serological evidence that humans have been infected from this source, possibly via the squirrel flea.

4. Reservoir—Humans are the reservoir and are responsible for maintaining the infection during interepidemic periods. Although not a major source of human disease, sporadic cases may be associated with flying squirrels.

5. Mode of transmission—The body louse, *Pediculus humanus corporis*, is infected by feeding on the blood of a patient with acute typhus fever. Patients with Brill-Zinsser disease can infect lice and may serve as foci for new outbreaks in louse-infested communities. Infected lice excrete rickettsiae in their feces and usually defecate at the time of feeding. People are infected by rubbing feces or crushed lice into the bite or into superficial abrasions. Inhalation of infective louse feces in dust may account for some infections. Transmission from the flying squirrel is presumed to be through the bite of the squirrel flea, but this has not been documented.

6. Incubation period—From 1 to 2 weeks, commonly 12 days.

7. Period of communicability—The disease is not directly transmitted from person to person. Patients are infective for lice during the febrile illness and possibly for 2-3 days after the temperature returns to normal. Infected lice pass rickettsiae in their feces within 2-6 days after the blood-meal; they are infective earlier if crushed. The louse invariably dies within 2 weeks after infection; rickettsiae may remain viable in the dead louse for weeks.

8. Susceptibility—Susceptibility is general. One attack usually confers long-lasting immunity.

9. Methods of control—

   A. Preventive measures:

      1) Apply an effective residual insecticide powder at appropriate intervals by hand or power blower to clothes and persons of populations living under conditions favoring louse infestation. The insecticide used should be effective on local lice.
      2) Improve living conditions with provisions for bathing and washing clothes.
      3) Treat prophylactically those who are subject to risk, by application of residual insecticide to clothing (dusting or impregnation).

B. Control of patient, contacts and the immediate environment:

1) Report to local health authority: Report of louse-borne typhus fever required as a Disease under Surveillance by WHO, Class 1 (see Reporting).
2) Isolation: Not required after proper delousing of patient, clothing, living quarters and household contacts.
3) Concurrent disinfection: Appropriate insecticide powder applied to clothing and bedding of patient and contacts; launder clothing and bedclothes. Lice tend to leave abnormally hot or cold bodies in search of a normothermic clothed body. If death from louse-borne typhus occurs before delousing, delouse the body and clothing by thorough application of an insecticide.
4) Quarantine: Susceptible persons infested with lice and exposed to typhus fever should ordinarily be quarantined for 15 days if possible after application of an insecticide with residual effect.
5) Management of contacts: All immediate contacts should be kept under surveillance for 2 weeks.
6) Investigation of contacts and source of infection: Every effort should be made to trace the infection to the immediate source.
7) Specific treatment: A single dose of doxycycline 200 mg will normally cure patients. When faced with a seriously ill patient with possible typhus, suitable treatment should be started without waiting for laboratory confirmation.

C. Epidemic measures: The best measure for rapid control of typhus is application of an insecticide with residual effect to all contacts. Where louse infestation is known to be widespread, systematic application of residual insecticide to all people in the community is indicated. Treatment of cases in an epidemic may also decrease the spread of disease. In epidemics, individuals may protect themselves by wearing silk or plastic clothing tightly fastened around wrists, ankles and neck, and impregnating clothes with repellents or permethrin.

D. Disaster implications: Typhus can be expected to be a significant problem in louse-infested populations in endemic areas if social upheavals and crowding occur.

E. International measures:

1) Telegraphic notification by governments to WHO and to adjacent countries of the occurrence of a case or an outbreak of louse-borne typhus fever in an area previously free of the disease.

2) International travellers: No country currently requires immunization against typhus for entry.
3) Louse-borne typhus is a Disease under Surveillance by WHO. WHO Collaborating Centres.

F. Measures in case of deliberate use: *R. prowazekii* has been produced as a possible bioweapon and used before World War II. It is infectious by aerosol with a high case-fatality rate. The initial reference treatment of any suspected case is a single dose of 200 mg of doxycycline.

II. ENDEMIC FLEA-BORNE TYPHUS FEVER ICD-9 081.0; ICD-10 A75.2
(Murine typhus, Shop typhus)

1. Identification—A rickettsial disease whose course resembles that of louse-borne typhus, but is milder. The case-fatality rate for all ages is less than 1% but increases with age. Absence of louse infestation, geographic and seasonal distribution and sporadic occurrence of the disease help to differentiate it from louse-borne typhus. For laboratory diagnosis, see section I, 1.

2. Infectious agents—*Rickettsia typhi* (*Rickettsia mooseri*); *R. felis*.

3. Occurrence—Worldwide. Found in areas where people and rats occupy the same buildings. Multiple cases may occur in the same household.

4. Reservoir—Rats, mice and possibly other small mammals. Infection is maintained in nature by a rat-flea-rat cycle where rats are the reservoir (commonly *Rattus rattus* and *R. norvegicus*) but infection is inapparent. A closely related organism, *Rickettsia felis*, has been found to pass from cat to cat flea to opossum or other animals in North America, Europe and Africa. Both rickettsiae are transmitted transovarially.

5. Mode of transmission—Infective rat fleas (usually *Xenopsylla cheopis*) defecate rickettsiae while sucking blood, this contaminates the bite site and other fresh skin wounds. An occasional case may follow inhalation of dried infective flea feces.

6. Incubation period—From 1 to 2 weeks, commonly 12 days.

7. Period of communicability—Not directly transmitted from person to person. Once infected, fleas remain so for life (up to 1 year) and transfer it to their progeny.

8. Susceptibility—Susceptibility is general. One attack confers immunity.

9. Methods of control—

  A. *Preventive measures:*

  1) To avoid increased exposure of humans, wait until flea populations have first been reduced by insecticides before instituting rodent control measures (see Plague, 9A2-9A3, 9B6).
  2) Apply insecticide powders with residual action to rat runs, burrows and harbourages.

  B. *Control of patient, contacts and the immediate environment:*

  1) Report to local health authority: Case report obligatory in most countries, Class 2 (see Reporting).
  2) Isolation: Not applicable.
  3) Concurrent disinfection: Not applicable.
  4) Quarantine: Not applicable.
  5) Immmunization of contacts: Not applicable.
  6) Investigation of contacts and source of infection: Search for rodents or opossums (North America) around premises or home of patient.
  7) Specific treatment: As for Rocky Mountain Spotted Fever.

  C. *Epidemic measures:* In endemic areas with numerous cases, use of a residual insecticide effective against rat or cat fleas will reduce the flea index and the incidence of infection in humans.

  D. *Disaster implications:* Cases can be expected when people, rats and fleas are forced to coexist in close proximity, but murine typhus has not been a major contributor to disease rates in such situations.

  E. *International measures:* WHO Collaborating Centres.

III. SCRUB TYPHUS   ICD-9 081.2; ICD-10 A75.3
(Tsutsugamushi disease, Mite-borne typhus fever)

1. Identification—A rickettsial disease often characterized by a primary "punched out" skin ulcer (eschar) corresponding to the site of attachment of an infected mite. An acute febrile onset follows within several days, along with headache, profuse sweating, conjunctival injection and lymphadenopathy. Late in the first week of fever, a dull red maculopapular eruption appears on the trunk, extends to the extremities and disappears in a few days. Cough and X-ray evidence of pneumonitis are common. Without antibiotherapy, fever lasts for about 14 days. The case-fatality rate in untreated cases varies from 1% to 60%, according to area, strain of infectious agent and previous exposure to disease; it is consistently higher among older people.

Definitive diagnosis is made by isolation of the infectious agent by inoculating the patient's blood into mice. Serological diagnosis is complicated by antigenic differences of various strains of the causal rickettsia; the IF test is the preferred technique, but EIAs are also available. Many cases develop a positive Weil-Felix reaction with the Proteus OXK strain.

2. **Infectious agent**—*Orientia tsutsugamushi* with multiple serologically distinct strains.

3. **Occurrence**—Central, eastern and southeastern Asia; from southeastern Siberia and northern Japan to northern Australia and Vanuatu, as far West as Pakistan, to as high as 3000 meters (10 000 feet) above sea level in the Himalaya Mountains, and particularly prevalent in northern Thailand. Acquired by humans in one of innumerable small, sharply delimited "typhus islands," (some covering an area of only a few square feet), where infectious agent, vectors and suitable rodents exist simultaneously. Occupational infection is restricted mainly to adult workers (males more than females) who frequent overgrown terrain or other mite-infested areas, such as forest clearings, reforested areas, new settlements or even newly irrigated desert regions. Epidemics occur when susceptibles are brought into endemic areas, especially in military operations in which 20%–50% of troops have been infected within weeks or months.

4. **Reservoir**—Infected larval stages of trombiculid mites; *Leptotrombidium akamushi*, *L. deliensis* and related species (varying with area) are the most common vectors for humans. Infection is maintained by transovarian passage in mites.

5. **Mode of transmission**—Through the bite of infected larval mites; nymphs and adults do not feed on vertebrate hosts.

6. **Incubation period**—From 6 to 21 days , usually 10–12 days.

7. **Period of communicability**—No direct person-to-person transmission.

8. **Susceptibility**—Susceptibility is general. An attack confers prolonged immunity against the homologous strain of *O. tsutsugamushi* but only transient immunity against heterologous strains. Heterologous infection results in mild disease within a few months but produces typical illness after a year or so. Second and even third attacks of naturally acquired scrub typhus (usually benign or inapparent) occur among people who spend their lives in endemic areas or who have not been completely treated (see below). No experimental vaccine has been effective.

9. **Methods of control—**

   A. *Preventive measures:*

   1) Prevent contact with infected mites through personal pro-phylaxis against the mite vector, achieved by impregnating clothes and blankets with miticidal chemicals (permethrin and benzyl benzoate) and application of mite repellents (diethyltoluamide) to exposed skin surfaces.
   2) Eliminate mites from the specific sites through application of chlorinated hydrocarbons, such as lindane, dieldrin or chlor-dane, to ground and vegetation in environs of camps, mine buildings and other populated zones in endemic areas.
   3) In a small group of volunteers in Malaysia, the administration of 7 weekly doses of doxycycline (200 mg/week in a single dose) was an effective prophylactic regimen.

   B. *Control of patient, contacts and the immediate environment:*

   1) Report to local health authority: In selected endemic areas (clearly differentiated from murine and louse-borne typhus). In many countries, not a reportable disease, Class 3 (see Reporting).
   2) Isolation: Not applicable.
   3) Concurrent disinfection: Not applicable.
   4) Quarantine: Not applicable.
   5) Immmunization of contacts: Not applicable.
   6) Investigation of contacts and source of infection: None (see 9C).
   7) Specific treatment: One of the tetracyclines orally in a loading dose, followed by divided doses daily until patient is afebrile (average 30 hours). Chloramphenicol is equally effective and should be given if tetracyclines are contraindicated (see section I, 9B7). If treatment is started within the first 3 days of illness, recrudescence is likely unless another course of antibiotic is given after an interval of 6 days. In Malaysia single doses of doxycycline (5 mg/kg) were effective when given on the 7th day, and in the Pescadores Islands (China, province of Taiwan) when given on the 5th day; earlier administration was associated with some relapses. Azithro-mycin and rifampicin have also been used successfully in pregnant patients.

   C. *Epidemic measures:* Rigorously employ procedures described in this section, 9A1–9A2 above, in the affected area; daily observation of all people at risk for fever and appearance of primary lesions; institute treatment on first indication of illness.

D. Disaster implications: Only if refugee centers are sited in or near a "typhus island."

E. International measures: WHO Collaborating Centres.

[D. Raoult]

WARTS, VIRAL   ICD-9 078.1; ICD-10 B07
(Verruca vulgaris, Common wart, Condyloma acuminatum, Papilloma venereum)

1. Identification—A viral disease manifested by diverse skin and mucous membrane lesions. These include: the common wart, a circumscribed, hyperkeratotic, rough-textured, painless papule, varying in size from a pinhead to large masses; filiform warts, elongated, pointed, delicate lesions that may reach 1 cm in length; laryngeal papillomas on vocal cords and the epiglottis in children and adults; flat warts, smooth, slightly elevated, usually multiple lesions varying in size from 1 mm to 1 cm; venereal warts (condyloma acuminatum), cauliflower like fleshy growths, most often seen in moist areas in and around the genitalia, around the anus and within the anal canal, which must be differentiated from condyloma lata of secondary syphilis; flat papillomas of the cervix; and plantar warts, flat, hyperkeratotic and often painful lenous of lesions of the plantar surface of the feet.

Both laryngeal papillomas and genital warts have occasionally become malignant. The warts in epidermodysplasia verruciformis occur usually on the torso and upper extremities, usually appearing in the first decade of life; they often undergo malignant transformation to squamous cell carcinomas in young adulthood.

The diagnosis is usually based on the typical lesion. If there is doubt, the lesion should be excised and examined histologically.

2. Infectious agent—Human papillomavirus (HPV) of the papovavirus group of DNA viruses (the human wart viruses). At least 70 HPV types have been associated with specific manifestations and more than 20 types of HPV can infect the genital tract. Most genital HPV infections are asymptomatic, subclinical, or unrecognized. Visible genital warts are usually caused by HPV types 6 or 11: they can also cause warts on the uterine cervix and in the vagina, urethra, and anus, and are sometimes symptomatic. Other HPV types in the anogenital region, types 16, 18, 31, 33, and 35, have been strongly associated with cervical dysplasia; they have been associated also with vulvar, penile, and anal squamous intraepithelial neoplasia (i.e. squamous cell carcinoma in situ, bowenoid papulosis, erythroplasia of Queyrat, or Bowen disease of the genitalia). Type 7 is associated with warts in meat handlers and veterinarians. Types 5 and 8 are associated with epidermodysplasia verruciformis.

3. **Occurrence**—Worldwide.

4. **Reservoir**—Humans.

5. **Mode of transmission**—Usually through direct contact. Warts may be autoinoculated, such as by razors in shaving; contaminated floors are frequently incriminated as the source of infection. Condyloma acuminatum is usually sexually transmitted; laryngeal papillomata in children are probably transmitted during passage of the infant through the birth canal. The viral types in the genital and respiratory tracts are the same.

6. **Incubation period**—About 2-3 months; range is 1-20 months.

7. **Period of communicability**—Unknown, probably at least as long as visible lesions persist.

8. **Susceptibility**—Common and flat warts are most frequently seen in young children, genital warts in sexually active young adults, and plantar warts in school-age children and teenagers. The incidence of warts is increased in immunosuppressed patients.

9. **Methods of control**—

   A. *Preventive measures:* Avoid direct contact with lesions on another person.

   B. *Control of patient, contacts and the immediate environment:*

      1) Report to local health authority: None, Class 5 (see Reporting).
      2) Isolation: Not applicable.
      3) Concurrent disinfection: Not applicable.
      4) Quarantine: Not applicable.
      5) Immunization of contacts: Not applicable.
      6) Investigation of contacts and source of infection: Sexual contacts of patients with venereal warts should be examined and treated if indicated.
      7) Specific treatment: Warts usually regress spontaneously within months to years. Treatment of the affected individual will decrease the amount of wart virus available for transmission. If treatment is indicated, use freezing with liquid nitrogen for lesions on most of the body surface; salicylic acid plasters and curettage for plantar warts; and 10%-25% podophyllin in tincture of benzoin, trichloroacetic acid or liquid nitrogen for readily accessible genital warts—except in pregnant females. For widespread genital lesions, 5-fluorouracil has been helpful. Intralesional recombinant interferon

alpha-2b has been effective in treatment of condyloma acuminatum and is approved for this use. Surgical removal or laser treatment is required for laryngeal papillomata. Caesarean section may be considered if genital papillomatosis is very extensive.

8) Microscopic examination of cells (Papanicolaou smears) is an effective method for detecting cellular abnormalities associated with malignancy in women. Surgical intervention for cervical cancer is curative if the intervention is done early in the disease.

C. Epidemic measures: Usually a sporadic disease.

D. Disaster implications: None.

E. International measures: None.

YAWS   ICD-9 102; ICD-10 A66
(Framboesia tropica)

1. Identification—A chronic relapsing nonvenereal treponematosis, characterized by highly contagious, primary and secondary cutaneous lesions and noncontagious, tertiary/late destructive lesions. The typical initial lesion (mother yaw) is a papilloma on the face or extremities (usually the leg), persisting for weeks or months, and painless unless secondarily infected. This proliferates slowly and may form a framboesial (raspberry) lesion, or undergo ulceration (ulceropapilloma). Secondary disseminated or satellite papillomata and/or papules and squamous macules appear before or shortly after healing of the initial lesion in successive crops, often accompanied by periostitis of the long bones (sabre shin) and fingers (polydactylitis), with mild constitutional symptoms. In the dry season, papillomatous crops are usually restricted to the moist skinfolds and papules/macular lesions predominate. Painful and usually disabling papillomata and hyperkeratosis on palms and soles may appear in early and in late stages. Lesions heal spontaneously; relapses may occur after periods of latency.

The late stage, with destructive lesions of skin and bone, occurs in about 10%–20% of untreated patients, usually 5 or more years after infection. Unlike what happens in syphilis, the brain, eyes, heart, aorta and abdominal organs are not involved. Congenital transmission does not occur; the infection is rarely if ever fatal, but can be very disfiguring and disabling.

Diagnosis is confirmed through darkfield or direct FA microscopic examination of exudates from primary or secondary lesions. Nontreponemal serological tests for syphilis (e.g. VDRL [Venereal Disease Research

Laboratory], RPR [rapid plasma reagin]) become reactive during the initial stage, remain so during the early infection and tend to become nonreactive after many years of latency, even in the absence of specific treatment; in some patients they remain reactive at low titre for life. Treponemal serological tests (e.g. FTA-ABS [fluorescent treponemal antibody absorbed], MHA-TP [microhemagglutination assay for antibody to Treponema pallidum]) usually remain reactive for life despite adequate treatment.

2. Infectious agent—*Treponema pallidum*, subsp. *pertenue*, a spirochaete.

3. Occurrence—Predominantly a disease of children living in rural humid tropical areas; more frequent in males. Mass penicillin treatment campaigns in the 1950s and 1960s dramatically decreased worldwide prevalence but yaws has re-emerged in parts of equatorial and western Africa, with scattered foci of infection persisting in Latin America, the Caribbean islands, India, southeastern Asia and some South Pacific islands.

4. Reservoir—Humans and possibly higher primates.

5. Mode of transmission—Principally through direct contact with exudates of early skin lesions of infected people. Indirect transmission through contamination from scratching, skin-piercing articles and flies on open wounds is probable but of unknown importance. Climate influences the morphology, distribution and infectiousness of the early lesions.

6. Incubation period—From 2 weeks to 3 months.

7. Period of communicability—Variable; may extend intermittently over several years when moist lesions are present. The infectious agent is not usually found in late destructive lesions.

8. Susceptibility—No evidence of natural or racial resistance. Infection results in immunity to reinfection and may offer some protection against infection by other pathogenic treponemes.

9. Methods of control—

    A. Preventive measures: The following apply to yaws and other nonvenereal treponematoses. Although present techniques cannot differentiate the infectious agents, differences observed among clinical syndromes are unlikely to result from epidemiological or environmental factors alone.

    1) General health promotion measures; health education of the public about the value of better sanitation, including liberal use of soap and water and the importance of improving social and economic conditions over a period of years to reduce incidence. Improve access to health services.

2) Organize intensive control activities on a community level suitable to the local problem; examine entire populations, and treat patients with active or latent disease. Treatment of asymptomatic contacts is beneficial, and WHO recommends treating the entire population when the prevalence rate for active disease is above 10%; if prevalence is 5%–10%, treat patients, contacts and all children below 15; if <5%, treat active cases plus household and other contacts. Periodic clinical resurveys and continuous surveillance are essential for success.

3) Serological surveys for latent cases, particularly in children, to prevent relapses and development of infective lesions that maintain the disease in the community.

4) Provide facilities for early diagnosis and treatment as part of a plan in which mass control campaigns (See 9A2) are eventually consolidated into permanent local health services.

5) Treat disfiguring and incapacitating late manifestations.

B. *Control of patient, contacts and the immediate environment:*

1) Report to local health authority: In selected endemic areas; in many countries not a reportable disease, Class 3 (see Reporting). Differentiation of venereal and nonvenereal treponematoses, with proper reporting of each, has particular importance in the evaluation and consolidation of mass campaigns.

2) Isolation: Avoid intimate contact and contamination of the environment until lesions are healed.

3) Concurrent disinfection: Care in disposal of discharges and articles contaminated therewith.

4) Quarantine: Not applicable.

5) Immmunization of contacts: Not applicable.

6) Investigation of contacts and source of infection: Treat all family contacts; those with no active disease should be regarded as latent cases. In low-prevalence areas, treat all active cases, all children and close contacts of infectious cases.

7) Specific treatment: Penicillin. For patients 10 years or older with active disease and contacts, a single injection of benzathine penicillin G, 1.2 million units IM; 0.6 million units for patients under 10 years.

C. *Epidemic measures:* Active mass treatment programs in areas of high prevalence. Essential features are: 1) examining a high percentage of the population through field surveys; 2) extending treatment of active cases to family and community contacts based on the demonstrated prevalence of active yaws; 3) surveys at yearly intervals for 1–3 years, as part of the established rural public health activities of the country.

D. Disaster implications: None observed, but potentially a risk in refugee or displaced populations in endemic areas without hygienic facilities.

E. International measures: To protect countries against risk of reinfection where active mass treatment programs are in progress, adjacent countries in the endemic area should institute suitable measures against yaws. Movement of infected people across frontiers may require supervision (see Syphilis, section I, 9E). WHO Collaborating Centres.

[G. Antal]

YELLOW FEVER   ICD-9 060; ICD-10 A95

1. Identification—Acute infectious viral disease of short duration and varying severity. The mildest cases may be clinically indeterminate; typical attacks are characterized by sudden onset, fever, chills, headache, backache, generalized muscle pain, prostration, nausea and vomiting. The pulse may be slow and weak out of proportion to the elevated temperature (Faget sign). Jaundice is moderate early in the disease and intensifies later. Albuminuria, sometimes pronounced, and anuria may occur. Leukopenia appears early and is most pronounced about the fifth day. Most infections resolve at this stage. Some cases progress after a brief remission of hours to a day into the ominous stage of intoxication manifested by hemorrhagic symptoms including epistaxis, gingival bleeding, hematemesis (coffee-ground or black), melaena, and liver and renal failure; 20%–50% of jaundiced cases are fatal. The overall case-fatality rate among indigenous populations in endemic regions is 5% but may reach 20%–40% in individual outbreaks.

Laboratory diagnosis is through isolation of virus from blood by inoculation (suckling mice, mosquitoes or cell cultures, especially mosquito cells); through demonstration of viral antigen in the blood by ELISA or liver tissue by use of labelled specific antibodies; and through demonstration of viral genome in blood and liver tissue by PCR or hybridization probes. Serological diagnosis includes demonstrating specific IgM in early sera or a rise in titre of specific antibodies in paired acute and convalescent sera. Serological cross-reactions occur with other flaviviruses. Recent infections can often be distinguished from vaccine immunity by complement fixation testing. The demonstration of typical lesions in the liver confirms the diagnosis.

2. Infectious agent—The virus of yellow fever, of the genus *Flavivirus* and family Flaviviridae.

3. Occurrence—Yellow fever exists in nature in 2 transmission cycles, a sylvatic or jungle cycle that involves *Aedes* or *Haemagogus* mosquitoes and nonhuman primates, and an urban cycle involving humans and mainly *Aedes aegypti* mosquitoes. Sylvatic transmission is restricted to tropical regions of Africa and Latin America, where a few hundred cases occur annually, most often among occupationally exposed young adult males in forested or transitional areas of Bolivia, Brazil, Colombia, Ecuador and Peru (70%–90% of cases reported from Bolivia and Peru). Historically, urban yellow fever occurred in many cities of the Americas; no outbreak of urban yellow fever has occurred for 50 years in North America.

Reinfestation with *Ae. aegypti* may put many cities at risk of renewed urban yellow fever transmission. In Africa, the endemic zone includes the area between 15°N and 10°S latitude, from the Sahara desert to northern Angola, the Democratic Republic of the Congo and the United Republic of Tanzania. There is no evidence that yellow fever has ever been present in Asia; in western Kenya, sylvatic yellow fever was reported in 1992–1993.

4. Reservoir—In urban areas, humans and *Aedes* mosquitoes; in forest areas, vertebrates other than humans, mainly monkeys and possibly marsupials, and forest mosquitoes. Transovarian transmission in mosquitoes may contribute to maintenance of infection. Humans have no essential role in transmission of jungle yellow fever, but are the primary amplifying host in the urban cycle.

5. Mode of transmission—In urban and certain rural areas, the bite of infective *Aedes* mosquitoes. In South American forests, the bite of several species of forest mosquitoes of the genus *Haemagogus*. In eastern Africa, *Ae. africanus* is the vector in the monkey population, while semidomestic *Ae. bromeliae* and *Ae. simpsoni*, and probably other *Aedes* species, transmit the virus from monkeys to humans. In large epidemics in Ethiopia, epidemiological evidence incriminated *Ae. simpsoni* as a person-to-person vector. In western Africa, *Ae. furcifer-taylori*, *Ae. luteocephalus* and other species are responsible for spread between monkeys and humans. *Ae. albopictus* has been introduced into Brazil and the USA and has the potential for bridging the sylvatic and urban cycles of yellow fever in the Western Hemisphere, even though no involvement of this species in yellow fever transmission has been documented.

6. Incubation period—From 3 to 6 days.

7. Period of communicability—Blood of patients is infective for mosquitoes shortly before onset of fever and for the first 3–5 days of illness. The disease is highly communicable where many susceptible people and abundant vector mosquitoes coexist; it is not communicable through contact or common vehicles. The extrinsic incubation period in *Ae. aegypti* is commonly 9–12 days at the usual tropical temperatures. Once infected, mosquitoes remain so for life.

8. Susceptibility—Recovery from yellow fever is followed by lasting immunity; second attacks are unknown. Mild inapparent infections are common in endemic areas. Transient passive immunity in infants born to immune mothers may persist for up to 6 months. In natural infections, antibodies appear in the blood within the first week.

9. Methods of control—

A. Preventive measures:

1) Institute a program for active immunization of all people 9 months or older who are exposed to infection because of residence, occupation or travel. A single subcutaneous injection of a vaccine containing viable attenuated yellow fever 17D strain virus, cultivated in chick embryo, is effective in almost 99% of recipients. Antibodies appear 7–10 days after immunization and may persist for at least 30–35 years, probably much longer, though immunization or reimmunization within 10 years is required by the *International Health Regulations* for travel from endemic areas.

Since 1989, WHO has recommended that at-risk countries in the endemic-epidemic belt of Africa incorporate yellow fever vaccine into their routine childhood immunization programs. Of the 33 at-risk countries, 17 have introduced YF in EPI; overall yellow fever average immunization coverage was 22% in 2002, with a range of 18% to 99% (Gambia and Ghana reached the recommended minimum of 80%). Many countries have only introduced YF vaccination recently and improvements are expected in coming years. The vaccine can be given any time after 6 months of age and can be administered with other antigens such as measles vaccine. The vaccine is contraindicated in the first 4 months of life and should be considered for those aged 4–9 months only if the risk of exposure is judged to exceed the risk of vaccine-associated encephalitis, the main complication in this age group. The vaccine is not recommended in the first trimester of pregnancy unless the risk of disease is believed to be higher than the theoretical risk to the pregnancy. There is no evidence of fetal damage from the vaccine, but lower rates of maternal seroconversion have been observed, an indication for reimmunization after delivery or termination. The vaccine is recommended for asymptomatic HIV seropositive individuals; there is insufficient evidence to permit a definitive statement on whether the vaccine would pose a risk for symptomatic individuals; it is not currently recommended in this case and a waiver clause therefore applies.

2) For urban yellow fever eradicate or control the vector; immunization when indicated.

3) Sylvan or jungle yellow fever, transmitted by *Haemagogus* and forest species of *Aedes*, is best controlled through immunization, which is recommended for all people in rural communities whose occupation brings them into forests in yellow fever areas, and for people who intend to visit those areas. Protective clothing, bednets and repellents are advised for those not immunized.

B. Control of patient, contacts and the immediate environment:

1) Report to local health authority: Case report universally required by *International Health Regulations*; Class 1 (see Reporting).

2) Isolation: Blood and body fluid precautions. Prevent access of mosquitoes to patient for at least 5 days after onset by screening the sickroom, by spraying quarters with residual insecticide, and by using insecticide-treated bednets.

3) Concurrent disinfection: The home of patients and all houses in the vicinity should be sprayed promptly with an effective insecticide.

4) Quarantine: Not applicable.

5) Immunization of contacts: Family and other contacts and neighbors not previously immunized should be immunized promptly.

6) Investigation of contacts and source of infection: Inquire about all places, including forested areas, visited by the patient 3–6 days before onset, to locate focus of yellow fever; observe all people visiting that focus. Search patient's premises and places of work or visits over the preceding several days for mosquitoes capable of transmitting infection; apply effective insecticide. Investigate mild febrile illnesses and unexplained deaths suggesting yellow fever.

7) Specific treatment: None.

C. Epidemic measures:

1) Urban or *Ae. aegypti*-transmitted yellow fever:

   a) Mass immunization, beginning with people most exposed and those living in *Ae. aegypti*-infected areas.

   b) Eliminate or treat all actual and potential breeding places.

   c) Spraying the inside of all houses in the community with insecticides has shown promise for controlling urban epidemics.

2) Jungle or sylvan yellow fever:

   a) Immediately immunize all people living in or near forested areas or entering such areas.
   b) Ensure that nonimmunized individuals avoid those tracts of forest where infection has been localized, and that those just immunized avoid the areas for the first week after immunization.

3) In regions where yellow fever may occur, a diagnostic postmortem examination service should be organized to collect small specimens of liver postmortem from fatal febrile illnesses of 10 days duration or less, provided biological safety can be ensured. Facilities for viral isolation or serological confirmation are necessary to establish diagnosis since histopathological changes in the liver are not pathognomonic.

4) In Central and South America, confirmed deaths of howler and spider monkeys in the forest are presumptive evidence of the presence of yellow fever. Confirmation by the histopathological examination of livers of moribund or recently dead monkeys or by virus isolation is highly desirable.

5) Immunity surveys through neutralization tests of wild primates captured in forested areas are useful in defining enzootic areas. Serological surveys of human populations are not useful where yellow fever vaccine has been widely used.

D. Disaster implications: Mass vaccination may be considered if an epidemic is feared.

E. International measures:

1) Telegraphic notification by governments to WHO and to adjacent countries of the first imported, first transferred, or first nonimported case of yellow fever in an area previously free of the disease; and of newly discovered or reactivated foci of yellow fever infection among vertebrates other than man.

2) Measures applicable to ships, aircraft and land transport arriving from yellow fever areas are specified in the *International Health Regulations* (1969), that are currently being revised.

3) Animal quarantine: Quarantine of monkeys and other wild primates arriving from yellow fever areas may be required until 7 days have elapsed after leaving such areas.

4) International travel: A valid international certificate of immunization against yellow fever is required by many countries for entry of travellers coming from or going to recognized yellow fever zones of Africa and South America; otherwise, quarantine measures are applicable for up to 6 days. WHO recommends immunization for all travellers to areas other than major cities in countries where the disease occurs in humans or is assumed to be present in nonhuman primates. The *International Certificate of Vaccination against Yellow Fever* is valid for 10 years from 10 days after date of immunization; if reimmunization occurs within that period, valid 10 years from date of reimmunization.

[C. Roth/R. Shope]

YERSINIOSIS	ICD-9 027.8
INTESTINAL YERSINIOSIS	ICD-10 A04.6
EXTRAINTESTINAL YERSINIOSIS	ICD-10 A28.2

1. Identification—Infection caused by enteropathogenic *Yersinia* typically manifested by acute febrile diarrhea with abdominal pain (especially in young children). Other clinical manifestations (extraintestinal or otherwise) include acute mesenteric lymphadenitis mimicking appendicitis (especially in older children and adults) and systemic infections. The most common post-infectious complications are erythema nodosum (about 10% of adults, particularly women), and reactive arthritis. Bloody diarrhea occurs in up to one-fourth of patients with *Yersinia* enteritis; diarrhea may be absent in up to a third of *Y. enterocolitica* infections. Ileitis is the characteristic lesion induced by *Y. enterocolitica*. *Y. pseudotuberculosis* causes an acute mesenteric lymphadenitis, clinically characterized by an appendicitis-like syndrome, sometimes with diarrhea. Specific *Y. pseudotuberculosis* syndromes (Izumi fever, Far East scarlet-like fever) have been reported in Japan and the Russian Federation.

Diagnosis is usually made through stool culture. Cefsulodin irgasan novobiocin (CIN) medium is highly selective and should be used if there is reason to suspect infection with *Yersinia*; it permits identification in 24 hours at 28°C (78.4°F). The organisms may be recovered on usual enteric media if precautions are taken to prevent overgrowth of fecal flora. Cold enrichment in buffered saline at 4°C (39°F) for 2–3 weeks can be used but this procedure usually enhances the isolation of non-pathogenic species. *Yersinia* can be isolated from blood with standard commercial blood culture media. Serological diagnosis is possible (agglutination test or ELISA), but availability is generally limited to research settings.

2. Infectious agents—Gram-negative bacilli. *Y. pseudotuberculosis* has 15 serotypes with 10 subtypes; over 90% of human and animal infections are due to O-group I. *Y. enterocolitica* has over 50 serotypes and 5 biotypes, many of them non-pathogenic. Strains pathogenic for humans are those of biotypes 1B, 2, 3 and 4; they are pyrazinamidase-negative. Biotype 1A strains are non-pathogenic whereas the very rare strains of biotype 5 have been isolated from hares. The distribution of pathogenic *Y. enterocolitica* varies in different geographic areas; biotype 4 (serotype O3) accounts for most of the cases in Europe, followed by bioserotypes 2 (serotypes O9 and O5,27). Biotype 1B strains were responsible for most outbreaks in the USA but bioserotype 4/O3 emerged in the 1990s and is now the most common type there.

3. Occurrence—Worldwide. *Y. pseudotuberculosis* is primarily a zoonotic disease of wild and domesticated birds and mammals, with humans as incidental hosts. In some countries such as Japan or the Russian Federation, *Y. pseudotuberculosis* is the main cause of human yersiniosis. Globally, *Y. enterocolitica* is the species most commonly associated with human infection, up to 1%–3% of acute enteritis in some areas. This species has been recovered from a wide variety of asymptomatic animals. The most important documented source of *Y. enterocolitica* 4 (serotype O3) infection is pork, as the pharynx of pigs may be heavily colonized by *Y. enterocolitica*. Approximately two-thirds of *Y. enterocolitica* cases occur among infants and children; three-quarters of *Y. pseudotuberculosis* cases are aged 5 to 20. Human cases have been reported in association with disease in household pets, particularly puppies and kittens.

The highest isolation rates have been reported during the cold season in temperate climates, including northern Europe (especially Scandinavia), North America and temperate regions of South America. Vehicles implicated in outbreaks attributed to *Y. enterocolitica* include soybean cake (tofu) and pork chitterlings (large intestines) in the USA, and the feeding of raw pork to infants in Europe. Contamination through milk (including pasteurized milk, where postpasteurization contamination is more likely than resistance of the agent to the pasteurization process) is less common. Studies in Europe suggest that many cases are related to ingestion of raw or undercooked pork. Since 20% of infections in older children and adolescents can mimic acute appendicitis, outbreaks can sometimes be recognized by local increases in appendectomies.

4. Reservoir—Animals. The pig is the main reservoir for *Y. enterocolitica* 4 (serotype O3). Asymptomatic pharyngeal carriage is common in swine, especially in winter, and bioserotype 2 (serotype O9) has been isolated from ovine, bovine and caprine origins. *Y. pseudotuberculosis* is widespread among many avian and mammalian hosts, particularly rodents and other small mammals.

5. Mode of transmission—Fecal-oral transmission through consumption of contaminated food or water, or through contact with infected people or animals. *Y. enterocolitica* has been isolated from many foods; pathogenic strains most commonly from raw pork or pork products. *Y. enterocolitica* can multiply under refrigeration and microaerophilic conditions, and there is an increased risk of infection by *Y. enterocolitica* if uncured meat that was stored in plastic bags is undercooked. *Y. enterocolitica* (usually non-pathogenic strains) has been recovered from natural bodies of water. Nosocomial transmission has occurred, as has transmission by transfusion of stored blood from donors who were asymptomatic or had mild GI illness.

6. Incubation period—Probably 3–7 days, generally under 10 days.

7. Period of communicability—Secondary transmission appears rare. There is fecal shedding at least as long as symptoms exist, usually for 2–3 weeks. Untreated cases may excrete the organism for 2–3 months. Prolonged asymptomatic carriage has been reported in both children and adults.

8. Susceptibility—Gastroenterocolitis (diarrhea) is more severe in children, postinfectious arthritis more severe in adolescents and older adults. Male adolescents are particularly prone to infection with *Y. pseudotuberculosis*; *Y. enterocolitica* equally attacks men and women. Reactive arthritis and Reiter syndrome occur more often in people with the HLA-B27 genetic type. Septicaemia occurs most often among people with iron overload (hemochromatosis) or immunosuppression (through illness or treatment).

9. Methods of control—

   A. Preventive measures:

   1) Prepare meat and other foods in a sanitary manner, avoid eating raw pork and pasteurize milk; irradiation of meat is effective.
   2) Wash hands prior to food handling and eating, after handling raw pork and after animal contact.
   3) Protect water supplies from animal and human feces; purify appropriately.
   4) Control rodents and birds (for *Y. pseudotuberculosis*).
   5) Dispose of human, dog and cat feces in a sanitary manner.
   6) During the slaughtering of pigs, head and neck should be removed from the body to avoid contaminating meat from the heavily colonized pharynx.

B. Control of patient, contacts and the immediate environment:

1) Report to local health authority: Case reporting obligatory in many countries, Class 2 (see Reporting).

2) Isolation: Enteric precautions for patients in hospitals. Remove persons with diarrhea from food handling, patient care and occupations involving care of young children.

3) Concurrent disinfection: Of feces. In communities with modern and adequate sewage disposal systems, feces can be discharged directly into sewers without preliminary disinfection.

4) Quarantine: Not applicable.

5) Immmunization of contacts: Not applicable.

6) Investigation of contacts and source of infection: A search for unrecognized cases and convalescent carriers among contacts is indicated only when a common-source exposure is suspected.

7) Specific treatment: Organisms are sensitive to many antibiotics, but are generally resistant to penicillin and its semi-synthetic derivatives. Treatment may be helpful for GI symptoms; definitely indicated for septicemia and other invasive disease. Agents of choice against *Y. enterocolitica* are the aminoglycosides (septicemia only) and trimethoprim-sufamethoxazole. Newer quinolones such as ciprofloxacin are highly effective. Both *Y. enterocolitica* and *Y. pseudotuberculosis* are usually sensitive to tetracyclines.

C. Epidemic measures:

1) Any group of cases of acute gastroenteritis or cases suggestive of appendicitis must be reported at once to the local health authority, even in the absence of specific causal identification.

2) Investigate general sanitation and search for common-source vehicle; pay attention to consumption of (or possible cross-contamination with) raw or undercooked pork; look for evidence of close contacts with pet dogs, cats and other domestic animals.

D. Disaster implications: None.

E. International measures: None.

[E. Carniel]

ZYGOMYCOSIS
(Phycomycosis)

Zygomycosis is the term encompassing a polymorphic disease of multiple etiology caused by rapidly growing moulds of the class Zygomycetes. Infections due to Mucorales or to Entomophthorales present distinct epidemiological, clinical and pathological forms. The mainly histopathological differences between them are the eosinophilic perihyphal material or Spendore-Hoeppli reaction seen in entomophthoromycosis.

INFECTIONS DUE TO MUCORALES   ICD-9 117.7; ICD-10 B46.0-B46.5

1. Identification—Infections caused by fungi of the order Mucorales leading to opportunistic disease. These fungi have an affinity for blood vessels, and cause thrombosis, infarction and tissue necrosis. The mycosis has an acute or subacute course. In debilitated persons it is the most fulminant fungal infection known. The 4 main systemic forms of the disease are the rhinocerebral, pulmonary, gastrointestinal and disseminated types. The underlying disease influences the portal of entry of the fungus. Rhinocerebral disease represents one-third to one-half of all cases and usually presents as nasal or paranasal sinus infection, most often during episodes of poorly controlled diabetes mellitus. Necrosis of the turbinates, perforation of the hard palate, necrosis of the cheek or orbital cellulitis, proptosis and ophthalmoplegia may occur. Infection may penetrate to the internal carotid artery or extend directly to the brain and cause infarction. Patients receiving immunosuppressive agents or deferoxamine are susceptible to either rhinocerebral or pulmonary zygomycosis. In the pulmonary form of disease, the fungus causes thrombosis of pulmonary blood vessels and infarcts of the lung. In the gastrointestinal form, mucosal ulcers or thrombosis and gangrene of stomach or bowel wall may occur. Disseminated type usually occurs in patients with hematological malignancy. Nosocomial cases have been reported.

Diagnosis is through microscopic demonstration of distinctive broad nonseptate hyphae on tissue section and through culture of biopsy tissue. Wet preparations and smears may be examined. Cultures alone are not diagnostic because fungi of the order Mucorales are frequently found in the environment. To be considered as an agent of the mycosis the fungus must survive and multiply at a temperature of 37°C (98.6°F).

2. Infectious agents—Some species of *Rhizopus*, especially *R. arrhizus*, have caused most of the culture-positive cases of zygomycosis. In addition to *Rhizopus*, *Mucor* and *Absidia*, human diseases due to

Rhizomucor, *Apophysomyces*, *Cunninghamella*, *Saksenaea* and *Syncephalastrum* spp. have all been identified.

3. Occurrence—Worldwide. Incidence may be increasing because of longer survival of patients with immunosuppression due to disease or medication, with diabetes mellitus and certain blood dyscrasias, especially acute leukaemia and aplastic anemia, as well as the use of deferoxamine for aluminium or iron overload in patients receiving chronic hemodialysis for renal failure.

4. Reservoir—Members of the order Mucorales are common saprophytes in the environment.

5. Mode of transmission—Inhalation or ingestion of fungal spores by susceptible individuals. Direct inoculation in IV drug users and at sites of IV catheters and cutaneous burns may occur.

6. Incubation period—Unknown. Fungus spreads rapidly in susceptible tissues.

7. Period of communicability—No direct person-to-person or animal-to-person transmission.

8. Susceptibility—The rarity of infection in healthy individuals despite the abundance of Mucorales in the environment indicates natural resistance. Corticosteroid use, metabolic acidosis, deferoxamine and immunosuppressive treatment predispose to infection. Malnutrition predisposes to the gastrointestinal form.

9. Methods of control—

   A. *Preventive measures:* Optimal clinical control of diabetes mellitus to avoid acidosis.

   B. *Control of patient, contacts and the immediate environment:*

      1) Report to local health authority: Official report not ordinarily justifiable, Class 5 (see Reporting).
      2) Isolation: Not applicable.
      3) Concurrent disinfection: Ordinary cleanliness. Terminal cleaning.
      4) Quarantine: Not applicable.
      5) Immmunization of contacts: Not applicable.
      6) Investigation of contacts and source of infection: Ordinarily not beneficial.
      7) Specific treatment: In the rhinocerebral form, clinical control of diabetes; amphotericin B and resection of necrotic tissue have been helpful.

   C. *Epidemic measures:* Not applicable; a sporadic disease.

D. Disaster implications: None.

E. International measures: None.

INFECTIONS DUE TO ENTOMOPHTHORALES
ICD-9 117.7 ICD-10 B46.0-B46.5

Entomophthoramycosis includes 2 histopathologically identical entities: basidiobolomycosis and conidiobolomycosis. These 2 infections have been recognized principally in tropical and subtropical areas of Asia, Africa and Latin America. They are not characterized by thromboses or infarction, do not usually occur in association with serious pre-existing disease nor cause disseminated disease, and seldom cause death.

BASIDIOBOLOMYCOSIS

Basidiobolus ranarum causes the subcutaneous form of entomophthoramycosis presenting as a granulomatous inflammation. The fungus is ubiquitous, occurring in decaying vegetation, soil and the gastrointestinal tract of amphibians and reptiles. The disease presents as a firm painless and sharply circumscribed subcutaneous mass, fixed to the skin, mainly in children and adolescents, more commonly in males. Common sites of infection are the buttocks, thighs and chest. The infection may heal spontaneously. Recommended treatment is oral potassium iodide.

CONIDIOBOLOMYCOSIS

Conidiobolus coronatus, occurring in soil and decaying vegetation, causes the mucocutaneous form of entomophthoramycosis. This usually originates in the paranasal skin or nasal mucosa and presents as nasal obstruction or swelling of the nose or adjacent structures. The lesion may spread to involve contiguous areas, such as lip, cheek, palate or pharynx. The disease is uncommon and occurs principally in adult males. Recommended treatment is oral potassium iodide or IV amphotericin B.

For both forms of entomophthoramycosis, incubation periods and modes of transmission are unknown. Person-to-person transmission does not occur.

A few cases of a rare primary visceral form of conidiobolomycosis due to *C. incongruus* have been reported in patients (immunocompromised or not) as lung infections spreading to contiguous organs.

[L.C. Severo]

Abbreviations and acronyms used in
Control of Communicable Diseases Manual

AAP	= American Academy of Pediatrics
ACIP	= Advisory Committee on Immunization Practices (CDC)
AFB	= acid-fast bacilli
AFP	= acute flaccid paralysis
AHC	= acute hemorrhagic conjunctivitis
AIDS	= acquired immunodeficiency syndrome
ALT	= alanine aminotransferase (was SGPT)
aP	= acellular Pertussis [vaccine]
AST	= aspartate aminotransferase (was SGOT)
AZT	= azidothymidine
BCG	= bacille Calmette-Guérin
BPF	= Brazilian purpuric fever
BSE	= bovine spongiform encephalitis
BSL	= biosafety level (i.e. BSL-1, -2, -3, -4)
ca	= circa
CAT	= computerized axial tomography
CD4	= antigen of T-helper lymphocytes
CDC	= Centers for Disease Control and Prevention
CF	= complement fixation
CIE	= counterimmunoelectrophoresis
CJD	= Creutzfeldt-Jakob disease
cm	= centimeter
CMV	= cytomegalovirus
CNS	= central nervous system
CRS	= congenital rubella syndrome
CSF	= cerebrospinal fluid
CTF	= Colorado tick fever
DAEC	= diffuse-adherence *Entamoeba coli*
DAT	= dried antigen test
DEC	= diethylcarbamazine citrate
DFA	= direct fluorescent antibody
DHF/DSS	= dengue hemorrhagic fever/dengue shock syndrome
DIC	= disseminated intravascular coagulation
DNA	= desoxyribonucleic acid
DT	= diphtheria/tetanus vaccine
DTaP	= diphtheria/tetanus toxoids and acellular Pertussis vaccine
DTP	= diphtheria/tetanus toxoids and whole cell Pertussis vaccine
EAggEC	= enteroaggregative *Entamoeba coli*

EBV	= Epstein-Barr virus
EEE	= Eastern equine encephalitis
EEG	= electroencephalogram
e.g.	= for instance
EHEC	= enterohemorrhagic *Entamoeba coli*
EIA	= enzyme immunoassay
EIEC	= enteroinvasive *Entamoeba coli*
EKC	= epidemic keratoconjunctivitis
ELISA	= enzyme-linked immunosorbent assay
EM	= electron microscopy—also erythema migrans
EMB	= ethambutol
ENL	= erythema nodosum leprosum
EPEC	= enteropathogenic *Entamoeba coli*
EPI	= Expanded Programme on Immunization, WHO
ERIG	= equine rabies immune globulin
ESR	= erythrocyte sedimentation rate
ETEC	= enterotoxic *Entamoeba coli*
FA	= direct fluorescent or immunofluorescent antibody test
FAO	= Food and Agriculture Organization of the United Nations
FEE	= Far eastern equine encephalitis
G6PD	= glucose-6-phosphate dehydrogenase
GBS	= Guillain-Barré syndrome
GI	= gastrointestinal
GSS	= Gertsmann-Staussler-Scheinker syndrome
HA	= hemagglutination
HAART	= highly active antiretroviral therapy
HAI/HI	= hemagglutination inhibition
HAV	= hepatitis A virus
HBV	= hepatitis B virus
HBcAg	= hepatitis B core antigen
HBIG	= hepatitis B immunoglobulin
HBsAg	= hepatitis B surface antigen
HCC	= hepatocellular carcinoma
HCV	= hepatitis C virus
HDCV	= human diploid cell rabies vaccine
HDV	= hepatitis D virus
HEPA	= high efficiency particulate air [filters]
HEV	= hepatitis E virus
HHV	= human herpesvirus
Hib	= *Haemophilus influenzae* type b
HIV	= human immunodeficiency virus
HPV	= human papillomavirus
HRIG	= human rabies immune globulin
HSV	= herpes simplex virus
HTLV	= human T-cell lymphotropic virus

HUS	=	hemolytic uremic syndrome
ICD	=	International Classification of Diseases
ID	=	intradermal
IEM	=	immune electron microscopy
IF	=	immunofluorescent testing
IFA/IFAT	=	indirect immunofluorescent antibody/assay
IG	=	immune globulin (serum)
IgA	=	immunoglobulin class A
IgG	=	immunoglobulin class G
IgM	=	immunoglobulin class M
IM	=	intramuscular
IND	=	investigational new drug
INH	=	isoniazid
IPV	=	inactivated poliovirus vaccine
IU	=	international unit
IV	=	intravenous
kg	=	kilogram
kGy	=	kiloGray
km	=	kilometer
KFD	=	Kyasanur Forest disease
KSHV	=	Kaposi sarcoma- associated herpesvirus
l	=	liter
LA	=	latex agglutination
lb	=	pound [weight]
LCM	=	lymphocytic choriomeningitis
LD	=	lethal dose
LTBI	=	latent TB infection
mEq	=	milliequivalents
mg	=	milligram
mIU	=	milli-IU (international units)
ml	=	milliliter
mm	=	millimeter
MDR	=	multidrug resistant
MDT	=	multidrug therapy
MOTT	=	*Mycobacteria* other than tuberculosis
MMR	=	measles-mumps-rubella [vaccine]
MR	=	measles-rubella [vaccine]
MRI	=	magnetic resonance imaging
MV	=	Murray Valley [fever]
NAG	=	non-agglutinable [vibrio]
NTM	=	nontuberculous mycobacteria
NGU	=	non-gonococcal urethritis
OHF	=	Omsk hemorrhagic fever
OPV	=	oral poliovirus vaccine
OspA	=	outer-surface protein A
PAHO	=	Pan American Health Organization
PCR	=	polymerase chain reaction

PE	=	Powassan encephalitis
PEP	=	postexposure prophylaxis
PO	=	oral (*per os*)
PPD-S	=	purified protein derivative-standard
ppm	=	parts per million
PZA	=	pyrazinamide
q.v.	=	see
RBC	=	red blood cell
RDS	=	respiratory distress syndrome
RIA	=	radioimmunoassay
RIF	=	rifampicin
RMSF	=	Rocky Mountain spotted fever
RNA	=	ribonucleic acid
rOspA	=	recombinant OspA
RSV	=	respiratory syncytial virus
RRV-TV	=	rhesus-based rotavirus vaccine
RT-PCR	=	retrotranscriptase PCR
RVA	=	rabies vaccine, adsorbed
RVF	=	Rift Valley fever
SARS	=	severe acute respiratory syndrome
SARS CoV	=	SARS coronavirus
SCBA	=	self-contained breathing apparatus
SC	=	subcutaneous
SI	=	Système International d'Unités (International System of Units)
SLE	=	St Louis encephalitis
sp.* or *spp.	=	species
subsp.	=	subspecies
STI	=	sexually transmitted infection
TB	=	tuberculosis
TCBS	=	thiosulfate-citrate-bile-sucrose [medium]
Td	=	tetanus and diphtheria toxoid
TIG	=	tetanus immune globulin
TLTBI	=	treatment of latent TB infection
TSS	=	toxic shock syndrome
TT	=	tetanus toxoid
TTP	=	thrombocytopenic purpura
UNAIDS	=	Joint United Nations Programme on AIDS
UNDP	=	United Nations Development Programme
USA	=	United States of America
USPHS	=	US Public Health Service
UV	=	ultraviolet
VAPP	=	vaccine-associated paralytic poliomyelitis
VCA	=	viral capsid antigen
vCJD	=	variant CJD
VEE	=	Venezuelan equine encephalitis
vs.	=	versus

VSV	= vesicular stomatitis virus
VZIG	= varicella zoster immunoglobulin
VZV	= varicella zoster virus
WEE	= Western equine encephalitis
WBC	= white blood cell
WHA	= World Health Assembly
WHO	= World Health Organization
wP	= whole pertussis [vaccine]
YF	= yellow fever
ZDV	= zidovudine

EXPLANATION OF TERMS
Technical meaning of some terms used in CCDM
(not binding definitions)

1. **Carrier**—A person or animal that harbours a specific infectious agent without discernible clinical disease and serves as a potential source of infection. The carrier state may exist in an individual with an infection that is inapparent throughout its course (commonly known as **healthy** or **asymptomatic carrier**), or during the incubation period, convalescence and postconvalescence of a person with a clinically recognizable disease (commonly known as an **incubatory** or **convalescent carrier**). Under either circumstance the carrier state may be of short or long duration (**temporary** or **transient carrier**, or **chronic carrier**).

2. **Case-fatality rate**—Usually expressed as the proportion of persons diagnosed as having a specified disease who die within a given period as a result of acquiring that disease. In communicable disease epidemiology, this term is most frequently applied to a specific outbreak of acute disease in which all patients have been followed for a period of time sufficient to include all deaths attributable to the given disease. The case-fatality rate, where the numerator is "deaths from a given disease in a given period" and the denominator is "number of diagnosed cases of the disease during that period" must be differentiated from the **disease-specific mortality rate**, where the denominator is "total population" (Synonyms: fatality rate, fatality percentage, case-fatality ratio).

3. **Chemoprophylaxis**—The administration of a chemical, including antibiotics, to prevent the development of an infection or the progression of an infection to active manifest disease, or to eliminate the carriage of a specific infectious agent in order to prevent transmission and disease in others. **Chemotherapy** refers to use of a chemical to treat a clinically manifest disease or to limit its further progress.

4. **Cleaning**—The removal by scrubbing and washing, as with water, soap, antiseptic or suitable detergent or by vacuum cleaning, of infectious agents and of organic matter from surfaces on which and in which infectious agents may find favourable conditions for surviving or multiplying.

5. **Communicable disease**—An illness due to a specific infectious agent or its toxic products that arises through transmission of that agent or its products from an infected person, animal or inanimate

source to a susceptible host; either directly or indirectly through an intermediate plant or animal host, vector or the inanimate environment. (Synonym: infectious disease)

6. **Contact**—As regards communicable diseases, a person or animal that has been in such association with an infected person or animal or a contaminated environment as to have had an opportunity to acquire the infection.

7. **Contamination**—The presence of an infectious agent on a body surface, in clothes, bedding, toys, surgical instruments or dressings, or other inanimate articles or substances including water, milk and food. Contamination of a body surface does not imply a carrier state. **Pollution** is distinct from contamination and implies the presence of offensive, but not necessarily infectious, matter in the environment.

8. **Disinfection**—Killing of infectious agents outside the body by direct exposure to chemical or physical agents. **High-level disinfection** may kill all microorganisms with the exception of high numbers of bacterial spores; extended exposure is required to ensure killing of most bacterial spores. High-level disinfection is achieved, after thorough detergent cleaning, through exposure to specific concentrations of certain disinfectants (e.g., 2% glutaraldehyde, 6% stabilized hydrogen peroxide and up to 1% peracetic acid) for at least 20 minutes. **Intermediate-level disinfection** does not kill spores; it can be achieved through pasteurization (75°C [167°F] for 30 minutes) or appropriate treatment with approved disinfectants.

   Concurrent disinfection is the application of disinfective measures as soon as possible after the discharge of infectious material from the body of an infected person, or after the soiling of articles with such infectious discharges; all personal contact with such discharges or articles should be minimized prior to concurrent disinfection.

   Terminal disinfection is the application of disinfective measures after the patient has been removed by death or transfer, or has ceased to be a source of infection, or after hospital isolation or other practices have been discontinued. Terminal disinfection is rarely practised; terminal cleaning generally suffices (see **Cleaning**), along with airing and sunning of rooms, furniture and bedding. Steam sterilization or incineration of bedding and other items is sometimes recommended after a disease such as Lassa fever or other highly infectious diseases.

   Sterilization involves destruction of all forms of microbial life by physical heat, irradiation, gas or chemical treatment.

9. **Disinfestation**—Any physical or chemical process serving to destroy or remove undesired small animal forms, particularly arthro-

pods or rodents, present upon the person, the clothing, or in the environment of an individual, or on domestic animals. (See **Insecticide** and **Rodenticide**.) Disinfestation includes delousing for infestation with *Pediculus humanus*, the human body louse. Synonyms include the terms **disinsection** and **disinsectization** when only insects are involved.

10. **Endemic**—A term denoting the habitual presence of a disease or infectious agent within a given geographic area or a population group; may also refer to the usual prevalence of a given disease within such area. **Hyperendemic** expresses a habitual presence at all ages at a high level of incidence, and **holoendemic** (a term applied mainly to malaria) a high level of prevalence with high spleen rates in children, lower rates in adults. (See also **Zoonosis**.)

11. **Epidemic**—The occurrence, in a defined community or region, of cases of an illness (or an outbreak) with a frequency clearly in excess of normal expectancy. The number of cases indicating the presence of an epidemic varies according to the infectious agent, size and type of population exposed, previous experience or lack of exposure to the disease, and time and place of occurrence; epidemicity is thus relative to usual frequency of the disease in the same area, among the specified population, at the same season of the year. A single case of a communicable disease long absent from a population or the first invasion by a disease not previously recognized in that area requires immediate reporting and full field epidemiological investigation; 2 cases of such a disease associated in time and place are sufficient evidence of transmission to be considered an epidemic. (See **Report of a Disease** and **Zoonosis**.)

12. **Food irradiation**—A technique that provides a specific dose of ionizing radiation from a source such as a radioisotope (e.g., cobalt 60), or from machines that produce accelerated electron beams or X-rays. Doses for irradiation of food and material are: low, 1 or less kiloGrays (kGy), used for disinfestation of insects from fruit, spices and grain and for parasite disinfection in fish and meat; medium, 1-10 kGy (commonly 1-4 kGy), used for pasteurization and the destruction of bacteria and fungi; and high, 10-50 kGy, used for sterilization of food as well as medical supplies (including IV fluids, implants, syringes, needles, thread, clips and gowns).

13. **Fumigation**—A process by which the killing of animal forms, especially arthropods and rodents, is accomplished by the use of gaseous agents. (See **Insecticide** and **Rodenticide**.)

14. **Health education**—The process by which individuals and groups of people learn to behave in a manner conducive to the promotion, maintenance or restoration of health. Education for health begins with people as they are, with whatever interests they may have in

improving their living conditions. Its aim is to develop their own sense of responsibility for health conditions, as individuals and as members of families and communities. In communicable disease control, health education commonly includes an appraisal of what is known by a population about a disease, an assessment of habits and attitudes of the people as they relate to spread and frequency of the disease, and the presentation of specific means to remedy observed deficiencies. (Synonyms: patient education, education for health, education of the public, public health education).

15. **Herd immunity**—The immunity of a group or community. The resistance of a group to invasion and spread of an infectious agent, based on the resistance to infection of a high proportion of individual members of the group.

16. **Host**—A person or other living animal, including birds and arthropods, that affords subsistence or lodgement to an infectious agent under natural (as opposed to experimental) conditions. Some protozoa and helminths pass successive stages in alternate hosts of different species. Hosts in which a parasite attains maturity or passes its sexual stage are **primary** or **definitive** hosts; those in which a parasite is in a larval or asexual state are **secondary** or **intermediate** hosts. A **transport host** is a carrier in which the organism remains alive but does not undergo development.

17. **Immune individual**—A person or animal that has specific protective antibodies and/or cellular immunity as a result of previous infection or immunization, or is so conditioned by such previous specific experience as to respond in a way that prevents the development of infection and/or clinical illness following re-exposure to the specific infectious agent. Immunity is relative: a level of protection that could be adequate under ordinary conditions may be overwhelmed by an excessive dose of the infectious agent or by exposure through an unusual portal of entry; protection may also be impaired by immunosuppressive drug therapy, concurrent disease or the ageing process.

18. **Immunity**—A status usually associated with the presence of antibodies or cells having a specific action on the microorganism concerned with a particular infectious disease or on its toxin. Effective immunity includes both **cellular immunity**, conferred by T-lymphocyte sensitization, and/or **humoral immunity**, based on B-lymphocyte response. **Passive immunity** is attained either naturally through transplacental transfer from the mother, or artificially by inoculation of specific protective antibodies (from immunized animals, or convalescent hyperimmune serum or immune serum globulin [human]); it is of short duration (days to months). **Active humoral immunity**, which usually lasts for years, is attained

either naturally through infection with or without clinical manifestations, or artificially through inoculation of the agent itself in
killed, modified or variant form, or of fractions or products of the
agent.

19. **Inapparent infection**—The presence of infection in a host without recognizable clinical signs or symptoms. Inapparent infections
are identifiable only through laboratory means such as a blood test
or through the development of positive reactivity to specific skin
tests. (Synonyms: asymptomatic, subclinical, occult infection).

20. **Incidence**—The number of instances of illness commencing, or of
persons falling ill, during a given period in a specified population.
The **incidence rate** is the ratio of new cases of a specified disease
diagnosed or reported during a defined period of time to the
number of persons at risk in a stated population in which the cases
occurred during the same period of time (if the period is one year,
the rate is the **annual incidence rate**). This rate is expressed,
usually as cases per 1000 or 100 000 per annum, for the whole
population or specifically for any population characteristic or
subdivision such as age or ethnic group. (See **Prevalence rate**.)

Attack rate, or **case rate**, is a proportion measuring cumulative
incidence for a particular group, over limited periods and under
special circumstances, as in an epidemic; it is usually expressed as
a percentage (cases per 100 in the group). The numerator can be
determined through the identification of clinical cases or through
seroepidemiology. The **secondary attack rate** is the ratio of the
number of cases among contacts occurring within the accepted
incubation period following exposure to a primary case to the total
number of exposed contacts; the denominator may be restricted to
the numbers of susceptible contacts when this can be determined.
The **infection rate** is a proportion that expresses the incidence of
all identified infections, manifest or inapparent (the latter identified
by seroepidemiology).

21. **Incubation period**—The time interval between initial contact
with an infectious agent and the first appearance of symptoms
associated with the infection. In a vector, it is the time between
entrance of an organism into the vector and the time when that
vector can transmit the infection (**extrinsic incubation period**).
The period between the time of exposure to an infectious agent
and the time when the agent can be detected in blood or stool is
called the prepatent period.

22. **Infected individual**—A person or animal that harbours an infectious agent and who has either manifest disease or inapparent
infection (see **Carrier**). An **infectious** person or animal is one from
whom the infectious agent can be naturally acquired.

23. **Infection**—The entry and development or multiplication of an infectious agent in the body of persons or animals. Infection is not synonymous with infectious disease; the result may be inapparent (see **Inapparent infection**) or manifest (see **Infectious disease**). The presence of living infectious agents on exterior surfaces of the body, or on articles of apparel or soiled articles, is not infection, but represents contamination of such surfaces and articles. (See **Infestation** and **Contamination**.)

24. **Infectious agent**—An organism (virus, rickettsia, bacteria, fungus, protozoan or helminth) that is capable of producing infection or infectious disease. **Infectivity** expresses the ability of the infectious agent to enter, survive and multiply in the host. **Infectiousness** indicates the relative ease with which an infectious agent is transmitted to other hosts.

25. **Infectious disease**—A clinically manifest disease of humans or animals resulting from an infection. (See **Infection**.)

26. **Infestation**—For persons or animals, the lodgement, development and reproduction of arthropods on the surface of the body or in the clothing. Infested articles or premises are those that harbour or give shelter to animal forms, especially arthropods and rodents.

27. **Insecticide**—Any chemical substance used for the destruction of insects; can be applied as powder, liquid, atomized liquid, aerosol or "paint" spray; an insecticide may or may not have residual action. The term **larvicide** is generally used to designate insecticides applied specifically for the destruction of immature stages of arthropods; **adulticide** or **imagocide**, to those destroying mature or adult forms. The term insecticide is used broadly to encompass substances for the destruction of all arthropods; **acaricide** is more properly used for agents against ticks and mites. Specific terms such as **lousicide** and **miticide** are sometimes used.

28. **Isolation**—As applied to patients, isolation represents separation, for a period at least equal to the **period of communicability**, of infected persons or animals from others, in such places and under such conditions as to prevent or limit the direct or indirect transmission of the infectious agent from those infected to those who are susceptible to infection or who may spread the agent to others. Universal precautions should be used consistently for all patients (in hospital settings as well as outpatient settings) regardless of their bloodborne infection status. This practice is based on the possibility that blood and certain body fluids (any body secretion that is obviously bloody, semen, vaginal secretions, tissue, CSF, and synovial, pleural, peritoneal, pericardial and amniotic fluids) of all patients are potentially infectious for agents such as HIV, HBV and other bloodborne pathogens. Universal precautions

are intended to prevent parenteral, mucous membrane and nonintact skin exposures of health care workers to bloodborne pathogens. Protective barriers include gloves, gowns, masks and protective eyewear or face shields. A private room is indicated if patient hygiene is poor. Local and state authorities control waste management. Two basic requirements are common for the care of all potentially infectious cases:

i) hands must be washed after contact with the patient or potentially contaminated articles and before taking care of another patient;

ii) articles contaminated with infectious material must be appropriately discarded or bagged and labelled before being sent for decontamination and reprocessing.

Recommendations made for isolation of cases in section 9B2 of each disease may allude to the methods that had been recommended as category-specific isolation precautions, based on the mode of transmission of the specific disease, in addition to universal precautions. These categories are as follows:

- *Strict isolation*: To prevent transmission of highly contagious or virulent infections that may be spread by both air and contact. The specifications, in addition to those above, include a private room and the use of masks, gowns and gloves for all persons entering the room. Special ventilation requirements with the room at negative pressure to surrounding areas are desirable.
- *Contact isolation*: For less highly transmissible or less serious infections, for diseases or conditions that are spread primarily by close or direct contact. In addition to the 2 basic requirements, a private room is indicated, but patients infected with the same pathogen may share a room. Masks are indicated for those who come close to the patient, gowns if soiling is likely and gloves for touching infectious material.
- *Respiratory isolation*: To prevent transmission of infectious diseases over short distances through the air, a private room is indicated, but patients infected with the same organism may share a room. In addition to the basic requirements, masks are indicated for those who come in close contact with the patient; gowns and gloves are not indicated.
- *Tuberculosis isolation (AFB isolation)*: For patients with pulmonary tuberculosis who have a positive sputum smear or a chest X-ray that strongly suggests active tuberculosis. Specifications include use of a private room with special ventilation and closed door. In addition to the basic requirements, those entering the room must use respirator-type masks. The use of gowns will

prevent gross contamination of clothing. Gloves are not indicated.

- *Enteric precautions:* For infections transmitted by direct or indirect contact with feces. In addition to the basic requirements, specifications include use of a private room if patient hygiene is poor. Masks are not indicated; gowns should be used if soiling is likely and gloves used when touching contaminated materials.

- *Drainage/secretion precautions:* To prevent infections transmitted by direct or indirect contact with purulent material or drainage from an infected body site. A private room and masking are not indicated. In addition to the basic requirements, gowns should be used if soiling is likely and gloves used when touching contaminated materials.

29. **Molluscicide**—A chemical substance used for the destruction of snails and other molluscs.

30. **Mortality rate**—A rate calculated in the same way as an **incidence rate**, by dividing the number of deaths occurring in the population during the stated period of time, usually a year, by the number of persons at risk of dying during the period or by the mid-period population. A **total** or **crude mortality rate** refers to deaths from all causes and is usually expressed as deaths per 1000. A **disease-specific mortality rate** refers to deaths due to a single disease and is often reported for a denominator of 100 000 persons. Age, ethnicity or other characteristics may define the population base. The mortality rate must not be confused with the **case-fatality rate** (Synonym: death rate).

31. **Nosocomial infection**—An infection occurring in a patient in a hospital or other health care facility in whom the infection was not present or incubating at the time of admission; or the residual of an infection acquired during a previous admission. Includes infections acquired in the hospital but appearing after discharge, and also such infections among the staff of the facility. (Synonym: hospital-acquired infection).

32. **Pathogenicity**—The property of an infectious agent that determines the extent to which overt disease is produced in an infected population, or the power of an organism to produce disease. Measured by the ratio of the number of persons developing clinical illness to the number of persons exposed to infection.

33. **Period of communicability/Communicable period**—The time during which an infectious agent may be transferred directly or indirectly from an infected person to another person, from an infected animal to humans, or from an infected person to animals, including arthropods.

In diseases (e.g., diphtheria and streptococcal infection) where mucous membranes are involved from the initial entry of the infectious agent, the period of communicability starts at the date of first exposure to a source of infection and lasts until the infecting microorganism is no longer disseminated from the mucous membranes, i.e. from the period before the prodromata until the termination of a carrier state, if the latter develops. Some diseases (e.g., hepatitis A, measles) are more easily communicable during the incubation period than during the actual illness.

In diseases such as tuberculosis, leprosy, syphilis, gonorrhoea and some of the salmonelloses, the communicable state may persist—sometimes intermittently—over a long period with discharge of infectious agents from the surface of the skin or through the body orifices.

For diseases transmitted by arthropods, such as malaria and yellow fever, the periods of communicability (or infectivity) are those during which the infectious agent occurs in the blood or other tissues of the infected person in sufficient numbers to permit infection of the vector. For the arthropod vector, a period of communicability (transmissibility) is also to be noted, during which the agent is present in the tissues of the arthropod in such form and locus as to be transmissible (infective state).

34. **Personal hygiene**—In the field of infectious disease control, those protective measures, primarily within the responsibility of the individual, that promote health and limit the spread of infectious diseases, chiefly those transmitted by direct contact. Such measures encompass:

- washing hands in soap and water immediately after evacuating bowel or bladder and always before handling food or eating;
- keeping hands and unclean articles, or articles that have been used for toilet purposes by others, away from the mouth, nose, eyes, ears, genitalia and wounds;
- avoiding the use of common or unclean eating utensils, drinking cups, towels, handkerchiefs, combs, hairbrushes and pipes;
- avoiding exposure of other persons to droplets from the nose and mouth as in coughing, sneezing, laughing or talking;
- washing hands thoroughly after handling a patient or the patient's belongings and keeping the body clean by frequent soap and water washing.

35. **Prevalence**—The total number of instances of illness or of persons ill in a specified population at a particular time (point prevalence), or during a stated period of time (period prevalence), without distinction between old and new cases. A **prevalence rate** (not to be confused with prevalence) is the ratio of prevalence to the population at risk of having the disease or condition at the stated

point in time or midway through the period considered; it is usually expressed per 1000, per 10 000 or per 100 000 population.

36. **Quarantine**—Restriction of activities for well persons or animals who have been exposed (or are considered to be at high risk of exposure) to a case of communicable disease during its period of communicability (i.e. **contacts**) to prevent disease transmission during the incubation period if infection should occur. The two main types of quarantine are:

Absolute or complete quarantine: The limitation of freedom of movement of those exposed to a communicable disease for a period of time not longer than the longest usual incubation period of that disease, in such manner as to prevent effective contact with those not so exposed. (See **Isolation**.)

Modified quarantine: A selective, partial limitation of freedom of movement of contacts, commonly on the basis of known or presumed differences in susceptibility and related to the assessed risk of disease transmission. It may be designed to accommodate particular situations. Examples are exclusion of children from school, exemption of immune persons from provisions applicable to susceptible persons, or restriction of military populations to the post or to quarters. Modified quarantine includes: *Personal surveillance*, the practice of close medical or other supervision of contacts to permit prompt recognition of infection or illness but without restricting their movements; and *Segregation*, the separation of some part of a group of persons or domestic animals from the others for special consideration, control or observation; removal of susceptible children to homes of immune persons; or establishment of a sanitary boundary to protect uninfected from infected portions of a population.

37. **Repellent**—A chemical applied to the skin or clothing or other places to discourage arthropods from alighting on and biting a person, or to discourage other agents, such as helminth larvae, from penetrating the skin.

38. **Report of a disease**—An official report notifying an appropriate authority of the occurrence of a specified communicable or other disease in humans or in animals. Diseases in humans are reported to the local health authority; those in animals, to the livestock, sanitary, veterinary or agriculture authority. Some few diseases in animals, also transmissible to humans, are reportable to both authorities. Each health jurisdiction declares a list of reportable diseases appropriate to its particular needs (see Reporting). Reports should also list suspected cases of diseases of particular public health importance, ordinarily those requiring epidemiological investigation or initiation of special control measures. When a person is infected in one health jurisdiction and the case is reported from another, the health authority receiving the report should notify the jurisdiction where infection presumably

occurred, especially when the disease requires examination of contacts for infection, or if food, water or other common vehicles of infection may be involved. In addition to routine report of cases of specified diseases, special notification is required of most epidemics or outbreaks of disease, including diseases not listed as reportable. (See **Epidemic**.) Special reporting requirements are specified in *International Health Regulations*.

Zero reporting (Syn: null reporting) consists in the explicit reporting of "zero case" when no cases have been detected by the reporting unit. This is a way of checking that the relevant data have not been forgotten or lost.

39. **Reservoir** (of infectious agents)—Any person, animal, arthropod, plant, soil or substance (or combination of these) in which an infectious agent normally lives and multiplies, on which it depends primarily for survival, and where it reproduces itself in such manner that it can be transmitted to a susceptible host.

40. **Rodenticide**—A substance used for the destruction of rodents, generally but not always through ingestion. (See also **Fumigation**.)

41. **Source of infection**—The person, animal, object or substance from which an infectious agent passes to a host. **Source of infection** should be clearly distinguished from source of **contamination**, such as overflow of a septic tank contaminating a water supply. (See **Reservoir**.)

42. **Surveillance of disease**—In communicable disease control, surveillance consists in the process of systematic collection, orderly consolidation, analysis and evaluation of pertinent data with prompt dissemination of the results to those who need to know, particularly those who are in a position to take action. It includes the systematic collection and evaluation of: 1) morbidity and mortality reports; 2) special reports of field investigations of epidemics and of individual cases; 3) isolation and identification of infectious agents by laboratories; 4) data concerning the availability, use and untoward effects of vaccines and toxoids, immune globulins, insecticides and other substances used in control; 5) information regarding immunity levels in segments of the population; 6) other relevant epidemiological data. A report summarizing the above data should be prepared and distributed to all cooperating persons and others with a need to know the results of the surveillance activities. The procedure applies to all jurisdictional levels of public health from local to international.

Serological surveillance identifies patterns of current and past infection using serological tests for antibody detection.

43. **Susceptible**—A person or animal not possessing sufficient resistance against a particular infectious agent to prevent contracting infection or disease when exposed to the agent.

44. **Suspect** —In infectious disease control, illness in a person whose history and symptoms suggest that he or she may have or be developing a communicable disease.

45. **Transmission of infectious agents**—Any mechanism by which an infectious agent is spread from a source or reservoir to a person. These mechanisms are as follows:

- *Direct transmission*: Direct and essentially immediate transfer of infectious agents to a receptive portal of entry through which human or animal infection may take place. This may be by direct contact such as touching, biting, kissing or sexual intercourse, or through direct projections (droplet spread) of droplet spray onto the conjunctiva or onto the mucous membranes of the eye, nose or mouth during sneezing, coughing, spitting, singing or talking (usually limited to a distance of about 1 meter or less). It may also occur through direct exposure of susceptible tissue to an agent in soil or through the bite of a rabid animal, or transplacentally.

- *Indirect transmission*:

  - Vehicle-borne—Contaminated inanimate materials or objects (fomites) such as toys, handkerchiefs, soiled clothes, bedding, cooking or eating utensils, surgical instruments or dressings; water, food, milk, and biological products including blood, serum, plasma, tissues or organs; or any substance serving as an intermediate means by which an infectious agent is transported and introduced into a susceptible host through a suitable portal of entry. The agent may or may not have multiplied or developed in or on the vehicle before being transmitted.

  - Vector-borne—(i) Mechanical: Includes simple mechanical carriage by a crawling or flying insect through soiling of its feet or proboscis, or by passage of organisms through its gastrointestinal tract. This does not require multiplication or development of the organism; (ii) Biological: Propagation (multiplication), cyclic development, or a combination of these (cyclopropagative) is required before the arthropod can transmit the infective form of the agent to humans. An incubation period (extrinsic) is required following infection before the arthropod becomes infective. The infectious agent may be passed vertically to succeeding generations (transovarian transmission); transstadial transmission indicates its passage from one stage of life cycle to another, as from nymph to adult. Transmission may be by injection of salivary gland fluid during biting, or by regurgitation or deposition on the skin of faeces or other material capable of penetrating through the bite wound or through an area of trauma from scratching or rubbing. This transmission is by an infected nonvertebrate host and not simple mechanical carriage by a vector as a vehicle. An arthropod in either role is termed a vector.

- *Airborne transmission:* The dissemination of microbial aerosols to a suitable portal of entry, usually the respiratory tract. Microbial aerosols are suspensions of particles in the air consisting partially or wholly of microorganisms. They may remain suspended in the air for long periods of time, some retaining and others losing infectivity or virulence. Particles in the 1-to 5-micrometer range are easily drawn into the alveoli of the lungs and may be retained there. Not considered as airborne are droplets and other large particles that promptly settle out (see **Direct transmission**).

  - Droplet nuclei—Usually the small residues that result from evaporation of fluid from droplets emitted by an infected host (see above). They may also be created purposely by a variety of atomizing devices, or accidentally as in microbiology laboratories or in abattoirs, rendering plants or autopsy rooms. They usually remain suspended in the air for long periods.

  - Dust—The small particles of widely varying size that may arise from soil (e.g., fungus spores), clothes, bedding or contaminated floors.

46. **Universal precautions**—See **Isolation**.

47. **Virulence**—The ability of an infectious agent to invade and damage tissues of the host; the degree of pathogenicity of an infectious agent, often indicated by case-fatality rates.

48. **Zoonosis**—An infection or infectious agent transmissible under natural conditions from vertebrate animals to humans. May be **enzootic** or **epizootic**. (See **Endemic** and **Epidemic**.)

INDEX

Immunization schedules

WHO's Expanded Programme on Immunization recommends the following proposed schedule for infants in developing countries. Whatever the national schedule, infants should be immunized as close as possible to the scheduled age with each vaccine in order to ensure the earliest possible protection against the target diseases. Specific epidemiological circumstances may lead to modifications in this schedule.

Vaccine	Birth	6 wks	10 wks	14 wks	9 mths
BCG	X				
Oral polio	X[1]	X	X	X	
DTP		X	X	X	
Hepatitis B Scheme A*	X	X			
Hepatitis B Scheme B*		X	X	X	
Haemophilus influenzae type b		X	X	X	
Yellow fever					X**
Measles					X***

[1]In polio-endemic countries

*Scheme A recommended where perinatal transmission of hepatitis B virus is common (e.g. southeastern Asia)

*Scheme B recommended where perinatal transmission of hepatitis B virus is less common (e.g. sub-Saharan Africa)

**Where yellow fever poses a risk

***A second opportunity of receiving measles vaccine to be provided for all children, as part of the routine schedule or in a campaign

The schedule proposed by the USA and applicable to most other industrialized countries is as follows:

Addendum to Influenza Data: Updated April 18, 2006

INFLUENZA   ICD-9 487; ICD-10 J10, J11

1. Identification—An acute viral disease of the respiratory tract characterized by fever, headache, myalgia, prostration, coryza, sore throat and cough. Cough is often severe and protracted; other manifestations are self-limited in most patients, with recovery in 2-7 days. Recognition is commonly by epidemiological characteristics (current rapid tests lack sensitivity); only laboratory procedures can reliably identify sporadic cases. Influenza may be clinically indistinguishable from disease caused by other respiratory viruses, such as common cold, croup, bronchiolitis, viral pneumonia and undifferentiated acute respiratory disease. GI tract manifestations (nausea, vomiting, diarrhea) are uncommon, but may accompany the respiratory phase in children, and have been reported in up to 25% of children in school outbreaks of influenza B and A (H1N1).

Influenza derives its importance from the rapidity with which annual epidemics evolve, the widespread morbidity and the seriousness of complications, notably viral and bacterial pneumonias. In addition, emergence among humans of influenza viruses with new surface proteins can cause pandemics ranking as global health emergencies (e.g. 1918, 1957, 1968) with millions of deaths (c50 million in 1918). Severe illness and death during annual influenza epidemics occur primarily among the elderly and those debilitated by chronic cardiac, pulmonary, renal or metabolic disease, anemia or immunosuppression. The proportion of total deaths associated with pneumonia and influenza in excess of that expected for the time of year (excess mortality) varies and depends on the prevalent virus type. The annual global death toll is estimated to reach up to 1 million. In most epidemics, 80%-90% of deaths occur in persons over 65; in the 1918 pandemic, young adults showed the highest mortality rates. Reye syndrome, involving the CNS and liver, is a rare complication following virus infections in children who have ingested salicylates.

While the epidemiology of influenza is well understood in industrialized countries, information on influenza in developing countries is minimal.

Reports from large outbreaks in Africa and recent studies from Thailand indicate that health implications from influenza (morbidity, hospitalizations) in developing countries may be comparable with health impact of the disease in developed countries. During the early febrile stage, laboratory confirmation is through isolation of influenza viruses from pharyngeal or nasal secretions or washings on cell culture or in embryonated eggs; direct identification of viral antigens in nasopharyngeal cells and fluids (FA test or ELISA); rapid diagnostic tests (these differ in the influenza viruses they detect); or viral RNA amplification. Demonstration of a specific serological response between acute and convalescent sera may also confirm infection.

2. Infectious agents—Three types of influenza virus are recognized: A, B and C. Type A includes 16 subtypes of which only 2 (H1and H3) are associated with widespread epidemics; type B is infrequently associated with regional or widespread epidemics; type C with sporadic cases and minor localized outbreaks. The antigenic properties of the 2 relatively stable internal structural proteins, the nucleoprotein and the matrix protein, determine virus type.

Influenza A subtypes are classified by the antigenic properties of surface glycoproteins, hemagglutinin (H) and neuraminidase (N). Frequent mutation of the genes encoding surface glycoproteins of influenza A and influenza B viruses results in emergence of variants that are described by geographic site of isolation, year of isolation and culture number. Examples are A/New Caledonia/20/99(H1N1), A/Moscow/10/99(H3N2)virus, B/Hong Kong/330/2001.

These relatively minor antigenic changes (antigenic drift) of A and B viruses, responsible for frequent annual epidemics and regional outbreaks, occur constantly and require almost annual reformulation of influenza vaccine. Emergence of completely new subtypes—at irregular intervals and only for type A viruses—results from antigenic shift in the HA gene, whereby genes from mammalian and animal viruses are exchanged during co-infection of the same cell (re-assortment); or from adaptive mutation of an entirely avian virus. Such completely new subtypes of the influenza A virus lead to global pandemics. A new formulation taking into consideration this drifted virus is required for vaccines to prevent pandemic influenza.

3. Occurrence—As pandemics (rare), epidemics (annual), localized outbreaks and sporadic cases. Clinical attack rates during epidemics range from 10% to 20% in the general community to more than 50% in closed populations (e.g. nursing homes, schools). During the initial phase of epidemics in industrialized countries, infection and illness appear predominantly in school-age children, with a sharp rise in school absences, physician visits, and pediatric hospital admissions. Schoolchildren infect family members, other children and adults. During a subsequent phase, infection and illness occur in adults, with workplace absenteeism, adult hospital admissions, and an increase in mortality from influenza related pneumonia. Epidemics generally last 3-6 weeks, although the virus is present in the community for a variable number of weeks before and after the epidemic. The highest attack rates during type A epidemics occur among children aged 5-9 years, although the rate is also high in preschool children and adults.

Epidemics of influenza occur annually, caused primarily by type A viruses, occasionally influenza B viruses or both. In temperate zones, epidemics tend to occur in winter; in the tropics, they often occur in the rainy season, but outbreaks or sporadic cases may occur in any month.

Influenza viral infections with different Influenza A subtypes also occur naturally in swine, horses, mink and seals, and in many other domestic

Amantadine or rimantadine is effective in the chemoprophylaxis of influenza A, but not influenza type B. Frequently, resistance occurs rapidly after treatment and resistant viruses are fully transmissible. Globally, resistance of type A against amantadine appears to be increasing. The CNS side-effects associated with amantadine in 5%-10% of recipients may be more severe in the elderly or those with impaired kidney function—the latter should receive reduced dosages that reflect the degree of renal impairment. Rimantadine is reported to cause fewer CNS side-effects. The use of these drugs should be considered in non-immunized persons or groups at high risk of complications, such as residents of institutions or nursing homes for the elderly, when an appropriate vaccine is not available or as a supplement to vaccine when immediate maximal protection is desired against influenza A infection. The drug will not interfere with the response to influenza vaccine and should be continued throughout the epidemic.

B. Control of patient, contacts and the immediate environment:

1) Report to local health authority: Reporting outbreaks or laboratory-confirmed cases assists disease surveillance. Report identity of the infectious agent as determined by laboratory examination if possible, Class 1 (see Reporting).

2) Isolation: Impractical under most circumstances because of the delay in diagnosis and virus excretion during incubation. In annual epidemics, because of increased patient load, it would be desirable to isolate patients (especially infants and young children) believed to have influenza by placing them in the same room (cohorting) in hospitals during the initial 5–7 days of illness.

3) Concurrent disinfection: Not applicable.

4) Quarantine: Not applicable.

5) Protection of contacts: A specific role has been shown for antiviral chemoprophylaxis with amantadine or rimantadine against type A strains (see 9A3). Neuraminidase inhibitors can be considered for influenza A and B.

Investigation of contacts and source of infection: Of no practical value during annual influenza epidemics.

Specific treatment: Neuraminidase inhibitors are effective against both influenza A and B viruses if treatment is begun within 48h after onset of clinical symptoms (oseltamivir: 75 mg a day for 5 days). Post-exposure prophylaxis (e.g. family

species in many parts of the world. Aquatic birds are a natural reservoir and carrier for all Influenza A virus subtypes. Interspecies transmission (mainly transitory) and re-assortment of influenza A viruses have been reported among swine, humans and some wild and domestic fowl.

Epidemiology of A(H5N1) outbreak, 1997 - March October 2006

Since 1997 sporadic zoonotic infections with avian influenza viruses of the A(H5N1) type have been identified in isolated human events, with high fatality. The first documented cases (18 cases, 6 deaths) occurred in Hong Kong, China in 1997. Two additional cases (1 death) occurred in Hong Kong in 2003. Beginning in end-2003, sporadic human zoonotic infections with high fatality have been associated with large and recurring outbreaks of A(H5N1) avian influenza in poultry in several Asian countries. Outbreaks in migratory birds in China in summer 2005 preceded rapid spread of H5N1 through Mongolia and Russia to many European, Middle Eastern and African countries. By end-March 2006 over 186 human cases had been reported from Azerbaijan, Cambodia, China, Egypt, Indonesia, Iraq, Thailand, Turkey and Viet Nam. Approximately half of these cases have been fatal (regular updates available at http://www.who.int/csr/disease/avian-_influenza/country/cases_table_2006_03_10/en/index.html). As of end-March 2006, species barrier between poultry and humans remained significant; the virus did not transmit easily from poultry to humans, and infection with A(H5N1) remained largely a disease of animals. Some instances of limited human-to-human transmission have occurred but there is no evidence as of end-March 2006 suggesting that there had been sustained and efficient spread of the virus among humans. When compared with viruses from 1997 and 2003, H5N1 viruses currently circulating in poultry in Asia survive longer in the environment and are more lethal to experimentally infected mammals. Like in all influenza viruses, several mutations occurred over time in human and animal H5N1 viruses circulating between 2003 and 2006. Although, the significance of these mutations in terms of virulence or transmissibility among humans is not fully understood, there is no evidence of increased transmissibility to humans of currently circulating H5N1 viruses The virus has significant pandemic potential.

Clinical features of human H5N1 influenza

Most patients infected with the influenza A(H5N1) virus show initial symptoms of fever (usually higher than 38° C) and an influenza-like illness, with symptoms in the lower respiratory tract. Upper respiratory tract symptoms may be present, but less commonly so. Diarrhea, vomiting, abdominal pain, pleuritic pain, and bleeding from the nose and gums may also occur early in the course of infection. Watery diarrhea is often present in the early stages of illness, and may precede respiratory symptoms by up to one week. One report has described two patients who presented with an encephalitis-like illness and diarrhea without apparent respiratory symptoms.

People with a possible exposure history should check for these signs (especially fever) each day for 14 days after the last exposure is thought to have occurred. The incubation period has generally ranged from 2 to 5 days. Longer incubation periods have been recorded, but these may arise from the difficulty of identifying a precise source of exposure, especially in areas where poultry outbreaks are widespread.

Lower respiratory tract manifestations develop early in the course of illness and are usually found at presentation. As illness progresses, almost all hospitalized patients develop clinically apparent pneumonia. Multi-organ failure with signs of renal dysfunction and sometimes cardiac compromise has been common.

4. Reservoir—Humans are the primary reservoir for human influenza viruses (H3; H1, B); birds and mammalian reservoirs such as swine are likely sources of new Influenza A human subtypes thought to emerge through genetic re-assortment or adaptive mutation.

5. Mode of transmission—Airborne spread and direct contact predominates among crowded populations in enclosed spaces; the human influenza virus may persist for hours, particularly in the cold and in low humidity, and transmission may also occur through direct contact. New subtypes may be transmitted globally within 3-6 months.

6. Incubation period—Short, usually 1-3 days.

7. Period of communicability—Probably 3-5 days from clinical onset in adults; up to 7 days in young children.

8. Susceptibility—Size and relative impact of epidemics and pandemics depend upon level of protective immunity in the population, strain virulence and extent of antigenic variation of new viruses. Infection produces immunity to the specific antigenic variant of the infecting virus; duration and breadth of immunity depend on the degree of antigenic similarity between viruses causing immunity and causing disease. Pandemics (emergence of a new subtype): total population is immunologically naive; in some pandemics children and adults have been equally susceptible, except for those who have lived through earlier pandemics caused by the same or an antigenically similar subtype.

Epidemics: population partially protected because of earlier infections; vaccines produce serological responses specific for the subtype viruses included, and elicit booster responses to antigenically related variant viruses with which the individual had prior experience.

Age-specific attack rates during an epidemic reflect persisting immunity from past experience with variant viruses related to the epidemic subtype, so that incidence of infection is often highest in school-age children.

9. Methods of control—Detailed recommendations for the preven-

tion and control of annual influenza epidemic are issued annually by national health agencies and WHO. WHO and many countries also have pandemic plans, outlining activities should a pandemic occur.

A. Preventive measures:

1) Educate the public and health care personnel in basic personal hygiene, especially transmission via unprotected coughs and sneezes, and from hand to mucous membrane.

2) Immunization with available inactivated and live virus vaccines may provide 70%-80% protection against infection in healthy young adults when the vaccine antigen closely matches the circulating strains of virus. Live vaccines, used in the Russian Federation for many years, have recently been licensed in the USA and other industrialized countries for intranasal application in healthy individuals aged 5-49. In the elderly, although immunization may be less effective in preventing illness, inactivated vaccines may reduce severity of disease and incidence of complications by 50%-60% and deaths by approximately 80%. Influenza immunization should preferably be coupled with immunization against pneumococcal pneumonia (see Pneumonia).

A single dose suffices for those with recent exposure to influenza A and B viruses; 2 doses more than 1 month apart are essential for children under 9. Routine immunization programs should be directed primarily towards those at greatest risk serious complications or death (see Identification) and those might spread infection (health care personnel and hous contacts of high-risk persons). Immunization of child long-term aspirin treatment is also recommended to development of Reye syndrome after influenza infect

The vaccine should be given each year before expected in the community; timing of immuniza based on the seasonal patterns of influenza in the world (April to September in the souther rainy season in the tropics). Biannual re vaccine components are based on the v circulating, as determined by WHO thro

Contraindications: Allergic hypersen other vaccine components is a cor swine influenza vaccine program in increased risk of developing Guil weeks after vaccination. Subsec other virus strains have not increased risk of Guillain-Bar

3) Inhibitors of influenza ne shown to be safe and ef ment of influenza A and B.

members) with same dose over 7-10 days was shown to be effective in reducing illness. Prophylaxis may last over 6 weeks (75 mg per day). Amantadine or rimantadine started within 48 hours of onset of influenza A illness and given for approximately 3-5 days reduces symptoms and virus titres in respiratory secretions. Dosages are 5 mg/kg/day in 2 divided doses for ages 1-9, 100 mg twice a day above 9 years (if weight less than 45 kg, 5 mg/kg/day in 2 doses) for 2-5 days. Doses should be reduced for those over 65 or with decreased hepatic or renal function.

Drug-resistant viruses may emerge late in the course of treatment and be transmitted to others; cohorting people on antiviral therapy should be considered, especially in closed populations with many high-risk individuals. Patients should be watched for bacterial complications and only then should antibiotics be administered. Because of the association with Reye syndrome, avoid salicylates in children.

C. Epidemic measures:

1) The severe and often disruptive effects of epidemic influenza on community activities may be reduced in part by effective health planning and education, particularly locally organized immunization programs for high-risk patients and their care providers. Surveillance by health authorities of the extent and progress of outbreaks and reporting of findings to the community are important.

2) Closure of individual schools has not proven to be an effective control measure; it is generally applied too late and only because of high staff and students absenteeism.

3) Hospital administrators must anticipate the increased demand for medical care during epidemic periods and possible absenteeism of health care personnel as a result of influenza. To prevent this, health care personnel should be immunized annually.

4) Maintaining adequate supplies of appropriate antiviral drugs would be desirable to treat high-risk patients and essential personnel in the event of the emergence of a new pandemic strain for which no suitable vaccine is available in time for the initial wave.

D. Disaster implications: Aggregations of people in emergency shelters will favor outbreaks of disease if the virus is introduced.

E. International measures: A disease under surveillance by WHO. The following are recommended:

1) Regularly report on epidemiological situation within a country to WHO (http://www.who.int/flunet).

2) Identify the causative virus in reports, and submit prototype strains to one of the WHO Centres for Reference and Research on Influenza in Atlanta, London, Melbourne and Tokyo (http://www.who.int/influenza). Throat secretion specimens, nasopharyngeal aspirates and paired blood samples may be sent to any WHO-recognized national influenza center (http://www.who.int/csr/disease/influenza/centres/en/index.html).

3) Conduct epidemiological studies and promptly identify viruses to the national health agencies.

4) Ensure sufficient commercial and/or governmental facilities to provide rapid production of adequate quantities of vaccine and antiviral drugs; maintain programs for vaccine and antiviral drug administration to high-risk persons and essential personnel.

Pandemic Influenza: The response to an influenza pandemic must be planned at the national and international levels; guidance is provided on the WHO website (http://www.who.int/csr/disease/avian_influenza).

{K. Stöhr}

ISBN 0-87553-034-6

9 780875 530345